Medical Imaging

For those who have loved or inspired us.
And friends we have found on our way.

Commissioning Editor: *Claire Wilson*
Development Editor: *Catherine Jackson*
Project Managers: *Anita Somaroutu/Shereen Jameel*
Designer: *Miles Hitchen*
Illustration Manager: *Jennifer Rose*

Medical Imaging
TECHNIQUES, REFLECTION & EVALUATION

Second Edition

Edited by

Elizabeth Carver BSc(Hons) DCR(R) FAETC

Deputy Director of Radiography,
Lead for Clinical Education,
Bangor University, Wales, UK

Barry Carver PgDipCT PGCE DCR(R)

Director of Radiography,
Bangor University, Wales, UK

Foreword by

Richard C. Price PhD MSc FCR

Head of School of Health and Emergency Professions,
University of Hertfordshire, UK

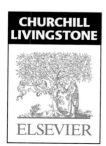

CHURCHILL
LIVINGSTONE

ELSEVIER

Edinburgh   London   New York   Oxford   Philadelphia   St Louis   Sydney   Toronto   2012

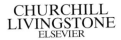

First edition 2006
Second edition 2012

ISBN 978 0 7020 3933 1

British Library Cataloguing in Publication Data
A catalogue record for this book is available from the British Library

Library of Congress Cataloging in Publication Data
A catalog record for this book is available from the Library of Congress

ELSEVIER your source for books, journals and multimedia in the health sciences
www.elsevierhealth.com

Working together to grow libraries in developing countries
www.elsevier.com | www.bookaid.org | www.sabre.org
ELSEVIER BOOK AID International Sabre Foundation

The publisher's policy is to use **paper manufactured from sustainable forests**

Printed in China

Contents

Contents

Foreword

The new edition of this now well established text, edited by Elizabeth Carver and Barry Carver, continues to provide an unparalleled and all-inclusive approach to the practice of radiography and medical imaging. As well as their own major inputs to the text, they have once again successfully integrated contributions from a range of experts within the field.

The book with its eight sections and 38 chapters provides a superb and comprehensive coverage of key topics. The reader will find a wealth of information from imaging principles and skeletal radiography to contrast studies, breast imaging, MRI, paediatrics, ultrasound and much more. The design of the chapters with well delineated sections on indications for examinations and pathologies, clearly labelled line diagrams and images and coloured prints provide clarity that the reader will value. However, the holistic approach to each chapter ensures that the book is not only about 'how to' position; it is much more than that. The book's subtitle 'Techniques, Reflection and Evaluation' reflects what the editors have set out to achieve. Adaptations to basic techniques are discussed, and criteria for assessing image quality are prominent features. If an image does not turn out as expected, the 'boxed' sections on common errors and possible reasons are particularly helpful. In Section 8 where CT, MRI, nuclear medicine and ultrasound are considered, equipment chronologies are presented. These are excellent features and provide important background and context to the stage of technology development today. The discussion sections in each chapter are well referenced, providing the reader with additional sources of reading which will be particularly helpful to students and researchers alike.

I am particularly pleased to see the chapter on Accident and Emergency. There is a clear focus on adaptations and the section on the mechanisms of injury related to examination requirements is innovative and clearly reflects the knowledge and understanding that radiographers need in the trauma setting today. The chapter stresses the advancing role of the radiographer and the fact that radiographers are key members of the multidisciplinary team. The radiographer, far from being merely the professional who acquires the image, is now someone who by education and training is able to evaluate images, comment on their findings and provide an interpretation to the referring clinician. The profession has taken a giant leap to reassert itself in image interpretation. Even 10 to 15 years ago it is highly unlikely that a chapter such as this one on Accident and Emergency would have been included in a radiography textbook. However, the chapter now rightly reflects 'the modernisation' of the profession and the giant leap it has made over a relatively short period. The editors deserve full credit for the chapter's inclusion.

In a world where technology development and diffusion continues to drive change there are a number of consequences: old equipment is replaced by new; old procedures are discarded and replaced by new techniques; and there is a shift in the definition of accepted practice. The impact of these changes is profound and more than ever radiographers must be able to evolve their practice and adapt to the demands of modern evidence-based health care. Students who join the profession do so from a different starting point than previous generations but their need to develop from a strong foundation for practice has not changed. This is a book that caters for students, learners and practitioners of all ages. The new edition provides that solid and reassuring platform which will give support and the confidence that students and practitioners alike seek in their professional journey. For the editors to produce a text that is cognisant of change and new development while providing the basic grounding for the practitioners of tomorrow is a challenge that has been met head-on. Elizabeth Carver and Barry Carver are to be complimented on the second edition of their book which will be sought by departments, institutional libraries and individuals wherever radiography is practised.

Dr Richard Price
Hatfield UK
March 2012

Preface to first edition

The role of practitioners in medical imaging has been developing for many years and professional practice now requires an evidence-based approach to this practice. In a rapidly expanding field this can seem overwhelming, especially for the undergraduate or newly qualified radiographer. No one can hope to reach advanced or consultant status as a diagnostic imaging professional without a reflective attitude.

Before even considering these requirements, professionals in medical imaging are required to acquire and implement skills that provide a safe, caring and efficient diagnostic service. Basically, we cannot expect professionals to be reflective if they do not first have access to information regarding the core requirements of medical imaging techniques. They have to know what their choices are before making their final choice on appropriate clinical practice, whilst considering the challenges that present themselves in a variety of guises: patient condition, the clinical question, image quality, dose from ionising radiation and related legislation, contraindications related to use of pharmaceuticals, contraindications related to the imaging modality in question and imaging principles. This list names but a few of the most relevant considerations, yet the concept of the reflective approach becomes even more complex when we realise that each one affects others in this important list and often we must consider a trade-off of one important consideration against another.

In order to cultivate this evidence-based approach we can no longer apply our skills without questioning the suitability of the techniques we employ. Most educators in medical imaging attempt to promote the reflective, evidence-based approach to all aspects of diagnostic imaging but it is often difficult for undergraduates, and even graduates, to continue this approach, especially during independent clinical practice or study.

Having considered these points it became clear to us that we needed to produce a resource which addressed these issues by providing information on a core of knowledge, sensibly presented and related to medical imaging techniques, whilst promoting the reflective approach. The result is this text, a project which has brought together contributions from radiographers, radiography lecturers, radiologists and other experts from the commercial sector of medical imaging, all selected for their clinical and academic expertise.

The first section of the book provides the basic information that is required to understand and initiate diagnostic imaging techniques, including implications for image quality and radiation dose related to exposure factors and image recording systems. Information is not merely descriptive; at times the authors consider and discuss published sources and relate this information to the concepts they present.

The next section has familiar aspects in that it offers descriptions of radiographic positioning and provides images of suggested patient positions and resulting radiographs, which also bear anatomical labelling. A step-by-step approach is used, making the requirements of each position easier to follow. Often a radiographer or student will only need to check a centring point or angle of central ray rather than read the whole position descriptor, and for this reason these sections are clearly identified under separate headings after the position descriptor. Often there are several methods described for one position requirement. These chapters are supplemented by a range of approaches:

- There is discussion, or even questioning, regarding suitability of projections or methods related to patient condition, practicality of the position used, radiation dose and imaging principles. References are used, either as a basis for reflection or to present an argument. At times questions are raised to promote further reflection by the reader.
- Tips for improved practical implementation are provided where relevant.
- Full image quality criteria for all radiographic projections are provided.
- Advice on causes and correction of common errors is given.

As an additional note, it should be mentioned that 'general radiography' is often considered as a non-specialist area, yet it relies so heavily on high level skills such as an understanding of human anatomy and related surface markings, an intuitive approach to communication which ensures patient concordance and compliance, and an understanding of the use of ionising radiation and its impact on image quality and human tissue. The editors acknowledge that general radiography still provides the higher proportion of a medical imaging service and stress that medical imaging professionals must not exclude general radiography as a specialist area in itself. By emphasising the reflective aspects of this section we hope to highlight this most clearly.

Moving on to other sections in the text, other non-contrast radiographic imaging is also covered in sections on mammography, accident and emergency, and paediatric imaging. A descriptive and reflective approach continues in these sections, which are again supported by references.

In the contrast examinations chapters, the descriptive and reflective philosophy continues. Improved imaging via complementary imaging methods posed a problem regarding what to include in this section; many angiographic examinations have been replaced by other methods such as computed tomography (CT) and magnetic resonance imaging (MRI) contrast studies and this is considered alongside descriptions of techniques used.

The final section on comparative imaging considers the basic principles and clinical applications associated with these techniques, also with some reflective content and considerations for future developments, thus complementing the other sections of the text to provide an all round medical imaging approach. Every attempt has been made to ensure that the information provided in this section is as up to date as is possible in the rapidly developing areas it covers, but the authors acknowledge that even the time in production between manuscript submission and publication may see developments beyond those described.

It would have been unrealistic to hope to provide a text which was all things to everyone, and for this reason the editors would urge that further reading is undertaken via up-to-date specialist texts or journal articles relating to physics, radiation science, imaging recording, CT, MRI, radionuclide imaging (RNI), ultrasound, accident and emergency, paediatrics, interventional radiology, gastrointestinal and genitourinary investigations, mammography and health psychology. However, we believe that this text will provide a good basis for a core of knowledge, leading to safe and holistic practice that is based on evaluation and reflection.

We conclude by mentioning that production of this text would not have been possible without a large number of people and institutions. The authors feature as key to its success and their names will obviously be associated with their chapters but others have helped with this project in various ways: provision of images or permissions to reproduce images from other authors' work, use of equipment in hospitals, modelling, providing advice or undertaking administrative tasks. A separate list of those we wish to acknowledge is given after this preface.

Elizabeth M. Carver
Barry Carver
Stoke-on-Trent, UK, 2006

Preface

The first edition of this text addressed vital aspects of the role of the radiographer: understanding theory, evaluating practice and using an evidence base in this evaluation. We are pleased to say that it was well received and considered to be a very relevant text for use on graduate courses. Of course this success demanded that we produce a second edition, a very necessary project in view of the rapidly changing field in which we work.

We have retained the broad aims of the first edition: to develop skills that provide a safe, caring and efficient radiographer who will subscribe to a quality diagnostic service. It still includes a logical approach to radiographic techniques and image evaluation, aspects that have proved very popular with readers. We continue to use experts in their field for our contributors, ensuring that information is kept up to date and retains credibility; we also welcome our new authors to the team. As a result we believe that we have again created a resource that provides a good basis for a core of knowledge that can be used at all levels of undergraduate study, and act as a basis for postgraduate study.

The project, again, has been huge and has taken over two years to complete. During that period we saw developments dictate changes in manuscripts on more than one occasion to ensure that the text remains as up to date as is possible in the publishing world.

Since the last edition was published we have been saddened by the death of Penny Nash. Penny played an important part in the first edition, both as an author and support mechanism as our manager in the Radiography department at Bangor University. Without her understanding the massive project that led to the success of the first edition would never have been completed. We will always remember her with much fondness, as will many in the Radiography profession, and the dedication on the opening pages of this edition has Penny in mind along with other important people in our lives.

We hope the resulting second edition will be as well received as the first and that it will be of value to those who choose to use it.

Elizabeth and Barry Carver
Stoke-on-Trent, UK, 2012

Acknowledgements

Acknowledgements are offered to the following, for their ongoing support for this project: Countess of Chester Hospital NHS Foundation Trust; Neuroradiology Department, King's College Hospital NHS Trust, London; Imaging Directorate, University Hospital of North Staffordshire NHS Trust; Delyth Hughes, Catherine Jackson, Maria Manfredi, Anita Somaroutu, Alice Turner, Claire Wilson and Shereen Jameel.

We are also grateful to those who have provided or given permission for use of images for this or the first edition: Accuray Inc., Phillip Ballinger and Eugene Frank, Stephen Eustace, Christine Gunn, Professor P Lauterbur, Linda Lee, Michelle McNicholas, Stephanie Ryan, Verdi Stickland, Robin Wilson, Anrew Evans, Professor Sir Peter Mansfield, Eric Whaites, Oncology Systems Ltd, Philips Medical Systems, TomoTherapy®, Toshiba Medical Systems, Xograph Medical Systems, Alexandra Unett-Stow, Graeme Stow, James Unett-Stow, Ultrasound Now Ltd.

For assistance with the MRI chapter, the author wishes to thank: Professor Sir Peter Mansfield for historical data and published papers; Professor Paul Lauterbur for his kind advice and help on the Xeugmatography Image; Philips Medical Systems for their commitment to furthering MRI education and their continuing support in providing images and advice; Karen Hackling Searle and her colleagues at Cobalt Imaging in Cheltenham UK for taking the time to proof-read and update the protocol section for this new edition.

For assistance with the paediatric chapter, the authors wish to thank: Dr Sue King, Consultant Paediatric Radiologist (Weston General Hospital) and Dr Mani Thyagarajan (Bristol Royal Hospital for Children) for their expert reviews; Miss Mary Smail, Clinical Scientist (Department of Medical Physics and Bioengineering, University Hospitals Bristol).

We are grateful to those who provided us with information or support for our first edition, valuable assistance that has underpinned information in this second edition: Neil Barker, Margaret Cliffe, Timothy Cox, Neil Deasy, Joanne Fairhurst, Chris Hale, Mark Hitchman, Mark Holmshaw, Lynn Gilman, Peter Groome, Leighton Hospital, Julie Mead, Gillian Phillips, Graham Plant, Jack Reese, Meryl Rogers, Claire Shacklestone, Christine Smith, Mike Tatlow, Ysbyty Maelor Wrexham, undergraduate radiographers and physiotherapists at St Martins University, Carlisle.

We wish to thank those authors who originated or assisted with some of the chapters in the first edition and whose work was used as foundation material for the second edition: Philip Cosson, Margot McBride, Jonathan McConnell, Susan Penelope Nash, Amanda Royle, Michael Stocksley.

The editors acknowledge the patience and commitment of the models who feature throughout the positioning sections of the text: Alexandra Unett-Stow, Danny Rhodes.

List of contributors

Julie Burnage, DCR DMU FETC
Director, Ultrasound Now Limited, UK

Barry Carver, PgDipCT PGCE DCR(R)
Director of Radiography,
Bangor University, Wales, UK

Elizabeth Carver, BSc(Hons) DCR(R) FAETC
Deputy Director of Radiography,
Lead for Clinical Education,
Bangor University, Wales, UK

Mark Cowling, BSc MBBS MRCP FRCR
Consultant Vascular and Interventional Radiologist,
University Hospital of North Staffordshire,
Stoke on Trent, UK

Susan Cutler, MSc HDCR PgCE
Senior Lecturer,
Teeside University,
Middlesbrough, UK

Donna Jane Dimond, MSc BSc DCR(D)
Senior Lecturer in Diagnostic Imaging, University of the West of England;
Formerly Superintendent Radiographer,
Bristol Royal Hospital for Children,
Bristol

Patricia Fowler, MMEd BSc(Hons) DCRR CertCI FHEA
Senior Lecturer, Faculty of Health and Social Care,
London South Bank University,
London

Peter Hogg
Professor, Diagnostic Imaging Research Programme Lead,
University of Salford, UK

David Wyn Jones, MSc DCR(R) DRI CRadP MSRP
Superintendent Radiographer,
Wrexham Maelor Hospital,
Wrexham;
Honorary Research Fellow,
University of Salford, UK

Judith Kelly, MSc PgC Cert Mammography DCR
Consultant Radiographer and Deputy Programme Director,
Chester Breast Unit;
Honorary Senior Research Fellow, University of Salford, UK

Andrew Layt, DCR(R)
Superintendent Radiographer, Neuroradiology,
King's College Hospital NHS Foundation Trust,
London, UK

Julian MacDonald, PhD MSc BSc
Head of Radioisotope Physics,
North Wales Medical Physics,
Betsi Cadwaladr University Health Board, North Wales, UK

Mark McEntee, BSc(Hons) PhD
Senior Lecturer in Medical Radiation Science,
Faculty of Health Sciences,
University of Sydney,
New South Wales,
Australia

Sara Millington, BSc(Hons) Cert Mammography
Advanced Practitioner (Mammography),
Countess of Chester Hospital NHS Trust,
Chester, UK

Colin Monaghan, DCR(R) Pg Cert
Superintendent Radiographer,
Liverpool Heart and Chest Hospital,
NHS Foundation Trust,
Liverpool, UK

Tim Palarm, MSc BSc(Hons) DCR(R)
Branch Manager (Ultrasound), Toshiba Medical Systems Ltd (UK);
Formerly Senior Lecturer in Diagnostic Imaging and Postgraduate Programme Leader in Medical Ultrasound,
University of the West of England,
Bristol, UK

List of contributors

Rita Phillips, MSc DMU FAETC DCR
Senior Lecturer, Medical Ultrasound,
University of the West of England,
Bristol, UK

Joanne Rudd, MSc PgCert BSc(Hons)
Lead Radiographer Practitioner in Gastrointestinal Imaging,
West Suffolk Hospital, NHS Foundation Trust,
Bury St Edmunds, UK

Michael Smith, DCR(R) PgCert
Advanced Practitioner in Gastrointestinal Imaging,
University Hospital of North Staffordshire, Stoke on Trent, UK

John Talbot, MSc DCR(R) PGC(LT) FHEA
Senior Lecturer, Medical Imaging,
Director www.mrieducation.com

Linda Williams, HDCR IHSM(Cert) PgCert (teaching in HE)
Radiology Services Manager, Directorate of Radiology,
Countess of Chester Hospital NHS Foundation Trust,
Chester, UK

Darren Wood, DCR(R) PgCert
Lecturer/Practitioner, BSc Diagnostic Radiography and Imaging,
Bangor University, UK

Abbreviations

2D	two-dimensional		CTDI	computed tomography dose index
3D	three-dimensional		CTLM	computed tomography laser mammography
4D	four-dimensional		CTPA	computed tomography pulmonary angiography
A&E	accident and emergency		CVA	cerebral vascular accident
AC	abdominal circumference		CVC	central venous catheter
ACR	American College of Radiology		CVP	central venous pressure
ADC	analogue-to-digital conversion/converter		CVS	chorionic villus sampling
AEC	automatic exposure chamber		CZT	cadmium zinc telluride
AED	automatic exposure device		D&C	dilatation and curettage
AFM	after fatty meal		DAP	dose–area product
ALARA	as low as reasonably achievable		DAS	data acquisition system
ALARP	as low as reasonably practical		DCIS	ductal carcinoma in situ
AO	anterior oblique		DDF	direct digital fluoroscopy
AP	anteroposterior		DDH	developmental dysplasia of the hip
ARAS	atheromatous renal artery stenosis		DDR	direct digital radiography
ARSAC	Administration of Radioactive Substances Advisory Committee		DGH	district general hospital
			DLP	dose length product
ASIS	anterior superior iliac spine		DNA	deoxyribonucleic acid
ATLS	advanced trauma and life support		DOBI	dynamic optical breast imaging
AVM	arteriovenous malformation		DP	dorsipalmar or dorsiplantar
BaFT	barium follow-through		DPO	dorsipalmar oblique or dorsiplantar oblique
BIR	British Institute of Radiology		DPT	dental panoramic tomography
BPD	biparietal diameter		DQE	detective quantum efficiency
BPH	benign prostatic hyperplasia/hypertrophy		DR	digital radiography
BPP	biophysical profile		DRL	diagnostic reference level
Bq	Becquerel		DSA	digital subtraction angiography
CAD	computer-aided detection		DTPA	diethylenetriamine penta-acetic acid
CBD	common bile duct		DVT	deep vein thrombosis
CC	craniocaudal		DW	diffusion weighted
CDH	congenital dislocation of the hip		EAM	external auditory meatus
CEMRA	contrast-enhanced MRA		EBCT	electron beam computed tomography
CFA	common femoral artery		ECG	electrocardiogram
CPR	cardiopulmonary resuscitation		EDD	estimated date of delivery
CR	computed radiography		EDE	effective dose equivalent
CRL	crown–rump length		EFOV	extended field of view
CRT	cathode ray tube		EOP	external occipital protuberance
CSE	conventional spin echo		EPI	echo-planar imaging
CT	computed tomography		ERCP	endoscopic retrograde cholangiopancreatography
CTA	computed tomography angiography		ESD	entrance surface dose or entrance skin dose
CTC	computed tomography colonography		EUS	endoscopic ultrasound

ESWL	extracorporeal shockwave lithotripsy
FAST	focused abdominal sonography for trauma
FB	foreign bodies
FDG	fluorodeoxyglucose
FET	field effect transistor
FFD	focus–film distance
FISH	fluorescence in situ hybridisation
FL	femur/femoral length
fMRI	functional MRI
FNA	fine needle aspiration
FNAC	fine needle aspiration cytology
FNST	fetal non-stress test
FO	fronto-occipital
FOOSH	fall onto outstretched hand
FOV	field of view
FRD	focus receptor distance
FSE	fast spin echo
FWHM	full-width half maximum
GCS	Glasgow Coma Scale
GI	gastrointestinal
GOJ	gastro-oesophageal junction
GOR	gastro-oesophageal reflux
GSV	gestational sac volumes
HC	head circumference
hCG	human chorionic gonadotrophin
HDP	hydroxymethylene diphosphonate
HIDA	hepatobiliary iminodiacetic acid
HIV	human immunodeficiency virus
HLA	horizontal long axis
HOCM	high osmolar contrast media
HRCT	high-resolution CT
HRT	hormone replacement therapy
HSG	hysterosalpingography
HU	Hounsfield unit
HyCoSy	hysterosalpingo-contrast sonography
IAM	internal auditory meatus
IARC	International Agency for Research on Cancer
ICH	intracranial haemorrhage
IOFB	intraocular foreign body
IV	intravenous
IVC	intravenous cholangiogram
IVC	inferior vena cava
IVF	in vitro fertilisation
IVU	intravenous urogram or urography
keV	kilo electron volt
KUB	kidneys, ureters and bladder
kVp	kilovoltage peak
LAO	left anterior oblique
LBD	light beam diaphragm
LCD	liquid crystal display
LCR	low-contrast resolution
LOCM	low osmolar contrast media
LNT	linear no threshold
LPO	left posterior oblique
lppm	line pairs per millimetre
LSJ	lumbosacral junction
LSO	lutetium oxyorthosilicate
MAA	macro-aggregated albumin
mAs	milliampere seconds
MCU	micturating cystourethrography
MDP	methylene diphosphonate
MI	mechanical index
MIP	maximum intensity projection
MIRD	medical internal radiation dose

MLO	mediolateral oblique
MML	meatomental line
MRA	magnetic resonance angiography
MRCP	magnetic resonance cholangiopancreatography
MR	magnetic resonance
MRI	magnetic resonance imaging
MRM	magnetic resonance mammography
MSD	mean sac diameter
MSP	median sagittal plane
MSS	maternal serum screening
mSv	milliSievert
mT	milliTesla
NAI	non-accidental injury
NCEPOD	National Confidential Enquiry into Perioperative Deaths
NHSBSP	National Health Service Breast Screening Programme
NICE	National Institute for Health and Clinical Excellence
NM	nuclear medicine
NMR	nuclear magnetic resonance
NMV	net magnetic vector
NOF	neck of femur
NRPB	National Radiological Protection Board
NST	non-stress test
NT	nuchal translucency
OF	occipitofrontal
OFD	object–film distance
OGD	oesophagogastric duodenoscopy
OI	osteogenesis imperfecta
OM	occipitomental
OMBL	orbitomeatal baseline
OPG/OPT	orthopantomography
ORD	object receptor distance
PA	posteroanterior
PACS	picture archiving and communication system
PCA	phase contrast angiography
PCNL	percutaneous nephrolithotomy
PD	proton density
PE	pulmonary embolism
PET	positron emission tomography
PID	pelvic inflammatory disease
PGMI	perfect, good, moderate, inadequate (system)
PMT	photomultiplier tube
ppm	parts per million
PSA	prostate-specific antigen
PSIS	posterior superior iliac spine
PSL	photostimulable luminescence
PSP	photostimulable phosphor
PTC	percutaneous transhepatic cholangiography
PW	perfusion weighted
QDE	quantum detection efficiency
RA	rheumatoid arthritis
RCR	Royal College of Radiologists
RF	radiofrequency
RNI	radionuclide imaging
RAO	right anterior oblique
RPD	renal pelvic dilatation
RPO	right posterior oblique
RSD	reflex sympathetic dystrophy
SA	short axis
SAH	subarachnoid haemorrhage
SBE	small bowel enema
SC	sternoclavicular

SFA	superficial femoral artery		TFT	thin film transistor
SFDM	small field digital mammography		TI	thermal index
SID	source image distance		TIA	transient ischaemic attack
SI	sacroiliac		TLD	thermo-luminescent dosimetry
SIJ	sacroiliac joint		TMJ	temporomandibular joint
SMV	submentovertical		TOF	time-of-flight
SNR	signal-to-noise ratio		TPN	total parenteral nutrition
SOL	space-occupying lesion		TR	time to repetition
SPET	single photon emission tomography		TS	transabdominal scan
SPECT	single photon emission computed tomography		TVS	transvaginal scan
SPR	scan projection radiograph		UAE	uterine artery embolisation
STIR	short tau inversion recovery		US	ultrasound
SUFE	slipped upper femoral epiphysis		UTI	urinary tract infection
SVC	superior vena cava		VDU	visual display unit
SXR	skull X-ray		VLA	vertical long axis
T	Tesla		VENC	velocity encoding
TAS	transabdominal scan		V/Q	ventilation/perfusion
TE	time to echo		w/v	weight to volume

Section | 1 |

Imaging principles

Chapter 1

Digital imaging

Mark McEntee, Barry Carver

INTRODUCTION

Film/screen systems are predictable as physical and chemical principles govern the exposure response of these systems. Digital systems, as a consequence of the technologies involved, do not have simple exposure–response relationships. It is not easy to transfer the old 'rules of thumb' to the new systems, causing difficulty in the use of these technologies in the radiography department.

Advantages of digital images

- *Image manipulation.* Digital images consist simply of a matrix of pixels; as each pixel has a numerical value it is very easy to apply mathematical formulae to these values. The effect of such formulae is to change the appearance of the image to enhance or subdue certain image features. Examples of image manipulation are edge enhancement, noise smoothing, subtraction or windowing.
- *Image transmission.* The numerical values of the individual pixels making up an image can be represented by pulses of electrical current, light, microwaves or radio waves. Consequently, images can be sent via an array of transmission media such as phone lines, optical fibre or satellite, enabling remote diagnoses regardless of where the image was acquired.
- *Image storage and compression.* Images can be easily archived as numerical data on an array of storage media. Storing clinical information on digital media enables easy access to all relevant patient data. Producing images in digital format allows for the compression of images, meaning that less storage space is required and images are more easily transmitted.
- *Image analysis or reconstruction.* A range of analyses can be performed on images in digital format. Images can also be reconstructed to produce images quite different from the original sequence, e.g. 3D reconstruction in computed tomography (CT).

There are two main types of system currently available, which can be considered as computed radiography (CR) and direct digital radiography (DDR).

COMPUTED RADIOGRAPHY

CR is a cassette-based digital radiography system that uses photo-stimulable phosphors (PSPs) in combination with a plate scanning system to produce a digital image. First introduced in 1983,[1] it became the dominant method of acquiring digital radiographs. Analogous to the rare earth phosphor screen technology of 1970–1990, CR uses alkaline-earth halides and alkaline halides as PSPs to record a latent image of any irradiated structure.

Components of a CR system

There are four basic components to any CR system: the imaging plate, the CR cassette, the image reader and the image display device.

The CR imaging plate

The layers that make up a typical CR plate are shown in Figure 1.1. The technology used is very similar to intensifying screen construction.

1. The top layer of the image plate is a thin protective layer. This layer is electron beam cured to reduce the amount of laser beam reflection that occurs during secondary excitation.
2. Directly beneath the protective layer is the PSP. The phosphor used is generally a barium fluorohalide with europium impurities, together known as europium-activated barium fluorohalide ($BaFX:Eu$). The most common of the halides used in storage phosphors are iodine and bromine (designated as X in the formula above). The thickness of the PSP layer and the flatness of the surface are factors associated with noise, noticed as mottle.[2]
3. The phosphor layer is attached to a dyed layer that is often described as the anti-halation layer. This layer stops or reduces the amount of laser light that is reflected back into the phosphor layer.
4. Underneath the anti-halation layer and part of the support polyurethane is a conductive layer which allows any static

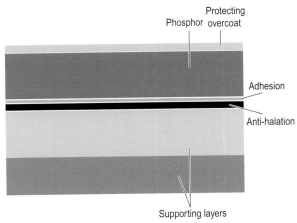

Figure 1.1 Cross-section diagram of typical imaging plate.

electricity to escape without causing damage to the image plate or stimulating the phosphor layer.

5. All of the above layers are supported by the support polyurethane backing layer, which provides rigidity for the whole structure. The polyurethane is also attached to a layer of laminate, which provides further support, and the complete image plate is stored inside a tough cassette for further protection.

The image plates are available in a range of standard sizes, and may be flexible or rigid. Flexible plates enable the plate reader to be made more compact, as the image plate can be transported into position underneath the laser via a system of rollers in a similar way to film being transported through a processor. The disadvantage of flexible image plates is that they are very prone to damage. Transporting an image plate through a system of rollers can cause scratches and cracks to appear in the phosphor surface. Rigid image plates are much less prone to damage caused by bending, but the image reader is less compact.

The CR cassette

The cassette in which the image plate is contained looks and feels similar to those used in film/screen radiography, which helps this technology to be accepted into existing work practices. CR cassettes are compatible with existing equipment such as cassette holders and trolleys, and will easily fit into cassette holder incorporated into mobile X-ray units. However, there are many differences between the two systems once the cassette cover is removed.

The body of a CR cassette, like any other used in radiography, must be very tough while at the same time being lightweight, with low X-ray attenuation. Polypropylene cassettes are warm to the touch, relatively inexpensive, and have a good level of flexibility; however, they have a higher attenuation coefficient than carbon fibre cassettes. Carbon fibre cassettes are more expensive but attenuate less radiation; they are also cold to the touch, which can be uncomfortable for patients, and relatively inflexible.

Outwardly one of the most noticeable differences between a film/screen cassette and a CR cassette is the missing identification window. There are several methods by which patient identification is associated with a cassette; whichever system is used it is essential that the patient information transferred to the image plate is accurate.

CR cassettes, like conventional film/screen cassettes, require back-scatter protection; this is of added importance when the sensitivity of PSP plates to scattered radiation is considered. The lead backing is typically 150 μm of lead.

An antistatic layer is present over the inside surface of the cassette; the material used provides a high degree of protection against electro-static charging and dust collection.

The image reader

The image reader is the device into which the cassette must be placed in order for the information on the image plate to be extracted. The design of the image reader can have implications for the ergonomics and workflow of the department. There are basically two designs: single plate image readers and multiple plate image readers.

- Single plate image readers allow the operator to insert one image plate at a time. The plate is scanned, the image is extracted, any residual information on the plate is erased and the image plate is returned to the operator before the next image plate may be scanned. The operator must be present to remove the scanned cassette and place the next image plate into the reader. Single plate image readers are best used to serve one X-ray room, one operator, or ward or theatre area.
- Multiple plate image readers incorporate a buffer system that allows multiple image plates to be scanned. These buffer systems usually accept up to 10 image plates of any size at any one time, and incorporate an automatic image plate loading system. The operator can thus leave the exposed image plates in the buffer and return to their patient while the image plates are being automatically read. Multiloader systems are usually centrally located in the X-ray department and may service multiple X-ray rooms.

CR image formation

The CR image formation process has basically four steps: primary excitation, secondary excitation, photomultiplication and digitisation.

1. Primary excitation: X-ray photons incident on the imaging plate interact with the storage phosphor layer. The impurities in the PSP, typically europium, cause the formation of electron traps; it is the electrons in these traps that form the latent image. The number of trapped electrons is directly proportional to the number of photons incident on the storage phosphor plate. These trapped electrons are relatively stable, but some may be prematurely released by receiving sufficient energy from sources such as background radiation or heating. Fading of the trapped signal will occur exponentially over time, so it is important to read the plate as soon as practicable after exposure.[3]
2. Secondary excitation: The image reader removes the image plate from its cassette and transports it to the laser. The laser stimulates the phosphors in the image plate providing enough energy to release the trapped electrons that form the latent image. These electrons, once released, drop immediately to their resting state. This drop in energy releases electromagnetic radiation in the form of light. Light leaving the phosphor plate is directed towards the photomultiplier tube via optical coupling. This is normally achieved through the use of fibreoptic bundles.
3. Photomultiplication and erasure: The photomultiplier tube (PMT) creates an electrical signal proportional to the light incident on the photocathode. This electrical signal is then

amplified and sent for digitisation. Once the laser has scanned the image plate and the photomultiplier has produced its signal, the image plate is then erased.

Erasure is essential to remove any residual image from the image plate and involves exposing the plate to high-intensity light. The energy imparted to the phosphors by this light releases any residual trapped electrons from the electron traps and prepares the image plate for further use.

4. Digitisation: The electrical signal generated by the PMT is digitised by an analogue-to-digital converter (ADC). The ADC does this by converting the continuous electrical signal into in a digital signal in two steps, called sampling and quantisation.

Sampling is about deciding the matrix size. The continuous signal from the PMT is broken up appropriately to form the required matrix. The size of the laser spot, the power of the laser beam and the plate read time are all critical to this choice. Quantisation assigns a grey scale value to each pixel according to the signal strength.

Advantages of CR vs film/screen radiography

Over the past 20+ years CR has proved to be an excellent method of producing digital images during projection radiography and can be easily adapted to an X-ray suite that has been used with conventional film/screen radiography. Nor do radiographic techniques need to change, as image plates are available in the same sizes and shapes as those used during conventional radiography.

The image reader can be placed centrally to facilitate multiple users. These image readers usually incorporate a buffer system that allows several cassettes to be processed without manual intervention, thus allowing a centralised architecture to be developed with the image reader in the centre of the department. Alternatively, image readers have also been developed in a small footprint format. This allows a complete CR system to be positioned inside the X-ray room, thus allowing the radiographer to complete the examination and process and view the images without having to leave the X-ray room or the patient.

The CR image plate is reusable and, if correctly maintained, can be used for many thousands of examinations. After each examination the image plate is simply erased and is then ready for reuse. The same image plate can be used for all examinations. The digital images produced by these systems require no costly and hazardous chemicals during processing.

CR produces a digital image which allows integration with a picture archiving and communication system (PACS), essentially improving data management. Many of the advantages of a PACS are not possible without the acquisition of information in digital format.

One of the most often cited advantages of CR is its resilience to over- and underexposure. The wide latitude of CR in comparison to film/screen radiography, combined with the post-processing capabilities of the system, means that repeat radiographs due to over- or underexposure can be virtually eliminated. This results in lower repeat rates and a reduction in radiation dose to the population as a whole. However, care must be taken to maintain the principles of dose minimisation to each individual patient. The wider latitude of CR can also be of benefit in situations where exposures cannot be easily controlled, such as in intensive or high care units, in theatre, or on the wards, where automatic exposure controls cannot be used and standardised optimum exposure conditions rarely exist.

Other advantages of the wider latitude include allowing soft tissue and bone to be visualised using only one exposure, and the use of lower exposure factors where in certain clinically justified examinations less dose is required. Although the radiation dose required with

CR is similar to that required with film/screen radiography systems, examinations that require visualisation of only gross details may be carried out with CR using less dose. Examples include radiographs for demonstration of orthopaedic fixation devices or joint replacement treatments; visualisation of a gross fracture for progress assessment; check-up and assessment of particular conditions such as scoliosis and kyphosis.

Disadvantages of CR vs film/screen radiography

Among the disadvantages of CR systems is the initial cost of purchasing and installing the system. This was initially prohibitive for many imaging departments, but as the cost of the systems dropped significantly it has become less of an issue. There is also some degradation in spatial resolution associated with these systems compared to film/screen radiography.

DIRECT DIGITAL RADIOGRAPHY

The practice of digital radiographic imaging is undergoing a dramatic change owing to a rapid proliferation of electronically readable X-ray detectors. These detectors provide rapid access to digital images and image quality exceeding that of both film/screen receptors and PSP CR systems.

The term direct digital radiography (DDR) is used in relation to a group of X-ray image acquisition devices that convert X-rays into an electrical signal without the need for a secondary excitation. DDR can be grouped into three specific technologies: charge coupled devices (CCD), large area flat panel detectors (FPD) and digital selenium drums. Within FPD there are two different technologies which will be considered here: amorphous silicon (aSi) and amorphous selenium (aSe).

Amorphous silicon (aSi) FPD

This system uses a caesium iodide-based phosphor (CsI:Tl), in much the same way as CR, coupled with an amorphous silicon/thin film transistor (aSi/TFT) array. The X-ray photons incident on the FPD cause the phosphor layer to produce light, the amount of which is proportional to the number of X-ray photons incident on the phosphor layer. An ultrathin ($2\ \mu m$) film of aSi, sensitive to this light, is attached to the thicker CsI:Tl phosphor. Phosphor thicknesses of up to $1000\ \mu m$ are used, with $500\ \mu m$ being common. The silicon is laid out in a fixed matrix of pixels: each pixel is a photodiode 'sensor' which acts as a receiver for electrons and records a separate signal. The TFT or field effect transistor behaves as a pixel switch to access the associated photodiode.

When light reaches the aSi photodiode, an electron-hole pair is created and an electric charge is generated. This charge is collected by the charge collectors and converted to an electrical signal. The signal is read by activating the electrodes in the TFT across each row. This electrical signal is amplified and converted to a digital signal via an ADC and sent to the computer, where it is processed and sent for display, archiving or printing.

The advantages to this system are the high sensitivity of CsI:Tl phosphor to X-rays and the relatively stable properties of amorphous silicon. These systems have the highest detective quantum efficiency of all digital systems. CsI:Tl is also used in fluoroscopy systems as it has a fast decay time, allowing for updated images at 30+ frames per second without noticeable lag.

Amorphous selenium (aSe) FPD

Selenium is a photoconductor, most sensitive to energies in the lower X-ray range. It is therefore able to directly convert X-ray photons to signal without a phosphor stage. The X-ray photons incident on the imaging plate are attenuated by the selenium, causing excitation of electrons throughout the aSe layer. This results in the generation of electron-hole pairs in proportion to the intensity of the incident X-rays. The charge is collected by the charge collecting electrodes and converted to an electrical signal via the TFT. This electrical signal is converted to a digital signal via an ADC.

The aSe is laid onto a predetermined matrix of TFTs, one for each pixel, and each pixel area records its signal on a capacitor. Normally pixel pitch is 140 μm, but 70–85 μm pixels can be used for mammography.

The advantage to this system is the lack of any light scattering in a phosphor layer. The aSe layer can be thick without the risk of increased noise, but the thicker the layer the larger the voltage required across it to capture the electrons. A practical limit would be 1000 μm, as this would require 10 000 volts (V). For lower photon energies, e.g. mammography, 200 μm thick detectors achieve 100% absorption with less than 5000 V. However, the requirement for a high-voltage system makes the detector relatively complex and bulky.

Developments in FPD

Wireless, cassette-based DDR systems are now available. The systems use a battery-based power supply which can be used for many exposures. This technology now enables an X-ray suite designed for film/screen or CR to be used for DDR without major building works or replacing the entire suite. This makes DDR more financially viable as an upgrade from film/screen, and largely eliminates the disadvantage of capital cost compared to CR.

DIGITAL IMAGE DISPLAY

Having captured a radiographic image, some form of display is required. The first characteristic of the visual system is that its performance is affected by the environment and changes over time: ambient lighting, fatigue and distraction are important factors. It is a mistake to specify a display technology without considering the whole reading environment. For example, the distance the eye is from the image will affect the resolution perceived. The angle at which the image is viewed can change the perception of patterns, and the background noise and heat of computer cooling fans can increase fatigue and distraction.

Display devices for medical use have higher quality requirements than the average domestic TV, with good spatial and brightness resolution and high performance graphics cards. The functions and characteristics of the graphics card and monitor affect the way in which images are displayed and viewed.

The main methods of displaying a soft copy image are the cathode ray tube (CRT) or the flat panel displays that include liquid crystal display (LCD), field emitting diodes, organic light-emitting diodes and plasma display. LCDs are currently the commonest method for displaying radiographic images in soft copy format.

Cathode ray tube (CRT)

CRTs have long been the dominant display technology, but have now largely been replaced by active matrix LCD panels. The diagnostic CRT has a high luminance of 700+ cd/cm^2, but this still does not approach that of a light box.

Disadvantages of CRTs are that they are large, heavy, have a high power (and hence heat) output, and a high quality assurance (QA) burden because luminance varies and deteriorates over time. There have also been fears regarding radiation output from workstations, although for a typical CRT there is no penetration of the glass screen front.

The use of a CRT reverses the process of analogue-to-digital conversion (ADC) in order to create an analogue signal from the digital data held in the computer; this extra step may produce signal distortion.

The required resolution of a CRT used for soft-copy reporting has been extensively debated. Generally it is thought that a medical CRT with a 1024 × 1024 pixel array (1K) with zooming capabilities is adequate for skeletal radiography whereas a 2048 × 2048 pixel (2K) monitor with zooming capability is adequate for thoracic radiography. The use of 4K monitors in mammography is still economically contentious. Once a spatial resolution of 5 lp/mm or higher is achieved across the field of view (with or without the use of zooming) and a luminance of 260 cd/cm^2 is used, primary diagnosis is not likely to be affected by the quality of the display.

LCD panels

An active matrix LCD panel uses similar technology to a DDR detector: a thin film semiconductor covers the surface with a predefined bitmap of pixels etched into it; these displays have a set maximum resolution. This technology does not require the size and space of a CRT. Although luminance is variable, the backlight can be changed and restored to original values very simply. Many systems have auto-calibration to account for this variability second by second. It is simple to site several LCD panels together to view many images at once.

Disadvantages of LCD panels are:

- Fixed resolution: zooming etc. requires resampling, which can cause aliasing artefacts.
- Angle of view can be limited or only single axis.
- Initial cost is greater than for CRT.

Image resolution

Resolution is typically expressed by identifying the number of pixels on the horizontal axis (rows) and the number on the vertical axis (columns); for an LCD monitor a typical value may be 1280 × 1024. This matrix size is very important to resolution: up to a point, the more squares on the matrix the better the image will look and the more the image can be modified.

A display device can normally support the spatial resolution of an incoming signal as well as several lesser resolutions. For example, a display with a physical grid of 1280 rows by 1024 columns can obviously support a maximum resolution of 1280 × 1024 pixels, but can easily support resolution of 800 × 600. Most commercially available medical monitors have 1024 (1K) or 2048 (2K) lines available on the horizontal and vertical axes. It may be tempting, if one has a 1K monitor, to assume that this is the maximum resolution of an incoming signal that can be displayed; however, one should remember that, as a result of magnification tools, part of the incoming signal can be displayed over the whole of the phosphor plate, thus facilitating display of all the incoming pixels. In reality, therefore, the spatial resolution of a digital image is generally limited by the spatial resolution of the image detector (camera, CCD or digital radiograph) rather than by the display system itself.

In PSP CR, the thickness of the phosphor layer is a limit to resolution, as is the size of the laser that reads them. In most DDR systems the size of the electronics required to amplify and transmit the signal

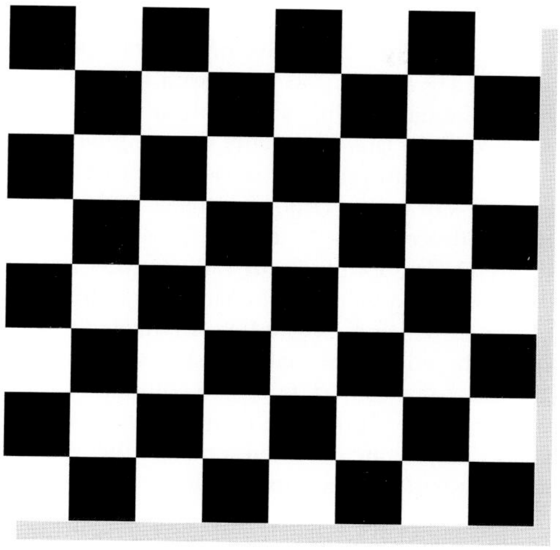

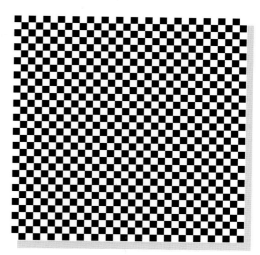

Figure 1.2 Standard chessboard: 8 × 8 matrix.

Figure 1.3 32 × 32 matrix.

from each pixel is finite, and no pixel can be any smaller than this. With either technology, to some extent the display technology limits the usefulness of very high-definition images, as radiographers and radiologists cannot work with small, zoomed areas of a larger image.

By far the biggest problem with minimising pixel size, however, is reduced signal strength, and hence problems with signal to noise ratio. As resolution is affected by noise as well as pixel size, increasing the matrix size often does not improve resolution without an increase in signal strength, i.e. an increase in the number of photons, and consequently radiation dose.

IMAGE STORAGE

Digital images can be stored as graphic files in a number of formats. Radiographs are generally stored as bitmap graphics, the common format being DICOM in medical archiving systems. Bitmapped graphics are stored as a series of numbers, rather than being described in terms of formulae as used in vector graphics (e.g. 'gif' files). Bitmaps are usually larger than vector graphics because areas of empty space must be recorded as well. Uncompressed they are the exact same size no matter what the image content.

A bitmap can be visualised by considering a chessboard pattern: each square ('pixel': picture element) is allocated a colour (in a bitmap this will be a numerical value to represent each shade) which best represents the contents of that square. The quality of the image produced will depend on the size of the 'chessboard', the number of squares (matrix), and the colours available (in radiography this will most often be shades of grey).

Changing the size of the image ('chessboard') will change the outer dimensions of the picture but not add any detail to it, just make each square bigger. When the squares are big and noticeable the image is said to be 'pixelated' (Fig. 1.2).

Increasing the number of pixels (squares on the chessboard) causes each to be smaller and therefore less noticeable. The Nyquist theory suggests that the smallest detail visible in any bitmap is twice the size of a pixel. This limit is referred to as the extended Kell factor.[4]

A smaller pixel size also makes the selection of the allocated 'colour' easier as each pixel is representing a smaller area of the image. As there can only be one colour covering each pixel, the closest match to the

average colour in that area of the image must be used. The smaller the area of the image and the more extensive the available colour selection (greyscale), the easier the choice and the more accurate the copy (stored image) (Fig. 1.3).

A standard chessboard has 8 rows and 8 columns of squares that form an 8 × 8 matrix, or array. The total number of pixels is 64. Each pixel is 50 mm square[5] and is adjacent to its neighbour, therefore a pixel pitch of 50 mm. A computer represents the colour of a pixel by storing a number, called the pixel value. In computing, numbers are stored in binary form, i.e. a series of 0s and 1s. Each numerical value is termed a bit; the number of values the computer can use for each pixel (i.e. number of bits) is called the bit depth. For example, if 6 bits were used, then binary values from 000000 to 111111 (0 to 63) would be available; that is, 64 grey shades (pixel values). Computers generally group bits into units of 8 (8 bits = 1 byte), hence images are generally stored as 8, 16, 24 or 32-bit files.

There are three ways to generate a radiological bitmap:

1. Computed tomography (CT), positron emission tomography (PET) and magnetic resonance imaging (MRI): The pixel values are found using a mathematical computation called Fourier back projection; the matrix is fixed (128, 256, 512, 1024). A variable called 'field of view' (FOV) determines how much of the scan area is used in the calculations and therefore displayed in the bitmap.
2. Analogue-to-digital conversion (ADC): The pixel values are found by scanning across a detector. The matrix size is fixed in the factory by the engineers who design the scan system, not the detector. Image intensifier fluoroscopy, ultrasound (with computation for radial scanning), PSP CR, transmission radiographic film scanners.
3. Scintillation detection/DDR/direct digital fluoroscopy (DDF)/gamma camera: The pixel values are directly detected within a fixed matrix, and are hard wired by the manufacturer of the detector.

Although there are fixed matrix sizes (as mentioned above), radiographers can alter the matrix size relative to the patient by altering:

- the detector (changing the CR plate size, or choosing DDR)
- the zoom or electrostatic focus of an image intensifier
- the FOV variable in CT and MRI.

DIGITAL IMAGE MANIPULATION

Perhaps the greatest advantage of digital imaging is the ability to duplicate, store, search and manipulate the acquired data.

In acquisition and display, the emphasis is on fidelity. Recording the radiographic contrast emerging from the patient as faithfully as possible is paramount, which means displaying the pixel values and locations accurately and consistently. The number one benefit of all digital projection radiography systems is the ability to deal with changing radiographic exposure parameters, even incorrect ones! In this case we want to change the data coming in before displaying it, because the pixel values are either too high (overexposed) or too low (underexposed). The computer achieves this adjustment by adding or subtracting an array from the stored bitmap before display.

This is a simplified example to show the benefit of changing the data in a controlled way. The initial data acquired is stored in a file called the RAW Data. Any manipulation should be on a copy of this, leaving the original intact. In some systems, after manipulation, only the new data is sent across the network to be viewed and stored; this can be with a reduced palette (14 becomes 12 bit). Although this might be seen as a disadvantage, it does emphasise the radiographer's role in QA informed by clinical indications. Poor decisions at the QA station can cause loss of diagnostic information.

Digital image processing

Different manufacturers have different names for certain processes; they may carry out tasks in a different order, and some have patented processes that are unavailable for scrutiny. This is a major cause for confusion in digital projection radiography at present, but there are several basic principles which should allow understanding of these disparate systems; these are:

- Histogram analysis
- Exposure control
- The characteristic curve and inherent response of the CR and DDR systems
- Digital system response and look up tables (LUT)
- Multifrequency processing.

Histogram analysis

Typically, one imagines a digital image as data that is displayed in a matrix that locates each pixel value in an X and Y location, but data does not have to be ordered in that fashion, it is just numbers. Another way to order data might be in size order. Consider an aerial view of a crowd at the Glastonbury festival: we can allocate each individual on the image a number representing their shoe size. We can then draw a graph of this data, but in size order rather than based on location (Fig. 1.4).

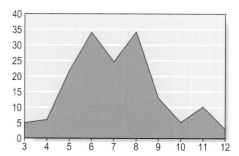

Figure 1.4 Shoe size graph.

Some educated guesses may be made using this data representation. For example, Glastonbury is an adult-only festival and the mean shoe size of the female UK population is 7. From this it may be inferred from the graphical data that this is a mainly adult female population, as the mean size is 7. This highlights the problem with graphical analysis. As with all assumptions, there is a risk that it is incorrect. In fact, Glastonbury is of course child friendly.

In CR, the first process that occurs is a histogram analysis. Various assumptions are made about how the radiographer exposed the PSP. Each manufacturer has a method of analysing the histogram, assuming various ways in which radiographers are likely to use the system, but this can be fooled by unusual exposure situations, e.g. using a large detector for a small object, failing to collimate, exposing several areas on one detector (splitting the field), gross over- or underexposure, and positioning the area of interest on an outer edge of a detector (because some systems use a combination of area and histogram analysis).

Manufacturers' software is becoming more and more sophisticated; some systems take note of the identity given to the image prior to histogram analysis, e.g. chest or hand X-ray. Errors are becoming fewer, but this is still a major cause of confusion for radiographers when using CR and DDR applications. Radiographers frequently have to 're-collimate' or 're-output' the image to provide guidance to the system as to which area of the exposed plate the histogram should be based on. When an apparent error has occurred this should be the first step to rectify it.

Exposure control

In digital systems a figure for exposure control must be indicated somewhere. Much has been made of the potential for over- and under-exposure in digital systems.

Several systems aim for a value of 2.0 (antilog 2.0 is 100, i.e. 100% of the expected value). Radiographers who produce a value of 2.3 seem within limits, but the antilog of 2.3 is 200%, i.e. double the expected value, and this is a considerable overexposure.

With such a system, an audit of pelvic examinations showed that 28% of images accepted had exposure levels of 2.6–2.8, possibly indicating endemic 400–600% overexposures.[6] Having said that, the exposure index or sensitivity is vital, but it may also be misleading.

The value is unpredictable, depending on collimation, positioning, time taken to develop the image, and background scatter present before exposure. Lehning et al.[7] showed a variation of up to a factor of 2 in sensitivity index values for the same exposure, depending on conditions prior to and after exposure and prior to reading of the plate. Examples of other such systems can be found in Chapter 3.

The characteristic curve and inherent response of CR and DDR systems

Radiographers should be familiar with the exposure response curve. Each film/screen system has a characteristic curve: this representation of exposure response is seldom used by engineers or physicists, as any exposure response is energy dependent and this is not represented on the graph. It is therefore difficult to find an exposure response graph in the literature for CR and DDR systems. Most systems are said to have linear exposure response.

In some ways the inherent response of the digital detector is not as relevant as with a film/screen system, but radiographers are used to the appearance of an image using a detector that has a typical 'S-shaped' response curve. This type of response to radiation differs from a linear response in its poorer sensitivity to low-energy radiation. Scattered radiation and extra focal radiation are both likely to be low energy and hence more likely to be detected by any CR/DDR system.

It is vital that all collimated areas are screened with lead and that CR plates are erased daily and used in strict rotation.

Digital system response and LUT

In the case of over- or underexposure of the imaging plate, the pixel value histogram will be shifted along the exposure axis. With a conventional film/screen system the characteristic curve is fixed, and the optical density histogram will therefore be severely affected. With digital systems another curve can be created with the aim of matching the pixel value histogram with the desired optical density histogram.

Modern systems can alter the response depending on the area of the image, enabling an effect similar to that of dual windowing in CT. This is useful to visualise C7 through the shoulders on a large patient, or view the lungs through the heart.

Multifrequency processing

Many systems now aim to reduce the complex content of the digital image into its constituent parts. Areas of mottle and noise are all very high frequency. Areas of clinically important detail, e.g. bony trabeculae, are said to be medium frequency. Areas of subtle shading over the whole image are said to be low frequency.

The low-frequency elements of the image can be digitally suppressed, as they are generally not felt to be helpful in image interpretation. This leads to an image with special properties that enhance fine details. Edge enhancement can be achieved through transforming the acquired data by applying a mathematical function to accentuate the difference between adjacent pixel values where one exists currently. This has the visual effect of enhancing any boundaries. These are high-frequency structures; statistical variation, such as noise, is also high frequency so becomes much more apparent. The most unsatisfying digital images visually are those with low exposure and high edge enhancement. However, this is what is preferred in situations such as central venous pressure line, long-line or chest drain locations; hence this is another important consideration for the radiographer, who must match appropriate manipulation to the clinical indication for the examination.

QUALITY ASSURANCE

Quality assurance (QA) is an all-encompassing term that includes acceptance testing and quality control; it is a programme that is intended, by its actions, to guarantee a standard level of quality. Quality control (QC) is the system by which the actual standard of quality is measured and maintained. The difference is that QA is process orientated and QC is product orientated. Both QA and QC can help with quality improvement; this is a systematic and continuous activity to improve all systems and processes to achieve optimal levels of performance.

Acceptance testing is formal testing carried out to determine whether or not a system satisfies its acceptance criteria and to enable the customer to determine whether or not to accept the system. Acceptance testing for DR systems usually involves user acceptance testing. The goal of acceptance testing is therefore to ensure that the system is functioning in accordance with the design and specifications of its manufacture.

QC tests are sometimes different, but they often use the results of the acceptance testing as a baseline to judge the performance of the system or to establish whether there has been a change in performance over time.

Quality control for CR

QC tests for CR can be split into two sections: acceptance testing and annual QC tests, and routine QC tests.

Acceptance testing and annual tests

The following tests should be performed for acceptance testing of the system when purchased and annually thereafter.

- Monitor and laser printer test [acceptance testing and annual]
- Erasure efficiency [acceptance testing and annual]
- Sensitivity index calibration and consistency [acceptance testing and annual]
- Uniformity [acceptance testing and annual]
- Scaling errors [acceptance testing and annual]
- Blurring [acceptance testing and annual]
- Limiting spatial resolution [acceptance testing and annual]
- Threshold contrast detail detectability [acceptance testing and annual]
- Dark noise [acceptance testing and annual]
- Moiré patterns [acceptance testing only]

Routine QC tests [performed every 3 months]

- General cassette condition check
- Sensitivity index monitoring
- Uniformity
- Threshold contrast detail detectability
- Limiting spatial resolution.

Note: The processing parameters that should be used during QC tests on a CR system will vary between manufacturers; consequently, there is the need to refer to their guidelines on processing parameters during QC. In general little or no image processing will be used.

Quality control for DDR

The QC tests that should be carried out for DDR are similar to those above for CR, but fewer tests are required:

- Monitor and laser printer set-up [acceptance testing and annual]
- Image retention [acceptance testing and annual]
- Sensitivity index consistency [acceptance testing and annual]
- Uniformity [acceptance testing and annual]
- Scaling errors [acceptance testing and annual]
- Blurring and stitching artefacts [acceptance testing and annual]
- Limiting spatial resolution [acceptance testing and annual]
- Threshold contrast detail detectability [acceptance testing and annual]
- Dark noise [acceptance testing and annual]
- Moiré patterns [acceptance testing only].

IMPLEMENTING A DIGITAL IMAGING SYSTEM

The transition from conventional methods of image acquisition to digital is fraught with pitfalls. No matter how much time is put into planning and training, issues will arise, largely due to the fact that digital imaging systems are not a development of old technology but rather a completely new method of image acquisition.

Digital radiography is not just a new type of film. It has been introduced in some departments on the basis that 'we have a new detector system, but nothing changes except that'. This is the wrong approach: digital radiography requires reconsideration of radiographic exposure, technique and protocols.

The installation of a digital radiography system will affect many staff, including radiographers, administrative staff and porters. An ongoing training programme is essential. Simple tasks necessary for the everyday completion of duties will be learned quickly, but more complicated tasks will require more sophisticated training.

All essential radiology equipment must be protected by an uninterruptible power supply (UPS). Digital radiology equipment such as the CR or DDR unit must have the facility to connect locally to the archive or film printer should the hospital network go down. This would ensure that even if images cannot be sent to the wards or to the reporting stations they can be archived or sent for printing. At the very least this will maintain the basic radiology service.

A system must be put in place to resolve a technical breakdown of the DDR system in an emergency. Hospitals who have adopted the 'big bang' approach to the installation of digital radiography with a single vendor will probably have a contract with that vendor for the maintenance and upgrade of the system. In this situation there will often be 24-hour support, at least in the early years. Hospitals who have adopted the phased approach to implementing digital radiography will most likely have purchased their equipment from multiple vendors. In this situation it would be too expensive to have a 24-hour service agreement with them all, so there may be an agreement with one or two of the most crucial.

Staff should have a good basic knowledge of problem solving with the DDR system; this is usually achieved through experience over a period of time and being provided with 'fix-it sheets' should things go wrong. Some hospitals have adopted the policy of selecting a limited number of radiographers to become specialists in problem solving. These specialists may provide effective technical support for other users.

When the argument is made to convert a film/screen radiography department to digital, the ability to eliminate or reduce the need for film will always be included as a potential saving. This may be true, but it may be some years until film is completely discarded in some departments. When initially installed, many digital radiography systems have been connected to a hardcopy printer; this can be expensive and is gradually becoming less common.

Common errors

Digital radiography is not an intelligent system: some of the most common human errors are not corrected by the digital radiography system. For example:

- Digital radiography will not correctly rotate an AP image processed as a PA.
- The system will not correct misidentification of an image, and, once archived, incorrectly identified images are difficult to retrieve unless the incorrect name placed on the image is known.
- The system will not correct processing errors. If the user puts a chest through the processor as a cervical spine the image will have the incorrect processing parameters applied. Unless the raw data of the image has also been stored the chances are high that the resultant image will not be diagnostic.
- The user must be aware that the diagnostic acceptability of an image must be judged on a monitor of diagnostic quality. The monitors provided with digital radiography systems for the initial appraisal of images are meant only as preview monitors for the assessment of gross positioning, inclusion of the region of interest, anatomical markers and identification.

CONCLUSIONS

Digital image acquisition has many benefits for an imaging department, particularly as more effective image and data management can be achieved. For every conventional imaging modality there is a digital image acquisition system on the market.

REFERENCES

1. Sonoda M, et al. Computed radiography utilizing scanning laser stimulated luminescence. Radiology 1983;148:833–8.
2. Nakano Y, et al. Improved computed radiography image quality from a BaFl:Eu photostimulable phosphor plate. Medical Physics 2002;29(4).
3. Mackenzie A. Effect of latent image decay on image quality in computed radiography.

Proceedings of UK Radiological Congress. BIR: London; 2004: 21.
4. Benson K, Fink D. HDTV: Advanced television for the 1990s. New York: McGraw-Hill; 1991.
5. Federation Internationale des Echecs Chessboard standard size. http://www.fide.com/official/handbook.asp?level=C02.

6. Field S, Blower C. Moving to CR – impact on radiography practice. Proceedings of UK Radiological Congress. BIR: London, 2004: 41.
7. Lehning L, et al. Exposure indicators in digital radiography: What is their relation to exposure? Proceedings of the European Congress of Radiology 2002; C-0746.

Chapter 2

Film/screen imaging

Barry Carver

INTRODUCTION

In Western Europe and North America in particular the advance of digital imaging technologies would appear to be irresistible. Indeed, although film/screen technology had been argued to offer some advantages in mammography,[1] digital imaging has now been shown to be at least comparable.[2] Consequently, film/screen systems are rapidly being replaced by digital technologies; indeed, in the UK, film/screen systems are largely a thing of the past.

This chapter is required for those regions in which this is not yet the case, and in the UK there is still a requirement for the teaching of this technology. It is helpful in order to evaluate digital technologies to have an understanding of the contribution of film/screen technology to medical imaging during the last century.

IMAGING PLATES

The first medical radiographic image receptors were silver halide-coated glass plates, which were placed in light-tight envelopes or cassettes. Junior staff often had the task of waxing the edges of the plates to prevent the emulsion from slipping off![3]

Although the value of photographic film was recognised, it was used sparingly prior to the 1920s. Once in regular use, however, the X-ray film soon proved its worth. It was quickly recognised that, unlike the early glass plates, a film could be coated on both sides. This had obvious advantages, particularly when used with intensifying screens. Because only about 1–2% of incident radiation was absorbed by the X-ray film alone, it was soon apparent that this wastefulness could be reduced by using light rather than X-rays to create the latent image on the film.[4]

INTENSIFYING SCREENS AND FILM EMULSION TECHNOLOGY

The introduction of fluorescent intensifying screens proved to be a significant development, enabling more of the incident X-rays to be absorbed by the phosphor material and emitted as light. In addition, the use of two intensifying screens meant that double emulsion films could be used, thereby instantly doubling the light absorption. However, the increase in density and contrast was partially counterbalanced by a decrease in resolution, and an increase in quantum noise in faster film/screen combinations. As always in radiography, there is a choice to be made when balancing image quality and patient dose.

During the remainder of the 20th century, film/screen technology continued to develop. Intensifying screens became more efficient when 'rare earth' phosphors were introduced in the 1970s, and the familiar globular silver halide crystals in the film emulsion were superseded by the 'tabular' variety.

The introduction of asymmetric film screen combinations with anti-crossover features provided greater visualisation with reduced image blur. In more recent years there were further developments in emulsion technology, but the undoubted success of the new digital technologies has mounted a serious challenge to traditional practices.

The X-ray cassette

The cassette is essentially a light-tight protective container for the film and intensifying screens. It is also designed to maintain uniform contact between the film and screens. A foam pressure pad behind the back screen helps to ensure this.

Various cassette materials, such as aluminium and plastic laminate, have been used. However, the ideal low-attenuation material for the cassette front is carbon fibre, as it represents a considerable reduction in patient dose. It is lightweight, durable, and relatively comfortable for the patient, but rather more expensive than other materials. The cassette back is lined with lead foil to reduce scattered radiation. A sliding aperture and lead blocker is incorporated into the design for use with patient identification systems.

Although the film/screen cassette is still relatively commonplace, older cassette types are less familiar sights in a modern imaging department. These include the multisection cassette, the formatter cassette and the photofluorographic cassette.[5]

RADIOGRAPHIC FILM

Film technology depends upon certain materials undergoing changes when subjected to electromagnetic radiation such as visible light or

X-rays. The main light-sensitive materials used are the halogens, e.g. bromine, iodine or chlorine. In radiographic film these are combined with silver to form, for example, silver bromide or silver idobromide.

Film manufacture

The manufacturing process is extremely stringent, as there must be no variation between batches of film. Solutions of silver nitrate ($AgNO_3$) and potassium bromide (KBr) are added to liquid gelatine. Potassium nitrate, which is soluble, is washed away in the process.[6]

There are usually four stages in the preparation of the emulsion layer. It is during the latter stages that the characteristics of the film are determined. For example, the speed and contrast of the film depend on the size of the silver halide grains. A high-contrast narrow-latitude film has a narrow range of grain sizes, whereas relatively large grains will produce a film of greater speed. In the final stage various additives are introduced, such as sensitisers, colour sensitisers, hardeners, plasticisers, fungicides, antistatic agents, wetting agents and anti-foggants.[5]

Impurities such as sulphur are deliberately added during the process in order to create imperfections in the crystal lattice. These imperfections create areas known as electron traps or sensitivity centres. These centres, coupled with excess bromine added to the mix, create the conditions necessary for the formation of the latent image.

Film construction (Fig. 2.1)

So that it can be used as a photographic material, the silver halide needs to be prepared in a form that can be coated on to a support or base.

Base

The material for the base is usually polyester, which has all the necessary characteristics required:

- strong but flexible
- dimensionally stable
- non-flammable
- unaffected by processing chemicals and high temperatures
- impermeable to water
- uniform colour tone and thickness.

Photographic emulsion

The silver halide crystals have to be suspended in a suitable binder to form a photographic emulsion. Gelatin has the properties required to act as a binding agent and suspension medium. It allows the silver halide crystals to grow. Gelatin is transparent and can exist as either a liquid or a solid, thereby allowing the crystals to be suspended evenly within the emulsion. It does not react chemically with the silver, but it allows the processing chemicals to penetrate the emulsion.

The emulsion layer is coated on to one or both sides of the base. A thin adhesive layer (substratum) binds the emulsion layer easily to the base. A supercoat or protective layer of clear gelatin protects the emulsion during processing and handling.[5,6]

Effect of exposure on silver halides

Silver halide crystals or grains may consist of a variety of shapes, although modern grains in X-ray applications are likely to be tabular. Tabular grains are flat and provide a greater surface area for latent image formation.

The latent image

The latent image is the hidden image created as a result of an interaction between X-ray or light photons and the silver bromide crystals. There are two theories of latent image formation: the Gurney–Mott and the Mitchell theories. These are the subject of some debate, but the Gurney–Mott theory seems to be preferred in radiographic imaging.[7]

The silver and bromine atoms are fixed in the crystal lattice in ion form: positive silver ions and negative bromine ions. In simple terms, the interactions between X-rays or light photons and bromine ions cause electrons to be released. These electrons migrate to the electron traps. The interstitial silver ions are attracted to the electrons in the electron traps (or sensitivity centres) and combine to form silver atoms.

As the process is repeated, other silver ions are attracted to the sensitivity centre and more silver atoms are created. The latent image centre is not visible, even microscopically: it is the developer that renders the image visible by acting as a chemical reducing agent and transforming the silver atoms into visible metallic silver.[7]

Types of film

Duplitised or double emulsion film is the standard film used for general applications (Fig. 2.2) The vast majority of these films are used with two intensifying screens. The exceptions are the intraoral dental film, which is a direct exposure film, and the radiation monitoring film, which is coated with two different emulsions and is used with various filters.

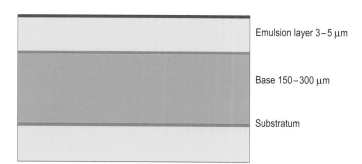

Emulsion layer 3–5 μm

Base 150–300 μm

Substratum

Figure 2.1 Diagrammatic representation of film structure (not to scale).

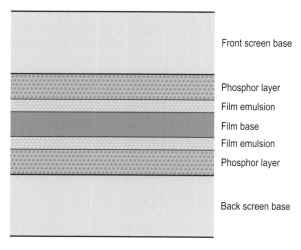

Front screen base

Phosphor layer

Film emulsion

Film base

Film emulsion

Phosphor layer

Back screen base

Figure 2.2 Cross-section of a duplitised film/screen combination.

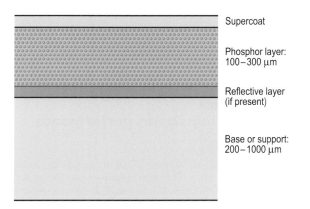

Figure 2.3 Diagrammatic representation of intensifying screen structure, not to scale.

Single emulsion film is used in mammography, where high resolution is the primary requirement. Laser imaging and duplication films are also coated with a single emulsion. Less frequently subtraction film and 100 mm photofluorographic single emulsion film may be seen.

INTENSIFYING SCREENS

In many ways the intensifying screen represents the most important component of the film/screen/cassette combination. Although X-rays do interact with the film emulsion, they contribute only approximately 1–3% to the latent image in a typical screen/film combination. On the other hand, about 30% of the incident X-rays interact with the screen.[6] Even though a considerable amount of the incident energy is lost, the process is much more efficient if intensifying screens are used. This results in a considerable dose reduction for the patient.

Screen construction (Fig. 2.3)

Base

The base or support consists of cardboard, plastic or polyester. It is usually up to 1 mm thick. Obviously the base must be robust and moisture resistant.

Substratum

The substratum is a bonding layer between the base and the phosphor layer. This may be reflective, absorptive or transparent. A reflective layer will reflect light back towards the film for maximum effect in faster film/screen combinations. Titanium dioxide is often the material used. The increase in speed, however, is achieved at the expense of increased image blur or lack of sharpness.[6] Alternatively, an absorptive layer contains a dye which will absorb light and therefore may be used in high-resolution screens. More commonly there may be a coloured pigment or carbon granules within the phosphor layer which serve the same purpose. Greater resolution is achieved at the expense of some loss of speed.[5,7]

Phosphor layer

The phosphor layer contains fluorescent crystals which emit light when bombarded by X-ray photons. The crystals are held in a clear binder such as polyurethane. This material protects the phosphor

material from moisture. This is important, as many phosphor materials are hygroscopic.

Luminescence

A luminescent material emits light as a result of external stimulation. The process is similar to the emission of characteristic radiation, but involving outer-shell electrons. There are many different types of luminescence but in radiography only three are relevant: fluorescence, phosphorescence and thermoluminescence. Thermoluminescent materials emit light when stimulated by heat. This process is used in thermoluminescent dosimeters.

Fluorescence (Fig. 2.4)

This occurs almost instantaneously and the emission of light ceases within 10–8 seconds.

Within the phosphor material there are three energy levels known as the conduction band, the forbidden band and the valence band. Incident X-ray photon energy is absorbed into the phosphor material by the photoelectric effect or Compton scattering. In the process high-energy secondary electrons are emitted. These collide with other electrons, knocking them from the valence band to the conduction band. Electrons already in the electron traps and electrons in the conduction band can fall into the holes created in the valence band, emitting light as they lose energy.[7]

Phosphorescence

If the phosphor continues to emit light after irradiation has ceased, then the process is known as phosphorescence. This is called afterglow or image lag, and is not desirable in an intensifying screen for obvious reasons. Afterglow, however, may occasionally be observed in older image intensifiers.

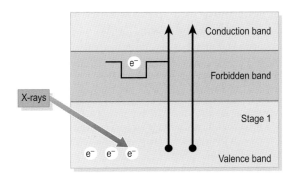

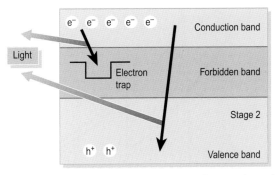

Figure 2.4 Fluorescence. Stage 1: X-rays remove electrons from the valence band. Stage 2: the electrons drop into the electron traps, or directly into the conduction band, emitting light energy as they do so.

Types of phosphor

Until the 1970s the most popular phosphor was calcium tungstate ($CaWO_4$). It was known as the universal phosphor and emitted ultraviolet light. Other phosphors included barium strontium sulphate and barium lead sulphate. Then rare earth phosphors were developed, such as gadolinium oxysulphide (Gd_2O_2S) and lanthanum oxybromide. Small quantities of activators such as terbium (Tb) are added during manufacture. The combination of phosphor and activator determines the colour and intensity of light emitted. These phosphors, combined with activators, had distinct advantages over $CaWO_4$, in particular higher quantum detection efficiency and improved conversion efficiency.

Quantum detection efficiency (QDE or absorption efficiency)

Rare earth phosphors are kVp dependent to a certain extent, but if used within recommended limits the QDE of rare earth phosphors is superior. The QDE is proportional to the atomic number of the rare earth phosphors. Consequently, these phosphors are usually more efficient at absorbing X-ray quanta, particularly between the K-shell absorption edge for rare earth elements and tungsten (Fig. 2.5).

The energy range extends from approximately 30 to 70 keV. For example, Gd_2O_2S:Tb has an absorption efficiency of 51% at 60 keV, compared to $CaWO_4$ at 13%. However, at 80 keV there is very little difference at 27% and 28%, respectively. Energy levels above or below this range will result in decreased QDE in rare earth phosphors.[5,6]

Conversion efficiency

The rare earth phosphors have an even greater advantage when X-ray photons are converted to light, approximately 15–20% being converted to light, compared to 3–5% for $CaWO_4$.[5]

Spectral sensitivity and spectral emission

Films are sensitive to all wavelengths of light, but during the manufacturing process certain types of X-ray film are designed to be particularly sensitive to certain wavelengths. Radiographic films are either monochromatic (blue/violet sensitive), orthochromatic (green sensitive) or panchromatic (red or infrared sensitive).

It is essential to match the spectral sensitivity of the film to the spectral emission of the intensifying screens. Calcium tungstate is known as a broadband emitter as it emits a continuous spectrum with a peak emission of approximately 440 nanometres (nm). Many rare earth phosphors emit narrow bands of wavelengths with peak emission of approximately 550 nm in the green area of the spectrum (Fig. 2.6). Spectral mismatching will occur if, for example, a green-emitting screen is used with a blue-sensitive film. The peak emission in the green region of the spectrum will be undetected by the film, and this will result in a considerable reduction in speed.[6]

Factors affecting screen performance

Crossover (Fig. 2.7)

The crossover effect can be detrimental to image quality owing to the increased image blur caused by light crossing from one screen as far as the opposite emulsion layer. The increased distance involved results in greater divergence of light and reduced sharpness.

Other factors

Speed will be increased if the following factors apply:

- larger phosphor crystal size and greater coating weight
- use of a reflective layer
- greater QDE
- greater conversion efficiency
- no anti-crossover layer.

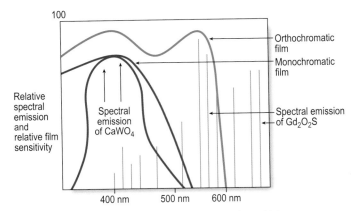

Figure 2.6 Relative spectral emission and spectral sensitivity.

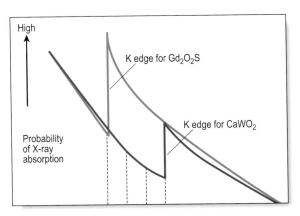

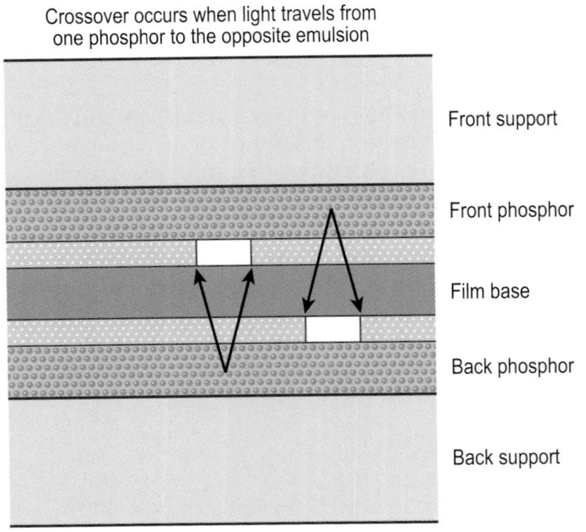

Figure 2.5 X-ray absorption spectra for calcium tungstate and gadolinium oxysulphide.

Crossover occurs when light travels from one phosphor to the opposite emulsion

Figure 2.7 Crossover.

The above factors will, however, reduce the sharpness of the image. Conversely, reducing the phosphor crystal size and coating weight, and adding a carbon granules or a dye to the phosphor layer, will reduce speed and increase sharpness.

COMPARISON OF FILM/SCREEN SYSTEMS

It is useful to be able to compare different systems easily in terms of speed, contrast and latitude. Manufacturers attach a number to their products in the same way as photographic films are identified. Par-speed $CaWO_4$ screens are assigned a value of 100. High-resolution screens are usually between 50 and 100, and others range from 200 to 1200.

The speed of a film/screen system is inversely proportional to the exposure required to produce a given density. Therefore, a 200-speed system will require half the mAs of a 100-speed system to produce the same density on the film (all other factors being constant).

Image quality deteriorates with very fast systems because quantum noise becomes unacceptable.

Purchasers of film/screen combinations do not make their choice on speed alone, however. Film contrast and latitude also need to be considered carefully before a system is selected for general or specialist use. In addition, processing requirements must not be forgotten.

Asymmetric screen/film systems

A dual receptor system uses asymmetric screens and dual emulsion films. The back screen contains a thicker phosphor than the front screen. The film has a high-contrast emulsion on the front surface and a wide-latitude emulsion on the back, and the film base is coated with

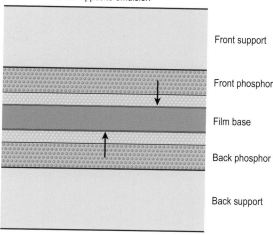

Anti crossover layer reduces crossover to the opposite emulsion

Front support

Front phosphor

Film base

Back phosphor

Back support

Figure 2.8 Asymmetric systems.

an anti-crossover layer (Fig. 2.8). This essentially means that two different images are superimposed.[4]

The result is that the final image has enhanced visualisation of the posterior mediastinum of the chest, for example, without losing detail of the lung fields. Asymmetric systems are not universally used, but are particularly valuable in chest and paediatric imaging. Research suggests that greater visualisation of anatomical structures is possible, although there do not seem to be particular advantages in identifying chest pathology.[8]

REFERENCES

1. Skaane P, et al. Population based mammography screening: comparison of screen-film and full-field digital mammography with soft copy reading. Radiology 2003;229(3):877–84.
2. Vinnicombe S, et al. Full-field digital versus screen-film mammography: comparison within the UK Breast Screening Program and systematic review of published data. Radiology 2009;251, 347–58.
3. Thomas A, et al. The invisible light: 100 years of medical radiology. Oxford: Blackwell Science; 1995.
4. Pizzutiello R, Cullinan J. Introduction to medical radiographic imaging. New York: Eastman Kodak; 1993.
5. Ball J, Price T. Chesney's radiographic imaging. 6th ed. Oxford: Blackwell Science; 1995.
6. Bushong S. Radiologic science for technologists. 8th ed. St Louis: Mosby; 2004.
7. Gunn C. Radiographic imaging: A practical approach. 3rd ed. Edinburgh: Churchill Livingstone; 2002.
8. Greaney T, Masterson J. Comparison of an asymmetric screen-film combination with a conventional screen-film combination for chest radiography in 51 patients. British Journal of Radiology 1997;70:929–32.

Chapter 3

Exposure factors, manipulation and dose

Barry Carver, Mark McEntee

IMAGE QUALITY

For accurate diagnosis we require high-quality radiographic reproduction of the patient area being examined. What is a high-quality image? Many factors need to be included in the assessment of an image to determine its quality: patient positioning and compliance will affect the resultant image, as will the image receptor and exposure used.

Density and contrast are the photographic properties that affect image quality, commonly combined (inaccurately) by students to form 'exposure'. Although density and contrast are inextricably linked they can be differentiated on the image and the effects of each manipulated to optimise image quality. Unsharpness includes many aspects of image geometry which also contribute to the quality of the result. Taken together these three factors may provide a means by which a radiographic image can be evaluated for 'technical quality'; other contributing factors, such as acceptability of positioning, will be discussed in the relevant chapters for each body part/technique.

Density

Density may also be referred to as optical or radiographic density. Density in radiography is a measurable quantity: in its simplest sense it is the degree of 'blackening' seen on the image. For film/screen systems, when thought of in this way density is easy to evaluate and correct: is the film too dark (decrease exposure) or too light (increase exposure)?

In the case of a radiographic film the density we can measure is the transmitted density (D); this is defined as the base 10 logarithm of the ratio of the light incident upon the film (I_o) to the light transmitted through the film (I_t):

$$D = \frac{I_o}{I_t}$$

The use of a logarithmic measure is appropriate as the response of the eye to visual stimulation is itself logarithmic.[1,2]

In order to be useful, the range of densities demonstrated on the image needs to be within the range for visual perception and differentiation, usually considered to be approximately $D = 0.25 \rightarrow 2.50$

(Figure 3.1).[3] Although a density of >2.5 may not be immediately differentiated by eye, densities of up to 4 may be recorded on film.[4] In effect, too much information has been recorded; it is sometimes (but not always) possible to use and view this information by use of increased illumination ('bright light') or photographic reduction.

Users of digital radiography systems need to be aware of the impact of over- and underexposure on the image. Underexposure of a digital radiographic image will not result in an image that has low density. In fact, the image will generally be manipulated by the system to be displayed with an adequate optical density of approximately 1.2 no matter how much or how little radiation the system receives.

Underexposure instead causes problems with the signal-to-noise ratio, and with underexposure the image will appear grainy as a result of quantum mottle. The image must be closely examined to recognise this appearance, as from a distance the image may appear diagnostic. In most cases where fine detail is required for diagnosis, low signal-to-noise ratio in the image will result in the image being repeated.

Overexposure will also not result in an image of high densities. Again, the optical density of the overexposed image will be approximately 1.2, but in this case overexposures (high patient doses) result in high signal-to-noise ratios and image quality will be increased. The temptation, especially when using digital techniques, is to overexpose, as the safety net of image manipulation will prevent the need for a repeat examination, but this practice leads to each individual exposure being higher than necessary for the individual patient. Clearly this is a temptation to be avoided, and professional standards in the application of the 'as low as reasonably achievable' (ALARA) principle need to be maintained: give the right exposure for the individual patient.

Variation of applied mAs is often given as the controlling factor for density,[5] although the effect of variation of kVp on intensity, and therefore density, must also be considered. However, in general it is considered better to use a fixed kVp for each examination, using variations of mAs to control required changes in density.[6]

Contrast

Image contrast is a combination of subject contrast, which is the contrast produced due to the anatomical area under examination, and the receptor (radiographic) contrast, which is the contrast produced as a result of the image receptor being employed; and may be

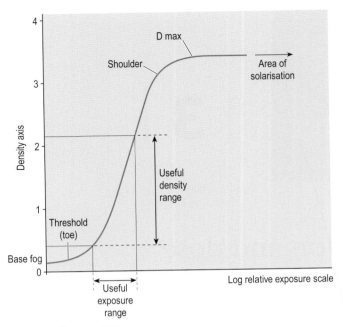

Figure 3.1 Characteristic curve.

reduction will also reduce the number of photons reaching the image receptor, and hence density, an appropriate increase in mAs is required to maintain the final image density.

For intrinsically high-contrast examinations such as the chest, the use of high kVp enables better visualisation of lung structures despite a reduction in overall image contrast. This is because at low energies the high subject contrast of the thorax, together with high radiographic contrast produced, makes the overall image contrast such that all structures cannot be demonstrated within the useful density range.

High contrast, lower kVp, can be referred to as 'short scale',[5] i.e. fewer shades of grey are represented within the image; consequently, fewer are available to represent the structures to be demonstrated. Use of a high kVp (120+)[9] reduces the radiographic contrast but enables all structures to be visualised within the useful density range. Low contrast produces a 'long scale' image,[5] with more shades of grey available for image depiction; the result is a 'flatter' image but with greater detail, particularly of lung parenchyma.

The 'flat' or grey appearance of such images does not suit all subjective tastes, and as such the technique is not universally accepted; however, this subjectivity is difficult to reconcile with accepted best practice, in terms of both image quality and dosimetry. Film readers need to educate themselves to accept these changes and embrace best practice,[7] the evidence for which is now long established.[9]

Subject contrast will be affected both by pathological processes, which may change the appearance from the expected 'norm', and the effects of scatter, which are discussed below.

As mentioned above, subjectivity in image viewing can be an important factor when considering image contrast, and 'subjective contrast' requires some consideration.

Not to be confused with subject contrast as described above, subjective contrast is due to the observer rather than inherent in the image,[10] but is nonetheless important to consider. The observer needs to be considered: eye strain and fatigue can have an effect on perception and several short viewing (or reporting) sessions are preferable to a single extended session; aids to visual acuity should be used as required (e.g. spectacles should be worn if they are needed!).

Viewing conditions need to be optimal. A dim viewing box in high ambient lighting, or holding a radiograph up to a window, are not ideal viewing conditions and will not enable accurate appreciation of either the radiographic density or the contrast demonstrated on the image. Viewing boxes should be matched for brightness and colour of illumination, checked on a regular basis, and used in appropriate conditions, i.e. in low ambient lighting.[11] Digital viewing stations should be of appropriate resolution and correctly adjusted.

As already stated, the amount of scatter reaching the image receptor will also affect image contrast. An increase in scatter reduces radiographic contrast by contributing a general increase in the overall image density, without any positive contribution to image definition.

Unfortunately, all examinations in the diagnostic range result in the production of scattered radiation, some of which inevitably reaches the image receptor. Consideration needs to be given to the most effective means by which scatter can be prevented from reaching the receptor in all circumstances.

Scatter production can only be effectively limited by using appropriate collimation: minimising the irradiated volume minimises the scatter produced. Maximum use of appropriate collimation should be applied to *all* projections undertaken, as there are also clear dose implications.

Given that some scatter will be produced, shielding the unused part of the image receptor by the use of lead rubber should be routine practice. This is particularly true when using film, as the unexposed area is rendered more sensitive when irradiated by scatter, further degrading the image when scatter from a second view is incident, which will then have a more severe effect on the final image. For

influenced by subjective contrast, which is the effect on contrast perception due to the observer or observing conditions.

The image itself is produced by means of differences in the attenuation of the X-ray beam within the patient. The differences thus produced in the transmitted beam are due to anatomical variations within the patient part under examination, in turn producing visible differences in density and contrast in the resultant image.

The contrast formed on the image in this way is termed 'subject contrast', due to the inherent 'contrast' which is the result of varying tissue types and densities of the body part under examination. Subject contrast can be influenced and manipulated by use of positive and negative contrast media, and the application of varying kVp techniques as described below.

Contrast can be shown to be inversely proportional to the applied kVp, hence in general at lower kVp values greater subject contrast is obtained. This is because, in the diagnostic range, the main interaction processes responsible for attenuation are photoelectric absorption and Compton scatter. Photoelectric absorption for a given beam energy is proportional to the cube of the atomic number and directly proportional to the density of the structure imaged, hence using the exposure ranges where photoelectric absorption is the dominant process (lower kVp) will maximise subject contrast. As digital systems manipulate the acquired image to produce a fixed image contrast (as described in Chapter 1), the direct relationship between kVp and subject contrast can be lost.

There is again a dose trade-off, as use of low kVp may increase skin dose. Several studies support the use of high kVp as a means of dose reduction. Guidelines for paediatric radiography recommend the use of 55–60 kVp, even for extremity work,[7] but the increase in kVp will reduce subject contrast and hence image definition.[8] Commonly forgotten in departments that have adapted this technique for adult use is the requirement for additional copper filtration to optimise the useful spectrum. Failure to use this additional filtration results in a reduction in image quality without the full benefit of the dose reduction intended.

kVp is the exposure factor by which contrast can be manipulated. If an image has adequate density but lacks contrast, even after digital manipulation, then kVp should be reduced; however, as kVp

digital systems it is important to reduce the amount of extra focal radiation reaching the receptor, as this may cause errors in histogram analysis; again, this is effectively achieved by the routine use of lead rubber shielding.

For larger body parts where higher beam energies are used and more forward scatter is produced which is more likely to reach the film, consideration should be given to the use of a grid. Placed between the patient and the image receptor, the grid will absorb scatter, but also to a degree primary radiation, leading to a requirement to increase exposure factors and consequently patient dose.

Careful thought needs to be given as to whether the use of a grid is required to produce the image quality required: for example when undertaking fluoroscopy the use of a grid should not be automatic.[12]

Unsharpness

Having the 'correct' density and contrast on the resultant image is important, but if the image produced is unsharp then detail is lost and the diagnostic quality of the image reduced.

- Such unsharpness may be due to several causes, which include system geometry (penumbra, photographic) and lack of patient cooperation due to voluntary or involuntary movement.
- As the anode target produces a finite effective focal spot size rather than the ideal point source, there is inevitably some penumbral effect produced, as shown in Figure 3.2.
- The penumbra causes geometric unsharpness within the resultant image. There are three ways in which this effect can be reduced:

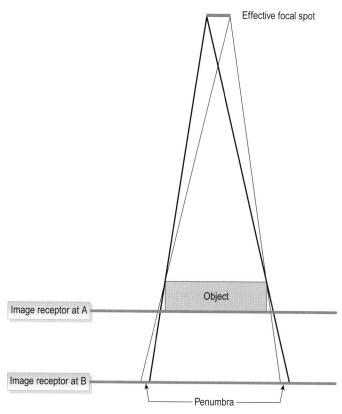

Figure 3.2 Penumbral effect: as ORD is increased the size of the penumbra produced can be seen to increase.

- Select the smallest useful focal spot size, which will minimise the size of the penumbra. Choice is limited in practice by tube loading considerations, but in general the smallest focal spot that enables the choice of the required exposure without compromise to tube life should be selected.
- Minimise object to receptor distance (ORD); as seen in Figure 3.2, increasing ORD increases the size and therefore the effect of the penumbra.
- If a broad focal spot is required and a large ORD cannot be avoided, e.g. when imaging a thick body part, consideration may be given to increasing focus receptor distance. Again this will lessen the penumbral effect due to the increase in focus object distance (FOD).

Unsharpness due to penumbral effects (geometric unsharpness) can be expressed as:

$$\text{Geometric unsharpness} = \frac{\text{ORD} \times \text{Focal Spot Size}}{\text{FOD}}$$

Photographic unsharpness is inherent to the receptor system resolution; it depends on the size of the detector and detection technique. (For DR/CR see Chapter 1.) For a film/screen system this will depend on the size of the light-emitting crystals in the intensifying screen and their distance from the film. Large crystals produce an image made up of large 'blocks' of information, and smaller crystals use smaller 'blocks' to build the image, which therefore appears sharper owing to its superior resolution.

As the distance between the crystals and the film increases the light emitted will diverge, causing a loss of resolution in the same way as described for the penumbral effect. Therefore, the requirement is for thin screens in good contact with the film.

Fine-grain screens with smaller crystals produce a sharper image but once again with a cost in terms of dose to the patient, so for most imaging a system with sufficient resolution produced with a reasonable dose is chosen.

Movement produces a blurred, unsharp image, and so steps should be taken to minimise patient movement. The risk of voluntary movement should be minimised by adequate explanation of the procedure, rehearsal of manoeuvres such as breath holding, and appropriate use of aids to immobilisation, such as radiolucent pads. The effect of involuntary movement should be minimised where appropriate selecting the shortest available exposure time.

Density, contrast and unsharpness are distinct elements which should in all cases be individually assessed and manipulated to produce images of optimal quality.

EXPOSURE FACTOR SELECTION

For skeletal radiography where areas with a relatively high subject contrast are being examined a fairly low-contrast film can be used to demonstrate the majority of structures within the useful density range. This selection will also provide a reasonably wide exposure latitude, which can lead to fewer repeats due to exposure errors. Digital systems generally have the advantage of offering wide latitude in all situations.

However, it should be noted that if a repeat is required and a wide-latitude film or a digital system is being used, small increments of changes in exposure factors are to be avoided. This is because small incremental changes (the 1 or 2 kVp change by the supervisor which so infuriates students, and is anyway useless) have no effect on the resultant image. A wide latitude means that within that range of exposures a similar resultant image is produced. For example, if a film image is considered too dark and a repeat is required, consideration should be given to halving the mAs to produce a more reasonable density.[3] Similarly, changes in kVp should be of the order of 15%.[5] If only a small change is required the question must be asked, should the film be repeated at all?

Computed radiography (CR) systems and direct digital radiography (DDR) systems are not inherently dose reducing except for the reduction in repeats.[13] In low tube voltage examinations it has been shown that CR and amorphous selenium (aSe) compare well with 200-class film/screen systems when exposed with equal mAs.[14] DDR amorphous silicon (aSi) systems using CsI:Tl phosphors have been shown to have higher detective quantum efficiency (DQE) than film/screen, BaF(X) photostimulable phosphor (PSP), and aSe systems. The thickness of these phosphors may allow lower than 400-class system exposure.[15] For all these systems, reducing exposure further will increase the appearance of noise and reduce image quality.

For digital imaging systems, the selection of kilovoltages has been debated by several authorities. Theoretically, any difference in the energy absorption spectra of CR and DDR detectors compared with film/screen systems could result in a different optimum kVp.

Data from Hubbell and Seltzer[16] and Nakano et al.[17] for BaF(X) based CR PSPs and aSi/CsI:Tl indirect digital systems suggests broadly similar responses to those of film/screen. aSe detectors, however, are highly kVp dependent and should always be used in the lower kVp range.

The ability to use signal processing techniques to amplify contrast can compensate for the reduced subject contrast available with high kVp techniques. This has led some authors to suggest increasing kVp to reduce patient dose. A thorough study of contrast detail detectability over the 60–120 kVp range concluded that BaF(X) based CR PSPs performed slightly better than 400-class film/screen systems in demonstrating low contrast detectability, but only when receiving a 200-class exposure level. This study concluded that patient dose savings could be made, but only through the use of increased tube filtration, as previously mentioned.[18]

There are many situations, however, where high-quality images are not required, such as the examination of a total hip replacement, limb length measurement, or any other examination where only gross image detail is required. In these situations digital radiography can produce the required image quality at 80% less dose than screen/film radiography. The quantity of radiation required must therefore be considered on an examination by examination basis. A sensible way to approach dose reduction with digital radiography systems is to define the image criteria that must be visualised for a given examination and reduce the dose systematically until it is as low as is reasonably achievable while maintaining diagnostic efficacy.

Because CR systems adjust the optical density to correct for under- and overexposure, inappropriate exposure technique may be disguised. For example, if the operator overexposes a film the resultant image is too dark, and the next time the operator will use less radiation; this is called negative feedback. No such negative feedback exists with CR. Increasing the radiation reaching the storage phosphor will reduce the quantum mottle and associated noise factors in the image. When too little radiation reaches the storage phosphor the image will not be too light; however, there may be insufficient data in the image to allow an accurate diagnosis to be made and the image will have a noisy or grainy appearance (quantum mottle) due to decreased signal-to-noise ratio.

As a result, an indicator of the average exposure on the imaging plate is necessary to verify proper exposure selection and to provide a method of feedback to the radiographer, thus keeping patient dose to a minimum. Exposure indicators used in CR indicate the dose reaching the image plate and provide no information as to the entrance surface dose received by the patient. For example, a patient of average size and body mass index will receive less radiation than a larger patient, even though the exposure indicator may be equal for both.

Exposure indicators are also affected by several other factors, including: radiation dose, kVp, mAs, focus receptor distance, patient position, patient size and composition, and equipment factors such as grid, table material and filtration.

Exposure indicators

Each system manufacturer has a different method for providing this information; some examples are discussed in the following sections.

System sensitivity: S number

Fuji CR systems use a system sensitivity number, which is the value sought by the computer during pre-processing in order to adjust the centre of the pre-processed histogram to the centre of the digital display range. The S number is calibrated in the factory settings and its relationship to dose is greatly influenced by beam energy. The digital system adjusts the sensitivity so that the mean optical density of the displayed image will always be 1.2. The sensitivity number is inversely related to the incident exposure.

As the S number is derived from exposure data recognition (EDR) processing it cannot be used as a direct exposure indicator, as the EDR depends on position and anatomy. However, if all things remain exactly the same, the S number will relatively reflect the exposure, i.e. double the dose, halve the S number.

Exposure index (EI)

Carestream systems use an exposure index (EI), which provides a value directly proportional to an average exposure across the entire image plate. This is a relative measure of the number of X-rays that reach the receptor and form the relevant portion of the image. This does not include background scatter or collimated areas.

The EI is directly proportional to the average log incident exposure on the plate. Keeping all other factors the same, double the screen exposure results in an increase of 300 in the EI value.

lgM

Agfa systems have a dose-monitoring tool that uses a relative exposure paradigm. The dose value is a log measurement (lgM) calculated for each scanned image and logged into a database. The database stores the lgM reading of the previous 100 exposures carried out for each specific radiographic examination. The mean is calculated and the current exposure compared against this value. The current exposure is determined as being overexposed (having an lgM greater than the average of the last 100 hundred exposures for that examination), underexposed or average.

When an image is presented to the radiographer a graphical indicator is displayed in the text fields indicating the statistical average mean exposure for the specific examination compared to the relative over- or underexposure level in the current image. If the exposure of the image plate exceeds the average of 100 exposures for the same examination the graph will indicate a red bar extending to the right; if the exposure is lower than the average the graph will indicate a blue bar extending to the left. The further the line extends to the left or to the right, the greater the deviation from the reference value.

DOSIMETRY

A full discussion on dosimetry is beyond the scope of this text. There are many resources, particularly for students, that discuss the issues of dose measurement and radiation protection.[1-4,6,9] The commonest measures used are effective dose equivalent (EDE quoted in milliSieverts, mSv), entrance surface dose (ESD quoted in milliGray, mGy) and dose-area product (DAP, quoted in mGy/cm²).

Optimisation of patient dose is a requirement of both European and international (ICRP) directive[19,20] and UK law,[21] each requiring doses to be kept 'as low as reasonably practicable'. IR(ME)R requires the setting of diagnostic reference levels; readings from DAP meters are often used to provide information for establishment of DRLs. ESD and EDE can also be used but require calculation from exposure factors or measurement with dose meters.

The current system for radiation protection uses the linear no threshold (LNT) model for assessment of the risk from medical exposures. This assumes a linear relationship between the exposure received and the risk of cancer induction. At high exposure levels (>200 mSv) there is evidence from epidemiological studies to show that this is the case; however, below this threshold there is little hard evidence. Current legislation, based on the LNT model, is a 'safe' approach assuming harmful effects from low doses in order to provide maximum protection to the public.[22]

It has been argued that individual molecular lesions may[23,24] or may not[25] induce cancer. There is a rising tide of opinion in favour of radiation hormesis, the argument being that there may in fact be beneficial effects associated with low doses. Our bodies have very efficient repair mechanisms which cope with the ever-present effects of background radiation, as well as the more significant effects of deoxyribonucleic acid (DNA) damage from biological sources. Feinendegen argues that the stimulation of these processes at low doses may in fact be beneficial.[26]

Deterministic effects encountered in radiotherapy are also found in diagnostic imaging, e.g. erythema has been observed,[27] and lens opacities may be induced in children from doses as little as 0.1 Gy[28] (a CT head scan can be 0.03–0.06 Gy in children).[29] These effects must also be taken into account when considering protection policy.

This is an extremely complex argument which is likely to continue for some time. Until proved otherwise, use of the LNT model as required by current legislation would seem to be a sensible approach. Research should continue – with an open mind: as Arthur Conan Doyle pointed out, 'premature assumption results in a tendency to interpret data to agree with the assumption'.[25] An appropriate quotation for application by all researchers at whatever level.

REFERENCES

1. Allisy-Roberts P, Williams J. Farr's physics for medical imaging. 2nd ed. London: Saunders; 2007.

2. Graham D, et al. Principles of radiological physics. 5th ed. Edinburgh: Elsevier; 2007.

3. Carlton R, Adler A. Principles of radiographic imaging. 4th ed. New York: Delmar; 2005.

4. Bushong S. Radiologic science for technologists. 9th ed. St Louis: Mosby; 2009.

5. Bontrager K, Lampignano J. Textbook of radiographic positioning and related anatomy. 6th ed. St Louis: Mosby; 2005.

6. Dowd S, Tilson E. Practical radiation protection and applied radiobiology. 2nd ed. Philadelphia: Saunders; 1999.

7. Cook JV, et al. Guidelines on best practice in the X-ray imaging of children. Bristol: Ian Allan Printing; 1998.

8. Pizzutiello R, Cullinan J. Introduction to medical radiographic imaging. Eastman Kodak; 1993.

9. European Guidelines on Quality Criteria for Diagnostic Radiographic Images, Rep. EUR 16260, 1996, Office for Official Publications of the European Communities, L-2985 Luxembourg.

10. Whitley AS, et al. Positioning in radiography. 12th ed. London: Hodder Arnold; 2005.

11. Brennan PC, et al. Ambient lighting: effect of illumination on soft-copy viewing of radiographs of the wrist. American Journal of Roentgenology 2007;188(2): 177–80.

12. Lloyd P, et al. The secondary radiation grid; its effect on fluoroscopic dose-area product during barium enema examinations. British Journal of Radiology 1998;71:303–6.

13. Field S, Blower C. Moving to CR – impact on radiography practice. Proceedings of UK Radiological Congress. BIR: London, 2004: 41.

14. Zähringer M, et al. Detection of porcine bone lesions and fissures. American Journal of Roentgenology 2001;177: 1397–403.

15. Borasi G, et al. On site evaluation of three flat panel detectors for digital radiography. Medical Physics 2003;30(7): 1719–31.

16. Hubbell J, Seltzer S. Tables of X-ray mass attenuation coefficients and mass energy-absorption coefficients (version 1.4), 2004. Online. Available: http://physics.nist.gov/xaamdi [6 Feb 2005]. National Institute of Standards and Technology, Gaithersburg, MD.

17. Nakano Y, et al. Improved computed radiography image quality from a BaFI:Eu photostimulable phosphor plate. Medical Physics 2002;29(4).

18. Lu Z, et al. Comparison of computed radiography and film/screen combination using a contrast detail phantom. Journal of Applied Clinical Medical Physics 2003;4(1):91–8.

19. European Union. Council directive 97/43 Euratom on health protection of individuals against the dangers of ionising radiation in relation to medical exposure. Official Journal of the European Communities 40; 1997.

20. European Commission Directorate-General for the Environment 2000.

Referral guidelines for imaging. Radiation protection 118.

21. The Ionising Radiation (Medical Exposure) Regulations. Statutory Instruments 2000, no. 1059. London: HMSO; 2000.

22. Martin C. UKRC 2004 debate: the LNT model provides the best approach for practical implementation of radiation protection. British Journal of Radiology 2005;78:14–6.

23. Chadwick K, Leenhouts H. UKRC 2004 debate: radiation risk is linear with dose at low doses. British Journal of Radiology 2005;78:8–10.

24. Anoopkumar-Dukie S, et al. Further evidence for biological effects resulting from ionising radiation doses in the diagnostic X-ray range. British Journal of Radiology 2005;78:335–7.

25. Cameron J. UKRC 2004 debate: moderate dose rate ionising radiation increases longevity. British Journal of Radiology 2005;78:11–3.

26. Feinendegen L. UKRC 2004 debate: evidence for beneficial low level radiation effects and radiation hormesis. British Journal of Radiology 2005;78:3–7.

27. Mooney R, et al. Absorbed dose and deterministic effects to patients from interventional neuroradiology. British Journal of Radiology 2000;73:745–51.

28. Wilde G, Sjöstrand J. A clinical study of radiation cataract formation in adult life following gamma irradiation of the lens in early childhood. British Journal of Ophthalmology 1997;81:261–6.

29. Shrimpton PC, et al. Doses from computed tomography (CT) examinations in the UK – 2003 review. NRPB W67.

Section | 2 |

Skeletal radiography

Chapter 4

Introduction to skeletal, chest and abdominal radiography

Elizabeth Carver

To avoid repetition within the text, some safety, terminological and technical issues can be addressed by the use of initial statements regarding projection names, patient preparation, selection and use of image recording media, dose reduction methods, image identification and anatomical markers. This information is covered in this chapter.

PROJECTION NAMES

Names of projections are always given as representations of the direction of beam, so that this gives the radiographer information on the initial patient position. This is in preference to a system which uses names for some projections that reflect the original describer of the projection (e.g. Towne's', 'Waters') but gives little or no information on the position. The UK system has for many years avoided overuse of named projections, and the use of position descriptors for projection titles is less confusing, making it unnecessary for the radiographer to learn eponymous titles. As a matter of interest, the editors of this text searched for all named projections in use, most popularly used in the US; the total number found was 200 (projections for all body areas, not exclusively relating to the head). Confusion caused by a lack of consistency in projection names/descriptors is further discussed in the chapter on facial bones, as it is a particularly relevant topic for that area.

In reality, one or two eponymous titles are still considered mainstream and heard in use by radiographers in the clinical setting; when such a name is very commonly used in everyday practice, the alternative will be given in brackets after the projection title.

PATIENT PREPARATION

For all examinations, patient preparation should always include:

- appropriate and effective communication methods which will ensure patient compliance or cooperation
- removal of items of clothing or artefacts overlying the relevant examination area; in cases of severe trauma it may not be advisable or even possible to remove some items

- accurate identification check
- assessing justification for request
- assessment of the possibility of pregnancy for examinations where this is required.[1]

IMAGE RECORDING (CR CASSETTES AND DIGITAL PLATES)

With the current situation of image recording, where there is a choice of computed radiography (CR), digital radiography (DR) and film/screen systems for use, it has been difficult to select a method of description that accurately embraces the use of all of these methods. It must be said that, in the UK, use of film/screen radiography is now almost obsolete. As CR uses cassettes similar in appearance to conventional film/screen systems, there would appear to be little change from film/screen methods for image receptor (IR) use; however, some notable differences regarding DR exist. It has therefore been decided that the term 'image receptor' will be used as an umbrella term. This is intended to include any of the recording systems that may be used by the radiographer. It should also be noted that use of lead rubber for masking is not advisable for CR and DR systems, although some of the positioning images do demonstrate this on a film/screen cassette.

Since the last edition of this book was published there have been significant developments in DR plates and increased use of these. Wireless plates are now widely available, which further improves the flexibility and range of uses for digital plates, with some manufacturers developing DR support units which are flexible in their positioning rather than being fixed vertically or horizontally. DR plates vary slightly in size and are usually square in shape, but generally do not come in the wider range of sizes found with film/screen or CR plates. They can be fixed under a stand or table surface, independent (wired or wireless), in a tray used under the table-top or pulled from the side of the table-top for extremity work.

As a result of the range of possibilities for receptor arrangement, the IR position will simply be referred to as horizontal or vertical and no IR sizes will be given.

DR plates do not require the centre of the body part to be placed coincident with the middle, unlike CR cassette radiography. For this reason, the positioning descriptors provided in this book assume that the radiographer will always ensure that the body part lies within the IR, or within an unexposed section if the IR is used for more than one projection. At times it will be necessary to centre the body part to the middle of the DR plate, e.g. when that body part is large (as in chest or abdomen radiography), and this will be advised in descriptors for some sections, in order to ensure that the whole of the body part is included in the image.

Another point to raise is the use of an antiscatter device (grid), which should be used in conjunction with the IR if scatter reduction is relevant. Their use will be indicated in descriptors when necessary.

CHANGE IN TERMINOLOGY FOR FOCUS FILM AND OBJECT FILM DISTANCES

With the disappearance of film/screen radiography it has become necessary to reconsider these radiographic terms in order to ensure accuracy of reference. It has been noted that different terminologies have been introduced in recent years in an attempt to address this issue, and US texts initiated the use of the terms 'source image distance' and 'object image distance' as long ago as 2005[2] in an attempt to use more appropriate terms that did not include the word 'film'. However, one must question the use of the word 'source': it is true that the tube target is a source of radiation but use of the word 'source' in a radiation environment does imply 'radioactive source', simply because 'source' is used more routinely when referring to radioactive materials (although it is not inaccurate to refer to electrically produced X radiation as a source of radiation). In addition, use of the word 'image' can be considered inaccurate, as the image is latent until digitally processed and displayed. As a result it has been decided to use the terms *focus receptor distance* (FRD) and *object receptor distance* (ORD) in this edition; we feel that these are more appropriate, especially as the terms only include one changed word from old terminology, making them more easy to adopt.

ANATOMICAL MARKERS

It is assumed that anatomical markers will *always* be placed within the field of primary beam, clear of the essential area of interest. Therefore, instruction for this will not be included for every description of projections. Unless otherwise specified, it will be assumed that AP (anteroposterior) markers will be applied. Use of posteroanterior (PA) markers will be referred to but the authors do acknowledge that some imaging departments do not use PA markers. Anatomical markers do not always appear in positioning images as often they are too small to reproduce on a small photograph.

It will also be assumed that the radiographer will always check accuracy of anatomical markers on the resulting images as this is an important medicolegal requirement; therefore the image quality criteria will not refer specifically to this requirement.

IMAGE IDENTIFICATION

Correct identification of the image will be assumed to be an area that the radiographer need not be reminded to assess during image quality assessment, since this is a vital medicolegal requirement. This is therefore not included in the image evaluation lists in the text.

EXPOSURE FACTORS – EVALUATION OF IMAGES

As digital radiography has brought the possibility of image manipulation, the image submitted for reporting is not always exactly as produced at the point of exposure, as it was with film/screen radiography. It is still possible to state required evaluation criteria for exposure factors in the way used in the first edition of this book, but recognition of faults, and suggested correction, may be less relevant if manipulation of images can successfully bring appearances in line with required standards stated. It is clear, though, that the possibility of manipulation is no excuse for poor attention to exposure factor selection, and balancing dose minimisation with high-quality appearance is of paramount importance.

DOSE REDUCTION METHODS

This refers to physical mechanisms for protection during the examination, rather than precautions such as avoidance of unnecessary irradiation of patient, fetus or personnel. The use of lead rubber will be specifically referred to in projection descriptors. Collimation is also commented upon, to:

- ensure that the required area of interest is definitely included on the image
- limit the radiation field to the area of interest as a dose limitation method
- reduce scatter in order to maintain image quality and reduce radiation dose.

The philosophy of the authors is that the use of lead rubber, wherever and whenever possible, must be a consideration for every patient and projection. Observations have shown that it is tempting to omit the use of lead rubber for extremity examinations that are low-dose and well collimated. However, because the only safe dose is *no* dose, the authors *always* recommend the use of lead rubber for protection. Consistent and habitual use of lead rubber, for every examination, will ensure that the radiographer never forgets to use it. Lead rubber protection will not always appear in positioning images, as at times its use may mask demonstration of the body position.

Other recommendations for dose reduction are:

- The patient's head should be turned away from the primary beam and examination area during exposure, if possible in the position described, in order to minimise radiation dose to the radiosensitive lenses of the eyes and thyroid.
- Legs are never placed under the table, to clear the femora and gonads from the primary beam, edge of collimation and scattered radiation.

Specific notes for Section 2: Skeletal radiography

Radiographic examination of the human skeleton may identify a range of pathologies or appearances that identify traumatically induced changes. Many of the conditions identified in this section are found generally throughout the skeleton or its articulations, and for this reason are listed before all sections describing skeletal examination techniques. Information related to specific areas of the skeleton will be included at the beginning of the appropriate chapter, or related to individual projections if more appropriate. Not all conditions listed are necessarily justification for plain radiographic examination, nor is plain radiography necessarily the initial imaging method of choice for each condition. The pathologies given here are by no means exhaustive, but comprise those conditions most commonly encountered.

COMMONLY ENCOUNTERED PATHOLOGIES THAT AFFECT THE SKELETON AND ITS ARTICULATIONS

Acromegaly

Overproduction of growth hormone due to a pituitary gland tumour may result in an increase in the size of the skeleton, even after full normal adult growth has been completed. The soft tissue of the heel outline shows an enlarged fat pad, whereas there is apparent increase in joint spaces, an increase in vertebral height, possible pituitary fossa enlargement and early arthritis.[3] Modern diagnostic methods have resulted in earlier detection of pituitary tumours, thereby significantly reducing the number of people suffering from increased growth. The radiographer will need to consider that patients with acromegaly often present with a larger skeleton than is considered average, and if CR plates are used an appropriate size relevant to the patient's size must be selected.

Ankylosing spondylitis

Most notably referred to as 'bamboo spine' in its advanced stages; inflammation of the fibro-osseous junctions leads to calcification of fibrous tissue. Eventually, vertebral bodies appear fused, with dense calcification that is wider than the bodies themselves. This gives the ridged appearance of the vertebral column, which is likened to a bamboo stick. Patients with ankylosing spondylitis are likely to have limited movement and may not be as able to cooperate with projectional requirements as easily as others.

Bone age

Although not technically seen as skeletal pathology, epiphyseal appearance and fusions will determine bone age.[3] This type of assessment is requested when a child's physical development or size does not fall within the range considered to be normal. Among areas included in bone age surveys are hand and wrist, knee, elbow and iliac crests. Bones selected for the bone age survey vary according to the chronological age of the child.

Chondrosarcoma

This aggressive lesion is the third most common primary bone tumour and arises from cartilaginous tissue. There may be a soft tissue mass at the site, usually with cortical destruction. Slow-growing lesions will show cortical thickening.[3]

Enchondroma

Enchondroma consists of hyaline cartilage found as an island in bone. A noticeable lesion, with some sclerosis and containing small calcifications, may be accompanied by pathological fracture. There may be some soft tissue outline changes, especially if accompanied by a visible mass. Often the lesion is asymptomatic and findings may therefore be incidental.

Gout

Crystals of monosodium urate monohydrate are deposited in synovial fluid, which results in inflammation and erosion of cartilage and articular surfaces of bone. Radiologically there are likely to be narrowed joint spaces, a soft tissue outline indicative of swelling around the joint, and small localised erosions over the bone surface.

Metastases

Metastases are malignant secondary tumours which spread to bone from a primary malignancy. They affect other tissue types in addition to the skeleton. In the skeleton lesions appear lytic, in some cases sclerotic (metastatic deposits from carcinoma breast and prostate); pathological fractures may be present.

Myeloma

This is a neoplastic condition arising from bone marrow. Lesions show as low-density lytic areas; they may appear as multiple lesions seen as clusters, which have a scalloped edge appearance.

Osteoarthritis

This wear-and-tear disease displays narrowed joint spaces which may show as asymmetry in weight-bearing joints; osteophytes; sclerosis and erosions. Bone density is likely to be preserved unless the patient is generally osteoporotic.[3-5] There may be increased bone density in the articulating parts of affected joints, and exposure factors should be modified to take this into account.

Osteochondritis

Osteochondritis is a condition affecting primary and secondary centres of ossification, leading to avascular necrosis of a portion of bone due to a cut in the blood supply. In children this is idiopathic; in adults it can be due to trauma or inflammation.[5,6] Appearances vary according to the locality of disease and include loose bodies apparent in joints, sclerosis of epiphyses, collapse of affected bone and soft tissue swelling.

Osteomalacia

This is low bone mineralisation causing low bone density, which may or may not be apparent radiologically. Vertebral bodies may collapse, causing a kyphosis seen on lateral spine radiographs. Small linear radiolucencies (Looser's zones) may appear and can develop into fractures that follow the same linear direction.

Osteomyelitis

Osteomyelitis is inflammation of the bone and bone marrow following soft tissue infection or, occasionally, injury. It most commonly, but not exclusively, affects children. In the acute stage radiological signs are not likely to appear for up to 10 days but, when present, will probably show as metaphyseal bone destruction and periosteal reaction. Radionuclide imaging is effective in early detection of the condition. More long-standing osteomyelitis can be very aggressive, leading to changes in the periosteum and even deformity of the bone.

Osteoporosis

Osteoporosis is bone demineralisation and mainly affects elderly women, but some elderly males may also suffer from the condition. The diagnostic route does not use plain radiography as the first choice as a significant percentage of demineralisation (approximately 30%) must occur before loss of bone density is shown on plain X-ray. Early diagnosis is made by osteoporosis screening methods. In addition to loss of bone density, plain images may reveal noticeable loss of cortical width and a wedge appearance of vertebral bodies. Patients with known osteoporosis will require a reduction of exposure factors for skeletal radiography, and possibly modification of technique if extreme kyphosis is present.

Osteosarcoma

Osteosarcoma is an aggressively malignant tumour which most often affects young patients. Soft tissue swelling is often seen on plain radiography.

Paget's disease

Increased bone density, which is a result of this disease, is often referred to as having a 'cottonwool' appearance. The inexperienced can confuse the signs with the moth-eaten appearance of metastatic deposits in bone, but the mottled appearance of both can be distinguished thus: metastases erode (reducing the density of areas of bone compared to normal bone) whereas Paget's disease has areas of increased density compared to normal bone. Exposure factors for skeletal radiography must be increased to take into account the increase in bone density.

Perthes' disease

This condition is categorised as an avascular necrosis of the head of femur and affects children. Radiologically there will be increased joint space at the hip, a flattened femoral head, a sclerotic appearance of the femoral epiphysis and areas of low density over the metaphysis.

Rheumatoid arthritis

This is a condition of unknown origin which may affect any of the synovial joints, most commonly in the hands and wrist. It results in synovial inflammation, joint articular destruction and deformity. Radiologically significant appearances include a soft tissue outline which indicates swelling at joints, osteoporosis, narrowing of joint spaces, joint deformity, subluxation and marginal erosions.[6-8] Reduction in bone density should be considered when selecting exposure factors for these patients.

Trauma

Most positive diagnoses involve fractures or dislocations, which are categorised as follows:

Avulsion fractures

These fractures occur as a result of hyperflexion, hyperextension or unnaturally forced lateral movement of a joint; they are often seen in examinations of the fingers and thumb.

Comminuted fracture

The fracture site consists of several fragments.

Compound fracture

The fracture site is accompanied by an open wound on to the surface of the affected body part.

Complicated fracture

Complications arise because of the involvement of the fracture with important functional sites of the body, usually a joint, vascular supply/drainage or nerves.

Dislocation

The articulating surfaces of bones are no longer normally aligned and within the normal joint capsule, showing as disruption of the normal radiographic appearance of the joint. This appearance varies according to joint type. Dislocation may occur at the site of any joint. Most commonly affected are the shoulder, hip and elbow. Incomplete dislocation is known as subluxation.

Depressed fracture

The fracture is caused by an impact or forced pressure on the vault of the skull. The fragments are forced to lie under the normal position of the dome of the vault (calvarium). Fragments may overlap and appear as hyperdense areas at sites of overlap. There may be a stellate appearance of fracture lines radiating from a central point.[8]

Displaced fracture

In this fracture fragments are separated, usually in more than one direction.

Epiphyseal injuries

Fracture and/or separation of the epiphysis can occur, with varying severity which ranges from the most simple (Salter–Harris class I), involving fracture along the epiphyseal line, to Salter–Harris V where the epiphysis is crushed[9] (Table 4.1).

Table 4.1 Salter–Harris types I–V	
Salter–Harris type I	The fracture line passes along the epiphyseal line, or physis. If there is no displacement of the epiphysis, effusion may be the only indication
Salter–Harris type II	The fracture line runs along the physis and then obliquely, taking a triangular fragment of metaphysis (this is the most common Salter–Harris classification injury found)
Salter–Harris type III	The epiphysis is split in a vertical direction with a fragment displaced along the epiphyseal line
Salter–Harris type IV	The fracture extends through the metaphysis, the epiphyseal line and the epiphysis
Salter–Harris type V	This is compression or crush of the epiphyseal plate, which may not be noticed radiologically. Axial loading injury typically causes this type of fracture. It is rare in occurrence and causes interruption or cessation of normal growth at the site. It is often undetected and only investigated after growth disturbance becomes apparent. Prognosis is poor

Salter–Harris types VI–IX are extremely rare and include injuries to the periosteum, which affect membranous growth, and injury to perichondral structures and injuries which may affect endochondral ossification.

Greenstick fracture

Greenstick fractures are almost exclusively found in the long bones of children and are frequently seen in the radius and ulna. This type of fracture does not traverse completely across the bone, which may appear bent rather than broken. A buckled appearance may be seen instead of an incomplete fracture, and this is known as a torus fracture. The torus fracture is most commonly found near the metaphysis of the bone, the most commonly affected bone being the radius.

Hairline fracture

This is a fine fracture which has no displacement or separation of the fragments.

Simple fracture

A simple fracture is a fracture of the bone, usually into two fragments, with no involvement of other structures and no displacement.

Spiral fracture

This is a fracture which travels along a bone shaft in a spiral direction. The fracture may be seen apparently travelling obliquely on each individual radiographic projection, rather than obviously demonstrated as a spiral in appearance.

Subluxation

Partial dislocation of a joint.

Torus fracture

See section on greenstick fracture above.

REFERENCES

1. The Ionising Radiation (Medical Exposure) Regulations. London: HMSO; 2006.
2. Bontrager K, Lampignano JP. Textbook of radiographic positioning and related anatomy. 6th ed. St Louis: Mosby; 2005.
3. Burnett S, et al. A-Z of orthopaedic radiology. London: Saunders; 2000.
4. Ryan S, et al. Anatomy of diagnostic imaging. 3rd ed. London: WB Saunders; 2010.
5. Helms CA. Fundamentals of skeletal radiology. 3rd ed. Philadelphia: WB Saunders; 2004.
6. Burgener F, et al. Bone and joint disorders. 2nd ed. New York: Thieme; 2006.
7. Manaster BJ. Handbook of skeletal radiology. 2nd ed. St Louis: Mosby; 1997.
8. Heller M, Fink A, editors. Radiology of trauma. Berlin: Springer; 2000.
9. Scally P. Medical imaging. Oxford: Oxford University Press; 1999.

Chapter 5

Fingers, hand and wrist

Elizabeth Carver

Descriptions of projections of the upper limb in this chapter will refer to aspects of the arm in relation to the human body, in the anatomical position (i.e. with arms abducted and palms facing anteriorly). This means that the aspect of the limb that would normally be orientated outwards (laterally) in this position will be referred to as the lateral aspect, even when the hand is in pronation. The aspect of the arm which is normally nearest the trunk in the anatomical position (medial aspect) will always be referred to as the medial aspect, even for projections with the hand in pronation.

THUMB

A common fracture affecting the thumb is the *Bennett's fracture,* an oblique fracture at the base of the first metacarpal causing dislocation of the first carpometacarpal joint. The mechanism of injury is usually forced abduction.

Anteroposterior (AP) thumb

Traditionally the AP thumb projection has been described with the patient seated,[1] but these positions create difficulties when trying to clear the hypothenar eminence from the field. Method 1 described here uses a position considered to be significantly more comfortable and achievable than others and may be at variance with the most commonly performed methods (methods 2 and 3). The idea for method 1 was originally researched with the patient in an erect position,[2] with the later suggestion that radiation protection and immobilisation might be more effective if the patient is supine.[3]

It is clear that the patient's thyroid and the lenses of the eyes are close to the primary beam and edge of collimation in method 1, but if the head is turned away efficiently, the image receptor (IR) is placed as far away as possible from the trunk and lead rubber is used effectively, risks can be minimised.

For all projections of the thumb the IR is placed horizontal unless otherwise specified.

Positioning

Method 1: Patient supine (Fig. 5.1A,B)

- The patient is supine with the affected arm flexed at the elbow and the dorsum of the hand initially in contact with the IR. Lead rubber is applied to the trunk
- The fingers are extended and separated from the thumb
- The anterior aspect of the thumb is placed in contact with the IR and adjusted until the long axis of the thumb is parallel to it; the hypothenar eminence is cleared from the thumb and thenar eminence
- As the dorsum of the hand is now not in contact with the IR, a radiolucent pad is used under the dorsum to aid immobilisation
- The head is turned away from the primary beam

Method 2: Patient seated alongside table (Fig. 5.2)

- The patient is seated with the affected side next to the table; lead rubber is applied to the waist
- The affected hand is externally rotated and the thumb cleared from the fingers
- The anterior aspect of the thumb is placed in contact with the IR; it may be necessary for the patient to lean towards the table in order to facilitate this
- A radiolucent pad is used under the dorsum of the hand to aid immobilisation
- Care must be taken to clear the hypothenar eminence from the first metacarpal
- The head is turned away from the primary beam

Method 3: Patient seated with back to table (Fig. 5.3)

- The patient is seated with their back to the table, with a lead rubber apron fastened behind the waist
- The affected arm is abducted posteriorly and medially rotated
- The anterior aspect of the thumb is placed in contact with the IR; the hypothenar eminence is cleared from the thumb and thenar eminence

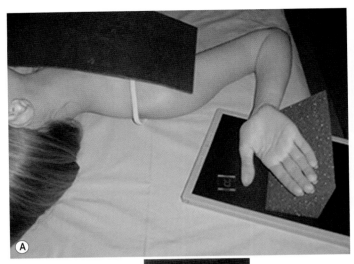

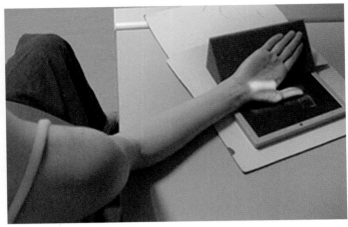

Figure 5.2 AP thumb with patient seated next to the table.

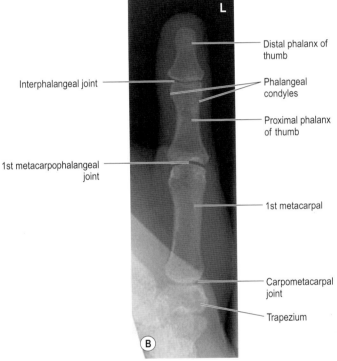

Distal phalanx of thumb

Interphalangeal joint

Phalangeal condyles

Proximal phalanx of thumb

1st metacarpophalangeal joint

1st metacarpal

Carpometacarpal joint

Trapezium

Figure 5.1 (A) AP thumb with patient supine; (B) AP thumb.

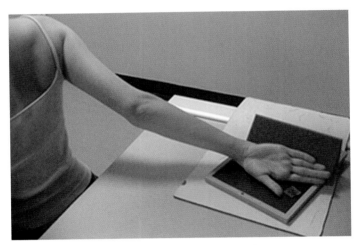

Figure 5.3 AP thumb with patient's back to the table.

- A radiolucent pad is used under the dorsum of the hand to aid immobilisation
- Care must be taken to clear the hypothenar eminence from the first metacarpal

For patients who are unable to achieve any of these positions, the posteroanterior (PA) projection should be used. Principles of radiographic imaging indicate that there will be some magnification of the thumb with this projection, thereby increasing unsharpness. However, an increase in the focus receptor distance (FRD) will compensate for and reduce the effects of this. An increase in mAs will also be necessary to account for reduction in radiographic density due to the inverse square law. However, this is likely to be minimal and the balance of benefit versus risk should be considered.

Popular opinion would suggest that the creation of an air gap between the thumb and the IR also requires an increase in mAs, in order to effect further film blackening as compensation for the reduction in scatter. For denser body areas requiring higher exposure factors than the thumb, this would be a relevant consideration. However, as this projection is performed with the selection of a relatively low kVp, the dominant interaction process is one of absorption rather than production of scatter. Therefore this negates the requirement for an increase in mAs (see Ch. 3). Possible other disadvantages of using the PA projection are the possibility of poor maintenance of position and immobilisation; use of immobilisation aids therefore becomes of paramount importance.

PA thumb (Fig. 5.4)

Positioning

- The patient is seated with the affected side next to the table; lead rubber is applied to the waist
- From a dorsipalmar (DP) position, the hand is externally rotated through 90° and the lateral border of the wrist placed in contact with the table

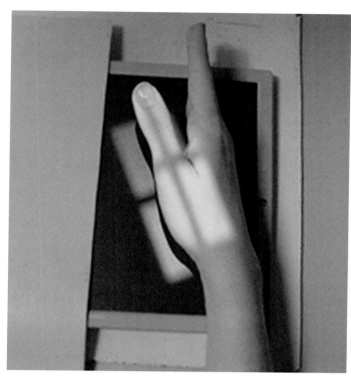

Figure 5.4 PA thumb. The immobilisation pad is removed to show position more clearly.

Common errors	Possible reasons
Interphalangeal joint space not clearly demonstrated	Long axis of thumb may not be parallel to IR
Asymmetry of phalangeal condyles	Transverse axis of thumb may not be parallel to IR
AP methods 1–3	
Shadow of hypothenar eminence superimposed over first metacarpal and trapezium	Inadequate rotation of hand; rotate hand further to clear
PA	
Shadow of thenar and hypothenar eminence superimposed over first metacarpal and trapezium	Thumb may be positioned too close to the rest of hand; clear thumb and first metacarpal from hand and fingers

- The fingers are extended and superimposed vertically; the thumb is extended and cleared away from the fingers
- The long axis of the thumb is supported in a horizontal position by a radiolucent pad
- The thumb and thenar eminence are cleared from the hypothenar eminence and palm of the hand

Beam direction and FRD (all AP methods and PA method)

Vertical, at 90° to the IR
100 cm FRD

Centring point

Over the first metacarpophalangeal joint

Collimation

All phalanges, first metacarpal, trapezium, soft tissue outlines including that of the thenar eminence

Criteria for assessing image quality (all AP methods and PA method)

- All phalanges, first metacarpal, trapezium and soft tissue outline are demonstrated and clear of the hypothenar eminence
- Clear interphalangeal and metacarpophalangeal joint spaces; symmetry of the phalangeal condyles
- Sharp image demonstrating soft tissue margins of the thumb and thenar eminence, bony cortex and trabeculae; adequate penetration of thenar eminence to demonstrate first metacarpal and trapezium

Lateral thumb (Fig. 5.5A–C)

Positioning

- The patient is seated with the affected side next to the table; lead rubber is applied to the waist
- In the DP position the thumb is cleared from the fingers and the hand is medially rotated until the thumb lies laterally, with its phalangeal condyles superimposed
- Because the medial aspect of the hand will be raised to achieve the correct position, a radiolucent pad is used under the palmar aspect of the hand to aid immobilisation
- An alternative method for immobilisation is to flex the fingers into the palm while maintaining separation of the thumb from the rest of the hand, and use the fist to support the dorsum in the required position (Fig. 5.5B)

Beam direction and FRD

Vertical, at 90° to the IR
100 cm FRD

Centring point

Over the first metacarpophalangeal joint

Collimation

All phalanges, the first metacarpal, trapezium, soft tissue outlines including that of the thenar eminence

Criteria for assessing image quality

- All phalanges, first metacarpal, trapezium and soft tissue outlines are demonstrated
- The thumb, first metacarpal and trapezium are cleared from the fingers and hand
- Superimposition of phalangeal condyles to clear interphalangeal and metacarpophalangeal joint spaces
- Sharp image demonstrating the soft tissue margins of the thumb and thenar eminence, bony cortex and trabeculae. The thenar eminence should be penetrated to adequately demonstrate first metacarpal and trapezium

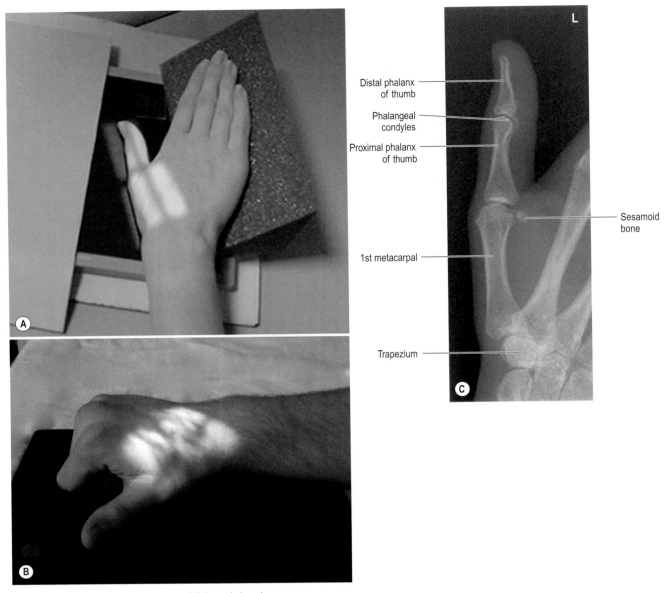

Figure 5.5 (A, B) Lateral thumb positions; (C) lateral thumb.

Common error	Possible reason
Poor joint space visualisation and non-superimposition of phalangeal condyles	Hand has not been rotated adequately; medial or external rotation of the hand will facilitate superimposition of phalangeal condyles

FINGERS

The most frequent reason for imaging of the fingers is to demonstrate the results of trauma to the area. Avulsion fractures, such as those accompanying *mallet finger*, are often seen, as are dislocations and foreign bodies.

Opinions on centring points and the area for inclusion in the primary beam vary for finger examinations. The radiographer has a medicolegal responsibility to ensure that the correct digit has been examined and that there is evidence to support this.

One way to ensure this is to include the adjacent finger or border of the hand in the field of collimation; comparison of size with the other fingers will ensure correct identification of the finger. Unfortunately this does involve irradiation of areas not required for examination and could theoretically be deemed to be in contravention of IR(ME)R 2006.[4] As a result, imaging department protocols should clearly identify the hospital's requirements for the radiographer, ensuring that there is uniformity of provision regarding finger images.

Centring points also vary, according to the area of interest required to be included in the field of radiation (see variation in descriptive section).

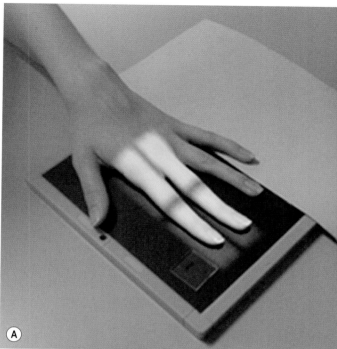

DP fingers (Fig. 5.6A,B)

For all projections of the fingers the IR is horizontal.

Positioning

- The patient is seated with the affected side adjacent to the table; lead rubber is applied to the waist
- The affected hand is pronated with the fingers extended, to facilitate visualisation of interphalangeal joint spaces, and slightly separated

Beam direction and FRD

Vertical, at 90° to the IR
100 cm FRD

Centring point

Method (a): Over the proximal interphalangeal joint *or*
Method (b): Metacarpophalangeal joint

Collimation

Centring method (a): All phalanges of the finger under examination; the metacarpophalangeal joint; adjacent finger/s to facilitate correct finger identification
Centring method (b): As above but to include associated metacarpal

Criteria for assessing image quality

- *Centring method (a):* All phalanges and the metacarpophalangeal joint are demonstrated
- *Centring method (b):* All phalanges, the metacarpophalangeal joint and the metacarpal are demonstrated
- Adjacent finger/s and soft tissue outline of the affected and adjacent fingers are demonstrated
- Symmetry of the phalangeal condyles
- The interphalangeal and metacarpophalangeal joint spaces are clearly visible and open
- Sharp image demonstrating the soft tissue margins of the finger, bony cortex and trabeculae

Common error	Possible reason
Interphalangeal joint spaces not clearly demonstrated	Fingers may be flexed; extend to clear

Lateral fingers

Lateral projections of some fingers can prove difficult to achieve and maintain in position, especially when attempting to separate and immobilise middle, ring and little fingers. The injured or arthritic patient may be even less cooperative. Small wedge-shaped radiolucent pads are efficient aids in separating fingers for radiographic examination.

Positioning

Index (first) finger (Fig. 5.7A,B)

- From the DP position the hand is internally rotated through 90° and the third and fourth fingers are flexed and held in position by the thumb
- The index finger is extended and positioned with its lateral aspect in contact with the IR
- The long axis of the index finger is separated from the palmar-flexed middle finger with a radiolucent pad

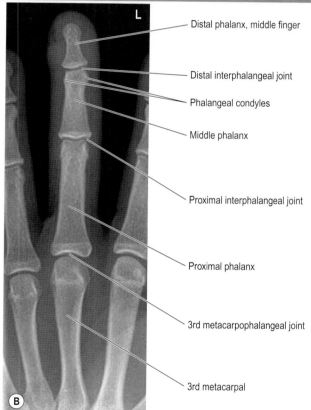

L
- Distal phalanx, middle finger
- Distal interphalangeal joint
- Phalangeal condyles
- Middle phalanx
- Proximal interphalangeal joint
- Proximal phalanx
- 3rd metacarpophalangeal joint
- 3rd metacarpal

Figure 5.6 (A) DP finger; (B) DP middle finger.

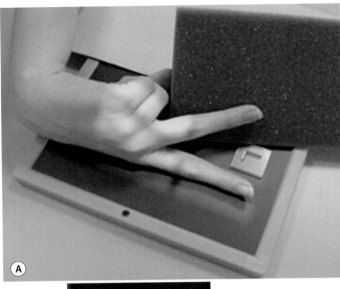

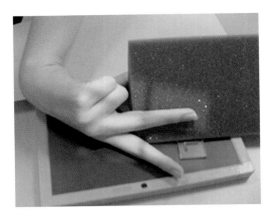

Figure 5.8 Lateral middle finger.

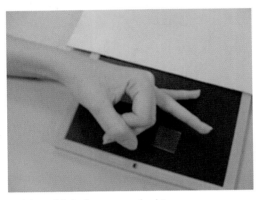

Figure 5.9 Ring and little finger – method 1.

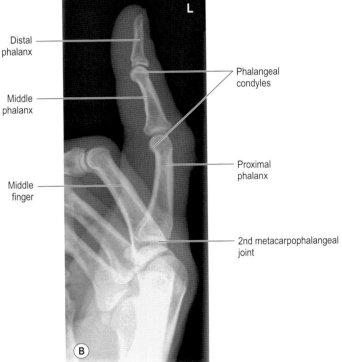

Distal phalanx

Phalangeal condyles

Middle phalanx

Proximal phalanx

Middle finger

2nd metacarpophalangeal joint

Figure 5.7 Lateral index finger.

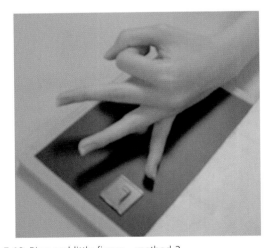

Figure 5.10 Ring and little finger – method 2.

Middle finger (Fig. 5.8)

- From the DP position, the hand is internally rotated 90° and positioned as for the lateral index finger projection
- The middle finger is extended and separated from the index finger with a radiolucent pad
- The middle finger is supported in a horizontal position by a radiolucent pad

Ring and little finger: method 1 (Fig. 5.9)

- From the DP position the hand is externally rotated through 90°
- The index and middle fingers are flexed and held by the thumb; the little finger remains extended, as does the ring finger

- The medial aspect of the fifth metacarpal is in contact with the IR
- The ring finger is slightly dorsiflexed to clear it from the little finger
- If under examination, the ring finger is supported in a horizontal position; in any event it is separated from the little finger by a radiolucent pad

Ring and little finger: method 2 (Fig. 5.10)

- From the DP position the hand is externally rotated through 90°
- The index finger is flexed and held by the thumb; the remaining fingers are slightly dorsiflexed and fanned out; their long axes remain horizontal

- If under examination, the ring finger is supported in a horizontal position; in any event it is separated from the other fingers by radiolucent pads

For all the fingers and positions

Beam direction and FRD

Vertical, at 90° to the IR
100 cm FRD

Centring point

Method (a): Over the proximal interphalangeal joint of the finger under examination *or*
Method (b): Metacarpophalangeal joint of the finger under examination

Collimation

Centring method (a): All phalanges, soft tissue outlines and the metacarpophalangeal joint. Evidence of the adjacent finger for confirmation of identification of the finger under examination
Centring method (b): All phalanges, soft tissue outlines and the associated metacarpal. Evidence of the adjacent finger for confirmation of identification of the finger under examination

Criteria for assessing image quality

- *Centring method (a):* All phalanges and the metacarpophalangeal joint are demonstrated, with the outline of adjacent finger/s
- *Centring method (b):* All phalanges, the metacarpophalangeal joint and the metacarpal are demonstrated with the outline of adjacent finger/s
- Clear interphalangeal and metacarpophalangeal joints are demonstrated, with phalangeal condyles superimposed
- Sharp image demonstrating the soft tissue margins of the finger, bony cortex and trabeculae of phalanges under examination

Common error	Possible reason
Poor joint space demonstration with non-superimposition of phalangeal condyles	Long axis of finger may not lie parallel to IR; reposition and support more effectively *or* angle beam to coincide with angle of interphalangeal joints if patient cannot comply

HAND

The *Boxer's fracture* (or *punch fracture*) is frequently seen on imaging requests from the A&E department. The mechanism of injury is that of impact on a clenched fist, hence the name of this fracture, which usually occurs in the fifth metacarpal. Usually there is anterior displacement of the distal bony fragment, particularly if the fracture occurs through the neck of the metacarpal (which is most common). Less commonly, the fourth metacarpal can be affected.

DP hand (Fig. 5.11A,B)

For all projections of the hand the IR is placed on the table-top.

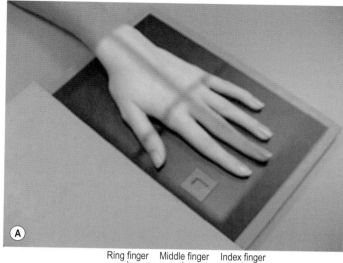

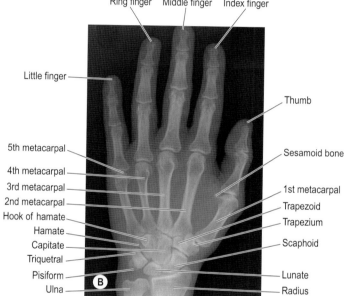

Ring finger   Middle finger   Index finger

Little finger

Thumb

5th metacarpal
4th metacarpal
3rd metacarpal
2nd metacarpal
Hook of hamate
Hamate
Capitate
Triquetral
Pisiform
Ulna

Sesamoid bone

1st metacarpal
Trapezoid
Trapezium

Scaphoid

Lunate
Radius

Figure 5.11 DP hand.

Positioning

- The patient is seated with the affected side next to the table; lead rubber is applied to the waist
- The hand is pronated and its palmar aspect placed in contact with the IR
- The fingers and thumb are extended and slightly separated

Beam direction and FRD

Vertical, at 90° to the IR
100 cm FRD

Centring point

Over the head of the third metacarpal

Collimation

All phalanges, soft tissue outline of the hand, wrist joint

Criteria for assessing image quality

- All phalanges, the wrist joint and the soft tissue outline of the hand are demonstrated
- The fingers are separated, and the interphalangeal and metacarpophalangeal joints are clear
- Symmetrical appearance of the heads of metacarpals 2–4
- Obliquity of thumb and the heads of metacarpals 1 and 5
- Sharp image demonstrating the soft tissue margins of the hand, bony cortex and trabeculae Adequate penetration to demonstrate the hook of hamate whilst showing distal phalanges

Common errors	Possible reasons
Superimposition of soft tissue outlines of fingers	Fingers are not separated adequately
Poor demonstration of joint spaces	Fingers may not be extended; extend fingers *or* examine with hand in supination to use obliquity of rays around centre of beam, to 'open out' joints

In this position it is to be noted that the fifth metacarpal and little finger are externally rotated into an oblique appearance. The concept of reducing this obliquity and the impact of this on the image has been discussed in the past,[5] yet it does not appear that there has been a widespread adoption of the measures suggested. Could this be because reporting radiographers and radiologists find that the projections of the fifth metacarpal provided by the DP and DPO positions are at sufficiently different angles? Or is familiarity with these more usual appearances enough to inspire confidence in outlining a report?

Dorsipalmar oblique (DPO) hand (Fig. 5.12A,B)

Positioning

- The patient is seated with the affected side next to the table; lead rubber is applied to the waist
- From the DP position the hand is externally rotated through 45°; the medial aspect of the hand remains in contact with the IR
- A radiolucent pad is placed under the lateral aspect of the hand as immobilisation and to keep the fingers extended and horizontal. An alternative is to allow the fingers and thumb to dorsiflex gently and rest on the IR for support
- The fingers are separated

Beam direction and FRD

Vertical, at 90° to the IR
100 cm FRD

Centring point

Over the head of the third metacarpal

Collimation

All phalanges, soft tissue outline of the hand, wrist joint

Previous descriptions of the DPO hand have shown the selection of a range of centring methods.[1,3] Originally, in the UK, centring for this projection was stated as over the head of the fifth metacarpal[6,7] in order to use the effect of the oblique rays which 'opened out' the spaces between the metacarpal heads. As the dose reduction culture gained influence in radiography, it became clear that this centring

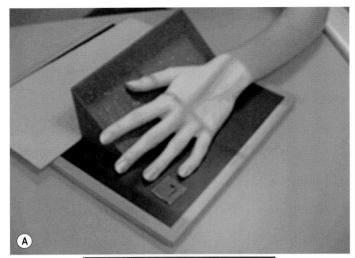

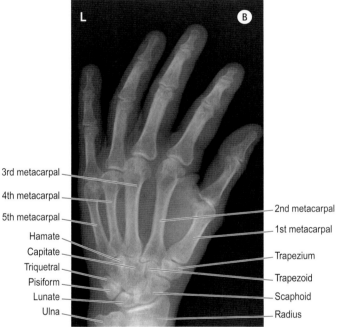

Figure 5.12 DP oblique hand.

point required an unacceptably large field of radiation, almost half of which was not usefully employed. The result was to suggest that centring should remain the same, with the addition of angulation across the dorsum of the hand until the central ray lay over the head of the third metacarpal. This would allow closer collimation around the hand, yet maintain the effects of the oblique rays afforded in the original centring point.

In principle, of course, this sounds a logical amendment. However, questions have arisen regarding this method.[3] Because the FRD for this projection lies at 100 cm and the distance between the heads of the fifth and third metacarpals is generally around 3 cm, the oblique rays referred to will actually be around 2° and possibly even less. How useful would such a small angle be? Can the human eye detect differences in images taken with or without this angle?

Why even consider 'opening up' the spaces between metacarpal heads when they are well separated on the DP image? Different projections in radiography are always used to give a different view of what is essentially a two-dimensional image medium, and adding angle onto a DPO projection will only serve to reduce the usefulness of the obliquity. If it is really essential (and the authors question whether or not this would actually be the case, bearing in mind the previous sentence) then why not utilise 2° less obliquity on the rotation of the hand? Could 2° even be assessed accurately by the human eye?

For these reasons, in this book the centring is selected as the head of the third metacarpal with a vertical central ray.

Criteria for assessing image quality

- All phalanges, wrist joint and soft tissue outline of the hand are demonstrated
- Separation of the shafts of the metacarpals but with some overlap of metacarpal heads 3–5
- Separation of the soft tissues of the fingers and intermediate phalanges and distal phalanges
- Joint spaces will not be demonstrated as clear
- Sharp image demonstrating the soft tissue margins of the hand, bony cortex and trabeculae

Common error	Possible reason
Overlap of shafts of metacarpals	Excessive external rotation of the hand

Lateral hand (Fig. 5.13A,B)

The lateral projection is most useful for demonstrating the direction of displacement in fractures of the metacarpals and is particularly useful to identify anterior displacement of distal bony fragments in the boxer's fracture. The fingers are superimposed and the adducted thumb overexposed, meaning that these structures are not well identified in this projection.

Positioning

- The patient is seated with the affected side next to the table; lead rubber is applied to the waist
- From the DP position, the hand is externally rotated through 90°
- The fingers are extended and superimposed vertically, and the thumb is extended and abducted from the hand
- The thumb lies horizontally and supported on a radiolucent pad

Beam direction and FRD

Vertical, at 90° to the IR
100 cm FRD

Centring point

Over the medial aspect of the head of the second metacarpal

Collimation

All phalanges, soft tissue outline of the hand, wrist joint

Criteria for assessing image quality

- All phalanges, the wrist joint and the soft tissue outline of the hand are demonstrated
- The fingers are superimposed, metacarpals 2–5 are superimposed and the thumb is cleared from other bones of the hand

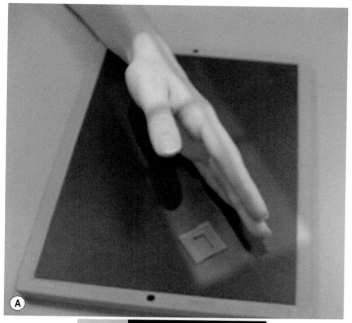

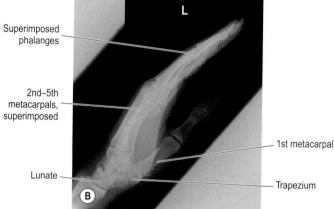

Figure 5.13 Lateral hand.

- Sharp image demonstrating the soft tissue margins of the hand, bony cortex and trabeculae of the lunate. Outlines of superimposed bones are demonstrated but not showing trabecular detail. Penetration to demonstrate individual carpal bones

Common error	Possible reason
Poor superimposition of phalanges and poor superimposition of metacarpals	Over- or under-rotation of the hand; ensure dorsum of hand is at 90° to IR

Palmar dorsal oblique examination of both hands for rheumatoid arthritis assessment (ball catcher's) (Fig. 5.14A,B)

Both hands are examined via the same single-exposure image. Hands are palm upwards with relaxed fingers and slight medial rotation. The hands appear as though the patient is poised ready to catch a ball, hence the alternative name 'ball catcher's projection'.

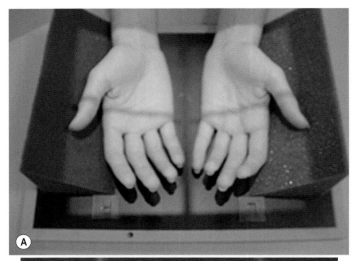

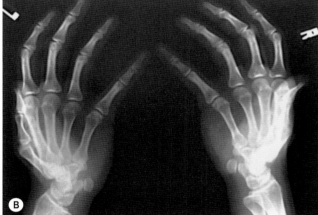

Figure 5.14 Ball catcher's.
(B) Reproduced with permission from Ballinger PW, Frank ED. Merrill's atlas of radiographic positioning and radiologic procedures. 10th edn. St Louis: Mosby; 2003.

Positioning

- The patient is seated alongside the table but it may be necessary to turn the trunk slightly towards the IR
- The arms are abducted forwards towards the IR and externally rotated to bring the region of the dorsum of the hands overlying the fifth metacarpal in contact with the IR
- The dorsum of the hands lie at 30° to the IR and the hands are supported in this position by radiolucent pads. The fingers are slightly relaxed

Beam direction and FRD

Vertical, at 90° to the IR
100 cm FRD

Centring point

Midway between the medial borders of the hand, level with the heads of the fifth metacarpals

Collimation

Both hands and wrist joints

Criteria for assessing image quality

- Both hands and wrist joints are demonstrated
- Clear metacarpophalangeal joint spaces 2–5
- Sharp image demonstrating bony detail in contrast with the joint spaces

WRIST

It has been estimated that some 17% of fractures encountered in A&E involve the distal radius,[8] making radiological assessment of this area a fairly common occurrence. A common fracture of the area is the *Colles' fracture*, which results from a fall onto an outstretched hand, leading to fracture of the radius (and possibly the ulna). There is posterior displacement of the distal fragments, which most frequently requires manipulation to reduce. Less frequently, fracture of the distal radius and ulna may show anterior displacement of the distal fragments. These cases are categorised as *Smith's fractures*. The mechanism of injury is usually falling onto the back of the hand.

Wrisnt examinations are often undertaken with the wrist in an immobilisation medium, which will have implications for selection of the exposure factor, according to density of the fracture immobiliser. If a dense medium is used, as in plaster of Paris, both kVp and mAs will need to be increased, although more modern immobilisers are less dense and require less or no increase in exposure factors. It should be noted that plaster of Paris is less frequently used than in the past. Any increase results in a higher radiation dose to the area.

PA wrist (Fig. 5.15A,B)

For all projections of the wrist the IR is horizontal.

Positioning

- The patient is seated with the affected side next to the table; lead rubber is applied to the waist
- The affected arm is flexed at the elbow and the wrist is internally rotated to pronate the hand
- The anterior aspect of the wrist is placed in contact with the IR; the fingers are relaxed to bring the forearm and wrist flat and in contact with the IR
- The radial and ulnar styloid processes are equidistant from the IR

Beam direction and FRD

Vertical, at 90° to the IR
100 cm FRD

Centring point

Midway between the radial and ulnar styloid processes

Collimation

Proximal third of metacarpals, carpals, distal third of radius and ulna, soft tissue outlines of wrist

Criteria for assessing image quality

- Proximal third of metacarpals, the carpals, distal third of radius and ulna, and soft tissue outlines of the wrist are demonstrated
- Clear demonstration of the distal radioulnar joint
- The radial and ulnar styloid processes seen on the lateral and medial margins of these bones

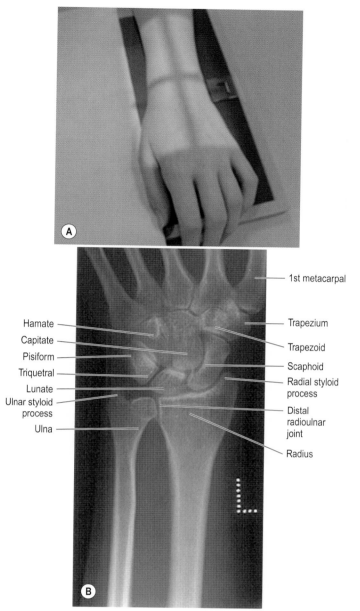

Figure 5.15 PA wrist.

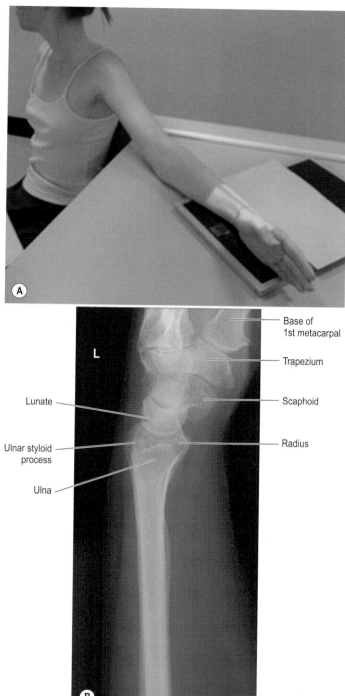

Figure 5.16 Lateral wrist.

- Sharp image demonstrating the soft tissue margins of the area, bony cortex and trabeculae. Adequate penetration will demonstrate hook of hamate clearly
- Good contrast is required over the soft tissue as there is evidence that changes in alignment and shape of the scaphoid fat pad, normally seen as a linear area of low density following the line of the medial edges of scaphoid and trapezium, can be an indicator of significant wrist injury. The fat pad sign alone cannot be considered unequivocal[9] and is not usually noted in patients under 12 years of age

Common error	Possible reason
Radial and ulnar styloid processes appear displaced from lateral and medial margins of these bones; superimposition of the radius and ulna over the distal radioulnar joint	Styloid processes are not equidistant from the IR

Lateral wrist (Fig. 5.16A,B)

Positioning

- The patient is seated with the affected side next to the table and a lead rubber sheet applied to the waist
- The wrist is externally rotated 90° from the PA position*

- The medial aspect of the wrist is placed in contact with the IR
- The wrist is externally rotated approximately 5° further, in order to superimpose the radial and ulnar styloid processes

*At this point it is important to discuss positioning for the lateral wrist, bearing in mind traditional approaches to this projection. Some texts have described the patient's position as with the arm abducted laterally, with a view to facilitate movement of the ulna to a position that is suggested to be at 90° to the PA,[3,9] and others describe a position involving external rotation from the PA position only.[7,10] The first method is believed to ensure that the ulna lies at 90° to its position in the PA by moving the arm at the shoulder and putting the humerus in a lateral position; at this point it is important to discuss this further.

Study of the movement of the forearm, for both methods, demonstrates that the outline of the ulnar styloid process on the image does not change between projections, whatever technique is used. The only way that a difference of 90° can be achieved is with the hand in supination as in an AP position, and with a lateral using *any* of the methods previously described[3,7-10] (Fig. 5.17A–F).

One can only wonder why wrist projections originated with two projections that provided images at 90° for only one of the bones required for demonstration, but a study of texts from the earlier days of radiography (over 70 years ago) show that the PA projection appears always to have been the projection of choice for this region.[11]

Beam direction and FRD

Vertical, at 90° to the IR
100 cm FRD

Centring point

Over the radial styloid process

Collimation

Proximal third of metacarpals, the carpals, distal third of radius and ulna, soft tissue outlines of wrist

Criteria for assessing image quality

- Proximal third of metacarpals, carpals, distal third of radius and ulna, soft tissue outlines of the wrist are demonstrated
- Superimposition of the distal radius and ulna; the lunate should have a crescent-shaped appearance; distal scaphoid superimposed over pisiform;[12] long axes of radius and third metacarpal are aligned[13]
- Sharp image demonstrating the soft tissue margins of the wrist, bony cortex and trabeculae. Penetration of carpus to demonstrate individual carpal bones while demonstrating pronator fat stripe within soft tissue, anterior to radius

Including the anterior fat stripe in collimation is recognised as necessary a it may be the only (subtle) indication of injury.[12] The area of reduced radiographic density lies approximately 0.6 cm from the anterior aspect of the radial outline and curves very slightly, following the distal radial outline in a proximal direction. Positional criteria given are simple descriptors of recurrently recommended criteria,[7,12] but more complex requirements have been described as 'the palmar cortex of the pisiform bone should overlie the central third of the interval between the palmar cortices of the distal scaphoid pole and the capitate head'.[14] Needless to say, deformities caused by severe trauma to the wrist and carpus may render it impossible to ensure that such positional criteria can be achieved.

Common errors	Possible reasons
Radius appears posteriorly in relation to ulna	Excessive external rotation
Ulna appears posteriorly in relation to radius	Inadequate external rotation

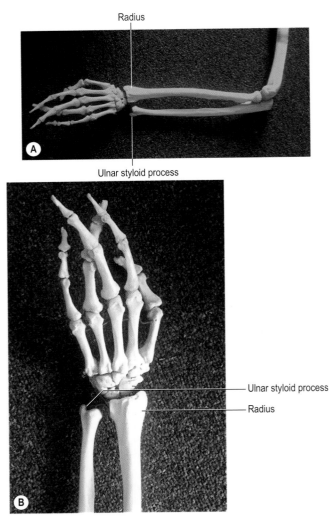

Figure 5.17 Changing position of ulna styloid process during forearm movements and rotation of the left wrist and forearm. (A,B) Ulnar styloid process position with the hand in pronation as in the PA wrist projection.

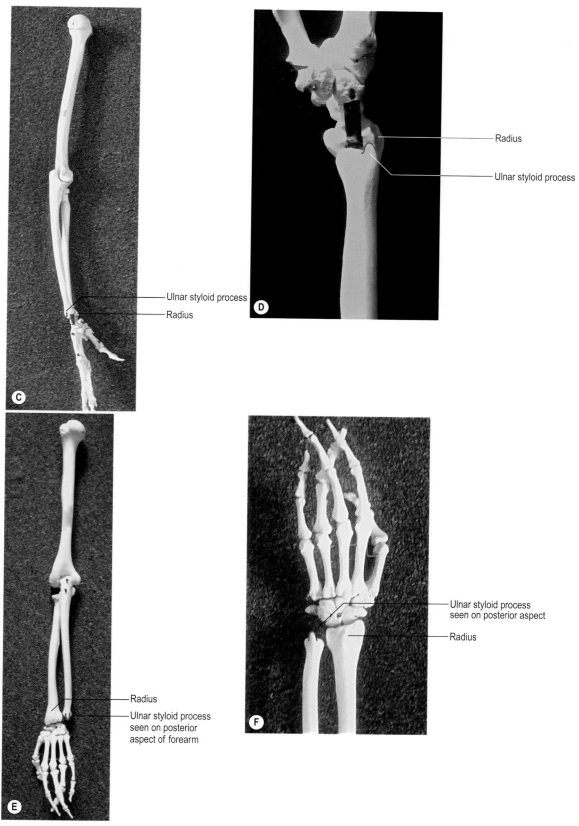

Figure 5.17, Continued (C,D) Ulnar styloid process position with the arm in the lateral position (as seen from the medial aspect in order to show the distal ulna; to show it from the lateral aspect would superimpose the radius over the ulna) – note that it appears as a mirror image compared to the lateral radiograph in Fig. 5.16B because the bone is shown from its medial aspect; (E,F) ulnar styloid process position seen from the posterior aspect when the arm is in supination, showing the ulnar styloid process has shifted in position when compared to Fig. 5.17A–D. This is the only position that will show the styloid process at 90° to the lateral.

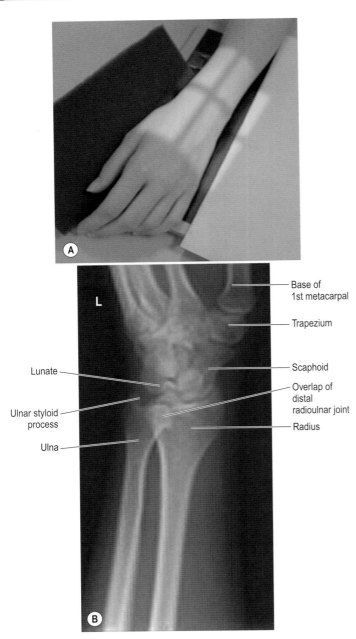

Figure 5.18 PA oblique wrist.

Base of 1st metacarpal

Trapezium

Scaphoid

Overlap of distal radioulnar joint

Radius

Lunate

Ulnar styloid process

Ulna

PA oblique wrist (Fig. 5.18)

Positioning

- The patient is seated with the affected side next to the table and a lead rubber sheet applied to the waist
- From the PA position the wrist is externally rotated 45°
- The wrist is supported in this position with a radiolucent pad or by slight flexion of the fingers until their tips rest on the IR or table to support the obliquity; there should be no dorsiflexion or palmar flexion at the wrist

Beam direction and FRD

Vertical, at 90° to the IR
100 cm FRD

Centring point

Midway between the radial and ulnar styloid processes

Collimation

Proximal third of metacarpals, carpals, distal third of radius and ulna, and soft tissue outlines of wrist

Criteria for assessing image quality

- Proximal third of metacarpals, carpals, distal third of radius and ulna, and the soft tissue outlines of the wrist demonstrated
- Overlap of the distal radioulnar joint
- Scaphoid and trapezium are clearly demonstrated
- Sharp image demonstrating the soft tissue margins of the wrist, bony cortex and trabeculae. Adequate penetration to demonstrate differentiation between overlapped carpal bones

SCAPHOID

Scaphoid fractures are difficult to detect radiographically immediately after injury and are best demonstrated after 10–14 days, when callus formation can be seen as increased bone density on radiographs. The scaphoid fat pad sign can be used to supplement bony information, but the fat pad sign cannot be used as standalone evidence of injury.[15]

However, because fractures of the radius and ulna must also be excluded at the time of injury, wrist projections are undertaken initially. Disruption of the single blood supply to the proximal end of the scaphoid may result in bony necrosis and onset of bony degenerative changes if the fracture is not treated; as a result, even in the event of negative findings for radius and ulna at the initial stage, the wrist is treated conservatively, with the use of immobilisation. At the end of the 10–14-day callus formation period immobilisation is removed and well-collimated scaphoid projections are requested. It is possible that plain radiographic imaging may not provide useful information, and it is possible that radionuclide imaging using technetium-99 (^{99m}Tc) will provide useful information on the location of injury, even if negative.[13]

Many projections that will demonstrate the scaphoid have been described and it is necessary to use the minimum that will provide the required information. Projections selected for description include ulnar deviation, to clear the scaphoid from adjacent carpal bones, and a 30° angle which has been shown to demonstrate fractures of the waist effectively. It may not be considered necessary to use all the projections described in one assessment of the scaphoid.

Descriptions include only those for the specifically centred, well-coned scaphoid assessment. In the PA wrist projection, where the centring point lies between the styloid processes, the scaphoid will be foreshortened owing to its orientation within the carpus.[12] Centring over the scaphoid reduces this effect and the scaphoid is likely to be more clearly demonstrated, with minimum distortion. However, in an attempt to consider this concept realistically, it should be asked whether this improved visualisation would be detected by the human eye, since the obliquity of X-rays around the central ray at 100 cm FRD will only be approximately 2° through the fracture.

Initial assessment, which includes the wrist, should be positioned as described in the section on wrist examinations but with ulnar deviation applied. When using this medial flexion on the wrist, care should be taken not to flex the joint anteriorly or posteriorly as this can distort the image of the scaphoid itself.[12]

In this book the term 'anatomical snuffbox' is used in centring point descriptions. The position of the scaphoid can be identified as lying under this 'snuffbox', a depression found on the lateral border of the carpus, between the base of the first metacarpal and the radius. It is particularly evident when the thumb is in lateral abduction.

For all projections of the scaphoid the IR is horizontal.

PA with ulnar deviation (Fig. 5.19)

Positioning

- The patient is positioned as for the PA projection of the wrist
- The 'snuffbox' is placed in the centre of the available space if an IR is used
- The hand is adducted towards the ulna; there should be no other flexion of the wrist. The thumb is in contact with the lateral aspect of the second metacarpal

Beam direction and FRD

Vertical, at 90° to the IR
100 cm FRD

Centring point

Over the 'snuffbox'

Collimation

Scaphoid, trapezium, trapezoid, lunate, first carpometacarpal joint, radiocarpal joint

Criteria for assessing image quality

- Demonstration of the scaphoid, trapezium, trapezoid, lunate, first carpometacarpal joint and radiocarpal joint
- Separation of the joint spaces around the scaphoid; adequate ulnar deviation will show long axis of the first metacarpal following that of the radius (if included in the image)
- Sharp image demonstrating bony cortex and trabeculae. Optimum penetration to demonstrate overlap of carpal bones and contrast to allow for demonstration of subtle scaphoid fat pat sign

Common error	Possible reason
Poor separation of joint space around scaphoid	Inadequate ulnar deviation

Scaphoid: PA oblique with ulnar deviation

(Fig. 5.20A,B)

Positioning

- The patient is positioned as for the PA oblique projection of the wrist
- The 'snuffbox' is placed in the centre of the available space if a IR is used
- A radiolucent pad is used under the wrist to aid immobilisation
- The hand is adducted towards the ulna; there should be no flexion of the wrist

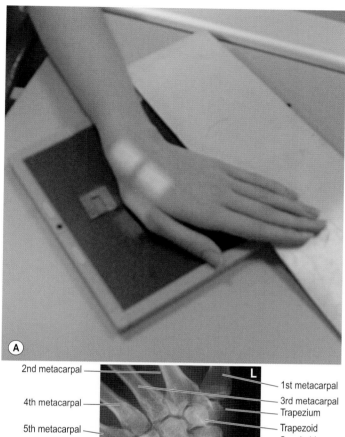

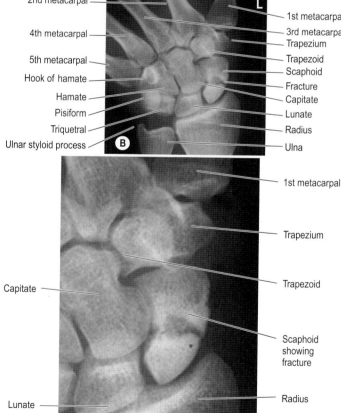

Figure 5.19 Scaphoid PA with (A) ulnar deviation, (B) showing fracture, (C) demonstrating close collimation.

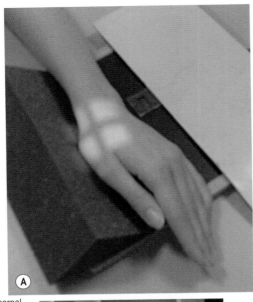

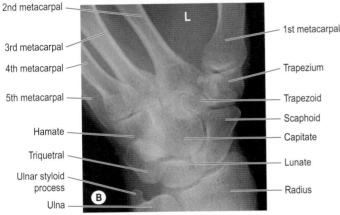

Figure 5.20 (A) Scaphoid PA oblique; (B) showing fracture.

Figure 5.21 AP oblique scaphoid.

Beam direction and FRD

Vertical, at 90° to the IR
100 cm FRD

Centring point

Over the 'snuffbox'

Collimation

Scaphoid, trapezium, trapezoid, lunate, first carpometacarpal joint, radiocarpal joint

Please note that Figure 5.19B shows less stringent collimation, to provide an example of the relationship of other carpal bones to the scaphoid.

Criteria for assessing image quality

- Demonstration of the scaphoid, trapezium, trapezoid, lunate, first carpometacarpal joint and radiocarpal joint
- Separation of joint spaces around the scaphoid

- Sharp image demonstrating bony cortex and trabeculae. Adequate penetration to demonstrate differentiation between overlapped carpal bones

Common error	Possible reason
Poor separation of joint space around scaphoid	Inadequate ulnar deviation

Scaphoid: AP oblique with ulnar deviation

(Fig. 5.21A,B)

Positioning

- The patient is positioned initially as for the lateral projection of the wrist
- The wrist is externally rotated 45° and a radiolucent pad is placed under the wrist to aid immobilisation

- The 'snuffbox' should be in the centre of the available space if an IR is used
- The hand is adducted towards the ulna; there should be no flexion of the wrist

Beam direction and FRD

Vertical, at 90° to the IR
100 cm FRD

Centring point

Over the 'snuffbox'

Collimation

Scaphoid, trapezium, trapezoid, lunate, first carpometacarpal joint, radiocarpal joint

Please note that Figure 5.20B shows less stringent collimation, to provide an example of the relationship of other carpal bones to the scaphoid.

Criteria for assessing image quality

- Demonstration of the scaphoid, trapezium, trapezoid, lunate, first carpometacarpal joint and radiocarpal joint
- The scaphoid seen above the radius, partially over lapping the lunate but clear of the pisiform and triquetral
- Sharp image demonstrating bony cortex and trabeculae. Adequate penetration to demonstrate differentiation between overlapped carpal bones

Lateral scaphoid (Fig. 5.22)

Positioning

- The patient is positioned as for a lateral projection of the wrist
- The 'snuffbox' is placed in the centre of the available space if an IR is used

Beam direction and FRD

Vertical, at 90° to the IR
100 cm FRD

Centring point

Over the 'snuffbox'

Collimation

Scaphoid, trapezium, lunate, first carpometacarpal joint, radiocarpal joint, radial and ulnar styloid processes

Please note that Figure 5.22B shows less stringent collimation, to provide an example of the relationship of other carpal bones to the scaphoid.

Criteria for assessing image quality

- Demonstration of the scaphoid, trapezium, lunate, first carpometacarpal joint, radiocarpal joint and radial and ulnar styloid processes
- The lunate projected as a crescent. The proximal end of the third metacarpal, capitate, lunate and distal radius should be in

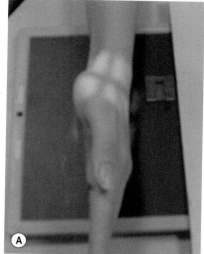
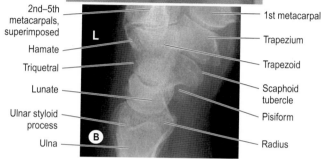

Figure 5.22 Scaphoid lateral.

alignment. The waist of the scaphoid should be superimposed over the pisiform, with the tubercle of scaphoid clear of the pisiform anteriorly on the palmar aspect of the wrist
- Sharp image demonstrating bony cortex and trabeculae. Adequate penetration to demonstrate differentiation between overlapped carpal bones

Scaphoid: PA with 30° angulation and ulnar deviation

Positioning

- Position is as for the PA scaphoid with ulnar deviation (Fig. 5.19A)
- The 'snuffbox' is positioned coincident with the centre of the available space if an IR is used

Beam direction and FRD

Initially vertical, then directed 30° towards the elbow
100 cm FRD

Centring point

Over the trapezium at base of thumb

Collimation

Scaphoid and surrounding joints

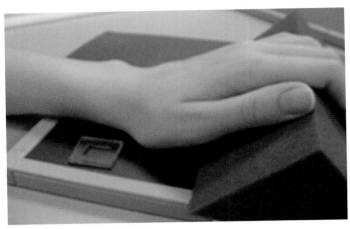

Figure 5.23 Scaphoid with wrist in dorsiflexion.

This projection should be undertaken with the forearm positioned parallel to the median sagittal plain (MSP), so that the central ray is not directed towards the trunk when angled towards the elbow. To achieve this, the patient's chair should be placed next to the longer dimension of the table rather than at the end, to allow easy and accurate angulation of the X-ray tube in the correct plane.

There are three alternative projections which will also place the scaphoid into a position where it will lie at 30° to the central ray, thus negating the need for angulation.

Wrist in dorsiflexion (Fig. 5.23)

- An initial PA wrist position is modified by dorsiflexing the hand at the wrist until it makes an angle of 30° with the IR
- The hand is supported on a radiolucent pad and the wrist is placed in ulnar deviation. The anterior aspect of the wrist remains in contact with the IR

Beam direction and FRD

Vertical, at 90° to the IR
100 cm FRD

Centring point

Over the 'snuffbox'

Collimation

Scaphoid and surrounding joints

Forearm raised 30° (Fig. 5.24)

- With the wrist in pronation, the forearm is raised 30° at the elbow
- The elbow remains in contact with the table
- The forearm and hand are supported on a radiolucent pad and the wrist is placed in ulnar deviation; the hand and forearm remain in the same plane

Beam direction and FRD

Vertical, at 90° to the IR
150 cm FRD, to reduce magnification caused by increased object receptor distance (ORD)

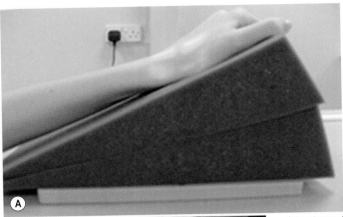

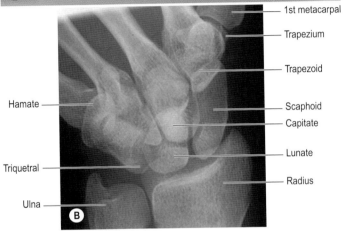

Figure 5.24 (A) Scaphoid with forearm raised 30°; (B) scaphoid–PA 30° image.

Centring point

Over the 'snuffbox'

Collimation

Scaphoid and surrounding joints

This projection option with the forearm raised 30° will cause a significant amount of magnification unsharpness, but this can be counteracted by placing pads under the IR to raise it by 30°; the forearm is then placed directly on the IR, thereby reducing ORD, and a vertical central ray is used instead of 30° angulation

Clenched fist with ulnar deviation

- With the wrist in pronation, the fist is fully clenched to raise the dorsum of the hand through 30°, as for the lateral thumb position seen in Figure 5.5B
- Ulnar deviation is applied to the wrist

Beam direction and FRD

Vertical, at 90° to the IR
100 cm FRD

Centring point

Over the 'snuffbox'

Collimation

Scaphoid and surrounding joints

Criteria for assessing image quality: all 30° projections

- The scaphoid and surrounding joints are demonstrated
- The scaphoid is cleared from other carpals due to ulnar deviation, with elongation due to 30° angle
- Sharp but elongated image demonstrating bony cortex and trabeculae of scaphoid (see Fig. 5.24B; please note that this image shows less stringent collimation, to provide an example of the relationship of other carpal bones to the scaphoid)

Common error	Possible reasons
Short appearance of scaphoid	Inadequate angle used or hand/ forearm not raised enough

CARPAL TUNNEL

Compression of the median nerve in the carpal tunnel on the anterior aspect of the wrist results in pain and paraesthesia of the fingers; the collection of these symptoms is known as carpal tunnel syndrome.[16]

Whenever possible, magnetic resonance imaging (MRI) should be the imaging modality of choice for symptoms suggestive of this condition. However, bony spurs which emanate from the carpus, impinging on innervation at the wrist, can be detected using plain film radiography. In addition, when there are valid reasons contraindicating the use of MRI it may still be necessary to undertake plain radiographic examination of the carpal tunnel.

Several methods of producing images of this region are available and implications of dose to radiosensitive organs, projectional principles and patient condition or capability should be considered when selecting the most appropriate. Method 1 is given priority for description, as it is considered to show the least magnification unsharpness and, with the trunk turned away from the primary beam, is most effective in reducing dose to radiosensitive areas (thyroid, gonads, breast, eye lens). Unfortunately, carpal tunnel syndrome is highly likely to impair the patient's ability to forcibly dorsiflex the wrist, and in these cases method 3 should be selected.

Method 1: superoinferior carpal tunnel – erect with patient facing away from the central ray (Fig. 5.25)

Positioning

- An IR at the edge of a table is required for this projection, placed horizontal and with its edge aligned with the edge of the table
- A lead rubber apron is fastened to the back of the waist
- The patient stands with their back to the table, which should be adjusted so that its height lies just below their waist
- The affected arm is internally rotated until the palm faces posteriorly, towards the table and IR
- The proximal half of the palm is placed in contact with the IR and the fingers are flexed around the edge of the receptor; the carpus should be as far away from the edge of the receptor as possible
- The patient effects dorsiflexion of the wrist in this position by leaning forward and exerting slight pressure on the forearm,

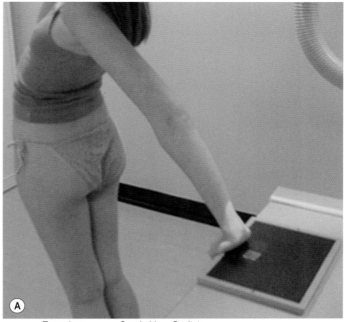

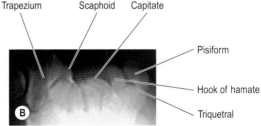

Figure 5.25 Superoinferior carpal tunnel (method 1) with (A) patient's back to X-ray beam; (B) carpal tunnel.

which is extended at the elbow to allow maximum effect. The forearm is cleared from the wrist and carpus

Method 2: superoinferior carpal tunnel – erect with patient facing the central ray

(Fig. 5.26)

Positioning

- IR is positioned as for method 1
- A lead rubber apron is fastened over the front of the waist
- The patient stands facing the table, which should be adjusted so that its height lies just below their waist
- The affected arm is externally rotated until the palm is in supination, facing anteriorly towards the table and IR
- The proximal half of the palm is placed in contact with the IR and the fingers flexed around the edge of the receptor; the carpus should be as far from the edge of the receptor as possible
- The patient effects dorsiflexion of the wrist in this position by leaning back and exerting a slight pressure on the forearm, which is extended at the elbow to allow maximum effect. The forearm is cleared from the wrist and carpus

Beam direction and FRD for methods 1 and 2

Vertical, at 90° to the IR
100 cm FRD

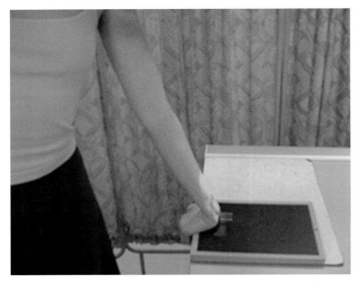

Figure 5.26 Superoinferior carpal tunnel (method 2) with patient facing X-ray beam.

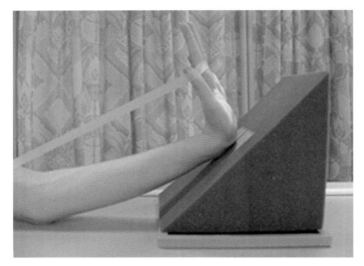

Figure 5.27 Inferosuperior carpal tunnel (method 3) with patient seated.

Centring point

Over the midpoint of the anterior part of the wrist, within the depression caused by the tunnel arrangement of the carpus

Collimation

Carpal bones, soft tissue of anterior aspect of wrist

Method 3: inferosuperior carpal tunnel – patient seated facing the table (Fig. 5.27)

Positioning

- The patient is seated at the table and a lead rubber sheet is applied to the waist
- The IR is horizontal, 30–40 cm from the patient, and there must be enough table or top space for the patient to rest their elbow for immobilisation and positioning

- A 45° radiolucent pad is placed onto the IR
- The patient places the flexed elbow of the affected side onto the table
- Whilst maintaining some elbow flexion, the hand is pronated and the forearm rested on the pad
- The wrist should lie over, but not in contact with, the IR
- The hand is dorsiflexed at the wrist and a bandage passed around the fingers; pulling this bandage gently will facilitate the extent of dorsiflexion required to clear the forearm from the carpus
- The patient maintains the dorsiflexion by holding and pulling the ends of the bandage; the elbow remains in contact with the table-top
- The head is turned to the side, away from the primary beam

Beam direction and FRD for method 3

Vertical, at 90° to the IR
150 cm FRD

Centring point

Over the midpoint of the anterior part of the proximal portion of the hand, within the depression caused by the tunnel arrangement of the carpus

Collimation

Carpal bones, soft tissue of anterior portion of distal hand

Criteria for assessing image quality (all methods)

- The carpal bones and soft tissue of the anterior portion of the wrist are demonstrated
- The carpal tunnel is seen as a curved, darker, soft tissue area anterior to the denser carpal bones
- The distal radius and ulna are cleared from the carpus to lie over the metacarpals
- The hook of hamate and pisiform are cleared from the rest of the carpus and on the medial aspect of the tunnel
- Sharp image demonstrating soft tissue of the carpal tunnel region, bony trabeculae of pisiform and hook of hamate. Optimum penetration to demonstrate these bones, whilst maintaining contrast with required soft tissue. Superimposed carpals will not be fully penetrated

Common errors	Possible reasons
Image overall appears pale with no distinguishable bony features	1. Inadequate penetration and exposure 2. Forearm may not have been cleared from carpus; improve dorsiflexion or consider examination using a method that may be more comfortable for the patient
Asymmetry of tunnel; fourth and fifth metacarpals are seen clear of forearm	Patient's arm is leaning towards radius; ensure forearm lies vertically over the hand and carpus
Asymmetry of tunnel; first and second metacarpals are seen clear of forearm	Patient's arm is leaning towards ulna; ensure forearm lies vertically over the hand and carpus

REFERENCES

1. Whitley AS, et al. Clark's positioning in radiography. 12th ed. London: Hodder Arnold; 2005.

2. Richmond B. A comparative study of two radiographic techniques for obtaining an AP projection of the thumb. Radiography Today 1995;61(696):11–15.

3. Unett EM, Royle AJ. Radiographic techniques and image evaluation. London: Chapman and Hall; 1997.

4. The Ionising Radiation (Medical Exposure) Regulations. London: HMSO; 2006.

5. Lewis S. New angles on radiographic examination of the hand. Radiography Today 1988;54(617):4–45, (618): 20–30, (619): 47–48.

6. Bell G, Finlay D. Basic radiographic positioning and anatomy. London: Baillière Tindall; 1986.

7. Clark KC. Clark's positioning in radiography. London: Heinemann; 1939.

8. Goldfarb CA, et al. Wrist fractures: what the clinician wants to know. Radiology 2001;219:11–28.

9. Carver E, Carver B, editors. Medical imaging: techniques, reflection, evaluation. Edinburgh: Churchill Livingstone; 2006.

10. Bontrager K, Lampignano JP. Textbook of radiographic positioning and related anatomy. 7th ed. St Louis: Mosby; 2010.

11. Sante LR. Manual of radiological technique. 2nd ed. Michigan: Edwards Brothers Inc; 1935.

12. McQuillen-Martenson K. Radiographic image analysis. 3rd ed. St Louis: Saunders; 2010.

13. Cooney W. The wrist: diagnosis and operative treatment. 2nd ed. Philadelphia: Lippincott Williams and Wilkins; 2010.

14. Goldfarb CA, et al. Wrist fractures: what the clinician wants to know. Radiology 2001 (April);219:11–28.

15. Nicholson DA, Driscoll PA. ABC of emergency radiology. Cambridge: BMJ Publishing Group; 1995.

16. Helms CA. Fundamentals of skeletal radiology. 2nd ed. Philadelphia: WB Saunders; 1995.

Chapter | **6** |

Forearm, elbow and humerus

Elizabeth Carver

FOREARM (RADIUS AND ULNA)

This region of the upper limb most usually presents for imaging as a result of trauma. The Colles' fracture is the most usual finding after trauma to radius and ulna; this is outlined in Chapter 5 (section on the wrist). Other fractures of these bones are much rarer. The *Galleazzi* fracture is more serious than the Colles', being a fracture of the distal portion of the radius accompanied by subluxation or dislocation of the distal radioulnar joint. The *Monteggia* fracture, conversely, is a fracture of the ulna accompanied by dislocation of the radius proximally.[1]

For all projections of the forearm the image receptor (IR) is placed horizontal unless otherwise specified.

Anteroposterior (AP) forearm (Fig. 6.1A,B)

Positioning

- The patient is seated with the affected side next to the table; lead rubber is applied to the waist
- The arm is extended at the elbow, abducted away from the trunk and externally rotated until the hand lies in supination
- The posterior aspect of the forearm is placed in contact with the IR, to include elbow and wrist joints
- The joints must lie in the same plane
- The humeral epicondyles and radial and ulnar styloid processes are equidistant from the IR
- The head is turned away from the shoulder of the side under examination, aiming to reduce scattered radiation to the lenses of the eyes and thyroid

Beam direction and focus receptor distance (FRD)

Vertical, at 90° to the IR
100 cm FRD

Centring

Midway between the wrist and elbow joints

Collimation

Elbow, wrist, shafts of radius and ulna, soft tissue outlines of forearm

Criteria for assessing image quality

- Wrist and elbow joints, radius, ulna and soft tissue outline of the forearm are demonstrated
- Partial superimposition of the radius and ulna at proximal and distal ends, with separation of the shafts. Radial tubercle should overlap the cortex of the ulnar shaft, but no further
- Humeral epicondyles equidistant from coronoid and olecranon fossae
- Radial styloid process seen on the lateral aspects of this bone
- Ulnar styloid process is shown in profile distally in the middle of the head of ulna
- Sharp image demonstrating soft tissue margins of the forearm, bony cortex and trabeculae. Adequate penetration to demonstrate overlap of olecranon over distal humerus while showing trabecular detail over shafts of radius and ulna

Common errors	Possible reasons
Radius cleared from ulna at the proximal end; radial head also shown clear	Externally rotated arm
Radial tubercle superimposed over shaft of ulna	Internally rotated arm
Shafts of radius and ulna show adequate contrast and density but elbow is 'thin', underpenetrated and shows poor contrast or bony detail	Inadequate kVp selected
Elbow joint shows adequate contrast and density but shafts of radius and ulna are dark, showing poor contrast and bony detail	Selected kVp too high

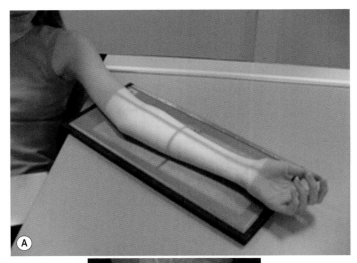

Lateral forearm (Fig. 6.2A,B)

Positioning

- The patient is seated with the affected side next to the table; lead rubber is applied to the waist
- The arm is flexed at the elbow, abducted away from the trunk and internally rotated at the wrist
- The medial aspect of the forearm is placed in contact with the IR, to include elbow and wrist joints
- The shoulder, elbow and wrist joints must lie in the same plane
- The humeral epicondyles are superimposed, as are the radial and ulnar styloid processes. Ensuring the shoulder lies in the same plane as the wrist and elbow will help facilitate this
- The head is turned away from the shoulder of the side under examination, aiming to reduce scattered radiation to the lenses of the eyes and thyroid

Beam direction and FRD

Vertical, at 90° to the IR
100 cm FRD

Centring

Midway between the wrist and elbow joints, on the medial aspect of the forearm

Collimation

Elbow, wrist, shafts of radius and ulna, soft tissue outlines of forearm

Criteria for assessing image quality

- The wrist and elbow joints, radius, ulna and soft tissue outline of the forearm are demonstrated
- Superimposition of posterior portion of radial head over coronoid process of ulna; superimposition of distal radius and ulna
- Shaft of the radius is seen anterior to that of the ulna
- There will be some superimposition of trochlea and capitulum of humerus. However, it may be unrealistic to expect to see full superimposition of these structures as the obliquity of the beam at its periphery is likely to pass through the elbow at around 3–4°
- Sharp image demonstrating soft tissue margins of the forearm, bony cortex and trabeculae. Adequate penetration to demonstrate overlap of radial head over the olecranon and distal radius over ulna, while showing trabecular detail over the shafts of the radius and ulna

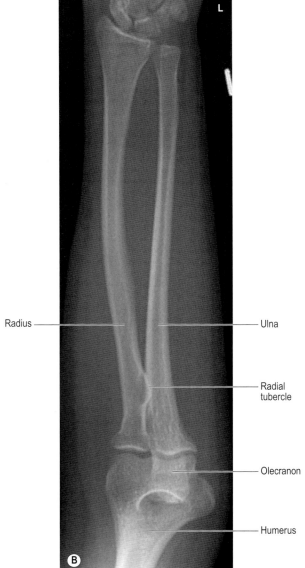

Radius — — Ulna

— Radial tubercle

— Olecranon

— Humerus

Figure 6.1 AP forearm.

Common errors	Possible reasons
Distal radius seen anteriorly in relationship to ulna	Wrist is medially rotated
Distal radius seen posteriorly in relationship to ulna; shafts of radius and ulna superimposed along most of their length	Wrist and elbow are externally rotated; this usually only occurs when the humerus does not lie in the same plane as the forearm and the shoulder lies above the table-top

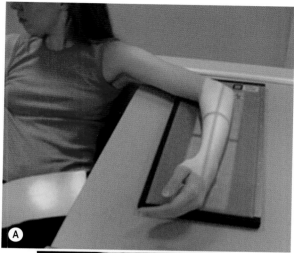

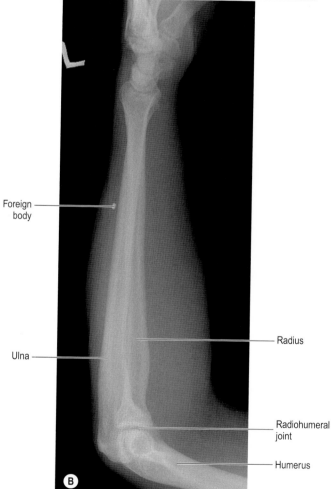

Figure 6.2 Lateral forearm.

ELBOW

Degenerative change and trauma are both major indicators for plain radiographic imaging. Dislocations at the elbow can be demonstrated radiographically and the head of the radius is the most likely part to be subluxed.

The *supracondylar fracture* of the humerus has many implications for the future of the patient's arm. The vasculature of the arm can be damaged, or existing damage can be exacerbated, by forced extension of the elbow joint; this can cause an ischaemic state in the lower arm resulting in paralysis of the hand and forearm and, long term, in what is known as a *Volkmann's ischaemic contracture*. It is therefore essential that the radiographer undertakes modified projections of the elbow which cannot be extended; these are outlined in Chapter 25 on accident and emergency (A&E) radiography.

For all projections of the elbow the IR is placed horizontal unless otherwise specified.

AP elbow (Fig. 6.3A,B)

Positioning

- The patient is seated with the affected side next to the table; lead rubber is applied to the waist
- The arm is extended at the elbow, abducted away from the trunk and externally rotated until the hand lies in supination
- The posterior aspect of the elbow is placed in contact with the IR
- The wrist, elbow and shoulder joints must lie in the same plane
- The humeral epicondyles are equidistant from the IR
- The head is turned away from the shoulder of the side under examination, aiming to reduce scattered radiation to the lenses of the eyes and thyroid

Beam direction and FRD

Vertical, at 90° to the IR
100 cm FRD

Centring

Midway between the humeral epicondyles

Collimation

Proximal radius and ulna, elbow joint, distal shaft of humerus, soft tissue outlines surrounding elbow joint

Criteria for assessing image quality

- The proximal radius and ulna, elbow joint, distal shaft of the humerus and soft tissue outlines surrounding the elbow joint demonstrated
- Partial superimposition of the radius and ulna at the proximal end (0.6 cm of radial head superimposed over ulna).[2] Radial tuberosity should overlap the cortex of the ulnar shaft, but no further
- Humeral epicondyles equidistant from the coronoid and olecranon fossae
- Sharp image demonstrating soft tissue margins around the elbow, bony cortex and trabeculae. Adequate penetration to demonstrate overlap of olecranon over distal humerus

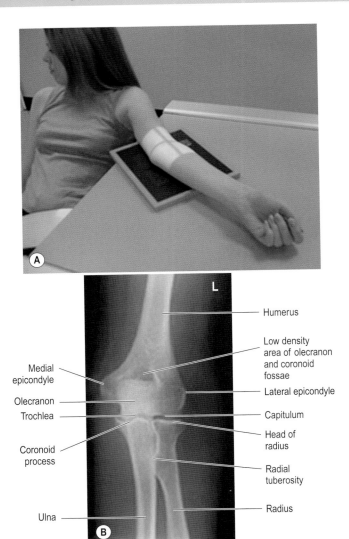

Figure 6.3 AP elbow.

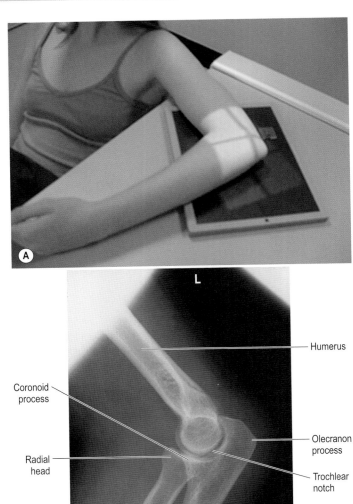

Figure 6.4 Lateral elbow.

Common errors	Possible reasons
Radius cleared from ulna; radial head also shown clear	Elbow is externally rotated
Radial head superimposed more than 0.6 cm over shaft of ulna	Internally rotated elbow
Radial head fully superimposed over ulna; distance between humeral epicondyles seems narrow	Hand may be in pronation rather than supination
Joint space between capitulum and radial head is closed; long axes of radius and ulna travel obliquely towards the lateral aspect of the arm away from the joint	Arm not fully extended at the elbow

Lateral elbow (Fig. 6.4A,B)

Positioning

- The patient is seated with the affected side next to the table; lead rubber is applied to the waist
- The arm is abducted from the trunk, internally rotated and flexed 90° at the elbow
- The wrist is externally rotated until the radial and ulnar styloid processes are superimposed
- The medial aspect of the elbow is placed in contact with the IR
- The shoulder, elbow and wrist joints must lie in the same plane
- The humeral epicondyles are superimposed. Ensuring the shoulder lies in the same plane as the wrist and elbow will help facilitate this more easily
- The head is turned away from the shoulder of the side under examination, aiming to reduce scattered radiation to the lenses of the eyes and thyroid

Beam direction and FRD

Vertical, at 90° to the IR
100 cm FRD

Centring

Over the lateral humeral epicondyle

Collimation

Proximal radius and ulna, elbow joint, distal shaft of humerus, soft tissue outlines surrounding elbow joint

Criteria for assessing image quality

- The proximal radius and ulna, elbow joint, distal shaft of the humerus and soft tissue outlines surrounding the elbow joint are demonstrated
- Superimposition of surfaces of trochlea and capitulum, with the posterior portion of the radial head shown over the coronoid process of ulna. Evidence of joint space of the elbow seen
- Shaft of the radius is seen anterior to that of the ulna
- Sharp image demonstrating soft tissue margins around the elbow, bony cortex and trabeculae. Adequate penetration to demonstrate overlap of radial head over the olecranon and superimposed epicondyles. Exposure factors must ensure that the anterior and supinator fat pads are shown in contrast with the surrounding soft tissue (the posterior fat pad will only be demonstrated if there is bony injury)

The importance of optimum exposure factor selection cannot be emphasised enough, especially in the case of the elbow radiograph requested after trauma. Information on both bone and soft tissue becomes even more vital in trauma cases. This is because personnel assessing and/or reporting on the radiograph need to inspect the image for evidence of the 'fat pad sign', an indication of presence of abnormal fluid (usually blood) outside the elbow's joint capsule. This sign suggests bony damage, often supracondylar or radial head fractures, which may or may not be evident on the radiograph. When significant trauma causes displacement of the pads there will be an appearance similar to a downturned rose thorn (seen as darker than the surrounding soft tissue) anterior and/or posterior to the distal humerus, just above the epicondyles. The normal positions of the fat pads are: supinator fat pad seen along the anterior aspect of the humerus; anterior fat pad seen anterior to the distal portion of humerus just above the coronoid fossa; the posterior fat pad is positioned within the olecranon fossa posteriorly.[1]

Flexion of the joint also affects fat pad appearance in the lateral elbow projection. Flexion <90° causes the olecranon to move towards the olecranon fossa, thereby displacing the posterior pad superiorly to a position which may be visible on the lateral radiograph. This may potentially mimic appearances suggestive of trauma and thus affect radiological comment.[2]

The injured patient often finds it difficult or impossible to extend the elbow joint, making it impossible for the radiographer to undertake routine projections of the area. Techniques must be modified, especially if there is a risk of Volkmann's ischaemic contracture after supracondylar fracture. These modifications are covered in Chapter 25 on A&E imaging.

HEAD OF RADIUS

A significant proportion of the radial head is superimposed over the proximal ulna in both the AP and the lateral projections of the elbow joint. As a result small fractures of the radial head may not be demonstrated by more routine projections. Modifications of these are recommended in order to provide the required information. These modified projections are undertaken in addition to AP and lateral projections.

Oblique head of radius: external rotation

(Fig. 6.5A,B)

This projection will also demonstrate the proximal radioulnar joint.

Positioning

- The patient is positioned initially as for the AP elbow projection
- The arm is externally rotated through approximately 20° to clear the radial head from the ulna. Asking the patient to lean sideways, towards the table and IR, will help facilitate this
- A radiolucent pad placed under the medial aspect of the forearm will aid immobilisation
- The head is turned away from the shoulder of the side under examination, aiming to reduce scattered radiation to the lenses of the eyes and thyroid

Beam direction and FRD

Vertical, at 90° to the IR
100 cm FRD

Centring

Over the middle of the crease of the elbow

Collimation

Proximal radius and ulna, elbow joint, distal shaft of humerus, soft tissue outlines surrounding elbow joint

Criteria for assessing image quality

- The proximal radius and ulna, elbow joint, distal shaft of the humerus and soft tissue outlines surrounding the elbow joint are demonstrated
- Radial head is cleared from the ulna, and the proximal radioulnar joint is clear
- Sharp image demonstrating soft tissue margins around the elbow, bony cortex and trabeculae

Common error	Possible reason
Radial head not cleared from ulna	Inadequate external rotation

Rotation as much as 45° has been suggested for demonstration of the radial head; this is significantly more than the 20° described here.[3] As 20° adequately demonstrates clearance of the head it seems excessive to expect the injured patient to aim for further rotation.

An alternative projection for clearance of the radial head from the ulna has been described as a *lateral with 45° lateromedial angulation of the primary beam*.[4] This projection is acknowledged to efficiently clear the radial head but will cause some significant distortion of the image

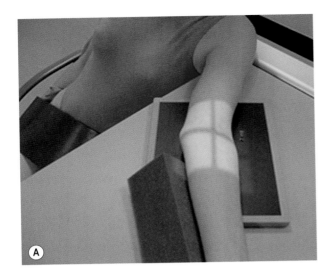

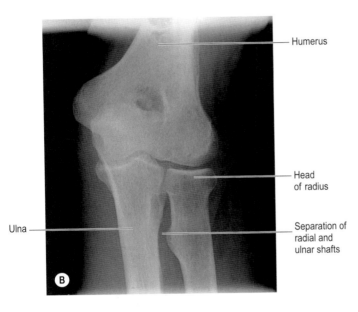

Humerus

Head
of radius

Separation of
radial and
ulnar shafts

Ulna

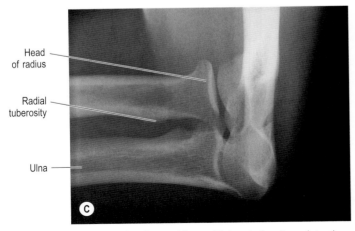

Head
of radius

Radial
tuberosity

Ulna

Figure 6.5 (A,B) Head of radius – oblique; (C) head of radius – lateral elbow with 45° lateromedial angulation to clear radial head from ulna. *(C) Reproduced with permission from Ballinger PW, Frank ED. Merrill's atlas of radiographic positioning and radiologic procedures. 10th ed. St Louis: Mosby; 2003.*

(Fig. 6.5C). Angulation of the beam towards the trunk also has implications for a potential increase in radiation dose to more radiosensitive areas of the body. However, severe elbow trauma may render the patient incapable of adequate elbow extension for the oblique projection, and the lateral with 45° angle may be the only suitable alternative – clearly a situation when a risk–benefit assessment must be made by the radiographer.

Lateral head of the radius (Figs 6.6A,B, 6.7A,B)

Although the externally rotated oblique projection for the radial head will clear it from the ulna to show more of its medial aspect, and its anterior aspect is seen on the lateral elbow projection, other aspects

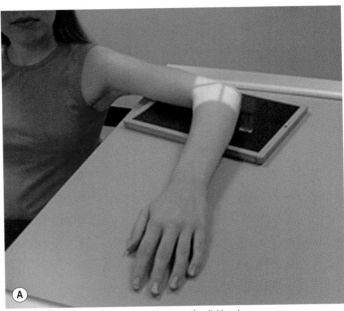

Radial tuberosity   Lateral aspect of radial head

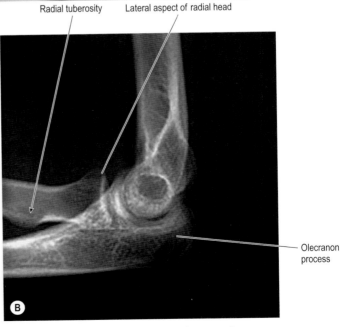

Olecranon
process

Figure 6.6 Lateral head of radius. Hand pronated. *(B) Reproduced with permission from Ballinger PW, Frank ED. Merrill's atlas of radiographic positioning and radiologic procedures. 10th ed. St Louis: Mosby; 2003.*

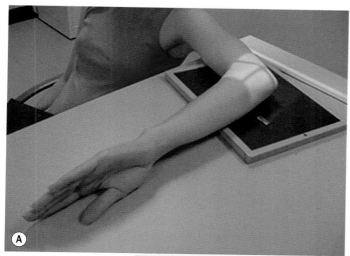

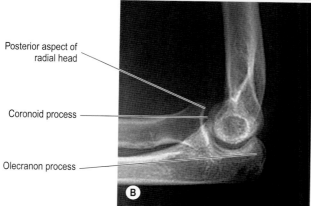

Posterior aspect of radial head

Coronoid process

Olecranon process

Figure 6.7 Lateral head of radius. Hand medially rotated.
(B) Reproduced with permission from Ballinger PW, Frank ED. Merrill's atlas of radiographic positioning and radiologic procedures. 10th ed. St Louis: Mosby; 2003.

of the head will not have been well demonstrated on any of the routine elbow images. As a result it is necessary to provide profile projections of the radial head. These are achieved with the elbow in a lateral position and as described below.

Positioning

- The patient is positioned initially as for the lateral elbow projection
- 1. *To demonstrate the lateral aspect of the radial head*: Rotate the forearm internally until the hand is in pronation and in contact with the table-top
- 2. *To demonstrate the posterior aspect of the radial head*: From the position described in 1 above, the forearm is rotated further until its medial aspect is in contact with the IR and table-top
- A legend is applied to each image to identify the palm position used
- The head is turned away from the shoulder of the side under examination, aiming to reduce scattered radiation to the lenses of the eyes and thyroid

Beam direction and FRD

Vertical, at 90° to the IR
100 cm FRD

Centring

Over the lateral humeral epicondyle (both forearm positions)

Collimation

Proximal radius and ulna, elbow joint, distal shaft of humerus, soft tissue outlines surrounding elbow joint

Criteria for assessing image quality

- As for the lateral elbow, plus demonstration of change in position of the radial tubercle as it moves with rotation at the elbow. With the hand pronated (position 1) it should be seen as a slight prominence on the radius, projecting into the space between radius and ulna. With the hand further rotated medially (position 2) the tubercle appears more prominent and its outline will be nearer the outline of the ulna

Olecranon and coronoid: AP oblique with internal rotation (Fig. 6.8A,B)

More detailed information of these areas on the ulna can be obtained by an internal oblique projection in cases where adequate AP and lateral projections cannot be undertaken because of the patient's condition.

Positioning

- The patient is positioned initially as for the AP elbow projection
- The forearm is pronated by rotation of the wrist, to effect crossover of the radius and ulna
- The whole arm is rotated medially through 45° at the shoulder
- A radiolucent pad placed under the lateral aspect of the forearm will aid immobilisation
- The head is turned away from the shoulder of the side under examination, aiming to reduce scattered radiation to the lenses of the eyes and thyroid

Beam direction and FRD

Vertical, at 90° to the IR
100 cm FRD

Centring

Over the middle of the crease of the elbow

Collimation

Proximal radius and ulna, elbow joint, distal shaft of humerus, soft tissue outlines surrounding elbow joint

Criteria for assessing image quality

- Proximal radius and ulna, elbow joint, distal shaft of the humerus and soft tissue outlines surrounding the elbow joint are demonstrated
- Proximal ulna appears as a 'spanner' with the olecranon process, trochlear notch and coronoid process shown in profile
- Olecranon process is superimposed over the olecranon fossa, the trochlear notch surrounds the outline of the trochlea and the coronoid process is shown clear of the radius
- Sharp image demonstrating soft tissue margins around the elbow, coronoid process in profile over soft tissue, bony cortex and trabeculae. Adequate penetration to demonstrate olecranon process overlying distal humerus

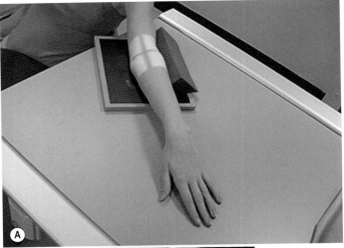

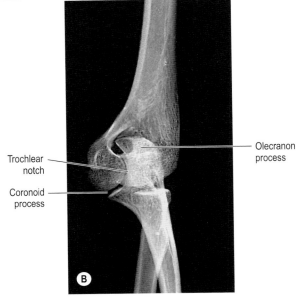

Trochlear notch

Coronoid process

Olecranon process

Figure 6.8 Olecranon and coronoid – AP internally rotated oblique. *(B) Reproduced with permission from Ballinger PW, Frank ED. Merrill's atlas of radiographic positioning and radiologic procedures. 10th ed. St Louis: Mosby; 2003.*

Common error	Possible reason
Coronoid process not cleared from radius	Inadequate medial rotation

Clearly this projection will not be possible in patients who cannot extend at the elbow joint, a common occurrence in cases of elbow trauma. An alternative has been suggested where the partially flexed elbow is positioned with the posterior aspect of the forearm in contact with the IR. A 45° central ray is then used and directed lateromedially, centred over the crease of the elbow. Appearance of the olecranon is similar to that in Figure 6.8B, in that the olecranon is seen as spanner-shaped. This position can also be used to demonstrate the radial head, used in conjunction with a mediolateral central ray, which projects the radial head laterally from the ulna. For cases where supination is also not possible, the arm (which is flexed at the elbow with the hand

in pronation) is abducted with the humerus at 45° from the trunk, the forearm is in contact with the table and the vertical central ray is centred over the lateral epicondyle;[5,6] this provides an image of the olecranon almost identical to that in Figure 6.8B but with less distortion, as the central ray is not angled. The issue of benefit versus risk is certainly relevant regarding the projections described that have the hand in supination, as it appears that the patient's legs may come close to the primary beam and their trunk is leaning towards it.

ULNAR GROOVE

The ulnar groove lies between the medial humeral epicondyle and the trochlea. It acts as a channel along which the ulnar nerve passes, down to the forearm from the humerus. Ulnar nerve compression at this point can cause paraesthesia and neuralgia. Because of its excellent capacity for imaging soft tissue, magnetic resonance imaging (MRI) is most suited to investigation of possible ulnar nerve compression and should be the imaging method of choice wherever possible.

Positioning (Fig. 6.9A)

- The patient is seated with the affected side next to the table; lead rubber is applied to the waist
- The arm is extended at the elbow, abducted away from the trunk and externally rotated until the hand lies in supination
- The posterior aspect of the elbow is placed in contact with the IR
- The elbow is fully flexed and the fist gently clenched. The wrist is also gently flexed, to bring the fingers and thumb in contact with the shoulder
- From a position when the humeral epicondyles are equidistant from the IR, the upper arm is externally rotated 45°. This is best achieved by asking the patient to lean over towards the affected side before effecting the external rotation. The fist remains in contact with the shoulder throughout

Beam direction and FRD

Vertical, at 90° to the IR
100 cm FRD

Centring

Over the medial epicondyle

Collimation

Olecranon process, distal humerus below shaft, soft tissue outlines around medial area of elbow

Criteria for assessing image quality

- Olecranon process, distal humerus below the shaft and soft tissue outlines around the medial area of the elbow are demonstrated
- Forearm is shown superimposed over the lateral portion of the distal humerus and clear of the medial epicondyle
- Olecranon process is seen distally in relationship to the humerus
- Ulnar groove is seen as a notch between the medial epicondyle and the trochlea
- Sharp image demonstrating soft tissue margins around the medial aspect of the elbow, bony cortex and trabeculae of the non-superimposed portion of the humerus (see Fig. 6.9B)

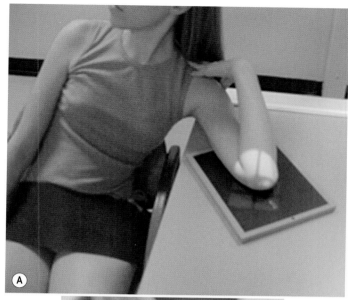

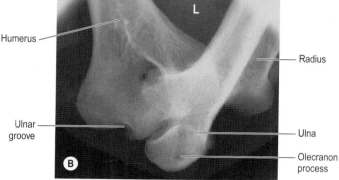

Figure 6.9 Ulnar groove.

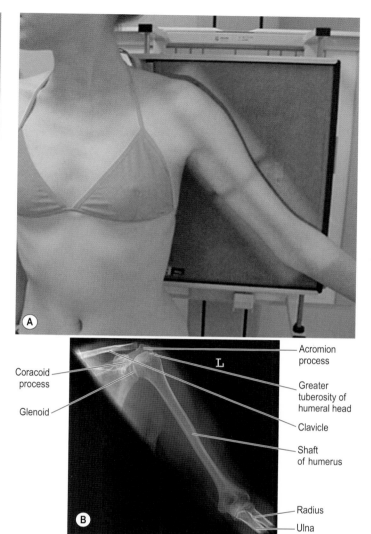

Figure 6.10 AP humerus.

Common error	Possible reasons
Groove not seen as a distinct notch between trochlea and medial epicondyle	Inaccurate external rotation. If accompanied by superimposition of forearm over the midline of the humerus, this indicates inadequate external rotation. Superimposition of trochlea over the groove also indicates this
	If the medial epicondyle appears flattened, there is over-rotation of the arm

HUMERUS

For all projections of the humerus the IR is placed vertical. If a patient presents supine, as on an A&E trolley, the IR can be used horizontally under the humerus, on the trolley top, for the AP projection.

AP humerus (Fig. 6.10A,B)

Positioning

- The IR is placed in the erect holder
- A lead rubber apron is applied to the patient's waist
- The patient stands erect facing the X-ray tube and the affected arm is extended and abducted from the trunk to avoid superimposition of the humerus and upper arm soft tissue over the soft tissue of the trunk
- The feet are slightly separated for stability
- The height of the IR is adjusted until its midpoint is coincident with the midshaft of the humerus
- Orientating the upper arm diagonally at 45° across the IR plate will maximise the available space for the area of interest which must include the shoulder and elbow joints on the image
- The palm faces forwards with the humeral epicondyles equidistant from the IR

Beam direction and FRD

Horizontal, at 90° to the IR
100 cm FRD

Centring

To the middle of the humerus, on the anterior aspect of the arm

Collimation

Shoulder joint, shaft of humerus, elbow joint, soft tissues surrounding the area

Aligning the light beam diaphragm housing along the long axis of the humerus before collimating will allow more effective collimation around the area of interest

Criteria for assessing image quality

- Shoulder joint, shaft of humerus, elbow joint and soft tissues are demonstrated
- Humerus is clear of the soft tissue of the trunk
- Greater tuberosity of humerus is in profile laterally on the head of humerus
- Humeral epicondyles are equidistant from coronoid and olecranon fossae
- Sharp image demonstrating soft tissue margins around the area of interest, bony cortex and trabeculae. Adequate penetration to demonstrate joints whilst maintaining trabecular detail over the humeral shaft

Common errors	Possible reasons
Pale shadow overlying medial aspect of the humerus and soft tissue of upper arm	Arm not abducted adequately from the trunk
Humeral epicondyles not shown as equidistant around coronoid and olecranon fossae; greater tuberosity projected over the humeral head	Arm is rotated. This is most frequently medial rotation, as this is a more comfortable position for the patient than with the rotation required for a true AP position of the humerus

Lateral humerus (Fig. 6.11A,B)

Positioning

- The IR is placed in the erect holder
- A lead rubber apron is applied to the posterior aspect of the patient's waist
- The patient stands erect facing the IR and the affected arm is extended and abducted from the trunk to avoid superimposition of the humerus and upper arm soft tissue over the soft tissue of the trunk
- The feet are slightly separated for stability
- The height of the IR is adjusted until its midpoint is coincident with the midshaft of the humerus
- Orientating the upper arm at 45° across the IR will maximise the available space for the area of interest, which must include the shoulder and elbow joints on the image
- The arm is medially rotated and the elbow flexed until the medial aspect of the hand comes into contact with the lower abdomen. The lateral aspect of the humerus is in contact with the IR. The humeral epicondyles are superimposed
- The head is turned away from the side under examination
- A PA anatomical marker is usually used for this projection

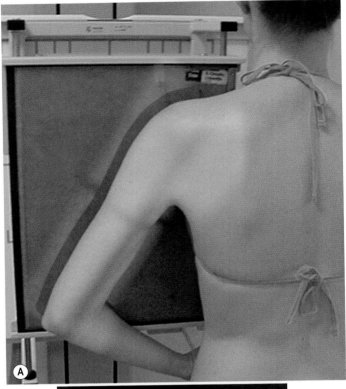

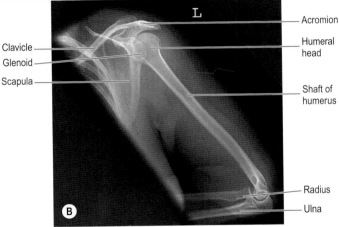

Figure 6.11 Lateral humerus.

The lateral humerus projection can also be undertaken with the patient facing the X-ray tube, in an AP position, and this should be adapted for the trolley-bound patient who is supine, rather than attempting a PA approach.

For the AP projection the arm is flexed at the elbow and the limb medially rotated to bring the medial aspect of the humerus in contact with the IR. The hand is placed on the hip to immobilise the arm. Unfortunately this position is somewhat difficult, even for the uninjured patient, especially as the movement required at the shoulder results in the scapula being positioned almost perpendicular to the IR; this in itself is not disadvantageous, but the position of the scapula does push the posterior aspect of the upper humerus away from the IR, making lateral representation of the image of the bone less accurate. The action of the hand resting on the hip also makes superimposition of the humeral epicondyles difficult.

Beam direction and FRD

Horizontal, at 90° to the IR
100 cm FRD

Centring

For patient in a PA position: to the middle of the humerus, on the medial aspect of the arm
For patient in an AP position: to the middle of the humerus, on the lateral aspect of the arm

Collimation

Shoulder joint, shaft of humerus, elbow joint, soft tissues surrounding the area

Aligning the light beam diaphragm housing along the long axis of the humerus before collimating will allow more effective collimation around the area of interest.

Criteria for assessing image quality

- Shoulder joint, shaft of humerus, elbow joint and soft tissues are demonstrated
- Humerus is clear of soft tissue of trunk and humeral head is cleared from the image of the scapula
- Greater tuberosity of humerus is seen over the middle of humeral head
- Superimposition of the trochlea and capitulum is ideal, but it must be remembered that oblique rays around the central ray are likely to impinge upon this area at around 5–8°, varying with humeral length. This obliquity will almost certainly affect the superimposition of trochlea and capitulum. If this area of the humerus is of particular interest then elbow projections should be undertaken
- Sharp image demonstrating soft tissue margins around the area of interest, bony cortex and trabeculae. Adequate penetration to demonstrate joints whilst maintaining trabecular detail over the humeral shaft

Common errors	Possible reasons
Pale shadow overlying the anterior aspect of the humerus (seen facing towards the thorax in this projection) and soft tissue of upper arm	Arm not abducted adequately from the trunk
Greater tuberosity appears towards or over the lateral margin of the humeral head	Arm is externally rotated. This can be avoided by ensuring that the entire length of the lateral aspect of the humerus is in contact with the IR; this encourages the patient to maintain the lateral position
Non-superimposition of trochlea and capitulum	Slight overlap, rather than full superimposition, can be explained by effects of obliquity of the beam around the central ray (see image quality criteria, above). However, when accompanied by incorrect appearance of the greater tuberosity (see point above) this may indicate external rotation of the humerus

INTERTUBEROUS SULCUS (BICIPITAL GROOVE)

The intertuberous sulcus lies on the anterior aspect of the humeral head, between the greater and lesser tuberosities; insertion of the long head of biceps lies here. Its position makes it difficult to image because it travels vertically and cannot be seen on an AP projection of the humerus or shoulder.

The projection aims to demonstrate the groove in profile, which is only possible in the superoinferior or inferosuperior directions. There are many problems associated with either of these approaches, the most obvious being implementation of either position with the bulky light beam housings commonly found today. Other important considerations are dose implications when directing a beam caudally (for superoinferior projection), and immobilisation.

The option of the superoinferior method does cause serious concern for patient dose, as the caudal ray required would almost certainly irradiate anterior structures of the trunk in addition to the upper humerus, thereby raising questions as to its suitability.

Therefore, an inferosuperior approach may fit with the requirement for the radiographer to use a technique that reduces the risk of irradiating radiosensitive tissues. Older texts describe an inferosuperior method which involves the patient leaning over a tube head which is directed vertically but in a cranial direction.[7] Use of the old long cones, which were replaced by modern collimators, meant that the patient could use the cone as an aid to immobilisation. The IR was supported by a special holder. The method described in this book uses an adaptation of this, with the patient supine. In the absence of the long cone, the patient is immobilised by lying supine; a specialist receptor support is not always necessary but does prove useful.

Inferosuperior bicipital groove: method 1

(Fig. 6.12)

Positioning

- The patient lies supine on the examination table and a lead rubber apron is laid over the top of the trunk
- The IR is supported vertically on the table with its tube side in contact with the superior aspect of the shoulder. Its centre is coincident with the humeral head
- The arm is abducted slightly from the trunk and externally rotated until the humeral epicondyles are approximately 45° to the table-top
- The greater and lesser tuberosities are palpated to ensure that the intertuberous sulcus is in profile superiorly
- The patient's head is turned away from the side under examination

Beam direction and FRD

Initially horizontal, with a 5° caudal angle
FRD may vary according to the size of the tube mounting but should be no less than 100 cm
A slightly longer FRD may be beneficial, as there may be a relatively long object receptor distance (ORD) in patients who have a significant amount of adipose or muscle tissue over the shoulder joint

Inferosuperior bicipital groove: method 2

(Fig. 6.13)

The IR is vertical.

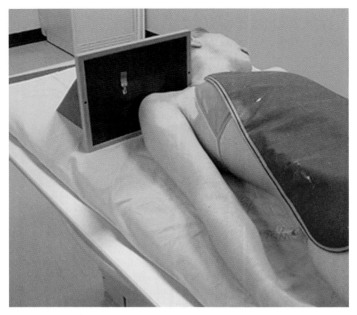

Figure 6.12 Inferosuperior bicipital groove – method 1.

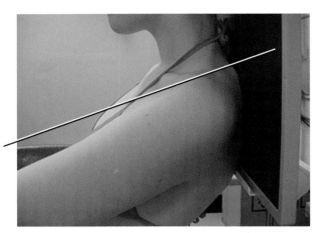

Figure 6.13 Inferosuperior bicipital groove – method 2.

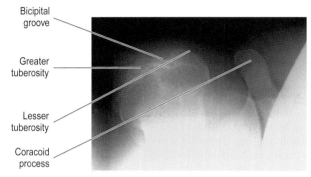

Figure 6.14 Bicipital groove.
Reproduced with permission from Ballinger PW, Frank ED. Merrill's atlas of radiographic positioning and radiologic procedures. 10th ed. St Louis: Mosby; 2003.

Positioning

- The patient sits facing the X-ray tube, their back approximately 30 cm away from the IR
- The patient leans back, approximately 30° from vertical, until they lean against the IR
- The arm is abducted slightly from the trunk and externally rotated until the humeral epicondyles are approximately 45° to the median sagittal plane
- The arm is elevated slightly to bring the long axis of the humerus to make an angle of approximately 30° with the floor (60° to IR)
- The greater and lesser tuberosities are palpated to ensure that the intertuberous sulcus is in profile superiorly
- The patient's head is turned away from the side under examination

Beam direction and FRD

Initially horizontal, with a 15–20° cranial angle
As for method 1, FRD may vary according to the size of the tube mounting but should be no less than 100 cm

Centring – both methods

Over the anterior aspect of the middle of the humeral head

Collimation

Anterior portion of humeral head, soft tissue overlying this area
Inclusion of the area within collimation can be ensured by checking that the outline shadow of the area lies within the light beam representation and the IR

Criteria for assessing image quality

- Anterior portion of humeral head and the soft tissue overlying it are demonstrated
- Bicipital groove is seen in profile as a notch superiorly over the outline of the anterior aspect of humeral head, between the greater and lesser tuberosities
- Sharp image demonstrating soft tissue margins above the area of interest, bony cortex and its outline over the sulcus (see Fig. 6.14)

Common errors	Possible reasons
Humeral head seen but sulcus not in profile	1. Sulcus projected medially or laterally due to inaccurate rotation of the limb *or*
	2. Extreme obliquity of the arm positions the sulcus obliquely, rather than perpendicular to IR
Dense soft tissue shadow overlying area of interest	Tube position too low; the soft tissues of the arm may be superimposed over the area of interest

REFERENCES

1. Scally P. Medical imaging. Oxford: Oxford University Press; 1999.
2. McQuillen-Martenson K. Radiographic image analysis. 3rd ed. St Louis: Saunders; 2010
3. Bontrager K, Lampignano JP. Textbook of radiographic positioning and related anatomy. 7th ed. St Louis: Mosby; 2010.
4. Greenspan A, Norman A. The radial head capitellum view; a useful technique in elbow trauma. American Journal of Radiology 1982;138:1186–8.
5. Tomás FJ, Proubasta IR. Modified radial head-capitellum projection in elbow trauma. British Journal of Radiology 1998;71:74–5.
6. Tomás FJ. Alternative radiographic projections of the ulnar coronoid process. British Journal of Radiology 2001;74:756–8.
7. Clark KC. Clark's positioning in radiography. London: Heinemann; 1939.

Chapter 7

The shoulder girdle

Linda Williams, Elizabeth Carver

The use of plain imaging is still an essential starting point when investigating shoulder trauma,[1] and basic diagnostic errors may occur if other imaging modalities are used alone, without the use of conventional plain radiography.[2] Guidelines still suggest that plain radiography is indicated for fractures, dislocations, shoulder instability and calcific tendonitis, with magnetic resonance imaging (MRI), ultrasound and computed tomography (CT) suggested for soft tissue injuries and 'more complex cases'. More specifically, ultrasound is recommended for rotator cuff injuries.[2]

Ultrasound can be used to assess disorders such as defects in the long head of the biceps tendon.[2] Subacromial and acromioclavicular joint impingement are dynamic processes and these can also be studied during ultrasound examination.

CT may be used in preoperative assessment of shoulder injuries, so that fractures are not underestimated (as can be the case in some instances with plain X-ray images) and 3D reconstruction is often used to fully demonstrate complex fractures and assist in surgical planning.[1]

MRI has become an increasingly important technique for evaluating rotator cuff disorders and joint instability,[1,2] its effectiveness being due to high contrast sensitivity and multiplanar imaging capabilities; therefore, diagnosis and appropriate management of the complex shoulder joint is established with greater confidence.

When imaging this region with plain radiography, radiation protection of the eyes and thyroid is an important consideration: the patient must always have their head turned away from the primary beam during exposure.

This area of high subject contrast has implications for overexposure of some structures involved in the joint. This is especially true of the acromioclavicular joint, which is often lacking in detail due to overexposure, whereas details of denser structures of the region (e.g. the humeral head or glenoid) are adequately demonstrated. Repeat examinations are often required as a result, and can be avoided in the first instance by using a wedge filter placed between the image receptor (IR) and the upper shoulder. The most effective type of filter for this is rubberised and boomerang shaped and can therefore sit comfortably and safely around and behind the upper shoulder. Use of a relatively high kVp and lower mAs can offer a solution in the absence of a filter, but the contrast of these images is somewhat reduced compared with those produced with a filter. Patients with very dense muscle (e.g. body builders and rugby players) will certainly need effective beam penetration.

INDICATIONS

Arthropathy

Erosions are a relatively late feature in patients with rheumatoid arthritis and the shoulder should only be examined by plain imaging if that joint is specifically affected. In patients with suspected osteoarthritis, X-ray is not indicated initially unless intervention is likely.

Fracture

This mostly affects the clavicle, humeral surgical neck, tuberosities of the humerus and scapula; fracture of the scapula is relatively uncommon, accounting for only 3–5% of shoulder injuries.

Fractures of the surgical neck of the humerus and the tuberosities have often been classified using Neer's method,[3] which considers the status and degree of displacement of the articular segment of the head of the humerus, the surgical neck of the humerus and the greater and lesser tuberosities. The reliability of such classification systems has been questioned and alternative classification methods suggested;[4] however, it must be mentioned that new methods, however reliable, need to be widely accepted so that they can be considered rigorous.

Dislocation

The shoulder joint is the most commonly dislocated joint in the human body,[5] with anterior dislocation most common; only up to 5% of dislocations occur posteriorly,[6] and an estimated 60–80% of these are missed on initial examination. As many as 50% of these uncommon dislocations can often be missed in A&E, highlighting the importance of an additional projection that can identify posterior dislocations.[7] Subluxation of the acromioclavicular joint can also occur.

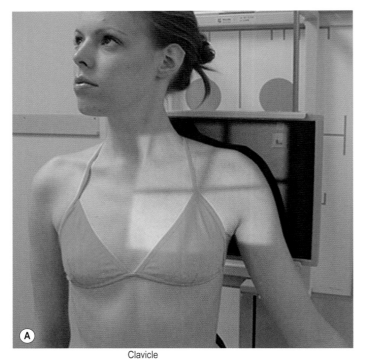

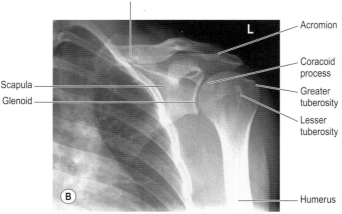

Figure 7.1 AP shoulder.

Anteroposterior (AP) shoulder (Fig. 7.1A,B)

This projection can be performed in the erect position, either standing or seated, depending on the patient's condition and ability. When examining a patient on a trolley, care should be taken to ensure either that the patient is in the fully erect position or the beam is accurately angled to compensate for any tilt on the trolley back rest; this will ensure that the central ray remains at 90° to the IR.

Positioning

- A lead rubber apron is applied to the patient's waist for radiation protection
- The patient sits or stands erect, with the posterior aspect of the shoulder under examination in contact with the vertical IR
- The arm is fully extended and slightly abducted with the palm of the hand facing forward to ensure the true anatomical position (with the greater tuberosity in profile on the lateral aspect of the humeral head)

- The patient's trunk is rotated approximately 20° towards the side under examination, to bring the scapula parallel to the IR
- The patient's head is turned away from the side under examination for radiation protection

Beam direction and focus receptor distance (FRD)

Horizontal at 90° to the IR
100 cm FRD

Centring point

To the coracoid process of the scapula, palpable anteriorly just below the lateral third of the clavicle and medial to the middle of the head of humerus

This centring point will bring the glenohumeral joint central to the IR but means that a large field of view is required to fulfil the image criteria for the area of interest. However, if the radiographic examination is for a general shoulder survey, the area of interest should be positioned to lie within the borders of the IR, with beam centring to the centre of the IR; this will ensure that the medial end of the clavicle, the whole of the scapula and the upper third of the humerus can be included in one image with the minimum field of radiation.

Collimation

The head and proximal third of humerus, scapula, clavicle, lateral soft tissues of proximal humerus

Criteria for assessing image quality

- Head and proximal third of humerus, clavicle, acromioclavicular joint and the inferior end of the scapula are demonstrated
- Greater tuberosity is seen in profile on the lateral aspect of the head of humerus
- Glenohumeral joint is obscured by head of humerus
- Acromion is demonstrated clear of the superior border of the humeral head
- Sharp image demonstrating the bony cortex and trabeculae of the head of the humerus in contrast with the shoulder joint and surrounding soft tissues; the acromioclavicular joint is seen clearly

The AP projection does not demonstrate the glenohumeral joint space clearly and orthopaedic departments may request either a 'True AP' or 'Grashey AP'[3] instead of, or to complement, the AP. This projection uses the same position and centring point as the AP described here but with an obliquity of the patient at 45° instead of 20°, to open the glenohumeral joint. The view shows the glenohumeral joint tangentially, but published work varies in assessment of its effectiveness in demonstration of direction of dislocation.[8–10]

Common errors	Possible reasons
Inferior end of the scapula not included on the image	The IR is often positioned in the 'landscape' position; putting it in the 'portrait' position will usually prevent this
Foreshortening of the clavicle	The patient is rotated too much towards the side under examination
The acromioclavicular joint is over-penetrated	This is due to the difference in subject contrast in this area; the use of a wedge filter will prevent this

AXILLARY/AXIAL PROJECTIONS OF THE SHOULDER

Evaluation of the shoulder joint, particularly for follow-up orthopaedic assessment, often requires an axillary projection to offer an image at 90° to the AP. Success of this projection will depend on the patient's condition and cooperation. Two methods are described here: method 1 is often difficult to implement or inappropriate, particularly in trauma, owing to the extent to which the arm must be abducted. Method 2 is the method of choice for a patient with restricted movement of the humerus as there is more scope for adaptation to suit the patient's condition. Method 2 is sometimes referred to as the Lawrence axillary.[11]

Method 1: superoinferior shoulder (Fig. 7.2A,B)

Positioning

- The IR is horizontal
- The patient sits with the side under examination next to and slightly away from the table
- For radiation protection purposes the legs are placed so they are not under the table and a lead rubber apron is worn around the waist
- The arm is abducted fully and the patient leans laterally over the IR; the hand is internally rotated and pronated. The axilla is positioned over the IR in a position that will ensure inclusion of the relevant anatomy, and with the axilla as close to it as possible
- The patient's head and neck are abducted away from the shoulder under examination as far as possible to clear them from the area of interest and reduce the radiation dose to these areas

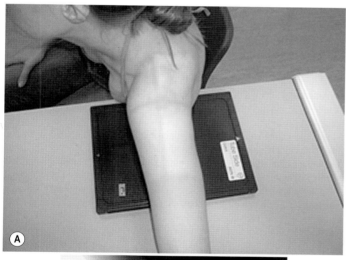

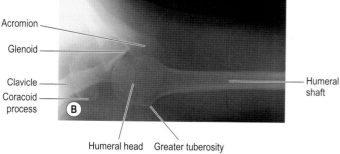

Acromion
Glenoid
Clavicle
Coracoid process
Humeral head   Greater tuberosity
Humeral shaft

Figure 7.2 Superoinferior shoulder.

Beam direction and FRD

Vertical at 90° to the IR
100 cm FRD

Centring point

To the superior aspect over the middle of the head of the humerus

Collimation

Head and proximal third of humerus, glenoid cavity, acromion, coracoid process, surrounding soft tissues

Criteria for assessing image quality

- Head and proximal end of humerus, glenoid fossa, lateral end of clavicle, acromion and coracoid process are demonstrated
- Head of humerus appears above the glenoid 'like a golf ball on a tee'[7]
- Greater tuberosity should be seen in profile anteriorly
- Acromion and lateral end of clavicle are superimposed on the superoposterior aspect of the head of humerus
- Coracoid process is demonstrated anterior to the head of humerus
- Sharp image demonstrating the soft tissue margins, bony cortex and trabeculae of the head of the humerus with adequate image density to demonstrate the bony detail of the humerus in contrast to the glenohumeral joint, acromion and clavicle

Common errors	Possible reasons
The glenohumeral joint is not demonstrated within the boundaries of the IR	The patient may not be stretching across the IR sufficiently. If the patient is capable of leaning further, try lowering the table-top to enable the patient to flex more at the waist
Magnification and unsharpness of the resulting image, probably accompanied by foreshortening of humeral head	The axilla is not in close enough contact with IR and the humerus may not be fully abducted, causing its shaft to lie at an angle with the IR. Try using a pad to raise the IR or consider increasing the FRD to compensate for the large ORD

Method 2: inferosuperior shoulder; 'Lawrence axillary projection' (Fig. 7.3)

Positioning

- The patient lies supine on the table
- A small radiolucent pad is placed beneath the shoulder to raise it slightly
- The head and neck are abducted as much as possible away from the side under examination to clear them from the area of interest and reduce radiation dose to these areas
- The IR is supported in the erect position, its tube side against the superior aspect of the head of the humerus and in contact with the neck
- The arm is abducted to 90° or as far as the patient's condition permits and the hand is supinated (although some internal rotation of the forearm is acceptable; supination acts mainly to help the patient maintain the correct relationship of the humerus to the IR)
- A lead rubber apron is placed over the patient's chest and abdomen for radiation protection

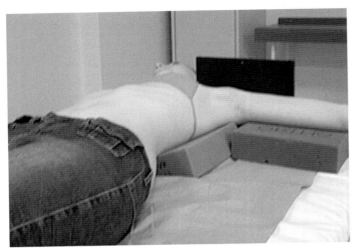

Figure 7.3 Inferosuperior shoulder.

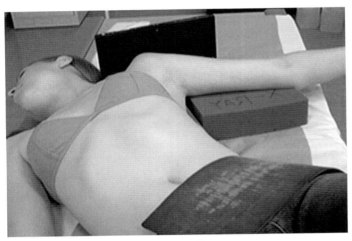

Figure 7.4 Modified inferosuperior shoulder.

Modern tube housings are usually too bulky to allow tube centring for this positioning. An alternative, *modified inferosuperior* is suggested, as follows:

This technique can be achieved with as little as 30° arm abduction,[3] but the tube needs to be brought in as close to the patient's body as possible. By lying the patient in a slightly diagonal position across the length of the table-top or trolley, access to the axilla is achievable (Fig. 7.4). Positioning the patient thus, diagonally across the table-top, requires consideration for the safety of the patient; this is directly related to table width and should only be considered in the relatively cooperative patient.

Beam direction and FRD (inferosuperior and modified inferosuperior projections)

Horizontal at 90° to the IR and coincident with the glenohumeral joint

100 cm FRD

The central ray must be at 90° to the IR and requires careful positioning to prevent a distorted image. To eliminate distortion, align the central ray with the patient first to ensure it is parallel to the glenohumeral joint, i.e. through the axilla, then position the IR until perpendicular to the central ray. This is suggested for both the inferosuperior and modified inferosuperior projections.

Centring point

Through the axilla

Collimation

Head and proximal third of humerus, glenoid cavity, acromion, coracoid process, surrounding soft tissues

Criteria for assessing image quality

- Head and proximal end of humerus, glenoid fossa, lateral end of clavicle, acromion and coracoid process should all be demonstrated
- Glenohumeral joint should be demonstrated
- Lesser tuberosity of humerus should be seen in profile
- Acromioclavicular joint will be superimposed on humerus
- Sharp image demonstrating the soft tissue margins, bony cortex and trabeculae of the head of humerus with adequate image density to demonstrate the bony detail of humerus in contrast to the glenohumeral joint

Common error	Possible reason
The glenohumeral joint is not demonstrated within the boundaries of the IR	The head and neck may not be sufficiently abducted away from the side under examination to enable the IR to be positioned correctly. Always ensure the IR is closely tucked into the neck

The inferosuperior projections can be adapted to demonstrate the classic Hill–Sachs compression fracture, seen in patients who have recurrent anterior dislocation of the shoulder.[1] This adaptation involves maximum external rotation of the arm, with the patient aiming to press the thumb down towards the table or trolley top. Unfortunately, this manoeuvre can be difficult for patients to achieve and the AP shoulder with maximum internal rotation can also demonstrate this lesion adequately.[2] In order to achieve the correct amount of rotation for this, the arm is medially rotated and flexed at the elbow; the dorsum of the hand is then rested on the waist. Yet another technique that can show Hill–Sachs lesions is the Stryker notch view, where the palm of the hand is placed on top of the head with the fingers toward the back of the head and the long axis of the humerus parallel to the median sagittal plane (MSP); a 10° cranial angle is centred over the coracoid process for this projection.[12]

Bankart lesions are also recognised as an effect of recurrent anterior dislocation[13] and are best seen on the true superoinferior view; clearly, superoinferior is recognised as difficult on the traumatised patient but feasible on patients with recovered range of shoulder movement following treatment.

30–45° modified superoinferior projection of the shoulder – 'apical oblique'[7] (Fig. 7.5A,B)

This projection has been described by Unett and Royle[11] and Raby et al.,[7] and a similar projection is described by Long and Rafert[3] but with more obliquity of the patient (i.e. the patient is rotated 45° onto the side under examination as opposed to bringing the scapula parallel to the IR; this is known as the 'Garth' apical oblique; see Fig. 25.16). Unett and Royle describe this as 'modified Wallace and Hellier', but the resulting image achieved with the 30–45° modified projection is much less magnified and distorted, which makes it easier to interpret. It is therefore probably a misnomer to use the term

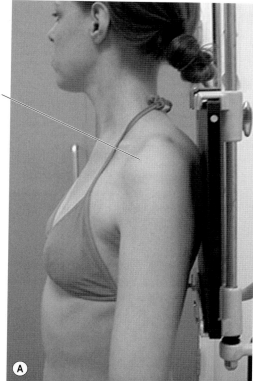

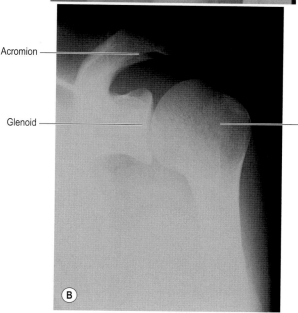

Acromion

Glenoid

Humeral
head

Figure 7.5 30–45° modified superoinferior shoulder.

the Velpau projection; this is similar to the Wallace and Hellier in that the IR is placed horizontally but the patient leans back 30° over it. A vertical central ray is used, which creates less distortion, but there is still a rather long object receptor distance (ORD); clearly the imaging implications for this projection are more favourable than for Wallace and Hellier, but it still has negative points in comparison to the 30–45° view.

It is easier to position the patient for the modified 30–45° view, as the patient position is identical to that for the AP shoulder, with the angle of central ray directed 30–45° caudally. The patient can satisfactorily be positioned supine or on a trolley or in a chair, and this is therefore a very useful technique for trauma patients. Raby et al. see the advantages of this method in terms of patient comfort and its ability to show small bony fragments easily; indeed, they state the only disadvantage as unfamiliarity due its infrequency of use. Despite the noticeable distortion caused by beam angulation, the humerus does still lie parallel to the IR, whereas in the Wallace and Hellier method the humerus lies at 90° to the IR and at 30° in Velpeau. In addition, Wallace and Hellier requires 45° caudal tube angulation; these combined factors cause more distortion than with the 30–45° AP shoulder.

The 30–45° projection demonstrates the glenohumeral joint in coronal profile, and therefore an assessment of dislocation or intra-articular fractures can be made. The radiographer only needs to understand the basic radiographic principles involving effects of angulation on the image in order to assess direction of dislocation. Basically, the structure lying closest to the IR will be less obviously displaced than structures further from it; therefore, a posterior dislocation will show the humeral head superimposed over the acromion, and anterior dislocation will show the humeral head well below the acromion and low compared to the glenoid position. The Wallace and Hellier method does not appear to provide more useful information than the 30–45° modified projection and therefore its use should be questioned, considering that it appears to have more disadvantages than any other projection of its type.

Positioning (as for AP shoulder)

- The IR is vertical or under/behind the patient's shoulder if supine or sitting on a trolley
- A lead rubber apron is applied to the patient's waist for radiation protection
- The patient can remain standing or be seated, with the posterior aspect of the shoulder in contact with the IR
- The arm is fully extended and slightly abducted with the palm of the hand facing forward to ensure the true anatomical position
- The patient is rotated approximately 20° onto the side under examination to bring the scapula parallel to the IR
- The patient's head is turned away from the side under examination for radiation protection

Beam direction and FRD

Erect: Initially horizontal, directed caudally at 30–45° to the IR
Supine: Initially vertical, directed 30–45° caudally
If the patient is semirecumbent: The beam is initially positioned perpendicular to the IR and then directed a further 30–45° caudally from this angle
100 cm FRD

Centring point

Above the coracoid process and slightly superior to the head of the humerus

'modified Wallace and Hellier' for this projection, as the similarity is only the use of a caudal angle. The Wallace and Hellier projection (often called the 'Wallace' view) cannot be undertaken on the supine or semi-recumbent patient, as it requires the patient to sit with their back against the table, but uses a horizontal IR; the affected limb is 90° to the IR. The air gap between shoulder and IR will require some increase in exposure, thereby increasing radiation dose in the Wallace and Hellier projection. Another well-known alternative projection is

Collimation

Head and proximal third of humerus, glenoid cavity, acromion process, surrounding soft tissues

Criteria for assessing image quality

- Head and proximal shaft of humerus, glenoid fossa, lateral end of clavicle and acromion process should all be demonstrated
- Greater tuberosity is demonstrated on the lateral aspect of humerus
- Elongation of the head of humerus, the position of which will vary if the humeral head is dislocated
- The glenoid fossa and head of humerus are projected clear of the lateral margin of the rib cage
- Sharp image demonstrating the head of humerus in contrast to the shoulder joint and surrounding soft tissues

'Y' view/true lateral (Fig. 7.6A,B)

This projection may be used in cases of suspected glenohumeral dislocation or fractures of the proximal humerus. It is similar to the basic lateral scapula projection but the humerus is not abducted in the same manner, to prevent it overlying the body of the scapula; in this case the humerus is adducted alongside the patient's trunk. It is relatively simple to position and requires little cooperation from the patient. The resulting image allows an assessment of fractures or glenohumeral dislocation, as the shoulder girdle is demonstrated in the true lateral position. Indeed, it has been claimed by some that the projection is superior to the axillary view for the demonstration of dislocation.[14] If the patient is presented on a trolley the technique can be performed in the AP position with the patient rotating approximately 25° towards the uninjured side.

This technique is considered to be superior to the modified supero-inferior or apical oblique (30–45° AP) described previously, as the modified axial can only help assess dislocations. This may then necessitate further radiographic examination. The 'Y' view is relatively simple to perform[15] and can be achieved satisfactorily even if the patient presents supine on a trolley or in a chair, and it is therefore recommended for trauma patients.[16–18] It is believed that it will show fractures of the humeral head, scapula and coracoid process, plus dislocation of the humeral head and the direction of this,[10] but can fail to demonstrate some intra-articular fractures well.[19]

In the normal shoulder the humeral head will be demonstrated superimposed on the glenoid process, as opposed to in the dislocated shoulder, where it will appear under the coracoid process in anterior dislocation and under the acromion in posterior dislocation.

Positioning

- A lead rubber apron is placed around the patient for radiation protection of the lower abdomen
- The patient stands or sits erect, facing the IR with their back to the X-ray tube
- From an initial posteroanterior (PA) position, rotate the patient approximately 25° to bring the side under examination closer to, and bring the body of the scapula 90° to, the IR
- The arm on the side under examination is adducted from the trunk, with the elbow flexed and hand resting on the side of the waist. Alternatively, the elbow may be flexed with the forearm resting across the chest and the hand resting on the shoulder of the opposite side (this may be more comfortable for the injured patient)
- The scapula is palpated to check the lateral and medial borders are superimposed
- The patient's head is turned as far as possible towards the unaffected side

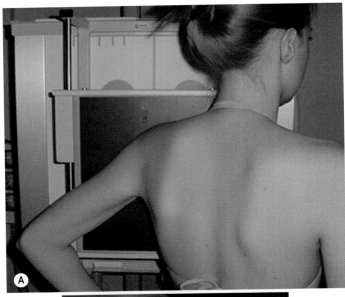

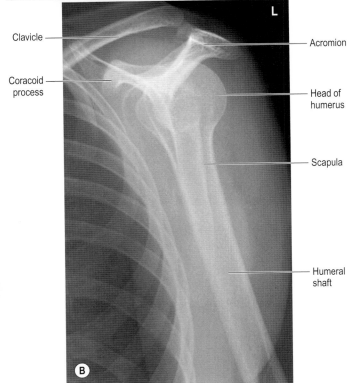

Figure 7.6 'Y' view. Note that the arm position in (A) may not be achievable in injury and the arm may be adductd across the trunk as an alternative.

If the patient is *supine*, this projection can be achieved by rotating their trunk 25° away from the side under examination, placing radiolucent pads under the trunk for support. The scapula should still lie at 90° to the IR. Although this will cause some magnification and have implications for scattered radiation exposure to the thyroid, eye lenses and female breasts, it is an acceptable alternative when a PA position is unsafe owing to the patient's condition.

Beam direction and FRD

Horizontal at 90° to the IR
100 cm FRD

Centring point

To the upper end of the palpable medial border of the scapula to pass through the glenohumeral joint

Collimation

Scapula, the head and proximal third of the humerus, surrounding soft tissues

Criteria for assessing image quality

- Scapula and the head and proximal third of humerus are demonstrated
- Superimposition of the medial and lateral borders of the scapula
- Body of scapula is projected clear of the thorax
- Glenoid process is seen en face with the humeral head superimposed over it (in the normal shoulder)
- Sharp image demonstrating the bony cortex and trabeculae of the scapula and upper shaft of humerus in contrast with the surrounding soft tissue

The above technique can also be used with a *caudal angle of 10–15°* from the horizontal in cases of *suspected impingement syndrome*. The acromiohumeral space will appear more open than the true lateral scapula to show abnormalities of this area. The projection is sometimes referred to as the 'shoulder outlet'.[3]

Common error	Possible reason
Scapula not cleared from the ribs and thorax; not seen in profile	Inaccurate obliquity of position; there is often a temptation to turn the patient more than is required, as the correct trunk position does appear to be close to a PA projection

CLAVICLE

PA clavicle (Fig. 7.7A,B)

This projection is the method of choice, as opposed to an AP projection, because the object is in closer contact with the IR, thereby reducing magnification and distortion of the clavicle. However, if the patient is injured or in a sling then positioning for the AP clavicle may be more readily achievable and more comfortable.

Positioning

- The IR is vertical
- A lead rubber apron is applied to the patient's waist for radiation protection, ensuring the posterior aspect is protected
- The patient sits or stands erect with the anterior aspect of the shoulder under examination in contact with the IR
- The arm is made comfortable and may remain in a sling if presented this way
- The patient is rotated approximately 15° away from the side under examination to bring the plane of the clavicle closer and parallel to the IR
- The patient's head is turned away from the side under examination for radiation protection

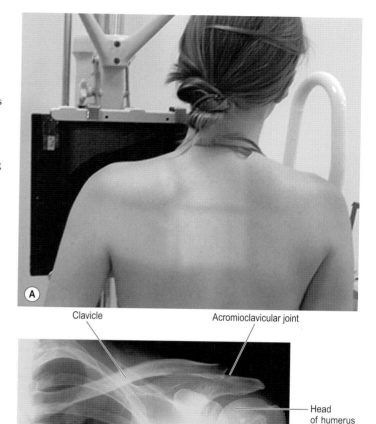

Clavicle   Acromioclavicular joint

Head of humerus

Figure 7.7 PA clavicle.

Beam direction and FRD

Horizontal at 90° to the IR
100 cm FRD

Centring point

To the centre of the IR so that the central ray exits the mid shaft of the clavicle

Collimation

Clavicle, acromioclavicular joint, sternoclavicular joint

AP clavicle (Fig. 7.8)

The clavicle is demonstrated in the true AP position when both the shoulders are equidistant from the table or vertical IR holder. Bontrager[20] and Ballinger and Frank[21] describe this positioning for the AP clavicle, but Swallow et al.[22] suggest a slight rotation towards the side under examination to ensure that the medial end of the clavicle is not superimposed onto the vertebral column (although this will place the clavicle into a more oblique position than the other methods).

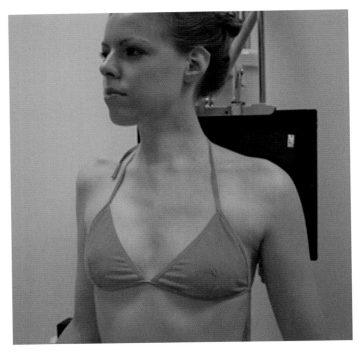

Figure 7.8 AP clavicle.

Common error	Possible reason
High contrast on image which demonstrates the clavicle but the acromioclavicular joint appears blackened	kVp insufficient to reduce the subject contrast

Inferosuperior clavicle

There are two methods described here to provide an inferosuperior projection of the clavicle. Method 1 is the easiest to achieve and is normally used to assess fracture union; method 2 can be used on the supine patient, e.g. when presented on a trolley, but only if a cassette type IR is available. The AP projection is most frequently used alone, as fractures are rarely severely displaced; immobilisation with a sling is usually quite effective as treatment. Occasionally the clavicular fracture may be so displaced that the fragments do not unify, and these cases will almost certainly require an additional inferosuperior projection prior to a decision being made about surgical intervention to pin the bone.

Method 1 (Fig. 7.9A,B)

Positioning

- The patient is seated and then positioned as for the AP clavicle projection
- The patient leans back by around 30°

Beam direction and FRD

Initially horizontal, angled cranially 30–45°; the maximum angle achievable will be governed by equipment variables
100 cm FRD

Centring point

Over the mid point of the clavicle

  The image of the clavicle will be projected superiorly to the ribs and lung apices compared to the AP or PA clavicle (Fig. 7.9B), because of the cranial angle used. Therefore, the IR should be displaced cranially to compensate for this.

Collimation

Clavicle, acromioclavicular joint, sternoclavicular joint

Criteria for assessing image quality

- The full length of the clavicle, including the acromioclavicular joint and the sternoclavicular joint, is demonstrated
- Clavicle is projected above the apex of the lung
- Acromioclavicular joint should be demonstrated
- Sharp image demonstrating the soft tissue, bony cortex and trabeculae of the clavicle. The clavicle should be demonstrated with even contrast along the length and without overexposing the medial and lateral ends

Method 2 (Fig. 7.10A)

Positioning

- The patient lies supine with their arms resting at their side
- The IR is placed vertically and in contact with the superior aspect of the shoulder
- The head and neck are abducted for radiation protection of the eyes and thyroid
- A lead rubber apron is applied to the patient's waist for radiation protection

Positioning

- The IR is placed in the vertical position
- A lead rubber apron is applied to the patient's waist for radiation protection
- The patient sits or stands erect with the posterior aspect of the shoulder under examination in contact with the IR
- The arm is made comfortable and may remain in a sling if presented this way
- The patient stands with their MSP perpendicular to the IR or is rotated slightly towards the side under examination to bring the medial end of the clavicle away from the vertebral column
- The patient's head is turned away from the side under examination for radiation protection

Beam direction and FRD

Horizontal at 90° to the IR
100 cm FRD

Centring point

Over the mid point of the clavicle

Collimation

Clavicle, acromioclavicular joint, sternoclavicular joint

Criteria for assessing image quality:
AP and PA projections

- Full length of the clavicle, including the acromioclavicular joint and the sternoclavicular joint, is demonstrated
- No or minimal distortion along the length of the clavicle
- Acromioclavicular joint should be demonstrated
- Sharp image demonstrating the soft tissue margins, bony cortex and trabeculae of the clavicle. The clavicle should be demonstrated with even contrast along the length and without overexposing the medial and lateral ends

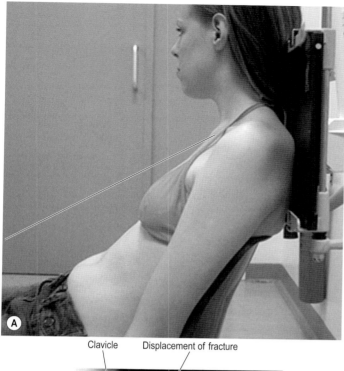

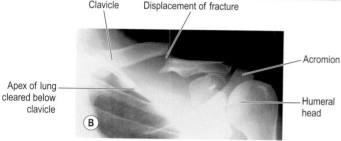

Clavicle   Displacement of fracture

Acromion

Apex of lung
cleared below
clavicle

Humeral
head

Figure 7.9 (A) Inferosuperior clavicle – method 1; (B) inferosuperior
clavicle.

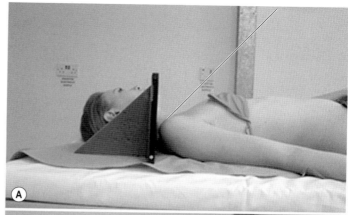

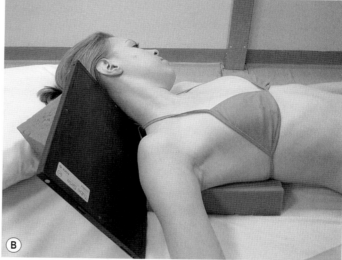

Figure 7.10 (A) Inferosuperior clavicle – method 2; (B) alternative
method for supine inferosuperior clavicle.

Criteria for assessing image quality

- Full length of the clavicle, including the acromioclavicular joint
  and the sternoclavicular joint, is demonstrated
- Clavicle is projected above the apex of the lung
- Acromioclavicular joint should be demonstrated
- Tubercle of the clavicle is visible on its under-surface at the
  junction of the middle and lateral portions
- Medial end of the clavicle is slightly superior to the lateral end
- Sharp image demonstrating the soft tissue, bony cortex and
  trabeculae of the clavicle. The clavicle should be demonstrated
  with even contrast along the length and without overexposing the
  medial and lateral ends

Beam direction and FRD

Initially vertical, angled at 45–60° towards the head, and 10–15°
mediolaterally. *Again, the angle achieved will depend on equipment
variables*
100 cm FRD

Centring point

Over the mid point of the clavicle

For the supine inferosuperior projection, it is often not possible to
position the X-ray tube low enough to achieve the required angulation
(as is often the case with units which have large tube and light beam
housing) and further modification may be necessary. The IR is placed
in contact with the posterosuperior aspect of the shoulder and tilted
backwards around 20° from vertical. The vertical central ray is then
angled cranially until it is perpendicular to the IR, and an angle of
approximately 10–15° mediolaterally away from the midline will
clear the clavicle towards the centre of the IR. Centre over the middle
of the clavicle (Fig. 7.10B).

Collimation

Clavicle, acromioclavicular joint, sternoclavicular joint

Common errors	Possible reasons
Clavicle not cleared from lung apices	Inadequate cranial angle used (both methods) *or*
	Patient not leaning back enough (method 1)
Pale, soft tissue shadow overlying some or all the area of interest	Thorax or abdomen lying in the path of the primary beam; this may be due to a large abdomen, large female breasts or too much angulation (method 1)

SCAPULA

AP scapula (Fig. 7.11A,B)

Positioning

- The IR is placed vertical
- A lead rubber apron is applied to the patient's waist for radiation protection
- The patient sits or stands erect with the posterior aspect of the shoulder under examination in contact with the IR
- The arm is fully extended and slightly abducted with the palm of the hand facing forward to lie in the true anatomical position
- The patient is rotated approximately 20° towards the side under examination, to bring the scapula parallel to the IR

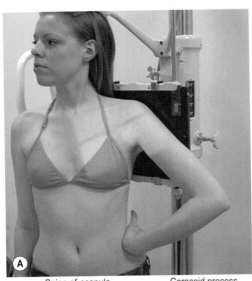

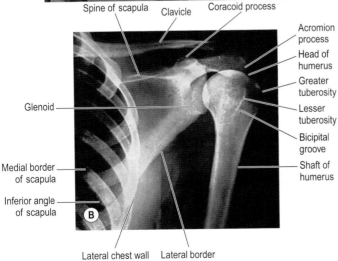

Spine of scapula · Clavicle · Coracoid process

Acromion process
Head of humerus
Greater tuberosity
Lesser tuberosity
Bicipital groove
Shaft of humerus

Glenoid

Medial border of scapula

Inferior angle of scapula

Lateral chest wall · Lateral border of scapula

Figure 7.11 AP scapula.
(B) Reproduced with permission from Ballinger PW, Frank ED. Merrill's atlas of radiographic positioning and radiologic procedures. 10th ed. St Louis: Mosby; 2003.

- The arm is flexed at the elbow and internally rotated, resting the dorsum of the hand on the patient's hip; this will move the scapula laterally away from the rib cage
- The patient's head is turned away from the side under examination for radiation protection

Beam direction and FRD

Horizontal at 90° to the IR
100 cm FRD

Centring point

To a point over the anterior chest (approximately 5 cm below the palpable coracoid process), to emerge over the mid-scapular area

Collimation

Scapula, the head and proximal third of humerus, the surrounding soft tissues

Criteria for assessing image quality

- Head of humerus, the acromioclavicular joint and the superior and inferior angles of scapula are demonstrated
- Glenohumeral joint is obscured by the head of humerus
- Scapula projected laterally, clearing as much of the rib cage from the medial border of the body as possible
- Acromion is demonstrated clear of the superior border of the humeral head
- Sharp image demonstrating the bony cortex and trabeculae of the scapula through the air filled thorax. The bony detail of the scapula should be seen in contrast to the lungs, axilla and other soft tissue structures

Lateral scapula (Fig. 7.12A,B)

Positioning

- The IR is vertical
- A lead rubber apron is placed around the patient for radiation protection of the lower abdomen
- The patient stands or sits erect, facing the IR with their back to the X-ray tube.
- From an initial PA position, rotate the patient approximately 25° to bring the side under examination closer to, and bring the body of the scapula 90° to, the IR
- The arm on the side under examination is flexed at the elbow, slightly abducted and the dorsum of the hand is placed on the hip; alternatively, the arm may rest across the chest with the hand resting on the shoulder of the opposite side (this may be more comfortable for the injured patient)
- The scapula is palpated to check the lateral and medial borders are superimposed

Beam direction and FRD

Horizontal at 90° to the IR
100 cm FRD

Centring point

To the middle of the palpable medial border of the scapula

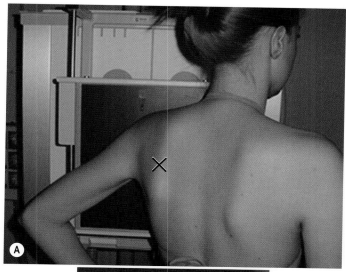

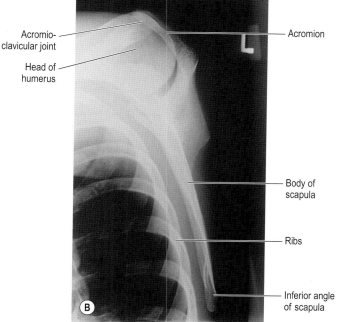

Figure 7.12 Lateral scapula.

Common errors	Possible reasons
Scapula not cleared from ribs and thorax; not seen in profile	Inaccurate obliquity of position; there is often a temptation to turn the patient more than is required, since the correct trunk position does appear to be close to a PA projection. Do not forget that the scapula will be moved into a position towards the lateral aspect of the thorax when the arm is placed in one of the required positions
Upper shaft of the humerus superimposed over the scapula	Arm not abducted or adducted sufficiently to clear the humerus from the body of scapula

ACROMIOCLAVICULAR JOINTS

These joints are normally examined to investigate subluxation of the joint following trauma. The radiographic examination should be requested following an orthopaedic assessment and not done routinely from A&E referrals, as clinical examination of the joint by an experienced orthopaedic surgeon often proves to be diagnostically accurate, as severe disruption of the joint is palpable,[23] thereby rendering radiographic examination unnecessary. Weightbearing projections may be performed to assess the degree of subluxation, although initial shoulder radiographs should be examined first to exclude fracture and because subluxation may be apparent without weights being given. However, research indicates that the weightbearing examination offers little in the diagnosis of subluxation[24-26] and therefore the technique is not described in this book. A fourth article[27] supports this research but does suggest a rather extensive series of radiographs for acromioclavicular joints, including:

- AP projection with arm in internal rotation
- AP with 10–15° cranial central ray (Zanca projection)[28]
- Axillary lateral (or lateral scapula or Wallace and Hellier projection if the axillary is unobtainable)

The full list of projections suggested by this article should not be routinely performed, particularly, as stated previously, clinical examination frequently offers sufficient diagnostic information and the axillary lateral shoulder is only helpful when assessing a possible posterior dislocation.[2] Comparative projections of both acromioclavicular joints should not be undertaken lightly, particularly in light of the requirements of IR(ME)R 2006,[29] and this practice should be discouraged.

AP acromioclavicular joint (Fig. 7.13A,B)

Positioning

- The IR is vertical
- A lead rubber apron is applied to the patient's waist for radiation protection
- The patient sits or stands erect with the posterior aspect of the shoulder under examination in contact with the IR
- The arm is made comfortable and may remain in a sling if presented this way
- The patient is rotated approximately 10° towards the side under examination to bring the plane of the acromioclavicular joint perpendicular to the IR
- The patient's head is turned away from the side under examination for radiation protection

Collimation

Scapula, the head and proximal third of humerus, the surrounding soft tissues

Criteria for assessing image quality

- Scapula, the head and proximal third of humerus are demonstrated
- Superimposition of the medial and lateral borders of the scapula
- Shaft of humerus should not overlie the body of the scapula
- The body of the scapula is projected clear of the thorax
- Sharp image demonstrating the bony cortex and trabeculae of the scapula in contrast with the surrounding soft tissue

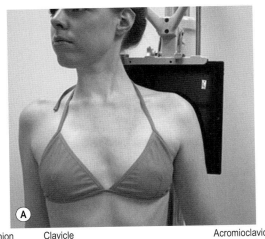

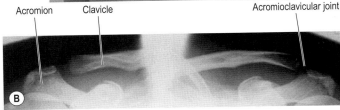

Acromion Clavicle Acromioclavicular joint

Figure 7.13 AP acromioclavicular joint.

Beam direction and FRD

Horizontal at 90° to the IR
100 cm FRD

Centring point

Over the acromioclavicular joint

Collimation

Acromioclavicular joint, acromion process, surrounding soft tissues

Criteria for assessing image quality

- Acromioclavicular joint, lateral end of the clavicle and soft tissue outlines are demonstrated
- If both joints are examined the images should be comparable in appearance
- Sharp image to demonstrate the bony trabeculae within the acromion and in contrast with the acromioclavicular joint and surrounding soft tissues

Common error	Possible reason
Dark image of joint with poor contrast between the joint and bones of the acromion and clavicle	Most obviously, exposure factors sets too high but poor collimation will allow scatter to overblacken the image or reduce contrast

REFERENCES

1. Royal College of Radiologists Working Party. Making the best use of a department of clinical radiology: guidelines for doctors. 6th ed. London: Royal College Of Radiologists; 2007.

2. Anderson JF, et al. Atlas of imaging in sports medicine. Sydney: The McGraw-Hill Companies; 1998.

3. Long BW, Rafert JA. Orthopaedic radiography. Philadelphia: WB Saunders; 1995.

4. Mora Guix JM, et al. Updated classification system for proximal humeral fractures. Clinical Medicine & Research 2009;7:1–2; 32–44.

5. Sanders T, Jersey S. Conventional radiography of the shoulder. Seminars in Roentgenology 2005;40(3):207–22.

6. Wilkinson K. Alternate trauma shoulder projection. Radiologic Technology Journal 2006;78:11–2

7. Raby N, Berman L, Lacey G. Accident & emergency radiology: A survival guide. 2nd ed. Philadelphia: Elsevier; 2005.

8. Schwartz D, Reisdorff E. Emergency radiology. New York: McGraw-Hill; 2000.

9. Vear V. Routine projections for the trauma shoulder. Radiographer Journal 1999;46: 36–40

10. Sanders T, Jersey S. Conventional radiography of the shoulder. Seminars in Roentgenology 2005;40(3):207–22.

11. Unett EM, Royle AJ. Radiographic techniques and image evaluation. London: Nelson Thornes; 1997

12. Ip D. Orthopedic traumatology: A resident's guide. 2nd ed. Berlin: Springer; 2008.

13. Magee D. Orthopedic physical assessment. 5th ed. St Louis: Saunders Elsevier; 2007.

14. Ianotti JP, Williams GR Jr. Shoulder diagnosis and management. 2nd ed. Philadelphia: Lippincott Williams and Wilkins; 2006.

15. Wilkie W. Back to basics: Trauma shoulder. Synergy Journal 2001;4:4–8.

16. Silverskoid JP, et al. Roentgenograph evaluation of suspected shoulder dislocation, a prospective study comparing the axillary and scapular Y view. Orthopaedics 1990;13(1):63–9.

17. Wilson FC, Lin PP. General orthopaedics. New York: The McGraw-Hill Companies; 1997.

18. Grainger RG, Allison D. Diagnostic radiology. 3rd ed. Edinburgh: Churchill Livingstone; 1997.

19. Edwards R, Jones H. Reporting on. shoulder trauma. Synergy Journal 2007;8:14–20.

20. Bontrager KL, Lampignano JP. Text book of radiographic positioning and related anatomy. 6th ed. St Louis: Mosby; 2005.

21. Ballinger PW, Frank ED. Merrill's atlas of radiographic positioning and radiologic procedures. 10th ed. St Louis: Mosby; 2003.

22. Swallow RA, et al. Clark's positioning in radiography. 11th ed. Oxford: Heinemann Medical Books; 1986.

23. Beim GM, Warner JJP. Clinical and radiographic evaluation of the acromioclavicular joint. Operative Techniques in Sports Medicine 1997;5(2):65–71.

24. Varnarthos WJ, et al. Radiographic diagnosis of acromioclavicular joint separation without weight bearing, importance of internal rotation of the arm. American Journal of Roentgenology 1994;162:120–2.

25. Bossart PJ, et al. Lack of efficacy of weighted radiographs in diagnosing acute acromioclavicular separation. Annals of Emergency Medicine 1998;17(1):20–4.

26. Yap JJL, et al. The value of weighted views of the acromion clavicular joint. American Journal of Sports Medicine 1999;27(6): 806–9.

27. Reeves PJ. Radiography of the acromioclavicular joint: a review. Radiography 2003;9:1–4.

28. Zanca P. Shoulder pain: involvement of the acromioclavicular joint (analysis of 1000 cases). American Journal of Roentgenology 1971;112(3):493–506.

29. The Ionising Radiation (Medical Exposure) Regulations. London: HMSO; 2006.

Chapter 8

Foot, toes, ankle, tibia and fibula

Linda Williams

When imaging the foot and ankle all artefacts should be removed, including socks, stockings and bandages. Extra care must be taken in cases of trauma.

Gonad protection should always be used and particular care should be taken with the direction of the central beam, as the gonads can easily be irradiated with the primary beam when examining the foot and ankle, particularly if a cranial angle is used. A lead rubber apron should always be applied when examining the lower limb extremities.

FOOT AND TOES

Indications

Examination of the foot for trauma should only be performed if there is true bony tenderness; the demonstration of a fracture rarely influences management.[1] Examination of the foot for hallux valgus is not indicated unless it is for preoperative assessment.

March fracture

March fractures are also known as fatigue or stress fracture of the metatarsals due to repetitive impact to this region; it is common for some new periosteal bone formation to be demonstrated on the images.

Lisfranc injuries

These are traumatic subluxations or dislocations at the base of the metatarsals at the tarsometatarsal joints, with or without fracture. This injury may involve some or all of the joints. The mechanism of injury can be from several incidents, such as the foot hitting the floor of a car in a road traffic accident, or missing a step or a kerb.[2]

Jones' fracture

This is a transverse fracture of the proximal fifth metatarsal, usually as a result of an inversion injury to the foot, the same mechanism that causes an ankle sprain.[2]

For all projections of the foot and toes the IR is horizontal (table-top) unless otherwise specified.

Dorsiplantar (DP) foot (Fig. 8.1A,B)

In both the DP and DP oblique positions, in order to enable the joint spaces between the tarsal bones to be demonstrated more clearly, a 15° cranial angle may be used.[3] When using this projection the tarsometatarsal articulations are demonstrated without as much bony overlap as when a perpendicular central ray is used. However, careful consideration must be given when directing the tube towards the gonads, and adequate radiation protection must be used. The same image can be produced by using a 15° foam wedge directly under the foot, the thickest end being placed at the toe end; this removes the necessity for angulation of the central ray directly towards the gonads, but the image of the metatarsals and phalanges will be magnified if used in this way, as the object to receptor distance will vary along the length of the foot. An alternative is to position the pad under the image receptor (IR), which does remove the problem of magnification.

Exposure for a foot requires the toes and the tarsal bones to be demonstrated on the one image and a suitable kVp should be selected, high enough to reduce subject contrast without over-penetrating the thinner end of the area. The use of a slim wedge filter, the thickest part of the filter being placed at the toes, will have the effect of reducing subject contrast. The wedge can be used under the foot, but some magnification of the metatarsals and phalanges will occur in a similar way to that mentioned above.

Positioning

- The patient is seated on the table with their legs extended and their hands are used to support themselves
- The patient's knee on the side under examination is flexed and the plantar aspect of the foot is placed in contact with the IR
- The opposite leg is abducted and a lead rubber sheet is placed over the abdomen and pelvis for radiation protection

Beam direction and focus receptor distance (FRD)

Vertical central ray, at 90° to the IR
100 cm FRD

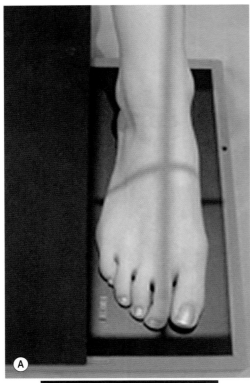

Centring point

Over the base of second metatarsal

Collimation

All phalanges, metatarsals, tarsals, soft tissues

Criteria for assessing image quality

- Demonstration of the phalanges, metatarsals, navicular, cuboid and cuneiform bones and soft tissue shadowing of the outline of the foot
- Adjacent phalanges should be demonstrated separately with exception of the bases of metatarsals 2–5, which will be slightly overlapped. Toes of patients with toe deformities are unlikely to all be separated
- Shafts of the metatarsals separated
- Tarsal bones should appear overlapped
- Talus and calcaneum should be superimposed over the tibia and fibula
- Sharp image demonstrating the soft tissue margins, bony cortex and trabeculae of the phalanges, metatarsals and tarsus. The proximal calcaneum and talus will not be penetrated sufficiently to be demonstrated

Common error	Possible reason
Superimposition of the lower leg over the tarsal bones	Knee may be too flexed, encouraging too much ankle flexion

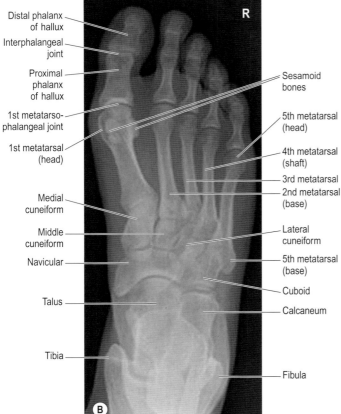

Figure 8.1 DP foot.

Dorsiplantar oblique (DPO) foot (Fig. 8.2A,B)

Positioning

- The plantar aspect of the foot is placed in contact with the IR
- From the DP position the patient's foot is internally rotated to bring the plane of the dorsum of the foot parallel to the IR
- A radiolucent pad is placed under the lateral plantar aspect of the foot for immobilisation
- The opposite leg is abducted and a lead rubber sheet is placed over the abdomen and pelvis for radiation protection

Beam direction and FRD

Vertical central ray, at 90° to the IR
100 cm FRD

Centring point

Over the base of third metatarsal

Collimation

All phalanges, metatarsals and tarsal bones, surrounding soft tissues

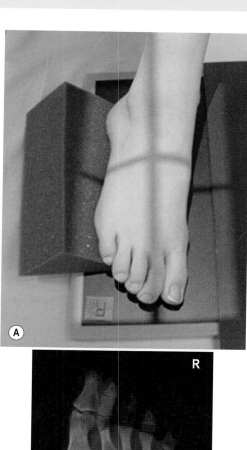

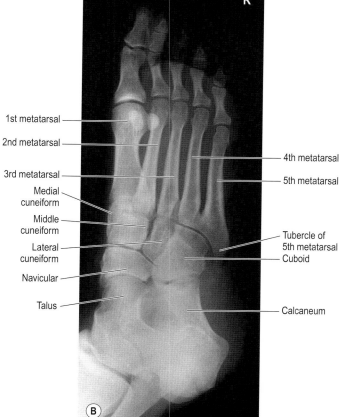

1st metatarsal

2nd metatarsal

3rd metatarsal

Medial cuneiform

Middle cuneiform

Lateral cuneiform

Navicular

Talus

4th metatarsal

5th metatarsal

Tubercle of 5th metatarsal

Cuboid

Calcaneum

R

Figure 8.2 DPO foot.

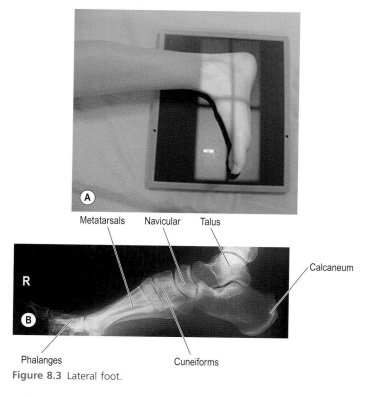

Metatarsals Navicular Talus

Calcaneum

R

Phalanges Cuneiforms

Figure 8.3 Lateral foot.

Criteria for assessing image quality

- Demonstration of the phalanges, metatarsals, navicular, cuboid and cuneiform bones and soft tissue shadowing of the outline of the foot
- Adjacent phalanges are not likely to all be separated, due to obliquity, especially in the case of patients with toe deformities (i.e. 'hammer toe')
- Shafts of metatarsals 2–4 separated
- Overlap of the bases of the first and second metatarsals
- Separation of the tarsal bones, although the medial and middle cuneiforms will appear superimposed, with some overlap of middle and lateral cuneiforms
- Talus and calcaneum are clear of the tibia and fibula
- Sharp image demonstrating the soft tissue margins of the foot, bony cortex and trabeculae of the phalanges, metatarsals and tarsus

Common errors	Possible reasons
Superimposition of the lower leg over the tarsal bones	Knee may be too flexed, or the foot may be under-rotated
Overlapping of metatarsals	Over-rotation of foot

Lateral foot (Fig. 8.3A,B)

Positioning

- With the leg extended, it is externally rotated until the lateral aspect of the foot is in contact with the IR. This may be more comfortable if the knee is slightly relaxed and not fully extended. The plantar aspect of the foot is 90° to the IR
- Radiolucent foam pads may be placed under the lower leg and foot for support in this position
- A lead rubber apron is placed over the abdomen for radiation protection

Beam direction and FRD

Vertical central ray at 90° to the IR
100 cm FRD

Centring point

Over the navicular cuneiform region

Collimation

All phalanges, metatarsals, tarsals, soft tissues

Criteria for assessing image quality

- Demonstration of the phalanges, metatarsals, navicular, cuboid and cuneiform bones and soft tissue shadowing of the outline of the foot
- Phalanges should be superimposed; the distal phalanges of the longest toe (hallux or second toe) will lie clear
- Metatarsals should be overlapped, with the first metatarsal lying most superiorly and the fifth inferiorly
- Sharp image demonstrating the superimposition of the phalanges and metatarsals and the bony trabeculae of the tarsal bones, navicular, talus and calcaneum

Weightbearing lateral foot (Fig. 8.4A,B)

This projection is usually performed as part of an orthopaedic assessment. It is important to include the whole length of foot on the image as the relationship between the joints of the tarsal bones and the metatarsals is an important indication of the degree of surgical intervention required following trauma. This is particularly important in Lisfranc injuries, where fracture dislocations are involved and a complete radiographic evaluation of the foot is required.[2]

A suitably designed platform is required for good radiography of this area. The platform should be made of radiolucent material, with a groove in the centre for positioning the IR vertically and to allow the IR to be placed at a level below the soft tissues of the plantar aspect of the foot to enable the soft tissues to be included on the image. The platform should be of a dimension to allow both feet to be placed comfortably on either side of the groove (Fig. 8.5). Most frequently these platforms are made as a bespoke design in hospital workshops, rather than obtained from commercial sources.

The IR is placed vertically in the groove of the support; this technique is only suitable when using a cassette type IR.

Positioning

- Stand the patient on the specially designed platform
- Ensure the patient is stable and suitable support is provided to allow even distribution of the weight of both feet
- Support the IR in the erect, transverse position in the groove of the platform on the medial aspect of the foot
- Use a sheet of lead or lead rubber between the back of the IR and the foot that is not under examination, for radiation protection
- The long axis of the foot should be parallel to the long axis of the IR
- A lead rubber apron is placed over the abdomen for radiation protection

Beam direction and FRD

Horizontal central ray, at 90° to the IR
100 cm FRD

Centring point

Over the tubercle of the fifth metatarsal

Collimation

The phalanges, metatarsals, tarsal bones, surrounding soft tissues

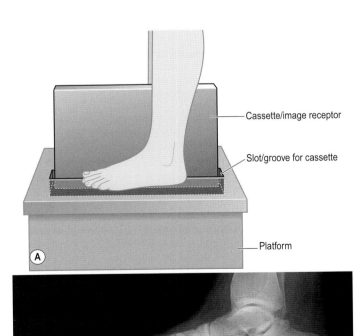

Figure 8.4 Weightbearing lateral foot.

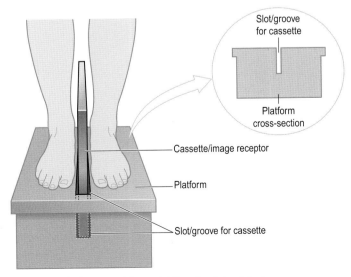

Figure 8.5 Platform used for weightbearing lateral foot.

Criteria for assessing image quality

- Distal phalanges, calcaneum, ankle joint and soft tissue outlines of the foot should all be demonstrated
- Phalanges should be superimposed, with the longest toe cleared as for non-weightbearing lateral
- Metatarsals should be overlapped as for the lateral foot
- Medial and lateral articular surfaces of the talus should be superimposed
- Sharp image demonstrating superimposition of the phalanges and metatarsals, bony trabeculae of the tarsal bones, navicular, talus and calcaneum. The soft tissue of the heel pad should not be over-blackened. kVp should be sufficient to reduce the subject contrast along the length of the foot

TOES

DP and DPO toes

It is often a requirement to examine all the toes, but most often toes 2–5, in one projection. Therefore, the description that follows gives the option to do this or to examine the toes individually. The practice of including other toes on an image is often used to establish which phalanx is being examined (see also the section on fingers in Ch. 5), but this involves irradiating areas that are not required for examination and it could be argued that this contravenes IR(ME)R 2006.[4] Collimation to include just part of the adjacent toe either side may be sufficient for identification purposes.[5]

DP toe/toes (Figs 8.6A,B, 8.7A,B)

Positioning

- The patient is seated on the table with their legs extended and their hands are used to support themselves
- The patient's knee on the side under examination is flexed and the plantar aspect of the toes is placed in contact with the IR
- The opposite leg is abducted and a lead rubber sheet is placed over the abdomen and pelvis for radiation protection

Beam direction and FRD

Vertical central ray, at 90° to the IR
100 cm FRD

Centring point

To the individual toe under examination at the metatarsophalangeal joint (Fig. 8.6A) or between the second and third metatarsophalangeal joints if all the toes are to be included (Fig. 8.7A)

Collimation

Distal half of metatarsals and phalanges of the relevant toe/toes

Criteria for assessing image quality

- All the phalanges and the distal half of the metatarsals should be included
- Symmetry of the phalangeal condyles
- Joint spaces of the interphalangeal joint spaces are demonstrated clearly. Separation of the toe or toes from the adjacent toes. Neither of these may be possible with patients with toe deformity
- Separation of adjacent metatarsal heads
- Sharp image demonstrating the soft tissue margins of the toe/toes, bony cortex and trabeculae of the phalange/s

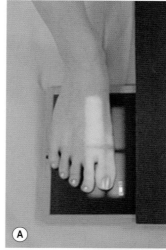

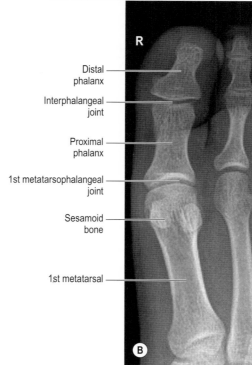

Figure 8.6 DP individual toe – hallux.

DPO toes (Fig. 8.8A,B)

Positioning

- The patient is seated on the table with their legs extended and their hands are used to support themselves
- The plantar aspect of the toes is placed on the IR
- From the DP position the patient's foot is internally rotated until approximately 30° to the IR
- A radiolucent pad is placed under the plantar aspect of the foot for immobilisation
- The opposite leg is abducted and a lead rubber sheet is placed over the abdomen and pelvis for radiation protection

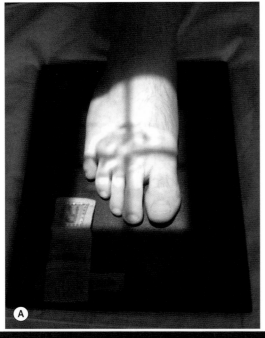

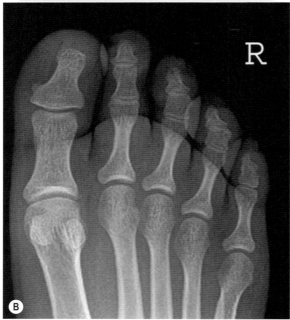

Figure 8.7 DP for all toes.

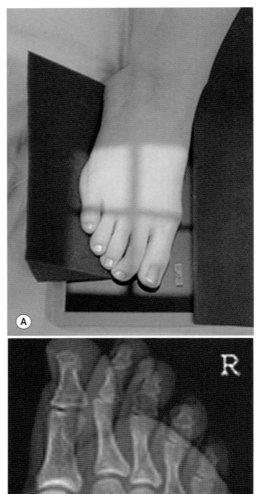

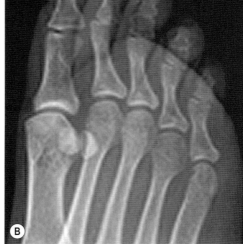

Figure 8.8 DPO toes.

Beam direction and FRD

Vertical central ray at 90° to the IR
100 cm FRD

Centring point

To the individual toe under examination at the metatarsophalangeal joint or between the second and third metatarsophalangeal joints if all the toes are to be included

Collimation

Distal half of metatarsals and phalanges of relevant toe/toes

Criteria for assessing image quality

- All the phalanges and distal half of the metatarsals should be included on the image
- As much separation of the phalanges as possible
- Sharp image demonstrating the soft tissue margins of the toe/toes, bony cortex and trabeculae of the phalange/s

The crepe bandage may be replaced by a piece of gauze between the toes. The radiographer should assess which is the most suitable method for the individual patient, depending on the flexibility of the patient's toes. It has been suggested that a tongue depressor/spatula can be used to separate the toes, but if the patient has suffered trauma to the region then this is not advisable. In any case, the use of a spatula will bring the patient's fingers closer to the primary beam. Also consider the use of a dental IR placed between the toes with the tube side of the IR in contact with the medial aspect of the toe under examination.

Beam direction and FRD

Vertical central ray, at 90° to the IR
100 cm FRD

Centring point

To the individual toe under examination at the proximal interphalangeal joint

Collimation

Distal half of metatarsals and phalanges of the relevant toe

Criteria for assessing image quality

- Relevant phalanges and the metatarsophalangeal joint demonstrated on the image
- Clear interphalangeal and metatarsophalangeal joints demonstrated with the phalangeal condyles superimposed
- Sharp image demonstrating the soft tissue margins of the toe and the bony cortex and trabeculae of the phalanges

Common error	Possible reason
Poor joint spaces with non-superimposition of the phalangeal condyles	Long axis of the toe may not lie parallel to the IR, or the leg may not be rotated sufficiently medially

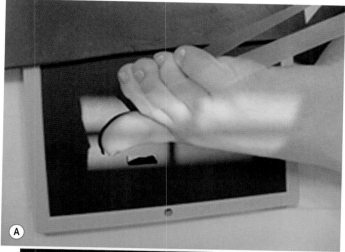

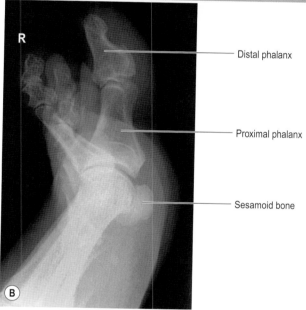

Distal phalanx

Proximal phalanx

Sesamoid bone

Figure 8.9 Lateral toe – hallux. Note that in (B) flexion of toes is opposite to that in (A).

Lateral hallux (Fig. 8.9A)

Positioning

- The patient is seated on the table with their legs extended and their hands used to support themselves
- The plantar aspect of the toes are placed on the IR
- From the DP position the patient's leg is internally rotated so that the medial aspect comes in contact with the table
- The patient is asked to assist with use of a crepe bandage to pull the toes that are not being examined away from the toe under examination in either (1) a plantar direction (Fig. 8.9A) or (2) a dorsal direction (Fig. 8.9B), depending on the patient and how their toes flex most easily
- The opposite leg is abducted and a lead rubber sheet is placed over the abdomen and pelvis for radiation protection

ANKLE

The ankle is a ring structure consisting of the tibia, talus and fibula, linked by the medial and lateral collateral ligaments and the interosseous ligament. A break in the ring is commonly associated with a second break in the ring elsewhere, which could be either ligamentous or bony.[1]

Most ankle fractures are a result of inversion or eversion injuries occurring with a combination of adduction, abduction, lateral rotation, or axial forces. Inversion injuries with supination and lateral rotation account for over half of ankle fractures.[2]

Fractured ankles can be complex and many attempts have been made to classify them according to the degree of injury. There is also an increasing element of dislocation with each degree of fracture. Pott's fractures are one such method of classification.

Pott's classifications

Abduction, external rotation type

Pott's I	A fracture of the lateral malleolus of the fibula
Pott's II	The fibular fracture, with also a transverse fracture of the medial malleolus and lateral subluxation of the talus
Pott's III	In addition to the fibular fracture, the posterior part of the medial malleolus is displaced upwards and the talus subluxed backwards

The above descriptions of the Pott's classifications are those most commonly found, but several more classifications are described for the more unusual adduction injury.

Adduction type

Pott's I	Vertical fracture of the medial malleolus
Pott's II	The fractured medial malleolus is accompanied by a transverse fracture of the lateral malleolus and medial subluxation of the talus
Pott's III	The talus is dislocated backwards. There is a fracture of the posterior part of the medial malleolus and a transverse fracture of the lateral malleolus

Ankle trauma in children and adolescents

It is much more likely for a child to suffer from an epiphyseal injury than a fracture or ligament tear because the ligaments in children are stronger than the physis. The distal tibial epiphysis is only second to the radius in the number of bony injuries occurring in children over the entire skeleton. The Salter–Harris classifications are used to describe these injuries; these are explained in the introductory section for skeletal radiography in Chapter 4.

The ankle joint may be examined for demonstration of the joint alone but is often examined for suspected fracture, and therefore the image usually requires inclusion of the lower third of tibia and fibula. To achieve this, collimation is required to be extended further up the tibia and fibula, but the centring point should remain the same as for the joint (midway between the malleoli). This will result in an excessive field of primary radiation below the plantar aspect of the foot and beyond the IR; to reduce the patient dose and prevent unnecessary scattered radiation reaching the IR (and thus improve image quality), place a sheet of lead rubber below the IR. Follow-up examinations need only include the affected area.

AP ankle (Fig. 8.10A,B)

The AP ankle is described in this book with the malleoli being equidistant from the IR. When the ankle is positioned in this way the distal tibia will be superimposed over the fibula and the distal tibiofibular joint will be obscured. The lateral aspect of the mortice, i.e. the fibiotalar joint, will be demonstrated ('mortice' refers to the appearance of the joint space around the upper talus, in the AP ankle projection, as it fits between the distal tibia and both malleoli; this is likened to the mortice joint used in carpentry). Some texts[5–7] describe this position as an oblique ankle and suggest that, for the AP, the intermalleoli line forms an angle of approximately 15–20° with the IR (with the lateral malleolus being closer to the IR than the medial malleolus). However, this positioning will obscure the most distal portion of the lateral mortice and demonstration of the distal fibula will be incomplete. Other texts[3,8,9] agree that, as described in this book, the malleoli should be equidistant from the IR. The AP is sometimes erroneously called the 'mortice' projection (see section on ankle obliques).

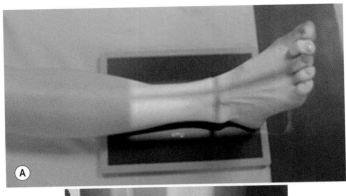

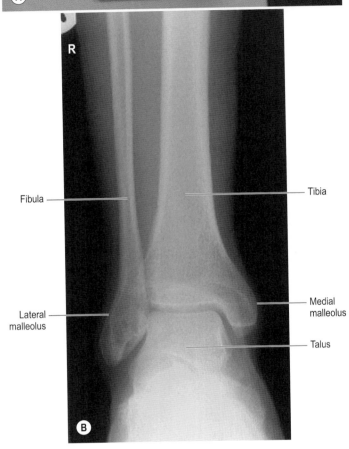

Figure 8.10 AP ankle.

Positioning

- The patient is seated on the table with their legs extended
- The leg under examination is adducted away from the opposite leg to offer protection from the main beam
- A lead rubber apron is worn to protect the gonads
- The posterior aspect of the lower leg is placed in contact with the IR
- The ankle joint is flexed to 90° (this is achieved by asking the patient to pull their toes towards their knee)
- The ankle is internally rotated to bring the medial and lateral malleoli equidistant from the IR
- The patient is immobilised in this position by using a 45° foam pad placed on the dorsal aspect of the foot with a sandbag resting on it

Beam direction and FRD

Vertical central ray, at 90° to the IR
100 cm FRD

Centring point

Midway between the malleoli

Collimation

Lower third of tibia and fibula, ankle joint, lateral and medial malleoli, talus, surrounding soft tissues

Criteria for assessing image quality

- Demonstration of the lower third of tibia and fibula, lateral and medial malleoli with soft tissue outlines
- Tibiotalar joint is well demonstrated, with equal space surrounding the superior aspect of the talus
- Talus and its articulation with the malleoli should be clearly demonstrated and free of superimposition
- Distal tibiofibular joint will be obscured
- Sharp image demonstrating the soft tissue margins, bony cortex and trabeculae of the distal tibia and fibula with the cortical margins of the superior aspect of the talus demonstrated

Common errors	Possible reasons
Joint space not demonstrated between the talus and fibula	The leg is not sufficiently internally rotated; make sure the malleoli are equidistant from the table-top
The tibiotalar joint is not clearly demonstrated	There is insufficient dorsiflexion of the foot

Lateral ankle (Fig. 8.11A,B)

To most easily achieve the best position for a lateral ankle, ask the patient to keep their leg extended and dorsiflexed at the ankle, and then roll over onto the side under examination. A common problem when performing the lateral ankle projection is that the patient tends to invert the foot, and it is difficult to rectify this once in the lateral position.

Positioning

- From the AP position the leg is externally rotated onto the side under examination until the malleoli are superimposed vertically
- The foot is dorsiflexed to bring the foot and tibia into an angle of 90°
- A small foam pad can be placed under the lateral border of the forefoot to support the patient in this position, as the lateral aspect of the forefoot will not be in contact with the table-top when the malleoli are superimposed

Beam direction and FRD

Vertical central ray at 90° to the IR
100 cm FRD

Centring point

Over the medial malleolus

Collimation

Lower third of tibia and fibula, talus, calcaneum, navicular, surrounding soft tissues

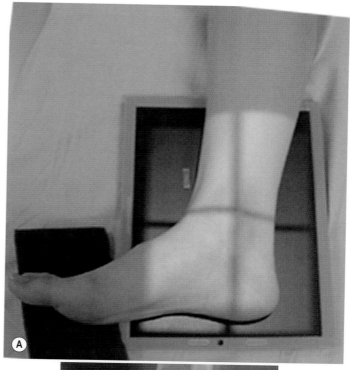

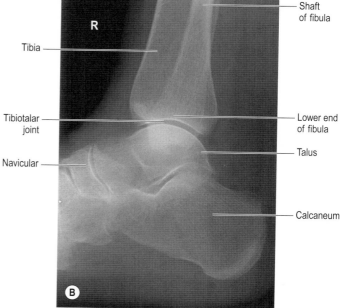

Figure 8.11 Lateral ankle.

Criteria for assessing image quality

- Lower third of tibia and fibula, talus, calcaneum, navicular and the surrounding soft tissues are demonstrated
- Medial and lateral borders of the talus are superimposed to give a clear joint space
- Extreme distal aspect of the fibula is superimposed centrally over the distal tibia, although the shaft becomes more posterior proximally
- Single line representing superior articulatory surface of the talus, with clear tibiotalar joint space
- Sharp image demonstrating the soft tissue, bony cortex and trabeculae of tibia, fibula and talus

Common errors	Possible reasons
Distal fibula projected posterior to the tibia	The leg is over-rotated laterally; make sure the malleoli are superimposed
Shaft of the fibula projected over the tibia	The leg is under-rotated
Loss of joint space and/or double edge to line representing superior articulatory surface of talus	Over- or under-rotation of the leg and/or inversion of the foot; poor flexion of the ankle

Ankle obliques

Obliques can be performed to further clarify or demonstrate any disruption to the joint, or to help in diagnosing a fractured malleolus. (a) Lateral/external and (b) medial/internal obliques with 45° rotation are usually required. In order to assess the distal tibiofibular joint, distal fibula, talus and its articulation with the lateral malleolus and tibia, the medial oblique has a reduced rotation of 30° (c). The 30° oblique projection is sometimes referred to as a *mortice* projection and it has been noted that some referring clinicians erroneously refer to the routine AP projection as 'mortice', thinking that the slight obliquity required to bring the malleoli into the correct position constitutes an oblique projection.

It must be mentioned, however, that magnetic resonance imaging (MRI) is the method of choice when provision of a visual account of the biomechanics of the ankle joint is required, although it is noted that some imaging centres advocate ultrasound as the imaging method of choice.

Positioning

(a) 45° lateral/external oblique (Fig. 8.12A,B)
- From the AP position the ankle is rotated 45° externally and a radiolucent foam pad is used to support the ankle in this position

(b) 45° medial/internal oblique (Fig. 8.13A,B)
- From the AP position the ankle is rotated 45° internally and a radiolucent foam pad is used to support the ankle in this position

(c) 30° medial/internal oblique (Fig. 8.14A,B)
- From the AP position the ankle is rotated 30° internally and a radiolucent foam pad is used to support the ankle in this position

Beam direction and FRD

Vertical central ray at 90° to the IR, although a 15° cranial angle will clear the distal fibula more efficiently
100 cm FRD

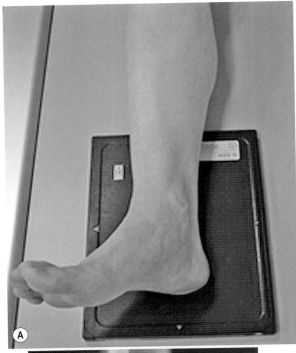

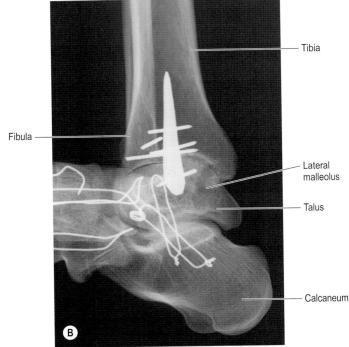

Figure 8.12 45° external oblique ankle.

Centring point

For all projections, midway between the malleoli

Collimation

Medial and lateral malleoli, distal tibia and fibula, talus, surrounding soft tissues

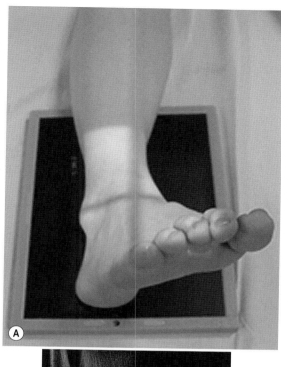

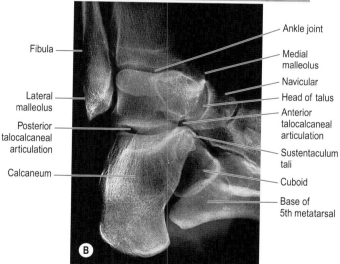

Fibula

Lateral malleolus

Posterior talocalcaneal articulation

Calcaneum

Ankle joint

Medial malleolus

Navicular

Head of talus

Anterior talocalcaneal articulation

Sustentaculum tali

Cuboid

Base of 5th metatarsal

Figure 8.13 45° internal oblique ankle.
(B) Reproduced with permission from Bryan GJ. Skeletal anatomy. 3rd ed. Edinburgh: Churchill Livingstone; 1996.

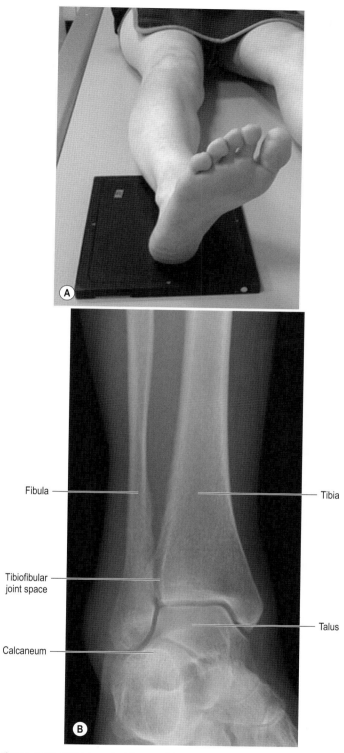

Fibula

Tibiofibular joint space

Calcaneum

Tibia

Talus

Figure 8.14 30° internal oblique ankle.

Criteria for assessing image quality

- *(a) 45° external rotation:* The malleoli should be superimposed on the talus. The lower end of fibula should be obscured by the anterior aspect of the distal tibia
- *(b) 45° internal rotation:* The lateral malleolus, lateral aspect of mortice and distal tibiofibular articulation should be well demonstrated. The medial aspect of the mortice will appear closed
- *(c) 30° internal rotation/mortice projection:* The tibiotalar joint should be well visualised and the medial and lateral aspects of the mortice should be open. The medial and lateral malleoli should be well demonstrated

SUBTALAR JOINT/TALOCALCANEAL JOINTS

The following projections are described here for completeness; however, it is now unusual to find them requested, as MRI will provide high contrast sensitivity and has multiplanar capabilities. It therefore facilitates superior demonstration of these articular surfaces.

Medial obliques, subtalar joint

Positioning

- As for 45° medial oblique (Fig. 8.13A)

Beam direction and FRD

1. *40° cranial angle* to show the anterior portion of the posterior talocalcaneal articulation
2. *30° cranial angle* to show the articulation between the talus and sustenaculum
3. *10° cranial angle* to show the posterior portion of the posterior talocalcaneal articulation

100 cm FRD

Centring point

All angulations – to a point beneath the lateral malleolus

Collimation

Distal end of the tibia and fibula, calcaneum, tarsal bones

Criteria for assessing image quality

- Distal end of tibia and fibula, calcaneum and tarsal bones are demonstrated
- (1) should demonstrate the anterior part of the posterior talocalcaneal articulation
- (2) should demonstrate the articulation between the talus and sustenaculum
- (3) should demonstrate the posterior part of the posterior talocalcaneal articulation. The sinus tarsi should be demonstrated as open on this projection
- Sharp image with adequate penetration to demonstrate the subtalar joint with visualisation of the bony cortex and trabeculae of the talus in contrast to the surrounding soft tissue margins

Lateral oblique subtalar joint

This demonstrates the posterior subtalar joint and will also confirm a fracture involving the joint surface[2] and disclose DP compression.

Positioning

- As for 45° external oblique projection (Fig. 8.12A)

Beam direction and FRD

15° cranial angle
100 cm FRD

Centring point

To a point just below and anterior to the medial malleolus

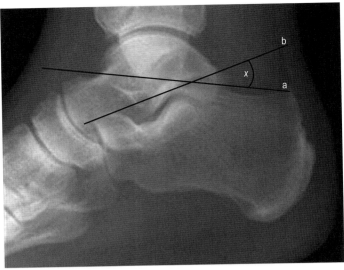

Figure 8.15 Bohler's angle. Bohler's angle is assessed by drawing two intersecting lines (a) from the highest point on the posterior aspect of the calcaneum to its highest midpoint and (b) from the highest midpoint to the highest anterior point. The lines are extended here to demonstrate the angle more accurately. If the angle x is less than 30° this suggests a calcaneal fracture with compression.

Collimation

Distal end of tibia and fibula, calcaneum, tarsal bones

Criteria for assessing image quality

- Distal end of tibia and fibula, calcaneum and tarsal bones are demonstrated
- Posterior subtalar joint should be well demonstrated, with the middle and anterior subtalar joint obscured by the inferior aspects of the talar neck and head
- Sharp image with adequate penetration to demonstrate the posterior subtalar joint with visualisation of the bony cortex and trabeculae of the talus in contrast to the surrounding soft tissue margins

CALCANEUM

The calcaneum is often examined when a patient presents after falling feet-first from height, but fractures of this area can result from a twisting injury. Some fractures will only become apparent when the Bohler's angle[1] is assessed; this angle is normally found to be between 30° and 40° and is reduced to below 30° when a fracture is present (Fig. 8.15). CT is useful for assessing the extent and involvement of fragments in the fractured calcaneum.

Lateral calcaneum (Fig. 8.16A,B)

For assessment of the calcaneal spur, the lateral projection only should be undertaken.

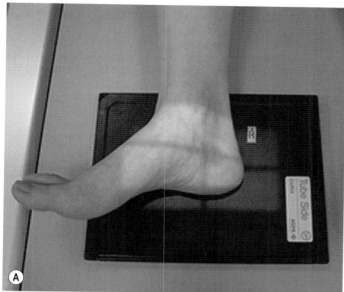

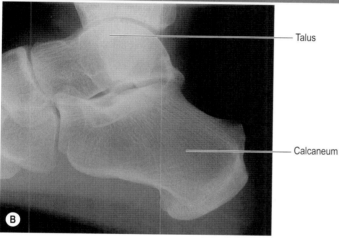

Talus

Calcaneum

Figure 8.16 Lateral calcaneum.

Positioning

- The patient is seated on the table, and the ankle of the side under examination is rotated externally
- The lateral aspect of the foot is brought into contact with the IR
- The ankle is dorsiflexed to 90° and the rotation of the leg adjusted until the malleoli are superimposed
- A lead rubber apron is worn to protect the gonads

Beam direction and FRD

Vertical central ray, at 90° to the IR
100 cm FRD

Centring point

To the middle of the calcaneum below the medial malleolus

Collimation

Calcaneum, ankle joint, navicular, surrounding soft tissues

Criteria for assessing image quality

- Calcaneum, talocalcaneal and cubocalcaneal joints and soft tissue outlines are demonstrated
- Distal fibula should be superimposed over the tibial malleolus
- Sharp image demonstrating the soft tissue margins, bony cortex and trabeculae of the calcaneum

Axial calcaneum

This projection can be achieved by several methods. It is commonly described with the patient seated on the table and the central ray directed 40° cranially towards the extended leg (method 4), but this has the X-ray beam directed towards the trunk and should only be used if the other methods described cannot be achieved due to the patient's condition.

Method 1 is easily achieved by the ambulant patient and methods 2 and 3 can be achieved in the less ambulant patient and most trolley patients. Methods 1–3 position the long axis of the calcaneum parallel to the IR, producing an image with minimal distortion. Method 4 positions the long axis of the calcaneum at 90° to the IR and produces maximum distortion to the image. All four techniques can be used to examine both calcanei simultaneously, with the X-ray beam centred between the heels, at the levels stated for the individual calcaneum. This will cause a degree of image distortion but will reduce the exposures made to one; two separate exposures will increase the radiation dose but will provide less distortion due to accurate centring over each heel in turn. Methods 1 and 2 are not suitable for use with a fixed plate detector.

Method 1: patient erect (Fig. 8.17A,B)

Positioning

- The patient stands in the erect position with their back to the X-ray tube and the plantar aspect of the heel under examination is placed directly on the IR
- The other leg is abducted to clear it from the radiation field
- A lead rubber apron is placed around the patient's waist to protect the gonads
- With the patient's knees slightly flexed the hands can be placed onto a table or chair in front for support. A vertical bucky stand can also be used
- The malleoli are checked until equidistant from the IR

Beam direction and FRD

Initially vertical, the beam is directed 30° towards the toes, i.e. 60° to the IR
100 cm FRD

Method 2: patient prone (Fig. 8.18)

A vertical IR is required for this method. Some digital IRs may not be suitable for this method.

Positioning

- The patient lies prone on the table with the toes projecting over the end of the table
- The IR is placed at the end of the table with the tube side of the IR facing the plantar aspect of the patient's feet
- Both legs are extended and the unaffected leg is abducted to clear it from the radiation field
- A lead rubber sheet is placed over the pelvis to protect the gonads
- The plantar aspect of the foot under examination is placed in contact with the IR
- The malleoli are equidistant from the IR

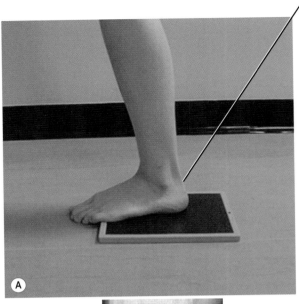

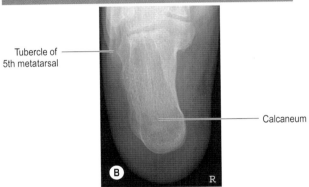

Tubercle of 5th metatarsal

Calcaneum

Figure 8.17 (A) Erect axial calcaneum; (B) axial calcaneum.

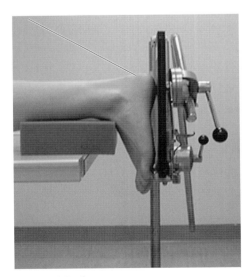

Figure 8.18 Prone axial calcaneum.

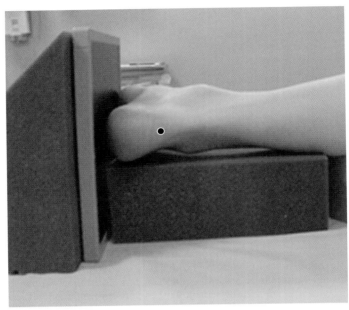

Figure 8.19 Axial calcaneum with patient on their side.

Beam direction and FRD

Initially horizontal, the X-ray tube is directed caudally towards the toes at approximately 30°, to create an angle of 60° with the IR
100 cm FRD

Method 3: patient lying on side (Fig. 8.19)

Positioning

- The patient lies in the lateral position on the side under examination
- The unaffected leg is abducted posteriorly and placed behind the side under examination
- The leg of the side under examination is supported above the table-top using foam pads and the IR is supported vertically, its tube side in contact with the plantar aspect of the heel
- The malleoli are equidistant from the IR
- A lead rubber sheet is placed over the hips for gonad protection

Beam direction and FRD

Initially the beam is horizontal, directed towards the posterior aspect of the heel and coincident with the long axis of the calcaneum, *and then*
The angle is approximately 30° caudally towards the toes to form an angle of 60° with the IR
100 cm FRD

Centring point for methods 1, 2 and 3

At the level of the malleoli, in the middle of the posterior aspect of the heel

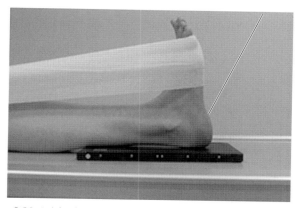

Figure 8.20 Axial calcaneum with patient seated.

Common errors – all methods	Possible reasons
Elongated long axis of the calcaneum	Over-angulation of X-ray beam
Foreshortening of long axis of the calcaneum	Not enough angulation on X-ray beam
Cubocalcaneal joint not demonstrated	Not enough dorsiflexion of the foot

TIBIA AND FIBULA

When examining the tibia and fibula both the knee and the ankle joint must be demonstrated. This is particularly important in the case of gross injuries in order to show general alignment and to be certain that a contracoup injury has not occurred. The fibula acts as a support for the tibia, and a fracture at one end of one bone often results in a fracture at the opposite end of the other. The ankle joint is often described as a bony ring, and this ring may be considered to extend into the knee. An external rotation injury of the ankle joint, resulting in a seemingly isolated fracture of the medial malleolus, may result in a fracture of the proximal fibula; this is called a Maisonneuve fracture.[1] In the case of spiral fracture the full length of the fracture may not be demonstrated if the full lengths of the tibia and fibula are not shown.

To ensure that the full lengths of the tibia and fibula are included it may be necessary to use two IRs per projection. However, most digital IRs are now 43 or 45 cm² or even 35 × 47 cm, and it may be possible to include the full length on one image for most patients.

AP tibia and fibula (Fig. 8.21A,B)

Positioning

- The patient is seated on the table and may support themselves by leaning on their hands
- Both legs are extended and the leg that is not under examination is abducted to clear it from the radiation field
- A lead rubber sheet is placed over the pelvis to protect the gonads
- The leg under examination is placed with its posterior aspect in contact with the IR
- The malleoli are positioned equidistant from the IR and the ankle is dorsiflexed; this position may be supported with use of a radiolucent pad and sandbag at the plantar aspect of the foot

Beam direction and FRD

A vertical central ray, at 90° to the IR
100 cm FRD

Centring point

Midway between the ankle and knee joint on the anterior aspect of the lower leg or, if both joints cannot be included on one image, in the middle of the area being exposed

Collimation

Tibia and fibula, ankle and knee joints, surrounding soft tissues

Method 4: patient seated (Fig. 8.20)

Positioning

- The patient is seated on the table with their legs extended and separated
- The posterior aspect of the heel under examination is placed on the IR with the inferior border of the heel pad at the lower edge
- A lead rubber sheet is placed over the pelvis to protect the gonads
- The foot is dorsiflexed; this position can be assisted and maintained by providing the patient with a bandage looped around the forefoot and pulled on towards the trunk. This is held by the patient
- The malleoli are equidistant from the IR

Beam direction and FRD

A vertical central ray is directed 40° cranially
100 cm FRD

Centring point

At a point midway on the plantar aspect of the heel, to pass through the malleoli

Collimation

Calcaneum, talocalcaneal and cubocalcaneal joints, the soft tissue outline

Criteria for assessing image quality

- Calcaneum, talocalcaneal and cubocalcaneal joints and the soft tissue outlines demonstrated
- Cubocalcaneal joint space clearly visualised without the metatarsals superimposed
- Lateral malleolus demonstrated on the lateral aspect of the calcaneum
- Calcaneum demonstrated without rotation and distortion
- Sharp image demonstrating the soft tissue margins and bony cortex and trabeculae of the calcaneum, cubocalcaneal joint shown adequately without over-penetration of the distal aspect of calcaneum

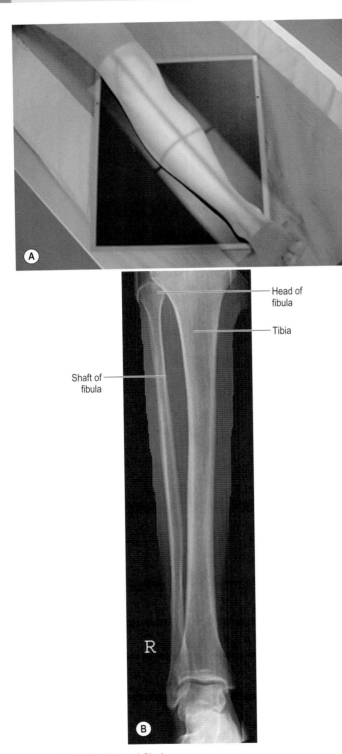

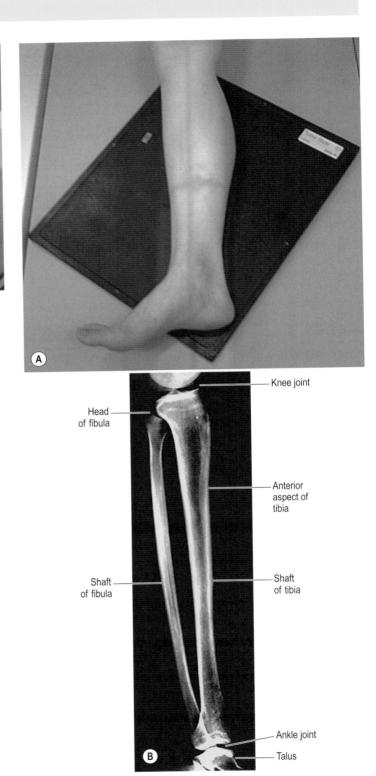

Figure 8.21 AP tibia and fibula.

Figure 8.22 Lateral tibia and fibula.
(B) Reproduced with permission from Bryan GJ. Skeletal anatomy. 3rd ed.
Edinburgh: Churchill Livingstone; 1996 and Gunn C. Bones and joints.
4th ed. Edinburgh: Churchill Livingstone; 2002.

Criteria for assessing image quality

- Tibia and fibula, ankle and knee joints and surrounding soft tissues are demonstrated
- Separation of the tibial and fibular shafts
- Proximal tibiofibular joint should show slight superimposition of tibia and fibula
- The distal tibiofibular joint should have slight superimposition of tibia and fibula
- Demonstration of the joint space between the medial and lateral borders of the talus and the medial and lateral malleoli, respectively
- Sharp image demonstrating the soft tissue margins, bony cortex and trabeculae of tibia and fibula with adequate penetration to demonstrate both the ankle joint and knee joint

Lateral tibia and fibula (Fig. 8.22A,B)

Positioning

- From the AP position the leg is externally rotated onto the side under examination
- The opposite leg is abducted to clear from the main beam
- A lead rubber apron is applied to the lower abdomen for gonad protection
- The lateral aspect of the leg is in contact with the IR, which is positioned to include the ankle and knee joint
- The long axis of the tibia and fibula should be parallel to surface of the IR
- The ankle is flexed and the malleoli are superimposed
- A small foam pad can be placed under the lateral border of the forefoot to support the patient in this position

Beam direction and FRD

Vertical central ray at 90° to the IR
100 cm FRD

Centring point

Midway between the ankle and knee joint on the medial aspect of the lower leg or, if both joints cannot be included on one image, in the middle of the area being exposed

Collimation

Tibia and fibula, ankle and knee joints, soft tissues

Criteria for assessing image quality

- Ankle, knee joints and soft tissue demonstrated
- Mid-shaft of fibula should project slightly posterior to tibia
- Proximal end of fibula should be slightly posterior to tibia with partial superimposition
- The distal end of fibula should be superimposed over the middle of the distal tibia
- Sharp image demonstrating the soft tissue margins, bony cortex and trabeculae of tibia and fibula with adequate penetration to visualise the ankle and knee joints. The kVp should be sufficient to reduce the high subject contrast along the length of the tibia and fibula

REFERENCES

1. Raby N, et al. Accident and emergency radiology, a survival guide. 2nd ed. London: Saunders; 2005.
2. Long BW, Rafert JA. Orthopaedic radiography. Philadelphia: WB Saunders; 1995.
3. Whitley AS, et al. Clark's positioning in radiography. 12th ed. London: Hodder Arnold; 2005.
4. The Ionising Radiation (Medical Exposure) Regulations 2006, London (HMSO).
5. Bontrager KL. Textbook of radiographic positioning and related anatomy. 5th ed. St Louis: Mosby; 2001.
6. McQuillen-Martenson K. Radiographic image analysis. 3rd ed. St Louis: Saunders; 2010
7. Eisenberg RL, et al. Radiographic positioning. 2nd ed. Boston: Little Brown and Company; 1995.
8. Unett EM, Royle AJ. Radiographic techniques and image evaluation. London: Nelson Thornes; 1997.
9. Bell GA, Finlay DBL. Basic radiographic positioning. Eastbourne: Baillière Tindall; 1986.

Chapter 9

Knee and femur

Linda Williams

The knee has a complex arrangement of ligaments, tendons and muscles which together provide stability to the joint. Because of the anatomical location and the complex biomechanics of the knee, it is susceptible to a variety of injuries.[1] The knee and femur are often investigated in the event of trauma; however, this should only be the case if there is a suspected fracture, as ligamentous and meniscal injuries may appear normal on plain images.[2] The knee should not be investigated for knee pain unless there is locking and restricted movement or a suspected loose body. Osteoarthritic changes are commonly found in the knee, and radiographic examination should only be undertaken if surgery is being considered.[3]

Plain radiography of the knee is undertaken less frequently in the 21st century as magnetic resonance imaging (MRI) is the method of choice for imaging the joint structures. This is because of its high contrast sensitivity and multiplanar imaging capabilities. It is particularly effective in investigating the effects of trauma to the anterior and posterior cruciate ligaments and menisci.[4] The images of non-bony parts of the joint obtained by MRI are far superior to, and carry more information than, plain radiographs, and diagnosis and appropriate management of this complex joint is established with greater confidence after MRI examination.[3]

Ultrasound is also used as a method of imaging some lesions of the knee joint, e.g. Baker's cyst; these can show as a vague mass behind the knee on plain X-ray images, but ultrasound will give a clear account of the full extent of the cyst.[4]

There is, however, still an important role for plain radiography of the knee for initial diagnosis in trauma and follow-up orthopaedic assessment.

FRACTURES AND INJURIES AFFECTING THE REGION OF THE KNEE AND FEMUR

Fractured shaft of femur

The shaft is usually fractured as a result of considerable force to the femur, commonly in road traffic accidents.

Supracondylar fracture

These are fractures superior to the femoral condyles; the gastrocnemius muscle may pull the distal fragments posteriorly.

Tibial plateau fracture

These fractures are often associated with considerable damage to the medial collateral or cruciate ligaments. The most common finding is depressed lateral tibial plateau caused by a car bumper injury; this is seen in 80% of cases.[1]

Patella fractures

Patellar comminuted fractures are usually the result of a direct blow. Muscle spasm (quadriceps), if severe enough, can cause transverse fractures. The bipartite patella (unfused secondary ossification centre) can be confused with a fracture, but these have well-defined margins. The patella may also be *dislocated* medially or laterally, and can be recurrent due to a shallow intercondylar groove. Dislocations usually occur following a twisting force, typically in sports injuries.

Anteroposterior (AP) knee – patient seated

(Fig. 9.1A,B,C)

IR is horizontal

Positioning

- The patient is seated on the table with their legs extended
- The posterior aspect of the knee under examination is placed over the image receptor (IR)
- The unaffected leg is abducted from the leg under examination to clear it from the field of radiation
- A lead rubber apron is worn for radiation protection of the lower abdomen
- The leg is rotated to bring the tibial condyles equidistant to the IR. The patella may appear centralised but this is not consistent for all patients

Orthopaedic requests may require this projection to be undertaken with the patient erect, weightbearing. This allows for assessment of

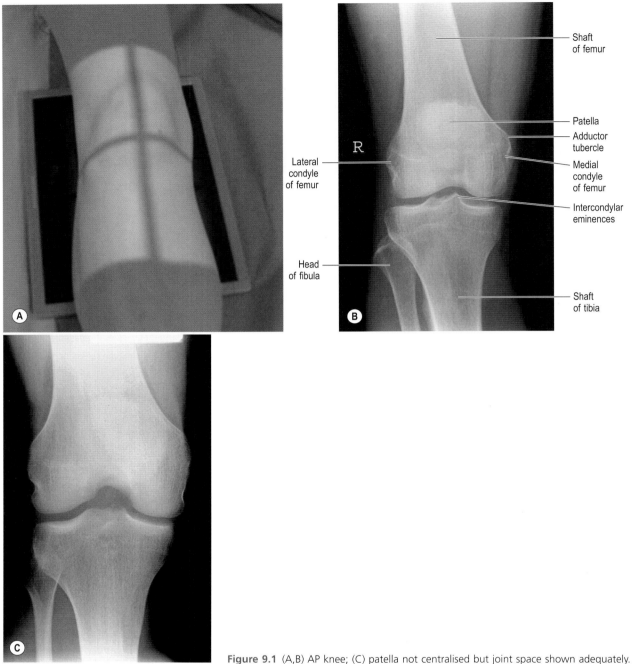

Figure 9.1 (A,B) AP knee; (C) patella not centralised but joint space shown adequately.

the joint space and alignment of the joint during weightbearing, prior to surgery.[1] Its use has become more widespread in that published evidence suggests that a weightbearing technique has advantages over the conventional sitting method, and that a PA rather than an AP approach may be even better.[5] Positioning for the erect AP remains the same as for the seated version, but with the patient standing with the back of their knee against the IR and still facing the X-ray tube. The stability of the patient should also be considered in the erect position and there should be a support for them to hold. The patient must be asked to distribute their weight evenly on both feet. Similarly, erect PA will require the patient to distribute their weight evenly, but with the patella in contact with the IR.

Beam direction and focus receptor distance (FRD)

Patient seated: Vertical central beam, at 90° to the IR *or* 90° to the long axis of the tibia (which will improve joint space demonstration if the patient cannot fully extend the knee)
Patient erect: Horizontal beam, at 90° to the IR *or* long axis of the tibia 100 cm FRD

Centring point

AP: On the anterior aspect of the knee in the middle of the joint space, midway between the tibial condyles

PA: On the posterior aspect of the knee in the middle of the joint space, midway between the tibial condyles

A point 2.5 cm below the apex of the patella is often cited as the centring point for AP of this joint, but this specific measurement does not allow for variations in patient build.

Collimation

Lower third of femur, knee joint, proximal third of tibia, head of fibula, surrounding soft tissues

Criteria for assessing image quality

- Distal third of femur, proximal third of tibia, head of fibula, patella and soft tissue outlines are demonstrated
- Medial and lateral epicondyles of the femur are demonstrated in profile
- Head of fibula should appear partially obscured by the tibia
- Shafts of tibia and fibula should be separated
- Joint space should appear clear and the upper margin of the tibial plateau should be shown in profile

Sharp image demonstrating the soft tissue margins, bony cortex and trabeculae of tibia, fibula, femur and patella, with sufficient penetration to visualise the bony trabeculae and cortical outline of the patella over the femur. Demonstration of the knee joint space in contrast to bony areas.

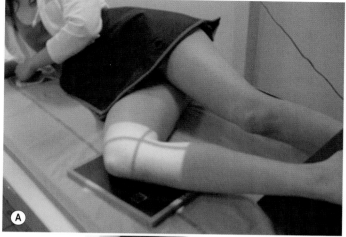
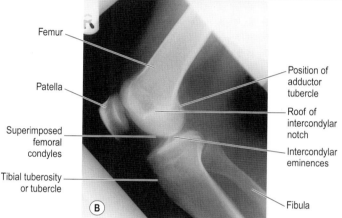

Figure 9.2 Lateral knee.

Common errors	Possible reasons
The patella appears medially in relation to the femur and the proximal tibiofibular joint is demonstrated. The joint space may appear narrowed or obscured, unilaterally or bilaterally. Part, or all, of the tibial plateau does not appear to be seen in profile	The leg is excessively internally rotated; ensure the tibial condyles are equidistant from the IR and the patella is centralised. However, take care to note whether the patient has a naturally medially positioned patella or knock knees before attempting repeat projection. *If the tibiofibular joint appears to be demonstrated correctly, and joint space shown clear, then it is likely that the patient's patella does not naturally lie centrally positioned; an example of this is shown in Figure 9.1C*
The patella is projected laterally in relation to the femur and the proximal tibiofibular joint is obscured by the tibia. The joint space may appear narrowed or obscured, unilaterally or bilaterally. Part or all of the tibial plateau does not appear to be seen in profile	There is excessive external rotation of the leg. Patellae are less likely to naturally lie on the more lateral aspect over the femur than medially, as above, but note should still be made to check if this is the case
There is no bony detail of the patella demonstrated – pale image of patella but femur may show trabecular detail outside the periphery of the patella	The radiograph is under-penetrated; increase kVp

Lateral knee (Fig. 9.2A,B)

IR is horizontal

Positioning

- The patient is seated on the table with their legs extended
- The patient is rotated laterally onto the side under examination and the hip and knee are flexed; the lateral aspect of the knee is in contact with the IR. Flexion of the knee should be at least 45°, to a maximum of 80°. Generally flexion through 60° (making an angle of 120° between the femoral and tibial shafts) is most commonly adopted
- The unaffected leg is abducted away from the knee under examination to clear it from the field of radiation; this may be posterior or anterior to the knee under examination. If cleared posteriorly, it is more comfortable if the unaffected leg remains extended; if cleared anteriorly it is more comfortable for the knee and hip to be flexed
- The ankle of the affected leg is supported with a sandbag to bring the long axis of the tibia parallel to the table-top

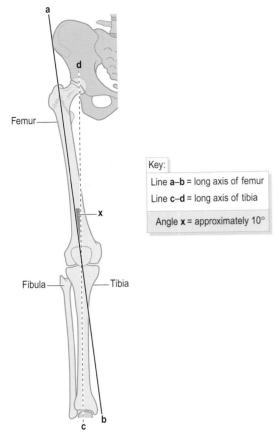

Key:

Line **a–b** = long axis of femur

Line **c–d** = long axis of tibia

Angle **x** = approximately 10°

Figure 9.3 Alignment of shafts of femur and tibia.

- The condyles of the femur are superimposed; this may be achieved by placing the middle finger on the lateral condyle and the thumb on the medial condyle, rotating the patient's femur until they are superimposed. Rotation at the pelvis may help with this adjustment
- The transverse plane of the patella is at 90° to the table-top
- A lead rubber apron is placed over the lower abdomen for radiation protection

Comments on superimposing the femoral condyles

Criteria for assessing the lateral knee radiograph require the knee joint to be demonstrated with the condyles of the femur superimposed. However, there is often difficulty in producing this as the femur and tibia do not follow a straight line. The femoral shaft angles medially through approximately 10° from hip to knee, yet the plane of the articular surface of the knee joint is at right-angles to the long axis of the tibia (Fig. 9.3); this means that there is an angle of approximately 170° between femur and tibia at the lateral aspect of the knee joint. Therefore, when the patient is placed on their side for the lateral knee position, it is unlikely that a vertical central ray would travel through the joint at 90° or superimpose the femoral condyles. To correct this the lower leg needs to be raised from the table-top, with pads or sandbags, to ensure the tibia lies parallel to, and the tibial plateau is perpendicular to, the IR.[6] Padding at the ankle end of the limb is likely to be most effective.

Without padding at the ankle the condylar surfaces will not lie in the same plane, and if padding is not used, some texts claim the solution is to apply a cranial angle of approximately 7° as compensation.[7,8] If this method is used the main beam will be directed towards the gonads. It has been noted that some radiographers adapt the above technique by centring lower, in conjunction with a vertical central ray, to achieve the same effect as applying a cranial angle, but this will necessitate a larger collimated field of radiation and this is also not recommended. Indeed, this practice must be actively discouraged and is in contradiction of the requirements of IR(ME)R 2006.

Beam direction and FRD

Vertical at 90° to the IR and coincident with the transverse axis of the joint

100 cm FRD

In cases of trauma horizontal beam laterals must be performed; this method will demonstrate any joint effusion displacing the suprapatellar bursa, which may contain fat released from the bone marrow following fracture.[2] A fat–blood effusion may be seen (lipohaemarthrosis), indicating a fracture even if not seen on the resulting radiograph. Use of a horizontal beam will also ensure that the unstable joint is not disrupted further, or fracture fragments further displaced. This is especially a risk in the case of transverse patellar fracture or fractures of the femoral shaft.

A mediolateral approach must be attempted if patient condition allows, with the unaffected leg raised away from the radiation field. This will most closely reproduce the routine lateral projection.

Centring point

Over the middle of the medial tibial condyle, through the middle of the knee joint

2.5 cm below and behind the apex of the patella has been described for the centring point for this projection but, as discussed in the AP knee projection description, this does not allow for variation in patient build.

Collimation

Lower third of femur, knee joint, proximal third of tibia, head of fibula, surrounding soft tissues

Criteria for assessing image quality

- Distal third of femur, proximal third of tibia, head of fibula and soft tissues should all be demonstrated
- Knee joint is demonstrated as clear, with the condyles of femur superimposed
- Patellofemoral joint space is demonstrated. However, if the patella is not naturally positioned centrally over the femur, the patellofemoral space will not be seen despite good superimposition of the femoral condyles. This is seen in Figure 9.2B
- Head of fibula is partly superimposed over tibia (approximately one-third to half of the head should be overlapped)
- Head of fibula is seen posteriorly in relation to tibia
- Sharp image demonstrating the soft tissue margins, bony cortex and trabeculae of femur, tibia, fibula and patella. Joint space is shown in contrast to denser bone

Common errors	Possible reasons
The condyles of the femur are not superimposed anteriorly and posteriorly and the patellofemoral joint space is not clear	Incorrect rotation but is the leg over-rotated or under-rotated? The *head of fibula* is a good indication of the direction to correct rotation: 1. If the *head of fibula* is excessively or completely superimposed over the tibia then there is insufficient rotation – further external rotation is required 2. If the proximal tibiofibular joint is shown clearly then there is excessive rotation – less rotation is therefore required
	The *adductor tubercle*, found on the posterior upper aspect of the medial femoral condyle, can also be used as an indicator when assessing knee rotation. In the correct position the tubercle is hardly discernible but in cases of incorrect rotation it becomes more apparent and can be used as follows: 1. If the tubercle lies anteriorly in relationship to the other condyle, the knee is over-rotated 2. If the tubercle lies posteriorly, the knee is under-rotated
	The *patellofemoral* joint space will clear once the rotation is corrected but it must be remembered that the patella may not be centralised naturally and this may result in unavoidable loss of joint space. If the condyles are superimposed and the patellofemoral space is not evident, this may be due to a naturally occurring non-centralised patella (this will also have been apparent when positioning for the AP projection)
	Another method for assessing direction of rotation is to estimate the relative *size of each condyle*; it is assumed that the outline of the apparently larger condyle will be that most remote from the IR (the medial condyle) since it will be more magnified than the lateral condyle. Unfortunately it is difficult to make this assessment when only part of the condyle lies clear of the other. Some patients also have one slightly flattened condyle (usually on its anterior aspect), which will never appear superimposed over the other, more normally curved, condyle
Femoral condyles not superimposed along the knee joint surface, i.e. nearest the upper surface of the tibial plateau	The tibia is not parallel to the table-top; usually this is due to a lack of attention to adequate padding of the lower leg. It is more difficult to assess correction requirements in this situation but estimation of size of condyles (as described above) may help. It is more likely that the lower leg is inadequately raised rather than excessively raised

INTERCONDYLAR NOTCH

Projections for this area are sometimes referred to as 'tunnel' projections, as the appearances are similar to that of a railway tunnel. It is commonly performed to investigate knee pain if there is locking, restricted movement and a suspected loose body. Three methods will be described here to achieve this projection; methods 1 and 2 are the methods of choice as the primary beam is not directly pointing towards the gonads. Method 3 will also provide a more distorted, magnified image. The third method should only be attempted in patients who are unable to achieve the positions required for methods 1 or 2.

Method 1 (Fig. 9.4A,B,C)

IR is horizontal

Positioning

- The patient kneels on the table with the knee of the leg under examination on the IR, their hands placed on the table for support
- The unaffected leg is separated from that under examination, to clear it from the radiation field
- The angle between the tibia and femur should be 120°
- The femoral condyles should be equidistant to the table-top and the patella centralised between them
- A lead rubber apron is worn for radiation protection to the lower abdomen, on its posterior aspect

Beam direction and FRD

1. Vertical central beam, at 90° to the long axis of the tibia
   This will demonstrate the posterior aspect of the notch. This is the only projection necessary to demonstrate loose bodies, as the whole of the notch can be visualised, with the exception of its anterior aspect.
2. Cranial angle at 70° to the tibia
   This will demonstrate the anterior aspect of the notch.

100 cm FRD

Centring point

In the middle of the crease of the knee

Method 2 (Fig. 9.5)

IR is horizontal

Positioning

- The patient lies prone on the table with the knee under examination in contact with the IR
- The unaffected leg is separated from that under examination, to clear it from the radiation field
- The knee is flexed until the tibia is at angle of 45° to the table-top and is supported in this position
- The femoral condyles are adjusted to centralise the patella
- A lead rubber apron is worn for radiation protection to the lower abdomen

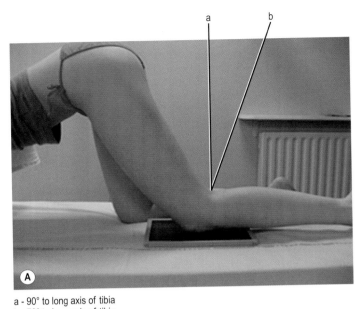

a - 90° to long axis of tibia
b - 70° to long axis of tibia

Loose body   Intercondylar notch   Anterior aspect of notch

Figure 9.4 Intercondylar notch – method 1; (B) with beam 90° to tibia; (C) with beam 70° to tibia.

Beam direction and FRD

1. Caudal central beam at 45° to the IR and femur. This will demonstrate the whole of the notch, with the exception of the anterior aspect
2. Caudal angle at 65° to the femur. This will demonstrate the anterior aspect of the notch

100 cm FRD

Centring point

In the middle of the crease of the knee

Method 3 (Fig. 9.6)

Positioning

- The patient is seated on the table with the leg under examination flexed through 60° until the angle between the tibia and femur is 120°
- The unaffected leg is separated from that under examination, to clear it from the radiation field
- The IR is supported on a pad under the flexed knee so that it is elevated high enough to ensure the upper and lower leg are in contact with it

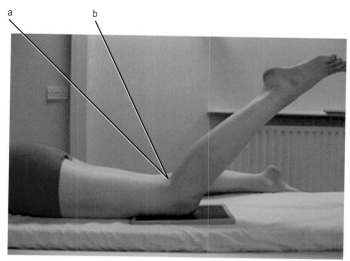

a - Beam 45° to femur
b - Beam 65° to femur

Figure 9.5 Intercondylar notch – method 2.

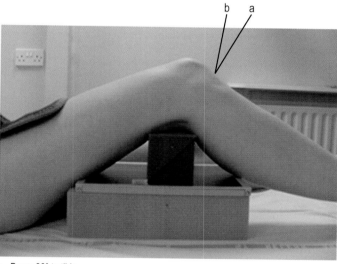

a - Beam 90° to tibia
b - Beam 110° to tibia

Figure 9.6 Intercondylar notch – method 3.

- The femoral condyles should be equidistant to the IR to centralise the patella
- A lead rubber apron is worn to protect the lower abdomen. This should be adjusted to lie between the thighs to ensure adequate protection to the gonads

Beam direction and FRD

1. Initially vertical, the central beam is angled cranially until at 90° to the long axis of tibia. This will demonstrate the whole of the notch, with the exception of the anterior aspect
2. Initially vertical, the central beam is angled until at 110° to the long axis of the tibia. This will demonstrate the anterior aspect of the notch

100 cm FRD

Angulation can be estimated accurately by initially positioning the tube housing or light beam housing parallel to the long axis of the tibia, then checking the angulation indicator on the unit before adding the required angulation to this reading.

Centring point

Immediately below the apex of the patella

Collimation

Femoral and tibial condyles

Criteria for assessing image quality

- Femoral and tibial condyles are included in the image
- Patella is cleared above the intercondylar notch and central between the femoral condyles
- Tubercles of the intercondylar eminences of tibia are visualised
- Tibiofemoral joint space should be clear
- *For the whole notch*: The notch should be seen as tunnel or 'n' shaped, with almost vertical lateral margins and an arched roof
- *For the anterior aspect of the notch*: The notch is shallower than required for the full notch, rather like an inverted 'v' with sloped lateral margins and narrow roof
- Sharp image demonstrating the soft tissue in the notch in contrast to the adjacent bone, intercondylar eminences and any loose bodies

Common error	Possible reason
Patella superimposed over notch	Beam angle not correctly set in relation to tibia (too much cranial angle in PA projections, methods 1 and 2; not enough cranial angulation in method 3, AP projection). Incorrect flexion can also cause this

PATELLA

Posteroanterior (PA) patella (Fig. 9.7A,B)

Although the PA is the preferred method for the patella projection, as it is in close contact with the IR, the patient may not be able to achieve the position because of injury or their general condition. In these cases a satisfactory image can be obtained by positioning the patient as for an AP knee projection, with a 10 kVp increase on exposure factors. Consideration must be given to increasing the FRD to compensate for the relatively large object–receptor distance.

IR is horizontal

Positioning

- The patient lies prone on the table with their legs extended and the affected patella in contact with the IR
- The unaffected leg is separated from that under examination to clear it from the radiation field
- A lead rubber apron is worn to protect the abdomen and pelvis
- The leg is rotated to align the patella between the femoral condyles and a small pad is placed under the tibia to prevent rotation of the leg

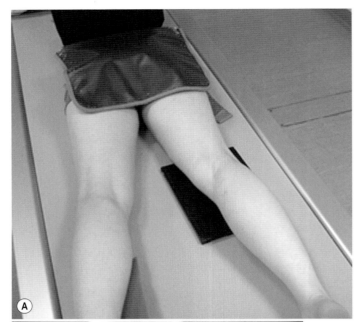

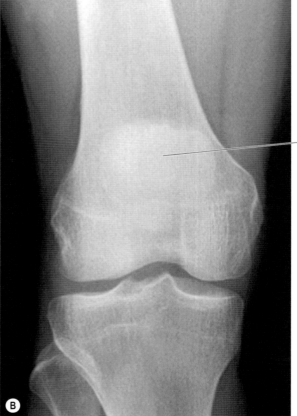

Figure 9.7 PA patella.

Beam direction and FRD

Vertical central beam, at 90° to the IR
100 cm FRD

Centring point

In the middle of the of the crease of the knee

Collimation

Femoral and tibial condyles, knee joint, surrounding soft tissues

Criteria for assessing image quality

- Distal third of femur, proximal third of tibia, head of fibula, patella and soft tissue outlines should all be demonstrated
- Patella is centralised over the femur
- Head of fibula should appear slightly obscured by tibia
- Shafts of tibia and fibula should be separated
- Sharp image demonstrating the bony cortex and trabeculae of patella in contrast to the femur

Inferosuperior patella

This projection is often undertaken to evaluate the patellofemoral joint in an orthopaedic assessment before and after knee surgery. It must not be attempted if there is a suspected fracture of the patella, as in the case of a transverse fracture, because the fragments can be further separated and thus exacerbate the effects of injury. However, if the patient presents with some flexion of the knee, method 3 may be considered.

There are several methods for achieving this projection and three will be described here. Method 1 is the preferred method as the central ray is not directed directly towards the gonads. In method 2, although the main beam is not directly towards the patient's abdomen, it is still aimed in the direction of the trunk. Method 3 is commonly described with the patient seated and supporting the IR themselves.[1,6,8,9] However, where the patient is supine[10] and the IR can be placed vertically, not only will greater radiation protection be achieved for the patient, i.e. the main beam will not be directed at the patient's torso and towards their fingers, but the risk of movement unsharpness from the patient holding the IR will be removed. Many digital radiography (DR) detectors are quite cumbersome and a computed radiography (CR) cassette may be preferable for this projection. In all cases the patient should wear a lead rubber apron for radiation protection.

To demonstrate the lateral movement of the patella if subluxation is suspected the projection can be performed with the knee at varying angles of flexion, e.g. 30°, 60° and 90°.[11]

Positioning

Method 1 (Fig. 9.8A,B)

IR is horizontal
- The patient lies in the prone position with the IR below the knee of the leg to be examined
- The unaffected leg is separated from the leg under examination, to clear it from the radiation field
- The knee is flexed through 60° and immobilised with the use of a bandage around the ankle; this is held by the patient. Alternatively, radiolucent pads and sandbags may be placed under the lower leg for support (although a significant depth of pad would be required for this)
- The patella is centralised over the femur

Method 2 (Fig. 9.9)

IR is vertical
- The patient lies on the side under examination with knee flexed through approximately 75°
- The unaffected leg is cleared backwards, away from the leg under examination, to clear it from the radiation field
- The patient's arms are used as support

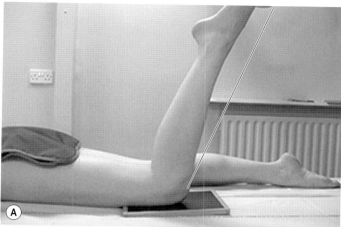

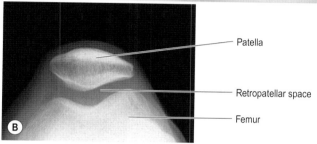

Figure 9.8 (A) Inferosuperior patella – method 1; (B) inferosuperior patella.

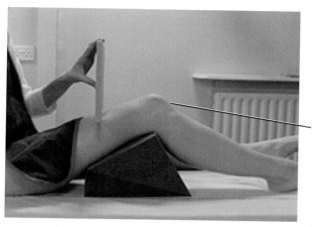

Figure 9.10 Inferosuperior patella – method 3.

- The unaffected leg is separated from the leg under examination, to clear it from the radiation field
- The IR is supported vertically, its lower edge in contact with the lower end of the femur and at 90° to the long axis of the patella (the tube side of the IR is towards the knee and feet)
- If no holder is available the IR must be supported by the patient, but this leads to an increased radiation dose, especially to the trunk and hands. There is also increased potential for movement unsharpness and distortion of image if the patient does not maintain the correct relationship of the IR to the patella

Beam direction and FRD

Method 1: Vertical, directed cranially (approximately 15°) to coincide with the long axis of the patella
100 cm FRD
Method 2: Horizontal, at 90° to the IR and to coincide with the long axis of the patella
Method 3: Horizontal, directed cranially up to approximately 15° and to coincide with the long axis of the patella

Centring point: all methods

Immediately below (behind) the apex of the patella

Collimation

Patellofemoral joint space, articular surfaces of the femur, anterior surface of the patella, surrounding soft tissues

Criteria for assessing image quality

- Patella is projected clear from the femoral condyles for a clear view of the patellofemoral joint space
- Sharp image demonstrating the joint space and surrounding soft tissues, in contrast to the bony cortex and trabeculae of patella

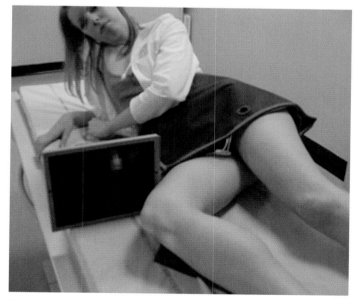

Figure 9.9 Inferosuperior patella – method 2.

- The IR is positioned in the vertical position on the table, tube side in contact with the lower end of the femur and at 90° to the long axis of the patella, or support using pads and sandbags

Method 3 (Fig. 9.10)

- The patient lies supine on the table with the affected knee flexed through 60°

105

FEMUR

The femur has a wide variation in subject contrast from the hip joint, through the shaft and down to the knee joint; to reduce this it is advisable to use a kVp of at least 75.

The increasing size of the population, particularly in the western world,[12] has not been reflected in the availability of significantly larger IRs and, unfortunately, average limb length has been seen to have increased even more than trunk length. This has implications for radiographic examination of the femur, which ideally should have only one exposure per projection, with the entire femur from hip to knee included. In reality, limitations of IR space very often require the radiographer to provide images of the upper and lower femur on two overlapping images of the same projection.

CR cassettes remain at a maximum 35 × 43 cm in size, but most DR IRs have a maximum size of 43 or 45 cm^2 or 35 × 47 cm. There will be increased space for the femoral length on the larger receptor if it is positioned diagonally, compared to the space available across the diagonal of the 34 × 43 cm cassette. Simple mathematical calculation of the length of the diagonal in the 43 cm^2 receptor shows it to be 60.8 cm, compared to 55 cm in the case of the 35 × 43 cm cassette, although it must be noted that this only relates to the extreme measurement from corner to corner. The 35 × 47 cm IR will facilitate even more of the body area.

If the femur really is too long for inclusion on one image, the leg should remain in the same position for both images used for the same projection, to assess the rotation of any fracture, and there should be overlap of the mid shaft of the femur on each image. Follow-up images taken for orthopaedic assessment only require demonstration of the fracture site and associated or nearest joint (unless there is a surgical prosthesis or pin present), thereby reducing the radiation exposure for these assessments to one projection.

Radiation protection is an essential consideration and the 28-day rule should be applied when the whole femur is to be demonstrated. Gonad protection is also essential, and careful positioning of this, to avoid covering the hip joint or upper femoral shaft, will prevent unnecessary repeats.

If it is considered that the gonad protection available may exclude part of the required information on the lateral projection of the upper femur, it should not be used. There is no reason for its use to be excluded when undertaking examinations of the lower femur.

AP femur (Fig. 9.11A,B,C)

IR is horizontal

Positioning

- The patient lies supine on the table with their legs extended
- The posterior aspect of the femur under examination is placed in contact with the IR and positioned to include the hip and knee joint if possible. If this is not possible, ensure that the knee is included if the lower two-thirds of the femur is required (Fig. 9.11A). If the upper third is required, the hip joint should be included
- The unaffected leg is separated from the leg under examination, to clear it from the radiation field
- The leg is internally rotated approximately 15° to bring the femur into the true AP position and the neck of the femur parallel to the IR
- A lead rubber apron is applied to the lower abdomen for radiation protection

Beam direction and FRD

Vertical at 90° to the IR
100 cm FRD

Centring point

Mid shaft, on the anterior aspect of the femur*

Collimation

Knee and hip joints, surrounding soft tissues*

*Note that the asterisked sections will require consideration for amendment if two images of the projection are required, when femoral length dictates this. Realistically, the *central ray* can be considered to be in the middle of the area covered by the IR space.

Criteria for assessing image quality

- Knee and hip joints, patella and all the soft tissue outlines should be demonstrated (or the area intended for inclusion if the whole femur cannot be included on the IR)
- Greater trochanter should be seen in profile on the lateral aspect of the upper femur and cleared from the neck
- Lesser trochanter, if included, should be seen on the medial aspect of the femur
- Sharp image demonstrating the soft tissue margins, bony cortex and trabeculae of femur; care should be taken in kVp selection to reduce the inherent contrast in the femur

Common errors	Possible reasons
Both joints not demonstrated	Inaccurate assessment of adequacy of receptor size or IR not positioned accurately. Patient simply may have long legs
Greater trochanter overlaps neck of femur	Inadequate internal rotation of leg

Lateral femur (Fig. 9.12A,B,C)

IR is horizontal

Positioning

- From the AP position the patient is rotated onto the side under examination with the opposite leg placed behind them, on the table-top
- With the knee and hip slightly flexed, the femur is positioned to include the hip and knee joint if possible. If this is not possible, ensure that the knee is included if the lower two-thirds of the femur is required (Fig. 9.12A). If the upper third is required, the hip joint should be included
- The femoral condyles are superimposed and a sandbag is placed under the ankle joint to help facilitate this. The more the hip is flexed, the easier it becomes to rotate the patient into a lateral position
- Foam pads may also be used to aid positioning and immobilisation, as for the lateral knee projection
- A lead rubber apron is place over the lower abdomen for radiation protection

Beam direction and FRD

Vertical at 90° to the IR
100 cm FRD

Centring point

Mid shaft, on the medial aspect of femur*

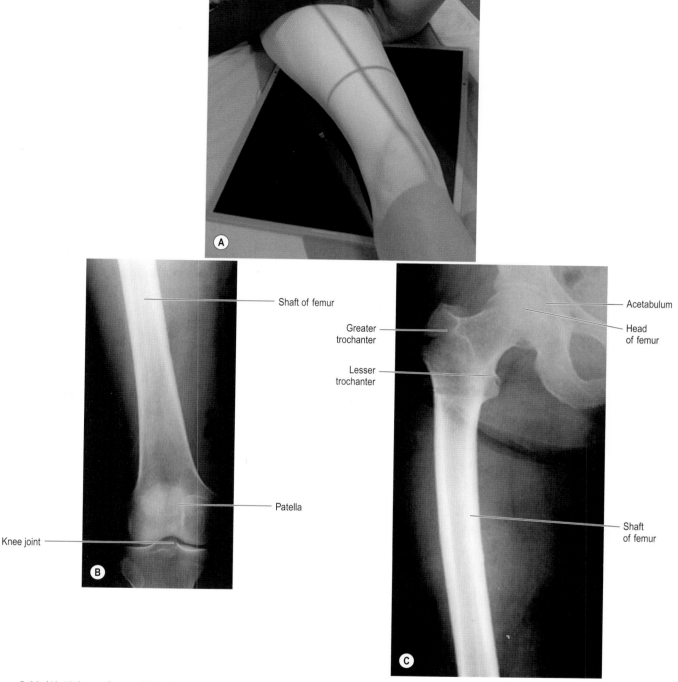

Figure 9.11 (A) AP lower femur; (B) AP lower femur; (C) AP upper femur.
(B) and (C) Reproduced with permission from Bryan GJ. Skeletal anatomy. 3rd ed. Edinburgh: Churchill Livingstone; 1996 and Gunn C. Bones and joints. 4th ed. Edinburgh: Churchill Livingstone; 2002.

Collimation

Hip and knee joints, surrounding soft tissues*

*As for the AP femur, these will vary according to the amount of femur that can be included on the image receptor.

Following *trauma* or *surgery* it may be necessary to undertake *horizontal beam lateral* projections. In either of these cases consider undertaking a horizontal beam lateral neck of the femur as described in Chapter 10, and horizontal beam lateral of the knee and lower two-thirds of the femur. To take this mediolateral approach, the opposite leg must be uninjured so that it can be raised. If this is not possible a lateromedial approach should be used for the lower two-thirds of the femur, with appropriate protection for the other leg, and a mediolateral oblique used as for the femoral neck lateral. This is described in Chapter 25 and in Figure 25.20.

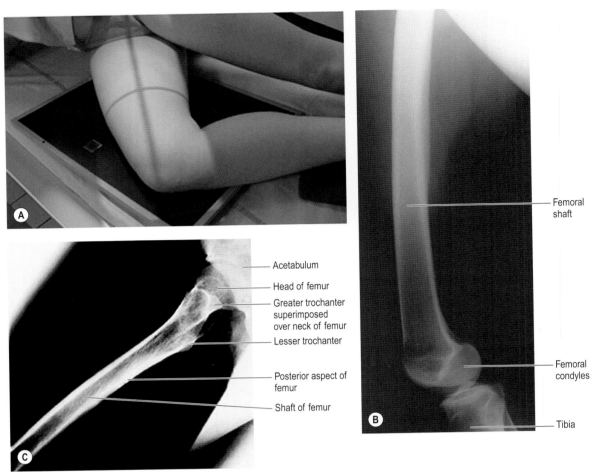

Figure 9.12 (A) Lateral femur; (B) lateral lower femur; (C) lateral upper femur.
(C) Reproduced with permission from Bryan GJ. Skeletal anatomy. 3rd ed. Edinburgh: Churchill Livingstone; 1996 and Gunn C. Bones and joints. Edinburgh: Churchill Livingstone; 2002.

Criteria for assessing image quality

- Hip, knee joint, patella and surrounding soft tissues are demonstrated, or the area intended for inclusion if the whole of the femur cannot be included on the image receptor
- Patellofemoral joint space is visualised (unless the patella is not naturally centralised on the individual patient)

- Greater trochanter is superimposed on the shaft of femur
- Lesser trochanter is seen in profile on the posterior aspect of the femur
- Sharp image demonstrating the soft tissue margins, bony cortex and trabeculae of femur; care should be taken in kVp selection to reduce the inherent contrast in the femur

REFERENCES

1. Long BW, Rafert JA. Orthopaedic radiography. Philadelphia: WB Saunders; 1995.
2. Raby N, et al. Accident and emergency radiology: a survival guide. London: Saunders; 2001.
3. Radiation protection 118 referral guidelines for imaging. European Commission Directorate-General for the Environment; 2000.
4. Burnett S, et al. A-Z orthopaedic radiology. London: WB Saunders; 2000.
5. Vince AS, Singhania AK. What knee X-rays do we need? A survey of orthopaedic surgeons in the United Kingdom. Knee 2000;7(2):101–4
6. Whitley AS, et al. Clark's positioning in radiography. 12th ed. Oxford: Hodder Arnold; 2005.
7. McQuillen-Martensen K. Radiographic image analysis. 3rd ed. Philadelphia: WB Saunders; 2010.
8. Eisenberg RL, et al. Radiographic positioning. 2nd ed. Boston: Little Brown and Company; 1995.
9. Bontrager KL. Textbook of radiographic positioning and related anatomy. 5th ed. St Louis: Mosby; 2001.
10. Bontrager KL, Lampignano JP. Textbook of radiographic positioning and related anatomy. 7th ed. St Louis: Mosby; 2010.
11. Unett EM, Royle AJ. Radiographic techniques and image evaluation. London: Nelson Thornes; 1997.
12. Cole TJ. Secular trends in growth. Nutrition Sociology 2000;59(2):317–24.

Chapter 10

Pelvis and hips

Linda Williams

Radiographic examination of the pelvis and hips must be undertaken with care as the region surrounds the radiosensitive reproductive organs. Gonad protection should be used in most cases and should be correctly positioned (Fig. 10.1A,B); an exception is made when examining the female pelvis in trauma, for an initial examination of a child, or when there is a non-specific region of pain in the first examination. The 28-day rule should always be used in women of reproductive capacity when examining this area.

INDICATION

The pelvis and hips may be examined for the following reasons:

Multiple myeloma

Osteolytic lesions may occur in the pelvis and the pelvis may be examined as part of a skeletal survey, although radionuclide imaging plays a greater role in this instance.

Osteoarthritis

The hip joints may degenerate in this condition, but radiographic examination should only be performed if the patient is likely to require hip replacement.[1]

Trauma

The pelvis and hips are commonly examined in the event of trauma, as this is most likely to establish whether a fracture or dislocation has occurred. As the pelvis consists of three bony rings, the main pelvic ring and the two secondary rings formed from the pubic and ischial bones, it is important to remember that a fracture of such a bony ring is usually associated with a fracture elsewhere in the ring (contracoup fracture).

Further reading on image interpretation is suggested at the end of the chapter.

Perthes'

A disorder of the upper femoral epiphysis, this manifests as osteonecrosis of the capital femoral epiphysis.[2] This is where the growing epiphysis shows ischaemic changes. It presents most commonly in children aged 4–9 years, and boys are four times more likely to be affected than girls.[3]

Slipped upper femoral epiphysis

The epiphysis is displaced, usually medially and posteriorly. The patient often presents with spontaneous pain in the groin. Thirty percent of patients suffering from this are obese, and the condition is possibly related to hormonal imbalance.[3]

Anteroposterior (AP) pelvis and hips
(Fig. 10.2A,B,C)

There are two methods for producing the AP pelvis: the first demonstrates the full pelvis and hip joints, the second is required for hips only. This second projection is usually requested for follow-up after hip replacement surgery and may be referred to as a 'low centred' pelvis. However, it is a valid and recognised projection, having been described in texts for many years.[4-7] Radiographers should not, therefore, assume that this is simply a 'mis-centred pelvis' and consider it to be a suboptimal procedure. Field size is as for the pelvis and hips AP, as it is often necessary to include a longer section of the femur to ensure the whole length of hip prosthesis is demonstrated (if relevant).

IR is horizontal, employed with antiscatter grid (for adults).

Positioning

- The patient lies supine on the table with their legs extended and their head resting on a pillow
- The median sagittal plane (MSP) is at 90° to the table-top and the anterior superior iliac spines (ASISs) should be equal distance from the table-top
- The arms are raised onto the pillow
- The legs are slightly internally rotated to bring the necks of femora parallel to the table-top
- Gonad protection is applied if appropriate. Exceptions are when examining the female pelvis in trauma, for a first examination of a child, or when there is a non-specific region of pain in the first examination

For this projection both feet are internally rotated slightly during positioning to bring them into the true anatomical position and allow the neck of femur (NOF) to lie parallel to the image receptor (IR).[4,7] This facilitates demonstration of the femoral neck with minimal fore-shortening, and also clears the greater trochanter from the femoral neck, the lesser trochanter appearing in profile medially. If the feet are excessively internally rotated the lesser trochanter will be obscured and if they are externally rotated, or even if the toes point in an upwards and vertical direction, the NOF will appear foreshortened on the resulting image, with the greater trochanter superimposed over the neck.[4,7]

In the case of trauma, foot position can provide an indication of a fractured NOF. The patient will present with the affected leg in noticeable external rotation, often with the lateral aspect of the foot in contact with the trolley top and apparent shortening of the leg. No attempt must be made to move or internally rotate this leg.[2]

A line known as Shenton's line (Fig. 10.3) follows the curve of the upper border of the obturator foramen and continues to travel inferiorly down the medial border of the femoral neck. This line can be used as a guide to compare the two sides when checking for injury, as a disruption in the normally smooth, curved line indicates subluxation, dislocation or change in femoral neck position as a result of fracture.

Overexposure of the greater trochanters can be a problem in this projection, particularly in thin patients who have little soft tissue in this region. This can be resolved by careful consideration of exposure factors: a reduction in mAs will reduce the degree of image blackening, and to cater for this a kVp of at least 70 will reduce the level of subject contrast.[4,7] It is suggested that a minimum of 70 kVp be used in all AP pelvis examinations.

Some patients will present with a body shape which is relatively slim over the legs and hip joint but larger over the pelvis and abdomen. This shape appears to occur most frequently in elderly women and can pose a problem in producing an image with a useful range of densities. The use of a kVp even higher than 70 may be useful in these cases, as the central region of the pelvis may appear underexposed when the hips appear correctly exposed (and vice versa) on the image when insufficient kVp is used. Use of an automatic exposure device can create problems in patients with this type of build: use of the outer chambers will result in termination of exposure related to thinner body tissue areas, therefore the central pelvic area will be of low radiographic density; use of the central chamber may mean that the area over the hips is over-blackened.

Beam direction and focus receptor distance (FRD)

Vertical at 90° to the IR
115–120 cm FRD

Note that the FRD suggested is longer than the traditional 100 cm used for the majority of radiographic projections. The buttocks elevate

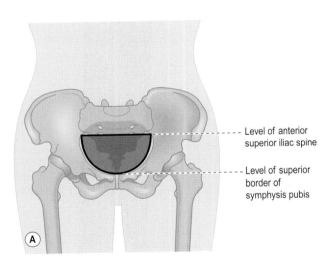

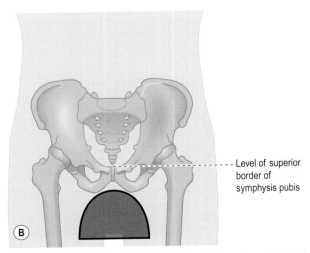

Figure 10.1 Position for gonad protection for (A) female patient and for (B) male patient.

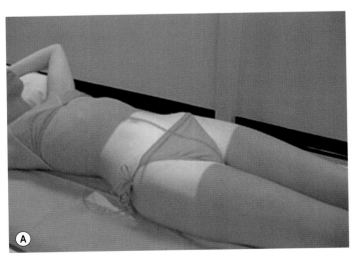

Figure 10.2 (A) AP position – pelvis and hips.

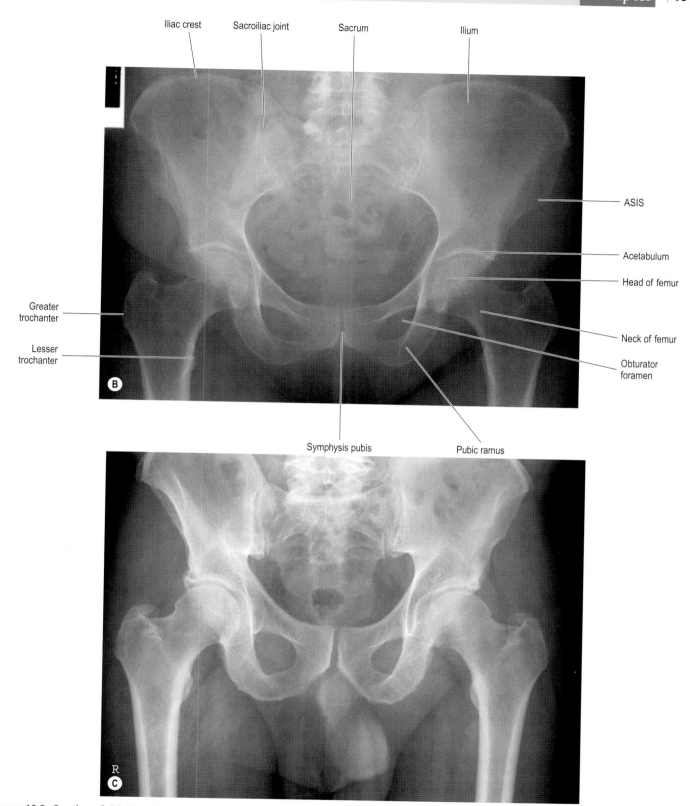

Figure 10.2, Continued (B) AP pelvis and hips; (C) centring the AP pelvis for hips.

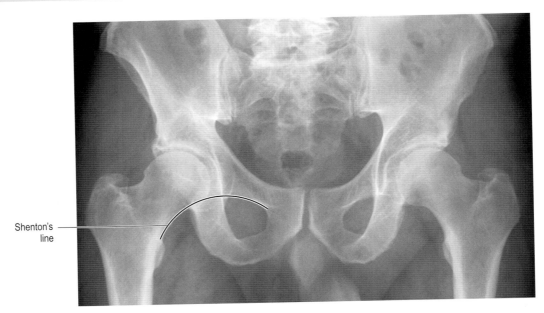

Shenton's
line

Figure 10.3 Shenton's line.

the pelvis, which is a relatively large structure, thereby increasing object–receptor distance (ORD) and magnification of the pelvis. The larger pelvis will potentially be less likely to be included within the perimeter of the IR; to overcome this, increasing the FRD reduces this magnification and improves on image sharpness.

Those patients with a noticeably larger amount of adipose tissue will, in effect, find their pelvis raised even higher above the IR than slimmer patients. Therefore, an FRD of 120 cm is recommended in these patients.

Centring point

For the pelvis and hips: in the midline, midway between the ASIS and the upper border of the symphysis pubis

While centring, it is wise to check that the tops of the iliac crests lie within the upper border of the IR; this will ensure that the maximum amount of anatomy distal to the iliac crests is demonstrated on the image.

For the hips: in the midline, 2.5 cm above the superior border of the symphysis pubis (the upper border of the symphysis pubis is located level with the greater trochanters)

Collimation

For the pelvis and hips: iliac crests, proximal portion of femora, greater and lesser trochanters

The IR may be aligned with the X-ray beam before examining the patient and, as originally suggested by Unett and Royle[4] and later by others,[7] collimation can be adjusted at this point. This avoids the temptation to open the collimators wider than necessary when X-raying a larger than average patient.

For the hips: acetabulae, greater and lesser trochanters, upper third of femur or full length of the prosthesis (if present)

If previous images are available it is recommended that they be viewed to establish the length of any surgical device that may be present in the hip/s to ensure that the IR is positioned correctly for their inclusion.

Criteria for assessing image quality

- Iliac crests and greater and lesser trochanters are demonstrated for full pelvis, acetabulae, trochanters and appropriate amount of femur for the hips only
- Iliac bones, heads and necks of femora and the greater and lesser trochanters and obturator foramina should be symmetrical
- Sharp image demonstrating the range of densities of the bony cortex and trabeculae of the pelvis and its soft tissues, hips and trochanters

Common errors	Possible reasons
Asymmetry of structures	MSP not 90° to table-top (rotated patient). This could be due to muscular atrophy or simply the patient lying awkwardly. Use of radiolucent pads may help correct this in the case of muscular atrophy. The notable features in the pelvis are the obturator foraminae and iliac bones; study of a rotated pelvis image will show a larger obtutator foramen (compared with the other obturator foramen) and narrowed ilium on the side that is raised from the table
Greater trochanters obscured and overlying the NOF	Feet are not internally rotated (this is unavoidable in patients with fractured NOF)
Overexposed image (see section after positioning, for overexposure of the greater trochanters and uneven exposure of hips and pelvis)	If an automatic exposure device (AED) has been used for a patient with hip prostheses the exposure will continue for longer than necessary to try to expose the hips correctly. There are other problems associated with AED use (see comments after the positioning section for the pelvis). Setting a manual exposure is a suitable solution in both events described here

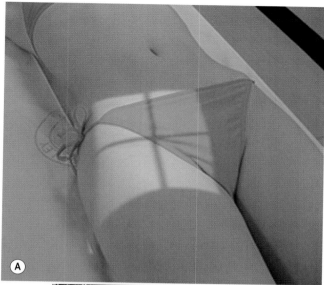

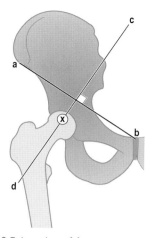

a–b = line from ASIS to upper symphysis pubis

c–d = bisects **ab** at 90°

x = femoral pulse 2.5 cm below where **cd** bisects **ab**

Figure 10.5 Location of femoral pulse.

Centring point

Over the femoral pulse

The femoral pulse (and therefore the centre of the head of femur) is located thus: draw an imaginary line from the ASIS to the upper border of the symphysis pubis; bisect this line perpendicularly and then locate a point 2.5 cm distally along this bisecting line (Fig. 10.5).

Collimation

ASIS, greater and lesser trochanters, proximal third of femur; full length of prosthesis if relevant.

Criteria for assessing image quality

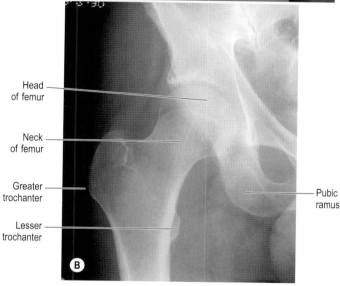

Head of femur

Neck of femur

Greater trochanter

Lesser trochanter

Pubic ramus

Figure 10.4 AP single hip.

* ASIS, proximal third of the femur and trochanters are demonstrated
* Greater trochanter is seen cleared from and laterally to the NOF, and slightly in profile
* Lesser trochanter is visible on the medial aspect of the femur
* Obturator foramen is seen 'open' and not obscured by the ischium
* Sharp image demonstrating the soft tissue margins, bony cortex and trabeculae of the distal ilium, ischium and proximal femora while demonstrating the greater trochanter

AP single hip (Fig. 10.4A,B)

This projection is most likely to be undertaken as a postoperative check after hip replacement surgery.

IR is horizontal, used with antiscatter grid

Positioning

* Initial positioning is as for the AP pelvis
* The leg of the side under examination is slightly internally rotated
* The unaffected leg is abducted to clear it from the radiation field
* Gonad protection is applied and should be clear from the hip joint

Beam direction and FRD

Vertical at 90° to IR
100 cm FRD

Common errors	Possible reasons
Length of hip prosthesis not fully demonstrated	Inaccurate centring or presence of prosthesis not known or considered. Ensure previous images are available to view and if necessary, use a larger IR or field
Greater trochanter obscured and overlying the NOF	Lack of internal rotation
Overexposed image	See discussion section under AP pelvis above, for overexposure of the greater trochanters and use of automatic exposure device (AED) for patients with hip replacement

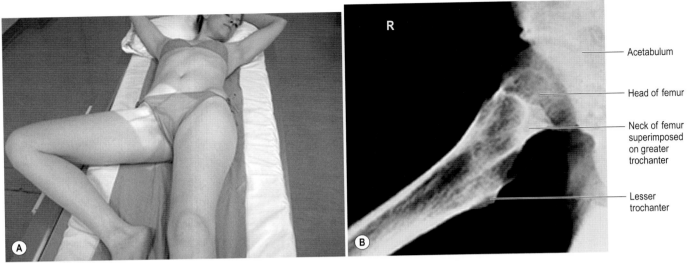

Figure 10.6 Lateral oblique single hip.
(B) Reproduced with permission from Bryan GJ. Skeletal anatomy. 3rd ed. Edinburgh: Churchill Livingstone; 1996 and Gunn C. Bones and joints. 4th ed. Edinburgh: Churchill Livingstone; 2002.

Labels on radiograph (B):
- Acetabulum
- Head of femur
- Neck of femur superimposed on greater trochanter
- Lesser trochanter

Lateral oblique single hip (Fig. 10.6A,B)

This projection must not be used in the case of trauma and is usually performed to supplement an AP pelvis when examining patients with non-specific hip pain. However, its use is rarely justified, as information gained is not significantly greater than that found on the AP hip projection.

IR is horizontal, employed with antiscatter grid

Positioning

- Initial positioning is as for the AP pelvis projection
- The MSP is 90° to the table; from this position the patient is rotated laterally through 45° onto the side under examination and supported in this position with foam pads
- The knee and hip are flexed and externally rotated to bring the lateral aspect of the thigh in contact with the table-top; the more flexion at the knee, the easier the patient finds it to achieve and maintain this position
- The arms are rested on the pillow
- Gonad protection is applied (because of the patient's position, care should be taken to prevent the gonad shield from slipping and hence obscuring essential anatomical structures)

Beam direction and FRD

Vertical at 90° to the IR
100 cm FRD

Centring point

Over the femoral pulse (see centring for AP single hip)

Collimation

ASIS, greater and lesser trochanters, anterior and posterior soft tissue outline of the femur

If, after positioning, the long axis of the femur lies obliquely across the table-top, consider rotating the light beam diaphragm to coincide with the long axis of the femur, to enable closer collimation.

Criteria for assessing image quality

- Acetabulum and proximal third of femur are demonstrated
- Greater trochanter is superimposed over the NOF
- Lesser trochanter is seen in profile on the medial aspect of the upper femur
- Ischium and pubic ramus will be superimposed
- Sharp image demonstrating the bony cortex and trabeculae of the proximal femora with sufficient penetration to demonstrate the acetabulum

Common error	Possible reason
Hyperdense area over the hip, increasing distally over the femoral shaft. Foreshortened femoral neck; the greater trochanter not superimposed over the NOF	Inadequate external rotation of the leg can cause these errors. The cause is usually inadequate flexion of the knee and insufficient rotation of the patient towards the side under examination; good knee flexion facilitates more comfortable and correct external rotation until the thigh is in contact with the table

Horizontal beam lateral for neck of femur (NOF) (Fig. 10.7A,B)

This projection must always be used if a lateral is required in cases of hip or pelvic trauma and following surgery to the hip. In these cases it is inadvisable to move the patient, but a projection at 90° to the AP projection is still often required. It is the most frequent lateral performed on the hip, despite being described in most texts as an adaptation to technique. Despite this extensive use, more recent discussion suggests that it need not be employed routinely in all cases of hip injury, suggesting that an AP alone may be sufficient.[8]

The NOF lies at 45° to the MSP and correct positioning of the IR, at 45° to the MSP and parallel to the NOF, will produce an image of the femoral neck at 90° to the AP hip image. The IR is best positioned using a 45° radiolucent pad placed next to the patient's thigh (see positioning section).

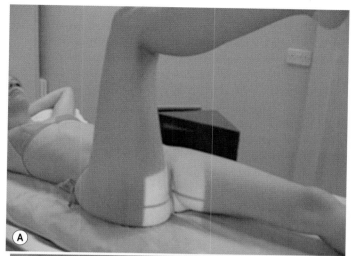

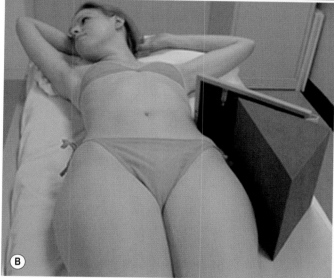

Figure 10.7 (A) Horizontal beam lateral for NOF – method 1; (B) cassette position for horizontal beam lateral hip.

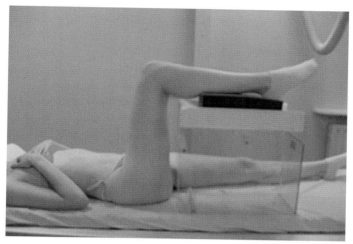

Figure 10.8 'Poole' leg support.

magnification. The method is advocated as a radiation dose-reducing technique.[9]

Positioning

Method 1 (Fig. 10.7A,B)

- The patient is supine on the A&E trolley, with the MSP perpendicular to the trolley top. The long axis of the trolley should be parallel to the ceiling track of the X-ray tube
- The MSP should also be coincident with the long axis of the trolley or parallel to the ceiling track of the X-ray tube if the patient is lying obliquely on the trolley

Method 2 (Fig. 10.9A,B)

- The X-ray tube is positioned next to the unaffected side, its light beam housing directed horizontally towards the patient
- The trolley is rotated to bring the leg on the patient's unaffected side nearer to the X-ray tube, until the patient's MSP is at 45° to the beam

Both methods

- The IR is placed vertically. The upper edge of the IR is adjacent to, and gently pushed into, the soft tissues immediately above the iliac crest on the affected side; it is then positioned at 45° to the MSP and parallel with the NOF (this must be done with great care to avoid discomfort to the patient). Note that, if using an air gap, the IR will not be in contact with the patient
- The use of a 45° foam pad between the patient and IR aids in correct assessment of receptor angle for this positioning (not particularly useful when an air gap is used)
- The holder is then adjusted to ensure that the IR and grid are pressed firmly down onto the mattress; this prevents the ischial tuberosity being omitted from the image. If using an air gap, ensure the area of interest will lie within the IR boundaries
- A leg support is placed on the table-top and the unaffected leg is flexed at the knee and hip to bring the anterior aspect of the femur as close to the trunk as possible (and at least into the vertical position to prevent superimposition of the thigh on the image)
- The ankle and foot are placed on the leg support. The greater the knee flexion, the more effective the clearance of the thigh from the hip under examination. If the patient's condition permits slight external rotation of the uninjured limb, this will clear the soft tissues of this thigh even more efficiently

As the projection requires the use of a medial approach to the hip, with horizontal beam, the unaffected leg must be cleared from the primary beam. This is achieved by the use of a leg support. This support should be radiolucent and with a comfortable lower leg and foot rest. One example of this is the 'Poole' leg support (Fig. 10.8). Great consideration for the maintenance of patient dignity and comfort is essential when positioning the leg on the support, as the position can be difficult to achieve, and revealing what is considered to be a very private area often proves embarrassing for patients.

Care should be taken when selecting exposure factors, as the inherent contrast of this area is high, from the dense hip joint down to the shaft of femur. The kVp chosen should be high enough to reduce this, and it is suggested that the range of 75–90 kVp is used.

Two initial approaches to positioning are given here, one to allow for tube angulation and the other to oblique the trolley as an alternative; both result in the same projection.

A grid is usually used with this technique to reduce scatter in image production, but studies have shown that a viable option may be to use an air gap between the IR and the patient, using method 2 for the trolley position and increasing FRD to counteract image

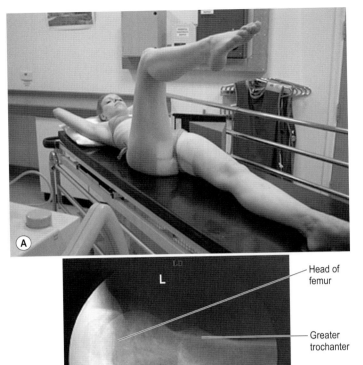

Figure 10.9 (A) Horizontal beam lateral for NOF – method 2;
(B) horizontal beam lateral. (B) Reproduced with permission from Ballinger P,
Frank E. Pocket guide to radiography. 5th ed. St Louis: Mosby; 2003.

Beam direction and FRD

Horizontal at 90° to the IR (the tube will require 45° rotational adjustment to achieve this in method 1 only)
100 cm FRD; 2 m FRD for air gap technique

Centring point

To the middle of crease of the internal and medial aspect of the groin of the affected leg

Collimation

Acetabulum, proximal femur, trochanters, anterior and posterior soft tissue outlines

Criteria for assessing image quality

• Head of femur and acetabulum clearly demonstrated
• Greater trochanter superimposed on neck of femur
• Lesser trochanter superimposed inferiorly on greater trochanter
• Soft tissue shadowing of raised thigh cleared from head and neck of femur
• Ischial tuberosity demonstrated posteriorly

• Sharp image demonstrating the soft tissue margins of the thigh, bony cortex and trabeculae of the head neck and proximal femur. The kVp chosen should be sufficient to demonstrate the acetabulum and head of femur, but the femoral neck should not be overpenetrated

Common errors	Possible reasons
The acetabulum and joint space not clearly demonstrated (dense soft tissue shadow overlying area)	The soft tissues of the opposite leg have obscured the area of interest and the exposure factors used were insufficient to penetrate them. Flex the knee and hip of the opposite leg to a greater degree
Part of the image has grid cut off	The grid is either not in a vertical position or the central ray is not at 90° to the grid
The acetabulum and joint space are clearly demonstrated but the NOF is overexposed	Incorrect exposure factors have been chosen; consider using a higher kVp and reducing the mAs, or use a filter
The image appears very grey and it is difficult to distinguish features	The collimation is insufficient and too much scattered radiation has reached the receptor. Collimate more closely and consider the use of lead rubber sheets over the anterior aspect of the patient's thigh on the side under examination

ACETABULUM

Acetabular fractures carry significant clinical sequelae but are difficult to assess in some cases, for example when the femoral head has pushed through the acetabulum but sprung back by the time the radiograph is taken, leaving only subtle soft tissue signs.[10] Reports show that as many as 57% of acetabular fractures are missed on plain radiography, and it is advisable to use computed tomography (CT) to accurately assess the existence, nature and extent of an injury to the acetabulum.[10] To some degree the extent of the injury can be established if the appropriate plain radiographic obliques of the acetabulum are undertaken.

The techniques described here are sometimes referred to as Judet obliques, first described by the brothers Judet in 1964;[2] they are also referred to as 'acetabulum en face' and 'profile' by Unett and Royle,[4] which are quite meaningful terms when considering the aspect of the acetabulum demonstrated by each projection. The projections, if taken in conjunction with an AP pelvis, allow for a more complete assessment of the acetabulum. Both obliques are necessary for a complete examination.

IR is horizontal, used with antiscatter grid, for both projections.

Acetabulum posterior rim/en face/obturator oblique position (Fig. 10.10A,B)

IR is horizontal, employed with antiscatter grid

Positioning

• The patient lies supine on the table with their legs extended and their head resting on a pillow
• Initially the MSP is 90° to the table; from this position the patient's trunk is rotated through 45°, away from the side under examination
• The raised side is supported in this position with radiolucent pads
• Gonad protection is carefully applied, avoiding the area of interest

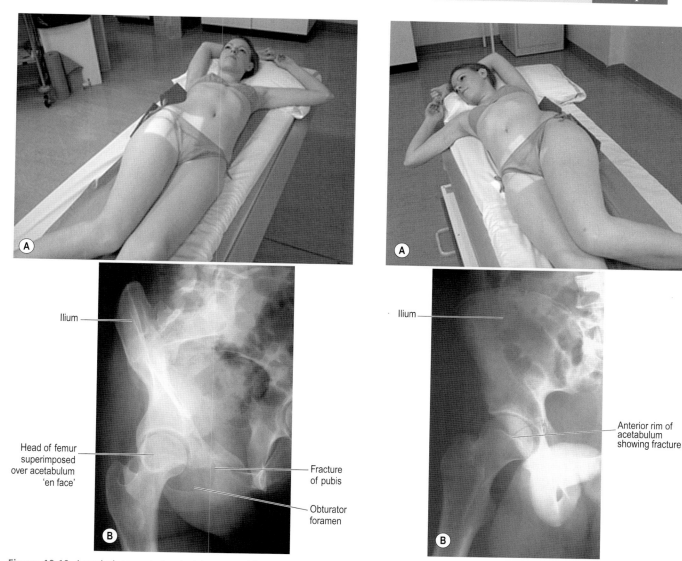

Figure 10.10 Acetabulum posterior rim/obturator oblique.

Ilium

Head of femur
superimposed
over acetabulum
'en face'

Fracture
of pubis

Obturator
foramen

Ilium

Anterior rim of
acetabulum
showing fracture

Figure 10.11 Acetabulum anterior rim/iliac oblique position.

Acetabulum anterior rim/profile/iliac oblique position (Fig. 10.11A,B)

IR is horizontal, employed with antiscatter grid

Positioning

- The patient lies supine on the table with their legs extended and their head resting on a pillow
- Initially the MSP is 90° to the table; from this position the patient's trunk is rotated through 45° towards the side under examination
- The raised side is supported in this position with radiolucent pads
- Gonad protection is carefully applied

Beam direction and FRD

Vertical at 90° to the IR
100 cm FRD

Centring point

Over the femoral pulse (Fig. 10.5)

Collimation

ASIS, ischium, pubic ramus

The obliques described should be undertaken when a complete orthopaedic assessment of the patient's pelvis has been carried out and it has been established that the pelvis is stable enough for movement. If not, and it is possible to lower the unaffected side of the pelvis, the projection for acetabulum en face can be undertaken as normal. For acetabulum in profile the patient remains in this position and the IR is supported vertically behind the raised side, using a horizontal central ray. Centre over the raised hip.

If injury to both acetabulae is suspected it is possible to examine one acetabulum in the en face position while the opposite one is in the lateral position, and vice versa with wider collimation. This will cut the number of exposures from four to two but, by centring in the midline, the accuracy of the resulting radiograph of each acetabulum will not be as accurate as performing separate well-centred projections. The central portion of the pelvis will also be irradiated, when it is likely that this area would not be irradiated if four well-coned exposures were made.

If there is access to a fluoroscopy suite with transverse C-arm rotational function, the injured patient can be moved across onto the table, using a suitable patient handling aid, and be examined using this equipment. The C-arm is rotated through 45° towards either side and this will achieve the same images as described above. This technique can be used with an ordinary X-ray tube and table, but problems with cross-gridding arise unless the bucky can be adjusted to bring the grid slats 90° to the long axis of the table-top. Using a stationary grid can allow the grid slats to be placed in the correct direction, but this method does require placement of the IR in a tray under the table or trolley, and will depend on the type of imaging system available.

Criteria for assessing image quality

Acetabulum posterior rim/en face/obturator oblique position

- The head and neck of femur are demonstrated with the acetabulum rim outlined as a circle ('en face')
- The posterior rim of the acetabulum is particularly well demonstrated
- The ilium is demonstrated in profile with the obturator foramen seen open
- Sharp image demonstrating the bony cortex and trabeculae of the head of femur and cortical outline of the acetabular rim

Acetabulum anterior rim/profile/iliac oblique position

- The anterior acetabular rim is superimposed across the head of femur
- The iliac wing is seen 'en-face' and without foreshortening
- The ischial spine is demonstrated in profile medial to the acetabulum
- Sharp image demonstrating the bony cortex and trabeculae of the head of femur and cortical outline of the acetabular rim

Lateral ilium and AP ilium

IR and positioning

Lateral ilium: As for the acetabulum posterior rim/obturator oblique position (Fig. 10.10A)
Ap ilium: As for the acetabulum anterior rim/iliac oblique position (Fig. 10.11A)

Beam direction and FRD for both projections of the ilium

Vertical at 90° to the IR
100 cm FRD

Centring point

Lateral ilium: over the ASIS of the raised side
AP ilium: midway between the midline and the ASIS of the raised side

Collimation

Sacroiliac joint, iliac crest, ischium, pubic ramus

Criteria for assessing image quality

Lateral ilium

- Iliac crest, symphysis pubis, sacroiliac joint and ASIS are demonstrated
- Ilium is demonstrated in profile
- Opening of the obturator foramen as compared to the AP pelvis
- Sharp image demonstrating the bony cortex and trabecular patterns of the ilium, pubis, acetabulum and femoral head

AP ilium

- Iliac crest, symphysis pubis, sacroiliac joints and ASIS are demonstrated
- Ilium demonstrated 'en face' with the iliac fossa seen without foreshortening
- Obturator foramen will appear closed
- Sharp image demonstrating the bony cortex and trabecular patterns of the ilium, acetabulum and femoral head

PELVIMETRY

The imaging examination of the maternal pelvis is known as pelvimetry. In circumstances when obstetricians need to decide whether a caesarean section is required, accurate measurements of the pelvic inlet and outlet are taken and compared with the biparietal diameter of the baby's skull, which has been measured during ultrasound examination. Any cephalopelvic disproportion can then be established. The examination is usually performed around the 38th week of pregnancy when the radiation risk to the viable fetus has been reduced. In some circumstances the examination is taken after a caesarean section to establish the mother's measurements for future pregnancy and delivery.

In the last decade of the 20th century, accurate CT became the method of choice for this assessment, superseding the traditional method of plain film pelvimetry. Although CT is seen as a high-dose examination, CT pelvimetry involves a relatively low-dose yet accurate technique compared to plain film pelvimetry.[11] One method uses AP and lateral scanogram/scout scans to identify the fovea over the femoral heads and a single axial CT slice to take the pelvimetric measurement. Alternatively, a single lateral scanogram from iliac crests down to include symphysis pubis may be used.

MRI has also evolved as a method of pelvimetry and has been suggested to be an excellent choice for this assessment,[12,13] especially as it avoids exposing mother and fetus to ionising radiation.

It is clear that plain radiographic pelvimetry need not and should not be undertaken. Indeed, descriptions of plain film pelvimetry have long been deliberately discontinued by some authors.[14]

REFERENCES

1. Radiation protection 118 Referral guidelines for imaging. European Commission Directorate-General for the Environment; 2000.

2. Long BW, Rafert JA. Orthopaedic radiography. Philadelphia: WB Saunders; 1995.

3. Burnett S, et al. A-Z of orthopaedic radiology. London: WB Saunders; 2000.

4. Unett EM, Royle AJ. Radiographic techniques and image evaluation. London: Nelson Thornes; 1997.

5. Kreel L, Paris A. Clark's positioning in radiography. 10th ed. London: Heinemann Medical Books; 1979.

6. Whitley AS, et al. Clark's positioning in radiography. 12th ed. London: Hodder Arnold; 2005.

7. Carver E, Carver B, editors. Medical imaging: techniques, reflection, evaluation. Edinburgh: Churchill Livingstone; 2006

8. Almazedi B et al. Another fractured neck of femur: do we need a lateral X-ray? British Journal of Radiology 2011;84:413–7.

9. Barrall T. Lateral hip air gap technique. Synergy: Imaging in Therapy and Practice. 2004; January:20–23.

10. Nicholson DA, Driscoll PA. ABC of emergency radiology. London: BMJ Publishing Group; 1995.

11. Gilstrap L et al. Operative obstetrics. 2nd ed. New York: McGraw-Hill; 2002.

12. Al-Ahwani S, et al. Magnetic resonance imaging of the female bony pelvis: MRI pelvimetry. Journal Belge de Radiologie 1991;74(1):15–8.

13. Kurjak A, Chervenak FA. Donald School textbook of ultrasound in obstetrics and gynaecology. Delhi: Jaypee Brothers; 2008.

14. Bontrager KL. Text book of radiographic positioning and related anatomy. 5th ed. St Louis: Mosby; 2001.

USEFUL READING

Ballard B. Reporting on the hip and pelvis. Synergy: Imaging in Therapy and Practice. 2010; December:16–21.

Chapter 11

Cervical spine

Barry Carver

REASONS FOR EXAMINATION

Trauma

Cervical spine injury is relatively common and is typically seen in association with road traffic accidents, falls from a height and sporting injuries. Most neck injuries are caused by transmission of force to the neck from force applied to the head. Consequently, evidence of head or facial trauma, particularly in the comatose patient, requires 'clearing the cervical spine'.[1] The overriding concern is of damage to the spinal cord, as this may result in varying degrees of paralysis or even death.

The tendency in the past has been to order plain X-radiography for all patients who have undergone trauma that might have involved the cervical spine, however minor. The positive yield of such examinations is extremely low, as injuries to the cervical spine have been found to occur in between 2% and 6.6% of patients suffering blunt trauma. Much work has been done, particularly in Canada and the USA (National Emergency X Radiography Utilization Study – NEXUS), to establish criteria for imaging referral.[2–7]

Application of these clinical criteria has been reported to have the potential to reduce requests for cervical spine radiography by up to 25%.[8] Significant savings could be made in staff and patient time, leading to financial savings as well as reductions in radiation dose to the patient.

A small but significant number of all victims of blunt trauma suffer injury to the spinal column, many of whom are young adults under the age of 40 years.[9] Damage to the spinal cord, secondary to spinal trauma and due to squeezing or shearing forces caused by displaced bone, herniated disc material or buckling of ligaments, is an important consideration in this group of patients. Despite the fact that at least three times as many spinal column injuries occur without neurological deficit as with neurological deficit, care must be taken and the cervical spine immobilised until the need for it is eliminated.[10] This caution must be observed as spinal cord injury without radiographic abnormality is a well-known phenomenon, most commonly described in children.[11] In addition, hyperextension injuries of the cervical spine may injure the spinal cord without apparent damage to the spine seen on radiographs.

Another cause of spinal cord injury is the 'whiplash' injury, which involves extremes of flexion and extension of the neck. This is most frequently the result of a road traffic accident. As the occupant of a vehicle and restrained by a seatbelt, the patient's head might be whipped backwards if the vehicle is struck from behind. Alternatively, the vehicle may stop abruptly, causing sudden forward flexion of the neck followed by forced extension. Most commonly muscular injury is seen, but in extreme circumstances quadriplegia may result from a violent whiplash injury.[10]

As stated above, all patients whose mechanism of injury is such that injury to the spinal column is suspected should be immobilised by the application of a spinal collar or similar device, until such time as the presence or absence of such injury is proven. Initial imaging must be obtained with minimal patient movement to avoid aggravating potentially unstable injuries.

Mechanism of injury is an important consideration, as symptoms of spinal injury may be masked by other distracting injuries,[12] or difficult to determine because of cranial or facial trauma.[13,14] Reliance on the mechanism of injury for referral criteria is controversial,[15] but there are specific mechanisms associated with high risk of injury, and work is ongoing in this field.[16,17]

Spinal clearance should, however, be achieved as promptly as possible, as there is significant morbidity associated with the prolonged use of spinal immobilisation in those who have undergone significant trauma.[18]

In the cervical spine lateral radiograph, a careful evaluation of the soft tissues may provide significant information about the location and extent of an injury. Even this can be the subject of debate. In adult patients it is said that the normal distance between the posterior aspect of the pharyngeal air column and the anterior vertebral margin measured at the body of C3 should be less than 7 mm;[19] however, in their study Herr et al.[20] quote less than 4–5 mm. The distance from the posterior aspect of the trachea to the anterior vertebral margin measured at the inferior aspect of C6 is more uniformly referred to as, 'should be less than 21 mm'.[19] An increase in these measurements is strongly indicative of the presence of a haematoma. Considering this information on evaluation of soft tissues, it is clear that inclusion of soft tissue is essential in the lateral projection.

Such prevertebral soft-tissue haematomas are common in patients with injury to the anterior spinal column, commonly avulsion fracture or hyperextension injury.[20] Ligament damage can occur without fracture; visualisation of the prevertebral haematoma will help

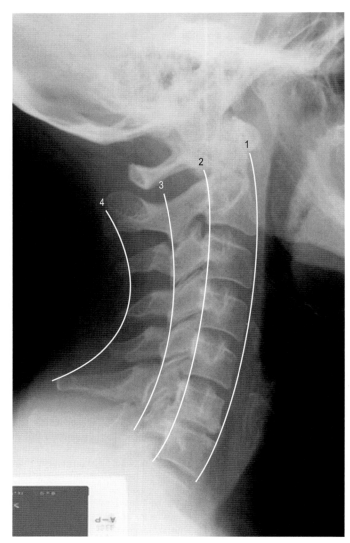

Figure 11.1 Assessing alignment of cervical vertebrae.

demonstrate the presence of such an injury, but is insensitive as a predictor of fracture or injury site.

Vertebral alignment can be demonstrated on the lateral cervical spine radiograph and is commonly assessed using examination of continuous convex lines as described below and shown in Figure 11.1.

Lines 1 and 2: The anterior and posterior spinal lines join the respective portions of the vertebral bodies.

Line 3: The spinolaminar line joins the anterior margins of the junction of the lamina and spinous processes.

Line 4: The fourth line joins the tip of the spinous processes.

Disruption of one or more of these lines can be indicative of injury. For example, if an upper vertebral body is anterior to the one below, this may be an indication of disruption of the posterior ligaments.

The cervical spine is normally lordotic in curvature; loss of lordosis has been said to be an indication of severe muscular spasm and is taken as a sign of cervical spine injury,[10] commonly seen in 'whiplash' type injuries. However, such loss of lordosis can be accentuated by neck position and may be a normal finding if the 'stiff neck' is held in a slightly flexed position during imaging. Hence it is not a reliable sign of definite injury.

Neck pain

Radiographic examination of the cervical spine is not recommended for the routine investigation of neck pain. However, cervical spine radiography may be useful where there is a history of trauma, or worsening/unresolved neurological symptoms, and in children where such pain is uncommon without a cause.[21]

Torticollis

This causes the neck to lie in abnormal lateral flexion with the head and neck rotated to the same side. This is usually caused following trauma by spasm in the sternocleidomastoid and trapezius muscles, and in isolation is not an indication for radiographic examination.

Degenerative disease processes

Symptoms of degenerative disease are commonly due to disk or ligamentous changes not demonstrated by plain film radiography.[21]

Rheumatoid arthritis

This can cause instability of the atlantoaxial joint. Subluxation may be demonstrated by a lateral view in flexion.[21]

Osteoarthritis

Osteoarthritis is not normally an indicator for radiography unless osteophytic impingement requires demonstration.

Neoplasia

See section on commonly encountered pathologies that affect the skeleton in Chapter 4.

Congenital processes

Klippel–Feil syndrome

Short neck and fused cervical vertebrae. This is not an indicator for cervical spine radiography but is seen as an incidental finding.

Cervical rib

This is an extra rib arising from C7. Cervical ribs vary in size and shape and clinical symptoms may bear little relationship to size. Its position relative to adjacent anatomy is the determining factor for severity of symptoms. It may cause compression of the subclavian artery or the brachial plexus.

RECOMMENDED PROJECTIONS

Imaging of the cervical spine, particularly in cases of trauma, has been the subject of worldwide debate for some considerable time. Although the cervical spine radiograph has long been the routine method for imaging this anatomical region, imaging department protocols vary widely as to the required 'routine' series to be undertaken. More recently, computed tomography (CT) has been used as an additional examination for equivocal findings, but there is a growing body of evidence to suggest that CT should be used as the first-line investigation.[2,15,22–24] This already tends to be the case where the patient has a head injury requiring CT,[25] owing to the correlation between major head injury and cervical spine injury, especially in the comatose patient. The increased capabilities of multidectector CT allow for better image detail and thereby enable the detection of injuries not seen on plain film.

Despite the growth in use of CT, in many centres the cervical spine is still most rapidly and most commonly initially assessed with plain X-radiography. The NEXUS study[4] has looked at its appropriateness for imaging and has proposed that there is no risk of cervical spine injury if 'low risk' criteria are met on patient examination. These criteria are:

1. No posterior midline tenderness
2. Not intoxicated
3. Normal level of alertness
4. No focal neurological deficit
5. No painful distracting injuries

As previously stated, imaging department protocols vary widely. Many centres perform a three-view series: lateral C1–C7 plus AP C3–C7 and AP C1–C2 ('odontoid process or peg'/'open mouth' view). Unfortunately there is no consensus in the literature as to what should be used. Harris et al.[26] reported that whereas 81% of Orthopaedic Trauma Association members responding to his survey used the three-view series, only 31% of the National Association of Spinal Surgeons respondents did so.

Studies such as that performed by West et al.[27] compared single-view to three-view screening, finding an increase in sensitivity from 81.8% to 83.3% in a comparatively small sample. A similar study in paediatrics by Baker et al.[28] found that a lateral view had a sensitivity of 79% for cervical spine injury, compared to 94% for the three-view series. MacDonald et al.[29] had similar findings to West and concluded that the three-view series alone was not always sufficient for adequate diagnosis.

There are other suggestions in the literature. Holliman et al.[30] suggest that the AP C3–C7 view adds little to the diagnostic ability of the series; Turetsky et al.[31] suggest its replacement by 30° trauma obliques. Doris and Wilson[32] advocate the use of obliques in a routine five-view series.

A problem with including oblique views as a five-view series is the question of 'which obliques?': 30° as above, 60° as advocated by Abel,[33] or something in between, such as 45°, as is a familiar suggestion in radiographic positioning texts.[34]

Daffner[35] goes further and discusses a routine six-view series: the five-view series as discussed above (but again with no mention as to the angle of obliquity) with the addition of a swimmer's view. It is interesting, from the perspective of a UK radiographer, to look at his results for plain X-radiography: examinations taking up to 46 minutes, with 13 radiographs being taken in one case, and 77% of patients requiring at least one repeat radiograph – standards related to radiation dose and patient care that would be unacceptable in the UK.

Following performance and evaluation of the lateral and such accessory views as may be required, the 'cervical spine series', including anteroposterior (AP), open mouth and oblique views, can be completed if no significant instability has been previously demonstrated.[36]

Some studies advocate the inclusion of flexion and extension radiographs[37] in the 'routine cervical spine series' (seven-view?), but care must be taken depending on the degree of suspicion of instability. Where a small subluxation is demonstrated, significant ligamentous injuries may be revealed by flexion and extension views. However, Pollack et al.[38] found that flexion and extension images failed to demonstrate any injuries not already demonstrated by other images; hence their usefulness must be questioned.

The cost and clinical efficacy of such protocols has also been called into question by Mirvis et al.[39] They query the use of 'routine' CT for clarifying areas of uncertainty, or non-visualised areas in asymptomatic patients, finding a less than 1% positive yield, and that finding was said to be a clinically unimportant injury. Careful clinical assessment of the patient is held to be more effective.

Also, information gained from the initial lateral image can be readily, if not necessarily fully, interpreted by the attending A&E doctor. This is less likely with CT examination, which requires radiological interpretation. CT has, however, been shown to be a more cost-effective option for imaging medium- to high-risk patients.[23]

Nunez et al.[40] found that 35% of fractures detected by CT were not seen on initial plain radiography in the most seriously ill group of patients, and that a third of these fractures were unstable, located mostly at C1/2 or C7/T1, again stressing the importance of adequate visualisation of C7. Suboptimal examinations were often found to be due to patient condition, and the suggestion is that CT be included for this most seriously injured patient group.

Lateral cervical spine

The image receptor (IR) is vertical.

Positioning

Method 1: patient standing/sitting erect (Fig. 11.2A,B)

- The patient is seated/standing with the lateral aspect of their shoulder resting against the IR
- The median sagittal plane (MSP) is parallel to the IR, with the neck extended to raise the jaw and prevent the angles of the mandible being superimposed over the vertebral bodies
- The shoulders should be relaxed and depressed as much as possible as they may obscure the lower cervical vertebrae and the cervicothoracic junction. It has been suggested that patients with broad muscular shoulders should be given a weight to hold in each hand to help project the shoulder masses below the level of C7.[34] However, this is often counterproductive, as patients frequently hunch their shoulders in an attempt to hold the weights firmly while keeping still. This is especially likely if what is being attempted is not carefully explained to the patient. Exposing the radiograph on arrested expiration may help.

Method 2: patient supine (Fig. 11.3)

This is a modification of method 1 to account for the change in patient position. This position is the one typically used in trauma, therefore movement of the patient for the performance of this projection is contraindicated. Before attempting the examination, it is always worth checking for necklaces beneath cervical collars that should have been, but often are not, removed at initial examination of the patient.

Superimposition of the shoulders can be more problematic in this position and several methods of applying shoulder traction have been described.[41,42] The key to success is again careful explanation to the patient to achieve their cooperation; traction should be applied above the elbow joints, and slowly to prevent the patient working against the application of traction.

The IR must be positioned to ensure that its inferior border is low enough to include the spinous processes of the cervical vertebrae.

- The trolley is positioned to ensure that the long axis of the cervical vertebrae is parallel to the wall or ceiling track of the X-ray tube
- 2 m focus receptor distance (FRD) is selected and the tube is centred approximately to the middle of the lateral aspect of the neck; approximate collimation to the neck should also take place at this point
- The IR is placed vertically at the side of the neck remote from the tube, its long axis parallel to the patient's MSP. Support for the IR may be via independent support designed for A&E examinations, erect holder as used for chest radiography, or sponge pads and sandbags

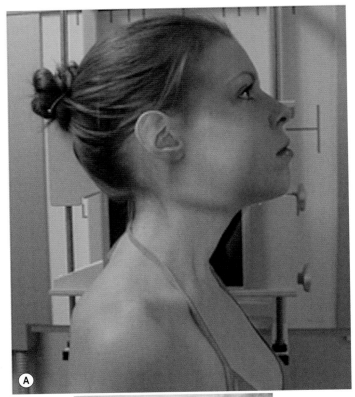

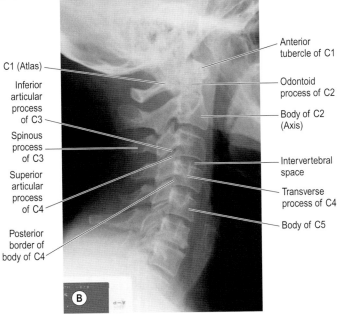

C1 (Atlas)

Inferior articular process of C3

Spinous process of C3

Superior articular process of C4

Posterior border of body of C4

Anterior tubercle of C1

Odontoid process of C2

Body of C2 (Axis)

Intervertebral space

Transverse process of C4

Body of C5

Figure 11.2 Lateral cervical vertebrae.

Beam direction and FRD: both methods

Horizontal, at 90° to the IR
200 cm FRD – to minimise magnification caused by object–receptor distance (ORD), which does, however, provide an air gap that reduces scatter reaching the IR

Centring point

In the middle of the neck at the level of the thyroid eminence

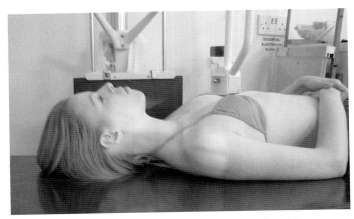

Figure 11.3 Lateral cervical vertebrae – supine (trauma) position.

A range of centring points are quoted for this examination. Fixed centring points, such as '2.5 cm posterior and inferior to the angle of mandible',[43] take no account of patient size or shape and in a larger than average person would lead to the beam being centred at soft tissues anterior to C2/3.

Collimation

Atlanto-occipital articulations, body of T1, cervical spinous processes, soft tissue structures of the pharynx

Soft tissues must be included, particularly in cases of trauma, where, as previously discussed, changes in appearance of the soft tissues can be a strong indicator of the presence of bony injury.[18,20]

Criteria for assessing image quality

- Atlanto-occipital articulations, body of T1, cervical spinous processes and soft tissue structures of the pharynx are included on the image
- Mandible should be cleared from the vertebral bodies, and the angles of the mandible in close approximation
- Left and right posterior borders of the vertebral bodies are superimposed to show no rotation
- There should be clear intervertebral joint spaces with no overlap of superior and inferior borders of vertebral bodies, to show no tilt of the cervical column
- Sharp image demonstrating soft tissue structures of the pharynx in contrast to bone and air in the trachea, detail of the bony cortex and trabeculae, the joint space between C7 and T1 and spinous processes of the cervical vertebrae

Common errors	Possible reasons
Posterior borders of the vertebral bodies not superimposed	Rotation of neck; MSP not parallel to IR (accuracy in positioning may be affected if the patient is supine and immobilised)
Superior borders of the vertebral bodies not superimposed; joint spaces may be obscured	Tilt of the neck in relationship to IR; MSP not parallel (accuracy in positioning may be affected if patient is supine and immobilised)
Superimposition of the mandible over vertebral bodies	Failure to raise the chin adequately – again may be difficult in the immobilised patient
Failure to demonstrate the body of T1	Usually due to superimposition of the shoulders over the field *or* insufficient kVp may have been used

Bony injury can manifest in many ways; fractures of the vertebrae may be obvious or very subtle, a typical example being the 'fat C2' sign, where the body of C2 appears wider than the body of C3 on a lateral radiograph.[44] This suggests the possibility of an oblique fracture of the body of C2, which may or may not be readily apparent on the lateral radiograph.

It has been estimated that, in acute cervical spine injury, up to 33% of fractures and dislocations have been missed,[10] hence the requirement for high-quality appropriate imaging. Given this figure, it is not surprising that there is a culture of ordering radiography on all possibly neck injured patients.

The American College of Radiology currently (in 2012) recommend routine CT scanning for all patients admitted after major blunt trauma.[15] However, where CT is not initially available a three-view series is recommended to include lateral cervical radiographs of C1–C7. Inclusion of C7 is vital, although not always easy! Unfortunately, the incidence of injuries at this level has been reported as up to 30% of patients with cervical spine injury, but C7 is not demonstrated in some studies in up to 40% of patients on 'cross-table' (horizontal beam) lateral radiographs.[10]

Modified projections to supplement the lateral

As previously mentioned, the cervicothoracic junction is often inadequately demonstrated on lateral projections of the cervical spine owing to superimposition of the shoulders. Where it is suspected that this may be the case, traction should be applied whenever possible (and safe) to help prevent superimposition; failure to do so inevitably results in a substandard and useless/unnecessary radiograph.

Should the body of T1 still not be demonstrated, alternatives such as the use of beam shaping filters or CT of the area should be considered. If neither is available the 'swimmers' view may be considered as a last resort. Despite the continued popularity of this projection,[45] there are concerns regarding its utility in terms of image quality and dose, with up to 45% of swimmers views failing to add to the patient's diagnosis.[46] CT is the best alternative; if unavailable, trauma oblique projections should be considered.

'Swimmers' view of C7/T1 junction

(Fig. 11.4A,B,C)

Consideration should be given to the suitability of this projection for trauma patients because of the movements required. Visualisation of the required anatomy is poor due to the overlying structures; this is exacerbated in larger patients owing to the significant increase in exposure factors required by the projection and their size. Scatter is also considerable. CT should now be the first option; if not available, alternatives such as obliques,[31–33,47] or methods for moving the shoulders down and clear from the C7/T1 junction[41,42] should be considered.

The IR should be vertical, using antiscatter device.

Positioning

- The patient should be seated/standing, or may be supine, with the lateral aspect of the shoulder resting against the IR; MSP parallel to it
- The centre of the IR is level with the heads of the humeri
- Without altering the relationship of the MSP to the IR, the arm furthest from the IR is raised and flexed at the elbow with the forearm resting across the top of the head
- The shoulder nearest the X-ray tube is lowered as far as possible

Beam direction and FRD

Horizontal at 90° to the IR
100 cm FRD

Centring point

Over the superior aspect of the head of humerus on the side nearest the tube (note that the superior aspect will lie inferiorly to the shaft when the arm is in the correct position)

Collimation

C6, T2, the anterior aspect of the vertebral bodies, the spinous processes

Criteria for assessing image quality

- C6–T2, the vertebral bodies and spinous processes are included on the image
- Right and left posterior, superior and inferior borders of the vertebral bodies are superimposed to show no rotation or tilt
- There should be vertical separation of the right and left shoulder masses enabling visualisation of the cervicothoracic junction
- Sharp image demonstrating detail of the bony cortex and trabeculae within the vertebral bodies of C6–T2, joint space between C7 and T1 and spinous process of seventh cervical vertebra

Common errors	Possible reasons
Failure to demonstrate the cervicothoracic junction – due to under/overexposed image	Exposure factors and their effect on image detail are the main problems in producing diagnostic radiographs of the cervicothoracic junction. This may be overcome with the use of an automatic exposure device with the centre chamber selected. Good collimation must be used to ensure correct exposure
Failure to demonstrate cervicothoracic junction – due to the humeri overlying vertebrae	The shoulders not adequately displaced: if due to patient condition consider other investigations to demonstrate the area (CT recommended)
Low-contrast 'grey' image	Strict collimation will significantly improve the quality of the image through a reduction in scatter

Lateral in flexion and extension

(Fig. 11.5A,B, Fig. 11.6A,B)

This projection is used to demonstrate abnormal movements or deformities such as atlantoaxial instability, and in cases of suspected ligamentous injury when the initial radiographic examination is normal; use of fluoroscopy is an alternative to the projections described below.[21]

Positioning

The principles of the technique are the same as described for the lateral projection above. The centre of the IR is coincident with the middle of the neck, with the long axis of the IR parallel to the long axis of the neck. For flexion the IR is most suitably orientated in a landscape orientation in the holder and extension with portrait orientation.

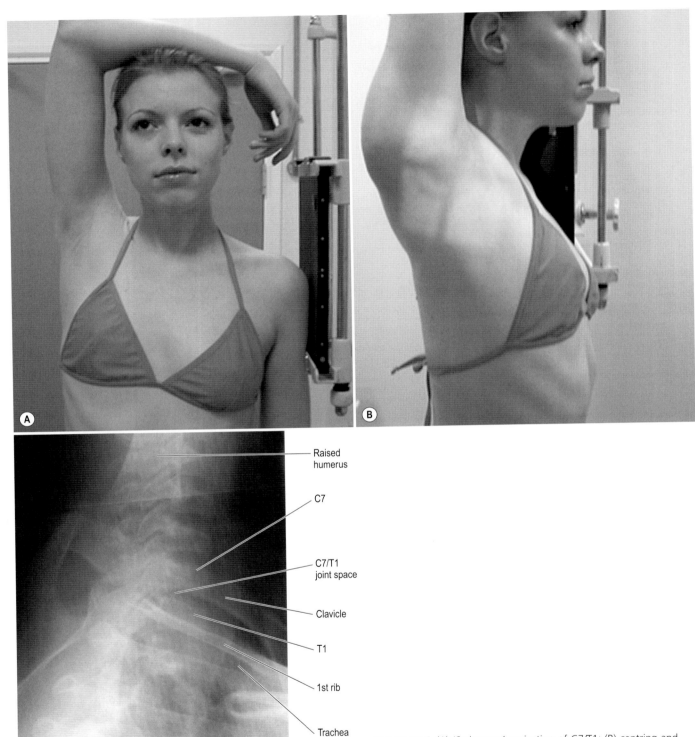

- Raised humerus
- C7
- C7/T1 joint space
- Clavicle
- T1
- 1st rib
- Trachea

Figure 11.4 (A) 'Swimmers' projection of C7/T1; (B) centring and collimation for swimmer's view; (C) swimmer's view.

Two exposures are made, one with the neck in full flexion and one in full extension; the degree of movement will be determined by patient condition and clinical indications, and should take place under medical supervision as required. The movements should not be forced and will be limited by the patient. This may be uncomfortable for the patient, so the position should be maintained for as short a time as possible.

Beam direction and FRD

Horizontal, at 90° to the IR
200 cm FRD

Centring point

To the middle of the neck at the level of the thyroid eminence

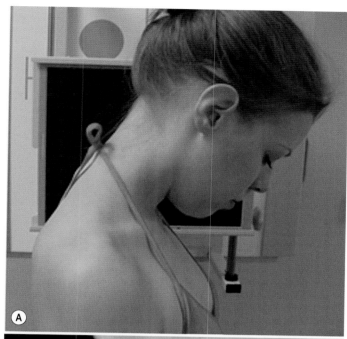

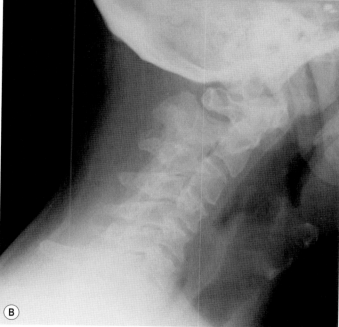

Figure 11.5 (A) Neck in flexion; (B) C-spine in flexion.

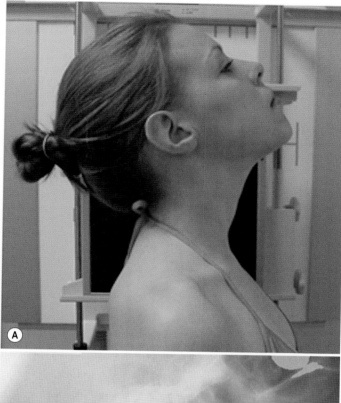

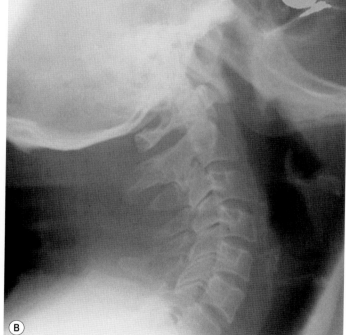

Figure 11.6 (A) Neck in extension; (B) C-spine in extension.

Collimation

Atlanto-occipital articulations, the body of T1, the anterior and posterior soft tissues

Criteria for assessing image quality

- Atlanto-occipital articulations, body of T1, anterior soft tissue structures of neck and spinous processes demonstrated

- Superimposition of right and left posterior, superior and inferior borders of vertebral bodies
- Sharp image demonstrating soft tissue structures of the pharynx in contrast to bone and air in the trachea, detail of bony cortex and trabeculae, joint space between C7 and T1 and spinous processes of cervical vertebrae

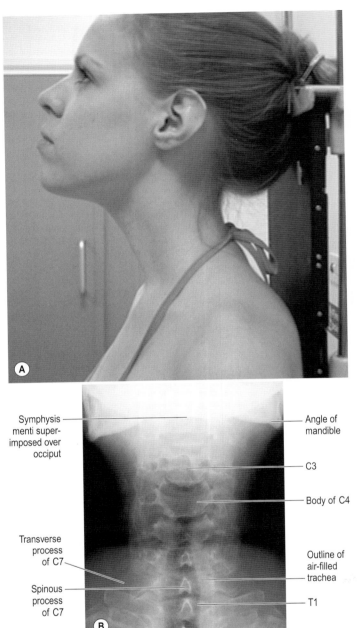

Figure 11.7 (A) AP C3–C7 with patient erect; (B) AP C3–C7.

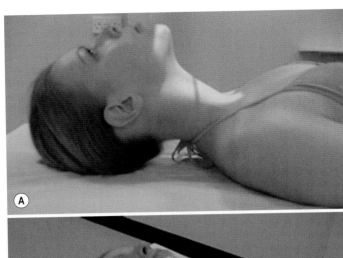

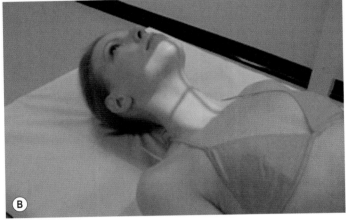

Figure 11.8 (A) AP C3–C7 with patient supine; (B) AP C3–C7 showing centring.

AP cervical spine: C3–C7 (Figs 11.7A,B, 11.8A,B)

Positioning

Method 1: patient standing or sitting erect (Fig. 11.7A)

The IR is vertical

- The patient is sitting or standing with the back of their neck resting on the IR
- The MSP is 90° to the IR
- The chin is slightly raised to superimpose the symphysis menti and the base of occiput to provide clear visualisation of C3

Method 2: patient supine (Fig. 11.8A,B)

This, as for the lateral cervical spine in method 1, is usual for trauma, where the patient will typically present on a trolley.

- The IR is placed beneath the neck or supported beneath the trolley on a tray. If placed beneath the neck then the lateral view *must* have been inspected prior to patient movement. If supported beneath the trolley in a tray effects of the increased ORD must be taken into account
- The MSP should be perpendicular to the IR wherever safely possible
- Superimposition of the symphysis menti and occiput is as for method 1, but this may not be possible with an immobilised patient

Beam direction and FRD: both methods

90° to the IR

100 cm FRD

Consider the effect of increased ORD if the patient is supine; a grid is not usually required but consideration needs to be given to patient size: a large patient may necessitate the use of a grid.

If the patient has undergone trauma and/or is in a cervical collar, or even has neck stiffness, it may not be possible to raise the chin; in which case a cranial angle should be applied to the X-ray beam; this should be sufficient to superimpose the lower mandible over the base of the occiput. The angle selected should equate to the line joining the symphysis menti to the occiput. Some neck immobilisation collars actually keep the chin elevated and superimpose the occiput over C3; in these cases a caudal angle should be employed. If angulation is used, it may be necessary to displace the IR to ensure the image falls within its boundaries.

Centring point

Over the MSP at the level of the thyroid eminence

Collimation

C2/3, T1, the transverse processes of all vertebrae included on the image

Criteria for assessing image quality

- C2/3 joint space, T1, and transverse processes are demonstrated
- Lower border of the mandible is superimposed on the base of occiput
- There is no rotation; the spinous processes are equidistant to the pedicles on each side
- Sharp image demonstrating air in the pharynx/trachea in contrast to the detail of the bony cortex and trabeculae; intervertebral disc spaces seen

Common errors	Possible reasons
Failure to visualise C3 – obscured by the mandible	Chin not raised sufficiently to superimpose the mandible over the base of occiput
Failure to visualise C3 – obscured by the occiput	Chin raised too much

Cervical rib

If it is suspected that a patient has a cervical rib, the AP cervical spine projection is modified as follows: the patient position is as described above but the central ray is directed over the sternal notch and collimation includes C3–T5 and the lateral soft tissues of the neck.

AP projection for C1/C2 (Fig. 11.9A,B)

Positioning

IR is vertical; antiscatter device is not necessary unless the patient is very large

- The patient initially is positioned as for the basic AP cervical spine position, erect or supine
- The patient opens their mouth as much as possible; if moving the head is an option it should be adjusted to bring the hard palate perpendicular to the IR. This may be achieved using the alatragal line (see Chapter 22), which lies parallel to the hard palate, as a guide. Positioning of the hard palate in this way superimposes the lower border of the upper incisors over the base of the occiput, thus clearing these structures from the odontoid process and C1/C2 joints
- The mouth is checked to ensure it is open far enough to adequately clear the teeth and mandible from the C2/C3 joint spaces

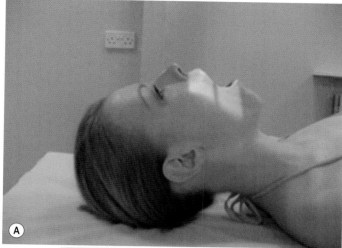

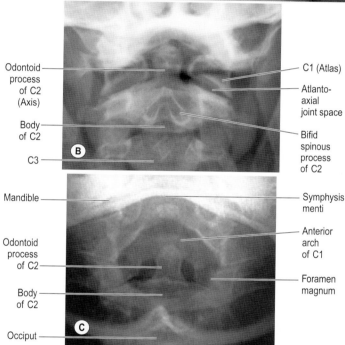

Figure 11.9 (A) AP C1–C2 (odontoid process); (B) AP C1–C2; (C) axial odontoid process.
(C) Reproduced with permission from Ballinger PW, Frank ED. Merrill's atlas of radiographic positions & radiologic procedures. St Louis: Mosby; 2003.

Beam direction and FRD

Parallel to the alatragal line
   This is especially useful as a guide for beam angulation in trauma cases where head movement is contraindicated.
100 cm FRD

Centring point

Through the open mouth at the level of the lower border of the upper incisors

Collimation

Atlanto-occipital joints, C2/C3 joint space, the transverse processes on each side

Criteria for assessing image quality

- Odontoid process, atlas, axis and atlantoaxial articulations are demonstrated and visualised symmetrically
- Upper teeth and base of the skull are superimposed
- Lower teeth are superimposed over the body of C3 but cleared from the C2/C3 joint space
- No rotation; the spinous processes are demonstrated centrally to the vertebral bodies
- Sharp image demonstrating the bony cortex and trabeculae, in contrast to adjacent soft tissues

Common errors	Possible reasons
Odontoid process obscured by upper teeth	Chin not raised sufficiently *or a* caudal beam angle is too great
Odontoid process obscured by the occiput	Chin raised too much *or a* cranial beam angle is too great
C1 and C2 not symmetrical *and/or* the lower teeth on one side obscure the C2/C3 joint space on one side	Rotation of the head
Lower teeth obscuring C2/C3 joint space bilaterally	Mouth not open sufficiently

The difficulty of obtaining the AP C1/C2 view in unconscious patients is emphasised by Blacksin and Lee,[48] who suggest CT of the craniocervical region in these patients.

For other (non-trauma) patients, for whom it is difficult to obtain an image of the odontoid process, and when the C2/C3 joint space has been adequately demonstrated, an axial odontoid peg projection can be undertaken. It is easier to undertake supine, as the chin is raised as much as possible and requires the patient to maintain this position. The central ray is then angled 25° cranially and directed midway between the angles of the mandible. The image produced shows the odontoid process through the foramen magnum (Fig. 11.9C).

OBLIQUE PROJECTIONS OF THE CERVICAL SPINE

For neurological referrals magnetic resonance imaging (MRI) examination of the neck is preferable to oblique projections of the cervical spine, which were used in the past to demonstrate the shape of the intervertebral foramina. The main use for obliques of the cervical spine is in trauma cases; obliques used are a modification of the 'routine' erect obliques and are described at the end of the section on obliques.

It should be noted that a wide variety of oblique projections have been described, the main variation being the tube angulation applied.[31,33,34,49] Which of the alternatives is used should be dependent on the pathology to be demonstrated, but those used are all too often selected from habit or protocol. For the sake of clarity and uniformity of approach, 45° neck obliquity (or 45° lateromedial tube angulation to produce appearances equivalent to 45° neck obliquity in the injured patient) is used throughout the following section, but this does not mean that it is necessarily the 'recommended technique'; reference must be made to the individual circumstances and the texts mentioned above before selecting the appropriate obliquity.

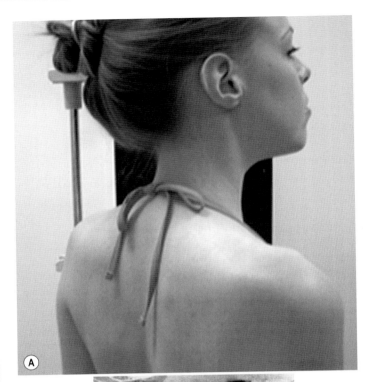

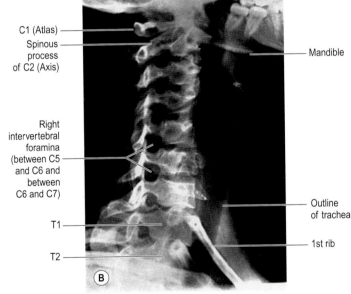

C1 (Atlas)
Spinous process of C2 (Axis)
Mandible
Right intervertebral foramina (between C5 and C6 and between C6 and C7)
Outline of trachea
T1
T2
1st rib

Figure 11.10 Anterior oblique cervical vertebrae.

Whatever obliquity is ultimately selected, the technique is broadly the same; to change from one to another simply insert the number of degrees required (not forgetting to displace the IR appropriately if using lateromedial angulation!).

Where practicable, posteroanterior (PA) obliques should be used in preference to AP obliques because of the potentially lower absorbed dose to the thyroid in this position.

Anterior obliques of the cervical spine

(Fig. 11.10A,B)

The *right anterior oblique* demonstrates the *right* intervertebral foramina.

The *left anterior oblique* demonstrates the *left* intervertebral foramina.

The IR is vertical

Positioning

- The patient is erect, facing the IR
- The patient is rotated away from the side under examination, until the MSP is at 45° to the IR. The head is turned a further 45° until the MSP of the head is parallel to the IR
- The chin is raised sufficiently to clear the mandibular rami from the upper vertebrae

Beam direction and FRD

Horizontal central ray
200 cm FRD

A 15° caudal angulation may be applied to better demonstrate the intervertebral foramina.

Centring point

To a point in the middle of the neck, at the level of the thyroid eminence

Collimation

Atlanto-occipital joints, T1, lateral soft tissue outlines

Criteria for assessing image quality

- Base of the occiput, the body of T1, and soft tissue outlines of the neck are demonstrated
- Mandible is cleared from the upper vertebrae
- Intervertebral foramina is demonstrated on the opposite side of the spine to the mandible; should be symmetrical ovoids
- Pedicles of the opposite side are projected centrally at the superior border of the vertebral bodies
- Spinous processes are demonstrated posterior to the intervertebral foramina
- Soft tissue structures of the neck are demonstrated anterior to the vertebral bodies
- Sharp image demonstrating detail of the bony cortex and trabeculae in contrast to the intervertebral foramina and adjacent soft tissue structures

Posterior obliques of the cervical spine

(Fig. 11.11)

This projection may be used as an alternative to the anterior oblique; however, it should be noted that this position will lead to increased absorbed dose in the thyroid gland.

This projection may be achieved in trauma cases with the patient supine, but the modified technique for trauma must be used, not the routine projection, as this requires patient movement, which would be contraindicated for the trauma setting.

The *right posterior oblique* (RPO) demonstrates the *left* intervertebral foramina.

The *left posterior oblique* (LPO) demonstrates the *right* intervertebral foramina.

IR is vertical

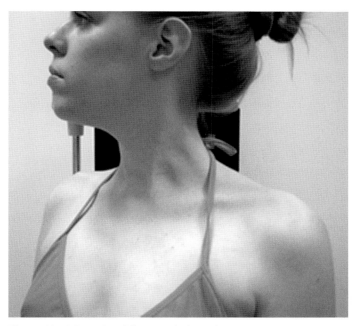

Figure 11.11 Posterior oblique cervical vertebrae.

Positioning

- The patient is erect, facing the X-ray tube and with their back against the IR
- The upper border of the IR is placed level with the top of the pinna of the ear
- The patient is rotated away from the side under examination, until the MSP is at 45° to the IR. The head is turned a further 45° until the MSP of the head is parallel to the IR
- The chin is raised sufficiently to clear the mandibular rami from the upper vertebrae

Beam direction and FRD

Horizontal central ray
200 cm FRD

A 15° cranial angulation may be applied to better demonstrate the intervertebral foramina.

Centring point

To a point in the middle of the neck at the level of the thyroid eminence

Collimation

Atlanto-occipital joints, T1, lateral soft tissue outlines

Criteria for assessing image quality

These are the same as for the anterior obliques.

Modified technique for trauma (Fig. 11.12 A,B)

Oblique projections of the cervical spine may be required as a supplementary examination in trauma cases where there is concern over the integrity of the facet joints.

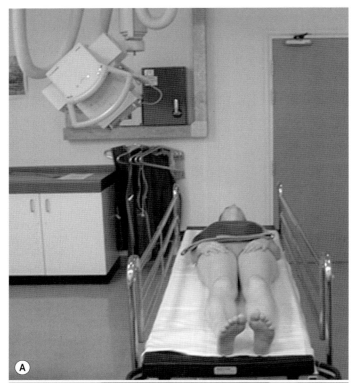

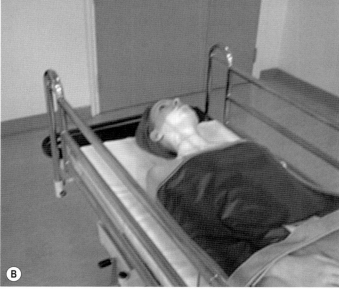

Figure 11.12 (A) Trauma cervical oblique; (B) trauma oblique showing collimation.

AP oblique projections can be undertaken without moving the patient, using lateromedial angulation to provide an apparently oblique neck image.
The *RPO* demonstrates the *left* facet joints and intervertebral foramina.
The *LPO* demonstrates the *right* facet joints and intervertebral foramina.

Positioning

- The patient is supine and the IR is supported beneath the trolley top
- The patient position is as close as possible to that for the AP cervical spine projection

Beam direction and FRD

The beam is angled 45° lateromedially across the patient from either side in turn. The IR should be displaced from the centre sufficiently to ensure that its centre is coincident with the central ray, allowing for the applied beam angulation 100 cm FRD, which may need to be increased if there is a long ORD (such as when an IR tray is used).

If a 15° cranial angulation is required, this may be obtained by rotating the X-ray tube 15° around its horizontal axis after the initial lateromedial angulation.

Centring point

To a point in the middle of the neck, at the level of the thyroid eminence, on the side nearest the X-ray tube

Collimation

Atlanto-occipital joints, T1, lateral soft tissue outlines

Criteria for assessing image quality

These are is the same as for the erect obliques.

Common errors – all methods	Possible reasons
Narrowed foramina	Under-rotation of the neck
Foreshortening of the pedicles	Over-rotation of the neck
The foramina distorted/disc space not demonstrated	Insufficient cranial/caudal tube angulation
Note that if lateromedial angulation is used, as for modified projections in trauma, this will cause more image distortion than projections using neck rotation	

OTHER IMAGING MODALITIES AND THE CERVICAL SPINE

Even though CT provides the most detailed evaluation of bony injuries, MRI has some clear advantages, being the most sensitive modality for the detection of intrinsic spinal cord pathology, and also providing the most detailed evaluation of the soft tissues. An added advantage is that there is no loss of resolution in areas such as the lower cervical spine, where the shoulders may interfere with visualisation, even with the use of CT.

It has been suggested that MRI should be available in the emergency department setting to be used as routinely as plain film radiography is currently;[50] however, even MRI is not without its disadvantages, particularly with the group of patients under consideration. Artefact can be a problem, from either the posterior fat pat in adults or the pulsatile flow of cerebrospinal fluid in children.[51] Studies have shown the effectiveness of using MRI in addition to CT,[2,52] particularly for diagnosis of ligamentous injury and cord impingement; however, it is unnecessary for diagnosis of unstable fractures,[53] as CT has been shown to have 100% sensitivity for this group of patients.[54]

There are other suggestions as to how imaging may be used in this group of patients. Brookes and Willett, researching in Oxford, proposed a protocol for spinal clearance involving dynamic screening of the cervical spine in unconscious trauma patients to enable rapid, safe discontinuation of spinal precautions.[18]

As with all debates in the field of medical imaging, it is not practicable to provide a concrete 'once and for all answer' to the question as to which of the above imaging methods is 'best'; the practice of medical imaging has changed dramatically in the latter decade of the 20th century and into the 21st, with a constant stream of new technologies that shows no sign of slowing down. CT has become unrecognisable from the slice-by-slice technology of the late 20th century, with the introduction of wide multidetector and dual-energy systems.

These advances are being driven by the rapid advances in computing and associated technologies. Already we can look to the image registration of various cross-sectional studies; for example, the registration of CT and MRI images may enable bony and soft tissue structures and their relationships to be better demonstrated than is possible with each individual modality.[55] As we are in such a state of flux we can only offer a snapshot and consider how to best use what is available today, but have a system with the flexibility to adapt to the changes tomorrow may bring.

REFERENCES

1. Anderson P, et al. Clearing the cervical spine in the blunt trauma patient. Journal of American Academy of Orthopaedic Surgeons 2010;18:149–59.

2. Menaker J, et al. Computed tomography alone for cervical spine clearance in the unreliable patient. Are we there yet? Journal of Trauma-Injury Infection & Critical Care 2008;64:898–904.

3. Hoffman JR, et al. Selective cervical spine radiography in blunt trauma. Annals of Emergency Medicine 1998;32(4):461–9.

4. Mower WR, et al. Selective cervical spine radiography of blunt trauma victims. Academic Emergency Medicine 1999;6(5):451.

5. Stiell IG, et al. Obtaining consensus for a definition of 'clinically important cervical spine injury' in the CCC study. Academic Emergency Medicine 1999;6(5):435.

6. Stolberg HO. The development of radiology guidelines in Canada. Canadian Association of Radiologists Journal 1999;50:83–8, 152–5.

7. Stiell IG, et al. Application of the NEXUS low-risk criteria for cervical spine radiography in Canadian Emergency Departments. Academic Emergency Medicine 2000;7(5):566.

8. Kerr D, et al. Implementation of the Canadian C-spine rule reduces cervical spine x-ray rate for alert patients with potential neck injury. Journal of Emergency Medicine 2005;28:127–31.

9. Hills MW, Dean SA. Head injury and facial injury: Is there an increased risk of cervical spine injury? Journal of Trauma 1993;34:549–54.

10. Melville GE, Taveras JM. Traumatic injuries of the spinal cord and nerve roots. In: Taveras J, Ferrucci J, editors. Radiology on CD-ROM. Lippincott; 2001.

11. Pang D, Pollack I. Spinal cord injury without radiographic abnormality in children – the SCIWORA syndrome. Journal of Trauma 1989;29:654–63.

12. Ullrich A, et al. Distracting painful injuries associated with cervical spinal injuries in blunt trauma. Academic Emergency Medicine 2001;8(1):25–9.

13. Link TM, et al. Substantial head trauma: value of routine CT examination of the cervicocranium. Radiology 1995;196:741–5.

14. Hackl W, et al. Prevalence of cervical spine injuries in patients with facial trauma. Oral Surgery Oral Medicine Oral Pathology Oral Radiology & Endodontics 2001;92(4):370–6.

15. Daffner R, Hackney D. ACR Appropriateness criteria on suspected spine trauma. Journal of the American College of Radiology 2007;4:762–75.

16. Thompson W, et al. Association of injury mechanism with the risk of cervical spine fractures. Canadian Journal of Emergency Medical Care 2009;11(1):14–22.

17. Stiell IG, et al. How important is mechanism of injury in predicting the risk of cervical spine injury? American Emergency Medicine 2001;8(5):456–7.

18. Brookes RA, Willett KM. Evaluation of the Oxford protocol for total spinal clearance in the unconscious trauma patient. Journal of Trauma 2001;50(5):862–7.

19. Matar LD, Doyle AJ. Prevertebral soft-tissue measurements in cervical spine injury. Australasian Radiology 1997;41:229–37.

20. Herr CH, et al. Sensitivity of prevertebral soft tissue measurement of C3 for detection of cervical spine fractures and dislocations. American Journal of Emergency Medicine 1998;16(40):346–9.

21. European Commission Directorate-General for the Environment 2000. Referral guidelines for imaging. Radiation protection 118.

22. Gonzalez-Beicos A, Nunez D. Role of Multidetector Computed Tomography in the Assessment of Cervical Spine Trauma. Seminars in Ultrasound, CT and MRI 2009;30(3):159–67.

23. Grogan E, et al. Cervical spine evaluation in urban trauma centers: lowering institutional costs and complications through helical CT scan. Journal of the American College of Surgeons 2005;200(2):160–5.

24. Harris T, et al. Clearing the cervical spine in obtunded patients. Spine 2008;33(14):1547–53.

25. Moppett I. Traumatic brain injury: assessment, resuscitation and early management. British Journal of Anaesthesia 2007;99(1):18–31.

26. Harris MB, et al. Evaluation of the cervical spine in the polytrauma patient. Spine 2000;15;25(22):2884–91.

27. West OC, et al. Acute cervical spine trauma: diagnostic performance of single view versus three view radiographic screening. Radiology 1997;204:819–23.

28. Baker C, et al. Evaluation of paediatric cervical spine injuries. American Journal of Emergency Medicine 1999;17:230–4.

29. MacDonald RL, et al. Diagnosis of cervical spine injury in motor vehicle crash victims: how many x-rays are enough? Journal of Trauma 1990;30(4):392–7.

30. Holliman CJ, et al. Is the anteroposterior cervical spine radiograph necessary in initial trauma screening? American Journal of Emergency Medicine 1991;9(5):421–5.

31. Turetsky DB, et al. Technique and use of supine oblique views in acute cervical spine trauma. Annals of Emergency Medicine 1993;22(4):685–9.

32. Doris PE, Wilson RA. The next logical step in the emergency radiographic evaluation of cervical spine trauma: The five view trauma series. Journal of Emergency Medicine 1985;3:371–5.

33. Abel MS. The exaggerated supine oblique view of the cervical spine. Skeletal Radiology 1982;8:213–9.

34. Unett EM, Royle AJ. Radiographic techniques and image evaluation. London: Chapman and Hall; 1997.

35. Daffner RH. Cervical radiography for trauma patients: A time-effective technique? American Journal of Roentgenology 2000;175:1309–11.

36. American College of Radiology. ACR standard for the performance of radiography of the cervical spine in children and adults. 1999. Online. Available: http://www.acr.org/departments/stand_accred/standards/dl_list.html.

37. Platzer P, et al. Delayed or missed diagnosis of cervical spine injuries. Journal of Trauma-Injury Infection & Critical Care 2006;61(1):150–5.

38. Pollack CV, et al. The utility of flexion-extension radiographs of the cervical spine in blunt trauma. Academic Emergency Medicine 2001;8(5):488.

39. Mirvis SE, et al. Protocol-driven radiologic evaluation of suspected cervical spine injury: efficacy study. Radiology 1989;170:831–4.

40. Nunez DB, et al. Cervical spine trauma: how much do we learn by routinely using

helical CT? RadioGraphics 1996;16:
1307–18.

41. Ballinger P. Merrill's atlas of radiographic
positions and radiologic procedures. 8th
ed. St Louis: Mosby; 1995.

42. Carver BJ, Roche D. An alternative
technique for visualisation of the C7/T1
junction in trauma. Supplement to British
Journal of Radiology 2000;73:73.

43. Swallow R, et al. Clark's positioning
in radiography. 11th ed. London:
Heinemann; 1986.

44. Pellei DD. The fat C2 sign. Radiology
2000;217:359–60.

45. Fell M. Cervical spine trauma radiographs:
Swimmers and supine obliques; an
exploration of current practice.
Radiography 2011;17(1):33–8.

46. Rethnam U, et al. The Swimmer's view:
does it really show what it is supposed to
show? A retrospective study. BMC Medical
Imaging 2008;8(2).

47. Kaneriya PP, et al. The cost-effectiveness of
oblique radiography in the exclusion of
C7–T1 injury in trauma patients. American
Journal of Roentgenology 1998;171:
959–62.

48. Blacksin MF, Lee HJ. Frequency and
significance of fractures of the upper
cervical spine detected by CT in patients
with severe neck trauma. American Journal
of Roentgenology 1995;165(5):751–4.

49. Woodford MJ. Radiography of the acute
cervical spine. Radiography 1987;53(607):
3–8.

50. Rogers LF. To see or not to see, that is
the question. American Journal of
Roentgenology 2001;176:1.

51. Westbrook C. Handbook of MRI
technique. Oxford: Blackwell Science;
1994.

52. Schoenfeld A, et al. Computed
tomography alone versus computed
tomography and magnetic resonance

imaging in the identification of occult
injuries to the cervical spine: a meta-
analysis. Journal of Trauma-Injury
Infection & Critical Care 2010;68(1):
109–14.

53. Tomycz N, et al. MRI Is unnecessary to
clear the cervical spine in obtunded/
comatose trauma patients: the four-
year experience of a level I trauma
center. Journal of Trauma-Injury
Infection & Critical Care 2008;64(5):
1258–63.

54. Hogan G, et al. Exclusion of unstable
cervical spine injury in obtunded patients
with blunt trauma: is MR imaging needed
when multi-detector row CT findings are
normal? Radiology 2005;237:106–13.

55. Panigrahy A, et al. Registration of
three-dimensional MR and CT studies of
the cervical spine. American Journal of
Neuroradiology 2000;21:282–9.

Chapter | 12 |

Thoracic spine

Linda Williams

The thoracic spine should not be routinely examined by radiography for pain without trauma, unless in the elderly when osteoporosis may cause sudden collapse of vertebrae. Magnetic resonance imaging (MRI) may be indicated if local pain continues.[1]

The clinical significance of wedge fractures should not be overlooked, as occasionally there may be fragments displaced within the spinal canal that could cause spinal cord compression.[2]

The 28-day rule should be applied when examining the thoracic spine in patients of reproductive capacity, as the inclusion of the lower thoracic vertebrae will also irradiate the medial portion of the upper abdomen.

INDICATIONS

Fracture

The most common reason for examining this area radiographically is trauma, either major or minor, involving the region. Fractures of the upper and middle sections of the thoracic spine do not occur as frequently as those of the cervical vertebrae and thoracolumbar region. However, with thoracic spine fractures there is a higher incidence of spinal cord injury.[3]

Osteomyeloma

The thoracic spine may be examined as part of a skeletal survey to stage the condition and assess which lesions may benefit from radiotherapy.[1]

Osteomyelitis

A two- to three-phase skeletal scintinogram is more sensitive than an X-ray examination,[1] so it is not routinely indicated, but in the later stages an area of porosis may be seen; the diagnosis at this stage can usually be made by blood cultures.[4]

Anteroposterior (AP) thoracic spine (Fig. 12.1A, B)

Much research has been undertaken on the advantages and disadvantages of the posteroanterior (PA) versus the AP projection of the lumbar spine, particularly in relation to dose reduction. Brennan and Madigan,[5] in their article analysing the PA projection of the lumbar spine, recommend the use of this procedure to facilitate dose reduction without loss of image quality. However, it must be remembered that, owing to the natural kyphotic curvature of the thoracic spine, oblique rays from the X-ray beam will be angled in the opposite direction to the intervertebral joint spaces. The resulting PA image is therefore not likely to demonstrate the intervertebral joint spaces as adequately as the AP projection. This is somewhat unfortunate, as the PA projection may reduce radiation dose to the breast, eyes and thyroid, all radiosensitive areas. However, breast shields may be used, and with good collimation this can significantly reduce the dose. Levy et al. have studied the use of the PA projection in examining the whole spine for scoliosis in adolescents.[6] Their work suggests that a PA study of the spine will effect a reduction in dose to the patient without any loss of image quality, and although the assessment for scoliosis using plain radiography has reduced significantly with the increased use of other imaging methods, their work indicates that PA thoracic spine examination may be a possibility in some cases.

A consideration when examining the thoracic spine is the variation in densities along the length of this section of the vertebral column, the upper end having the air-filled trachea superimposed and vertebrae 5–12 having the heart and great vessels superimposed. Abdominal contents are usually superimposed over T11 and T12 and the size of individual vertebrae increases gradually, with T1 being significantly smaller than T12.

Clearly this range of densities has implications for the choice of exposure factors to provide adequate contrast and density along the entire length of the region under examination. To achieve even density certain techniques may be employed, as follows:

1. A high enough kVp can be used to reduce the subject contrast along the length of the spine.
2. A wedge filter can be used with the thicker end at the upper region of the thoracic spine.
3. A flour filter can be used, consisting of flour inside a radiolucent bag (usually plastic, which is covered by a cotton bag that can be washed). The contents of the bag can be shaken to distribute the flour into a thicker layer at one end; this thicker end of the bag is then placed over the upper end of the sternum and the

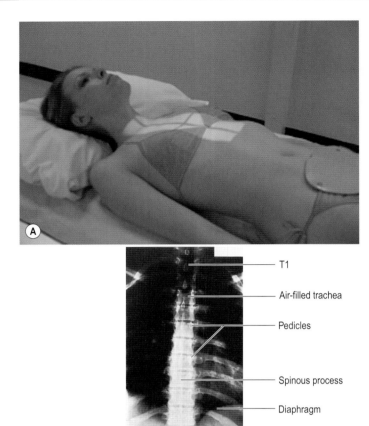

T1

Air-filled trachea

Pedicles

Spinous process

Diaphragm

Costovertebral
joint

T12

12th rib

Figure 12.1 AP thoracic spine.
*(B) Reproduced with permission from Bryan GJ. Skeletal anatomy. 3rd ed.
Edinburgh: Churchill Livingstone; 1996 and Gunn C. Bones and joints.
4th ed. Edinburgh: Churchill Livingstone, 2002.*

flour is patted by the radiographer until the thickness decreases
towards the lower end of the thoracic vertebrae. The filter
is therefore adaptable to any patient size, unlike set-size
aluminium filters. The filter can be made extremely cheaply
and requires no specialist attachment feature on the light beam
mounting, although manufacture of such a filter should only
be attempted after consultation with health and safety and
cross-infection specialists from the hospital where the filter is to
be used.

Some texts suggest the use of the anode heel effect to help reduce the
subject contrast along the length of the spine.[7,8] However, it must be
suggested that this is a somewhat outdated approach: anode targets
in modern X-ray tubes are set at such an angle that this effect will have
little or no difference on the resultant image.

When using an automatic exposure device (AED) for the thoracic
spine, accurate centring and good collimation are essential. If the
beam is not collimated sufficiently then the AED will end the exposure
before the required radiographic density of the image is achieved. This
is due to the effect of additional scatter from the excess irradiated
tissue lateral to the spine.

The AP thoracic spine is exposed on arrested inspiration to ensure
the diaphragm is lowered and a maximum number of thoracic vertebrae are demonstrated. However, it has also been suggested that the
use of arrested expiration to reduce the amount of air in the thorax
will provide a more uniform density over the thoracic spine, by
helping to reduce the subject contrast of the air-filled lungs against
the mediastinum and spine.[8,9] This is a questionable suggestion in that
there will always be air in the lung fields, even in expiration.

IR is horizontal, employed with antiscatter grid.

Positioning

- The patient is supine with their arms at their sides and legs
  extended
- A low radiolucent pillow or pad may be used to support the
  head, and the knees may be supported slightly with a pad for
  comfort
- A lead rubber apron is applied to the lower abdomen for gonad
  protection
- The median sagittal plane (MSP) is at 90° to the table-top and
  the coronal plane is parallel to the table-top

Note that this technique may be performed erect, either standing or
seated; the positioning is the same for each but a vertical IR is used.
The direction of the central ray is adjusted accordingly.

Beam direction and focus receptor distance (FRD)

Vertical central ray, at 90° to the IR
100 cm FRD

Centring point

In the midline approximately two-thirds of the distance between the
sternal angle and the xiphisternum, nearest the xiphoid end

Some texts quote the centring point for this projection as midway
between the sternal notch and the xiphisternum.[10,11] This point locates
the central ray over T6, i.e. numerically at the middle of the thoracic
vertebrae, and seems a logical selection; yet vertebrae T1–T6 are
shorter than T7–T12 and a centring point over T6 will therefore not
lie over the midpoint of the thoracic section of the vertebral column.
Indeed, it will be in a relatively high position in relation to the actual
midpoint of the area. Other texts quote a centring point as either
between the sternal angle and the xiphisternum, or 3–5 cm below the
sternal angle to a point over T7;[8,9,12] is this low enough to coincide
with the actual midpoint of the thoracic vertebrae? In the first edition
of this book it was thought necessary to reassess the situation and
consider AP thoracic spine radiographs in an attempt to see whether
there was a standard midpoint; in other words, which references suggested the most accurate midpoint of the thoracic spine? Several
images were studied by the author and it was been noted that the
actual halfway point between T1 and T12 lies, in fact, approximately
over T7/8 disc space. As anterior surface markings need to be used for
assessing this point, it has been identified, from skeletons and radiographs, that T7/8 junction lies two-thirds of the way down the sternum
itself (including xiphisternum) – hence the centring point chosen here
(Fig. 12.2).

Collimation

C7–L1, all transverse processes

Expose on arrested respiration

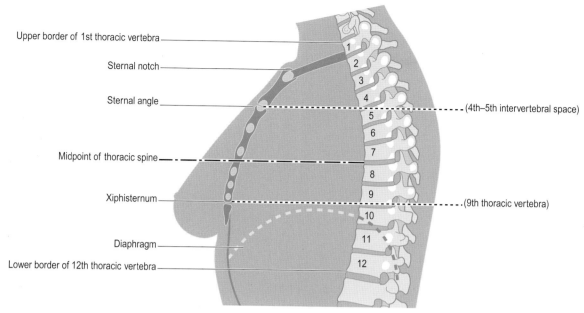

Figure 12.2 Level of midpoint of thoracic spine.

Criteria for assessing image quality

- C7 down to L1 and all their transverse processes are demonstrated
- The thoracic vertebrae are in the centre of the collimated area
- Spinous processes are centralised over the midline of the vertebral bodies
- Paraspinal line[2] should be clearly demonstrated
- Intervertebral joint spaces are demonstrated
- Sharp image demonstrating the bony cortex and trabeculae of the vertebral bodies of C7 down to L1, adequately penetrated through the denser mediastinal and upper abdominal structures without over-blackening of the upper vertebrae

Common errors	Possible reasons
Overexposure of the upper region or underexposure of the lower region	Failure to employ any of the techniques described above for even image density throughout
Superimposition of portions of the vertebral bodies vertically	The long axis of the spine is not near parallel to the table-top. Reducing the size of the head support and giving the patient a small pad beneath the knees for support can rectify this. (However, severely kyphotic patients may require two exposures with beam angled in each direction of the kyphosis)

Lateral thoracic spine (Fig. 12.3A,B)

As in the case of the AP projection, there also exists a range of densities along the area covered by the lateral thoracic spine projection. The more dense area in this case is the upper end of the thoracic region, as the average person is wider at the shoulders than they are lower down the thoracic region. The use of the filter described earlier in this chapter is used with the thicker end orientated in the opposite direction to that used for the AP, i.e. the thinner end at the shoulder end.

This will even out the densities encountered along the length of the spine.

There are two schools of thought when choosing exposure factors for the lateral projection. One that is commonly used is the breathing technique, using a low mA and long exposure time (2 seconds plus) to provide the required mAs. This technique is designed to blur rib shadows and lung markings that lie over the vertebrae, thereby enabling the viewer to see the vertebral bodies more clearly.[8,9,12,13] One suggestion regarding this is that, as the ribs are actually attached to the vertebrae, when using the breathing technique the rib shadow cannot be blurred without blurring the vertebrae also; in other words, what is actually happening is that, during breathing, the vertebral bodies are moving but to a lesser extent than the ribs. This gives the vertebral bodies an apparent sharpness owing to the differential sharpness between the ribs and the bodies themselves.

There is sometimes difficulty in demonstrating the intervertebral joint space of all the thoracic vertebrae on one image and this can be overcome by the use of a greater FRD (150 cm). This relatively long distance means there is less divergence of the beam around the central ray when it reaches the thoracic spine, and more chance of the joint spaces being demonstrated on the image, especially those at the extreme ends of the thoracic spine. Although this method has been used by many radiographers for many years it was not until 2003 that a study by Thomas provided evidence to support the practice, also showing that magnification and unsharpness are reduced.[14] This technique requires adjustment of exposure factors, with due attention to the inverse square law, unless an AED is used.

A lead rubber sheet placed behind the patient, next to the skin surface, will absorb some of the scattered radiation produced during exposure and enhance the image. Some research has disputed the necessity of placing lead rubber behind the patient for the lateral spine projection, arguing that the resulting radiograph is not enhanced by this practice. It also claimed that it is not necessary with the use of the accurate collimators available today which prevent any scatter reaching the IR. However, Thomas's 2003 study actually supports the use of lead rubber in this way, claiming that the resulting radiographic contrast is improved as a result of less scatter reaching the receptor.[14]

IR is horizontal, employed with antiscatter grid.

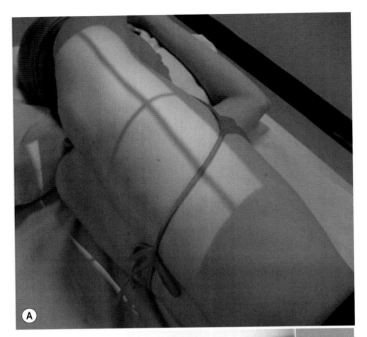

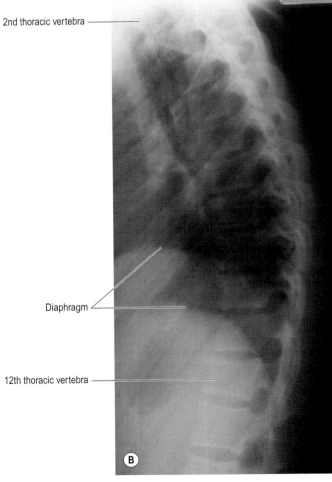

2nd thoracic vertebra

Diaphragm

12th thoracic vertebra

Figure 12.3 Lateral thoracic spine.

Positioning

- From the AP position the patient is turned 90° onto their side to bring the coronal plane 90° to the table-top and the MSP parallel to it, with their back to the radiographer for ease of positioning
- The patient's head is rested on a low radiolucent pad or pillow and the knees and hips are flexed for stability
- The patient's upper arm is placed stretched above their head to help bring the spine parallel to the table-top and clear the humerus and soft tissue of the arm from the field. The lower arm is raised onto the pad or pillow to clear it from the field
- A lead rubber apron is placed across the lower abdomen and pelvis for radiation protection
- The spinous processes are palpated and assessed to ensure that the long axis of the spine and the MSP are parallel to the table-top; this may require the use of a firm radiolucent pad under the lowered end of the thoracic spine if not parallel, but comments after the beam angulation section for this projection should also be noted before considering this. If the spine has a lateral curvature when the patient is lying on their side, with the curve appearing as a slight 'u' shape, it is usually not necessary to make adjustments to the central ray or to use pads. This is because the oblique rays around the central ray are likely to correspond with the obliquity of the intervertebral joint spaces. If a curvature appears as a slight 'n' shape, it will be more advantageous to turn the patient onto their opposite side for this projection. In any case, lateral curvature is often best assessed by viewing the AP projection before attempting the lateral position. If the vertebral column is straight, but not parallel to the IR, angulation will be required to ensure the central ray is perpendicular to the long axis of the spine (see beam direction below).

Beam direction and FRD

Vertical at 90° to the long axis of the thoracic spine

Reference has already been made to the use of radiolucent pads to help the spine lie parallel to the IR, but it must be remembered that the effectiveness of this will vary according to the weight of the patient (heavier patients will squash the pad more than slimmer patients, thereby reducing the effect of the pad). Variations in the anatomy of individual patients will require varying compensation to allow the thoracic column to lie parallel to the IR. Insertion of pads can also be somewhat difficult when a patient is elderly, obese, or suffering from back pain and lying in the lateral position. Angulation of the beam in a direction that will ensure the central ray strikes the long axis of the thoracic vertebrae at 90° can also be used as an alternative strategy. It is easier to use this, rather than the pad method, and beam angulation will more accurately facilitate the correct 90° beam–vertebral column relationship. Most frequently patients with broad shoulders present with the elevated end of the thoracic spine at their shoulder level, requiring cranial angle.

115–150 cm FRD

Note the range of FRDs offered; this is after consideration of the comments made in the introductory notes for this projection.

Centring point

At the level of T8 approximately 2–3 cm behind the mid-axillary line, and 7–9 cm anterior to the spinous process of T7.

Note that the spinous process of T7 lies level with the body of T8. T8 can also be located from the posterior aspect of the patient by palpating the inferior angle of the scapula, which lies level with T8, even when the arm is raised. Approximations in given measurements are due to the vast differences in patient shapes and sizes.

Collimation

C7 to L1, anterior vertebral bodies, spinous processes

Criteria for assessing image quality

- T2 should be demonstrated and not obscured by the upper arms and shoulders; the body of L1 should be included inferiorly (it is not usually possible to demonstrate T1 on the lateral projection because of the shoulder thickness; it may be necessary to take a supplementary projection of this area if the clinical history indicates a need for this)
- All anterior bodies and spinous processes are demonstrated
- There is superimposition of the posterior ribs and superimposition of the anterior and posterior borders of the vertebral bodies
- Superimposition of the inferior and superior borders of the vertebral bodies and intervertebral disc spaces is demonstrated
- There is blurring of the ribs and lung markings if the breathing technique is used
- Correct image density to demonstrate the bony cortex and trabeculae of all the vertebrae with sufficient penetration of the shoulder region to visualise the upper vertebrae, without over-blackening of the lower vertebrae

Common errors	Possible reasons
Collimation may result in some of the vertebral column being excluded from the image	Apart from poor centring and collimation, this may be caused by a kyphosis; this should be obvious on visual inspection of the patient and collimation must take the effects of kyphosis into consideration
The anterior and posterior borders of the bodies are not superimposed	The patient is either rotated too far forward or too far back; ensure the coronal plane is 90° to the table-top
The intervertebral joint spaces are not demonstrated; upper and lower borders of the vertebral bodies are not superimposed	The long axis of the spine is not parallel to the table-top. Care should be taken to ensure the spinous processes are all parallel to the table-top, with use of radiolucent pads if necessary, or the beam should be angled to strike the spine at 90° to its long axis

REFERENCES

1. Royal College of Radiologists Working Party. Making the best use of clinical radiology services: referral guidelines for doctors. 6th ed. London: Royal College of Radiologists; 2007.
2. Raby N, et al. Accident and emergency radiology, a survival guide. London: Saunders; 2001.
3. Long BW, Rafert JA. Orthopaedic radiography. Philadelphia: WB Saunders; 1995.
4. Duckworth T. Lecture notes on orthopaedics and fractures. UK: Blackwell Science; 1995.
5. Brennan PC, Madigan E. Lumbar spine radiology; analysis of the posteroanterior projection. European Radiology 2000;10: 1197–201.
6. Levy AR, et al. Reducing the lifetime risks of cancer from spinal radiographs amongst people with adolescent idiopathic scoliosis. Spine 1996;21(13):1500–7.
7. Eisenberg RL, et al. Radiographic positioning. 2nd ed. Boston: Little Brown and Company; 1995.
8. Bontrager KL. Textbook of radiographic positioning and related anatomy. 7th ed. St Louis: Mosby; 2010.
9. McQuillen-Martensen K. Radiographic critique. 3rd ed. Philadelphia: WB Saunders; 2010.
10. Unett EM, Royle AJ. Radiographic techniques and image evaluation. London: Nelson Thornes; 1997.
11. Bell GA, Finlay DBL. Basic radiographic positioning. Eastbourne: Baillière Tindall; 1986.
12. Ballinger PW, Frank ED. Merrill's atlas of radiographic positioning and radiologic procedures. 10th ed. St Louis: Mosby; 2003.
13. Whitley AS, et al. Clark's positioning in radiography. 12th ed. Oxford: Hodder Arnold; 2005.
14. Thomas A. Imaging the lateral thoracic spine. Synergy 2003;April:10–3.

Chapter 13

Lumbar spine

Barry Carver, Elizabeth Carver

CONDITIONS AFFECTING THE REGION

Trauma

Wedge fractures can occur when the anterior border of a vertebral body is crushed due to flexion or vertical pressure, i.e. a high fall landing on the feet or head. More serious bony injury can occur, including fracture and dislocation of vertebrae, which can cause misalignment of the vertebral column. Below the first lumbar vertebra (L1) the cauda equina is more resistant to injury than the spinal cord. Plain radiography is most likely to be undertaken in the acute setting when injury has been sustained.

Pars interarticularis fractures are shown on oblique lumbar spine projections; this type of injury can result in a spondylolisthesis (forward slippage of one vertebra in relation to the vertebra below), although plain radiography may not be the most appropriate investigative method. L5 slippage on the first sacral segment (S1) is most frequently found. These are often incidental findings on images and are not usually directly related to specific traumatic incidents.

Back pain

Lumbago

Low back pain; often no cause is found radiologically.

Sciatica

Pain radiating to the leg caused by compression of the lumbar nerve roots. This may be associated with a lumbar disc prolapse or spondylosis.

Back pain, whether acute or chronic, is not itself an indicator for plain radiography (except in the case of possible osteoporotic collapse);[1] however, back pain may be associated with more serious features, in which case magnetic resonance imaging (MRI) is the investigation of choice.[2]

Degenerative disease processes

Degenerative change is part of the normal ageing process. Among those affecting the lumbar region are spondylosis, spondylitis, spondylolisthesis, intervertebral disc collapse and osteoarthritis. In order to justify imaging, the potential to affect patient management must be considered.

Studies have shown that only a very small percentage of requests for plain radiography change patient management[3] and so they are not cost-effective.[4] The high radiation dose associated with lumbar spine radiography should not be used to provide patient reassurance, or indeed reassurance for the referrer.[5]

Metastatic disease

Metastatic disease is characterised by secondary deposits seen as lytic, and in some cases sclerotic, lesions; pathological fractures may be present. Nuclear medicine imaging or MRI are generally the most appropriate examinations for early detection.[2]

Congenital processes

Spina bifida

This is a congenital defect that usually occurs in the lumbosacral region. The laminae do not fuse, causing the vertebral arch to be incomplete posteriorly. Spina bifida has varying degrees of severity, as it may or may not be associated with protrusion of the meninges and spinal cord. Today, plain radiography is unlikely to be required as an initial investigation, as awareness of the existence of the abnormality is usually raised after routine prenatal ultrasound scanning. In spina bifida occulta the defect does not involve the meninges or spinal cord and is usually an incidental finding on an anteroposterior (AP) radiograph of the area.

Challenges of the lumbar spine examination

There are a number of challenges the radiographer will encounter when positioning a patient, not only due to the patient's physical shape and size but in judging the radiographic planes of the body in relation to the patient and X-ray table. The following tips may be helpful in overcoming difficulties that may be encountered.

Positioning tips

When initially studying a patient's X-ray request form, prior knowledge of their clinical history assists in the problem-solving and decision-making processes crucial for the optimum choice of positioning technique required, in order to achieve a high-quality diagnostic image. Initial clinical evaluation of the shape of the spine will assist in any positioning adjustment requirements when the patient is placed on the X-ray couch. This is particularly important for patients with abnormal configurations of the spine.

The patient should be made to feel comfortable and relaxed; tension can cause difficulty when attempting to move a patient into position. The examination gown should be adjusted if necessary to ensure that no folds will interfere with their movement into the required position and that the anatomical landmarks can be easily palpated. If the gown design includes a split, this must be at the back of the patient, to allow for visualisation of the spinal column while palpating its surface markings.

Palpation of the prime anatomical landmarks is important when adjusting the patient into the correct position for each projection. Clinical palpation is a skill which, if practised with reservations, can lead to mistakes. Physical contact involving the lower trunk, as required for lumbar spine examination, requires a degree of tact and diplomacy while using precision and gentleness but firmness.

A key requisite for accurate positioning of the lateral lumbar projections is to assess the position of the long axis of the vertebral column in relation to the image receptor (IR). The column should be palpated *and* visually assessed along the lumbar section, with the *eyes level with the vertebrae*. Radiographers often assess visually from a point that is higher than the spine; this does not give a true impression of the vertebral position. Palpation of the spinous processes is also essential and must be implemented in addition to visual assessment, as the muscles on the posterior aspect of the patient can sag (especially in the middle-aged and elderly), giving an inaccurate impression if visual assessment only is used.

For lumbar spine X-ray examinations the anatomical landmarks chosen during positioning set-up techniques are considered reasonably standard, although their position relative to the surrounding anatomical structures can vary due to osteological changes. Excessive fatty tissue can also cause difficulty in palpation techniques and there is a large variation in total body fat in individuals of varying age and between populations. Therefore, standardisation of the anatomical sites used for positioning and palpation is important.

AP lumbar spine (Fig. 13.1A,B)

IR is horizontal; an antiscatter grid is employed

Positioning

- The patient is supine with their arms placed on the pillow and legs extended
- The knees may be supported with a pad for patient comfort; to reduce the lumbar lordosis and enable better visualisation of the intervertebral joint spaces, the legs should be supported with the femora at 45° or more to the table-top
- The median sagittal plane (MSP) is 90° to the table-top and the coronal plane is parallel to the table-top
- Gonad protection should be applied to all patients; if it is correctly positioned it will not obscure any relevant detail, and is essential to reduce the dose to the gonads

Beam direction and focus receptor distance (FRD)

Vertical central ray, 90° to the IR
100 cm FRD

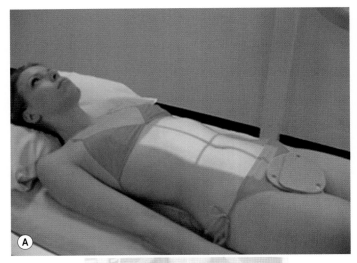

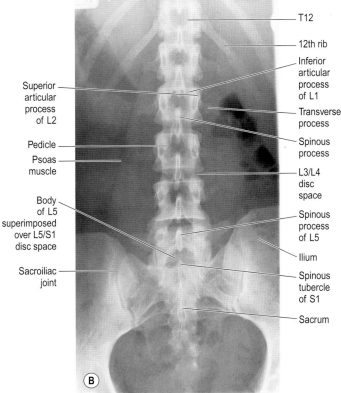

Figure 13.1 AP lumbar spine.

Centring

In the midline, at the level of the lower costal margin (level of L3)

Collimation

Psoas muscles, transverse processes of LV1–LV5, T12/L1 joint space, sacroiliac joints

Note that this technique may be performed erect, either standing or seated; the positioning is the same but a vertical IR and antiscatter device are used.[6] The central ray direction is adjusted accordingly.

Criteria for assessing image quality

- Psoas muscles, transverse processes of LV1–LV5, T12/L1 joint space, sacroiliac joints are demonstrated
- Spinous processes are in the centre of vertebral bodies, demonstrating no rotation
- L2/L3 and L3/L4 joint spaces are demonstrated; other intervertebral spaces will be projected obliquely due to lumbar curvature
- Sharp image demonstrating soft tissue of abdominal viscera in contrast to bone and air in the gastrointestinal tract; detail of bony cortex and trabeculae; spinous processes visualised through vertebral bodies

Common errors	Possible reasons
Spinous processes not in the midline of vertebral bodies	1. Rotation of the spine – MSP not perpendicular to the IR. Adjust the patient position so that the pelvis and shoulders are not rotated
	2. Scoliosis may cause this appearance and may not be improved upon. This is distinguishable from rotation due to position error by the distinct lateral curve of the column and potential variation of rotation down its length[7]
No intervertebral discs clearly demonstrated	Excessive lordosis – the direction of the primary beam can be adjusted so that the beam is directed through the required joint spaces (see comments below)

Expose on arrested respiration

Exposure is made on arrested respiration, to prevent blurring of abdominal contents. The respiratory phase is unimportant as the diaphragm will not move over the body of L1 in either phase. It is likely, though, that selection of exposure factors will be affected by opposite phases of respiration, as extreme inspiration will increase the volume and density of abdominal tissue overlying the lumbar area. This will be likely to necessitate an increase in exposure factors, which will result in an increase in radiation dose to the patient and a decrease in image contrast due to increased scatter from the greater tissue volume and density.

An alternative to demonstrate the transverse processes free from overlying gas shadows is to use a long exposure with the patient gently panting, using the effect of autotomography to prevent the gas obscuring bony detail.

It has commonly been believed that the curvature of the lumbar spine can be reduced by an angled pad being placed under the knees, enabling better visualisation of the intervertebral joint spaces by associated flattening of the lumbar lordotic curve.[8] The effectiveness of knee flexion is traditionally claimed to be felt by a simple experiment: if one lies supine with the legs extended a flat hand will slide easily under the arch made by the lumbar curve. When the knees and hips are flexed, the hand feels the lumbar area press down onto its dorsal aspect, suggesting a reduction in lumbar curve. The more the hips and knees are flexed, the more the curve appears to reduce. But is the movement felt by the hand merely muscular movement rather than reduction of lordosis? Would an increase in knee/hip flexion actually show a more significant lumbar curve reduction?

The effect has been disputed by Murrie et al.,[9] but this research was undertaken on a very small sample of seven examinations and this raises questions on the validity of the research. It is also noted that Murrie et al. flexed the knees over a pad, which may not offer adequate *hip* flexion to reduce the lumbar curve.

Further research on this topic was performed on a larger sample of 60 volunteers by Downing,[10] who found that the lumbar curve was effectively reduced by up to 64%, but that in order to be effective the femora should be at 45° to the table-top, as described in the technique description. Note that the key is the angle between the femora and the table-top, *not* the angle of flexion of the knees.

However, the question must be asked 'Do we require all joint spaces to be visualised on an AP?': information regarding intervertebral disc spaces is more readily available on the lateral view, and on MRI, which after all is the investigation of choice for most lumbar pathologies.

Posteroanterior (PA) or AP?

Owing to the anterior curvature of the lumbar spine it would seem reasonable that the PA projection could be preferable to AP, as in this position the diverging X-ray beam coincides more closely with the intervertebral joint spaces, enabling better demonstration.

This is not, however, a commonly adopted practice, reasons being the magnification and consequent unsharpness due to increased object–receptor distance (ORD). This could be compensated for by an increase in FRD and exposure factors.

Colleran[11] showed that the magnification produced does not cause a significant reduction in image quality and indeed recommends its adoption because of the superior demonstration of the sacrum, sacroiliac joints and intervertebral joint spaces. Her work has resulted in the adoption of the PA projection in a small number of imaging departments.

Lateral lumbar spine (Fig. 13.2A,B)

IR is usually horizontal; an antiscatter grid is employed

Erect weightbearing horizontal beam technique may be employed for this projection.[6]

Positioning

- From the AP position the patient is turned 90° onto their *left* side to bring the coronal plane 90° to the table-top and the MSP parallel to it, with their back to the radiographer for ease of positioning.
- The knees and hips are flexed for stability and comfort and the arms are rested on the pillow in front of the patient's head; this clears the patient's arms from the required area. A pad may be inserted between the knees to aid positioning, patient comfort and stability. Note that the choice of size is important: it should be of a size that ensures that the raised knee does not affect the parallel position of the MSP in relationship to the couch.
- A lead rubber apron is placed across the lower anterior aspect of the abdomen and pelvis for radiation protection, without obscuring the lower lumbar vertebrae and first sacral segment. A thin sheet of lead rubber may not be sufficient to absorb primary beam it impinges upon any aspect of the sheet, and should not be used.
- The spinous processes are palpated and assessed to ensure that the long axis of the spine and the MSP are parallel to the table-top; if not it will be necessary to angle the beam in a direction that will ensure the central ray strikes the long axis of

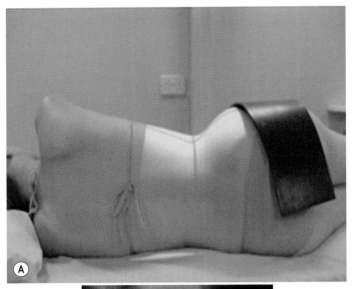

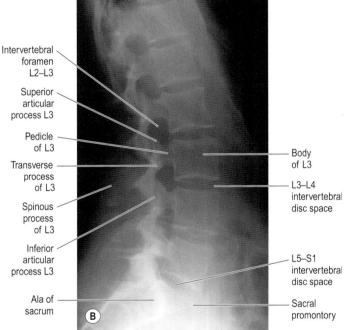

Intervertebral foramen L2–L3

Superior articular process L3

Pedicle of L3

Transverse process of L3

Spinous process of L3

Inferior articular process L3

Ala of sacrum

Body of L3

L3–L4 intervertebral disc space

L5–S1 intervertebral disc space

Sacral promontory

Figure 13.2 Lateral lumbar spine.

the lumbar vertebrae at 90°. Very often, the female pelvis causes the spine to tilt upwards towards the pelvic end of the vertebral column, whereas the male shoulders can cause the opposite effect (although this has more effect on the lateral thoracic spine projection). Radiolucent pads, placed under the lateral aspect of the lower end of the tilted vertebral column, can be used to address this problem. However, the accuracy and effectiveness of this is in question and beam angulation is likely to be more effective (see Ch. 12 regarding the lateral thoracic spine). The alignment of the spinous processes must be assessed with the eyes level with the spine to ensure accuracy, as previously discussed. Palpation of the posterior superior iliac spines (PSISs) to check their vertical superimposition will assure accurate lateral positioning of the pelvic end of the lumbar vertebrae. The

shoulder end of the column should also be assessed so that the posterior aspect of the patient's shoulders is vertical.

- If the spine has a lateral curvature when the patient is lying on their side, with L1 and L5 higher than the middle vertebrae, it is not usually necessary to make adjustments in the central ray or to use pads. This is because the oblique rays around the central ray are likely to correspond with the obliquity of the intervertebral joint spaces. If a slight curvature appears with L1 and L5 lower than the middle vertebrae (not commonly encountered), it will be more advantageous to turn the patient onto their opposite side for this projection. In any case, lateral curvature is often best assessed by viewing the AP projection before attempting the lateral position.

- If the patient has scoliosis, it is recommended that the side to which the largest curvature is more prominently demonstrated is placed nearest the X-ray couch. The central ray is then directed towards the lowest point of the convex shape of the curvature. This ensures that the oblique rays that penetrate each of the vertebral bodies produce an image which assists in reducing the superimposition of the vertebral bodies over intervertebral joint spaces, demonstrating the joint spaces as efficiently as is possible under the circumstances.

- A sheet of lead rubber is placed on the table-top behind the patient to prevent scatter reaching the receptor, thereby improving image quality. There has been some discussion as to the efficacy of lead rubber in this circumstance,[12] but its use has been shown to be effective and should be mandatory.[13]

Unless otherwise indicated, e.g. by scoliosis, the left lateral should be routinely performed as this results in up to 38% less effective patient dose.[14,15] However, there is some evidence that the right lateral may be preferable in paediatric patients owing to the greater radio-sensitivity of the liver in children.[16,17]

Beam direction and FRD

Vertical central ray 90° to the long axis of the lumbar spine
100–150 cm FRD

Consider using the longer FRD (e.g. 150 cm) to compensate for long ORD. This will also enable better visualisation of the intervertebral joint spaces, as shown in Figure 13.3A,B.

Centring point

At the level of the lower costal margin, which is coincident with L3

The beam is required to be directed through the vertebral body of L3; this can be located 7.5–10 cm anterior to the spinous process of L3, the distance varying with patient build.

Collimation

T12 to S1, anterior aspects of the vertebral bodies, spinous processes

It may be useful to include the aorta anteriorly in patients in whom calcification may indicate the presence of atheromatous degeneration in the aorta. Localised deviation (apparent bulge) of the calcified outline of the aorta is indicative of abdominal aortic aneurysm.

> Expose on arrested respiration
> The exposure is made on expiration, to ensure the posterolateral aspects of the diaphragms do not overlie L1.

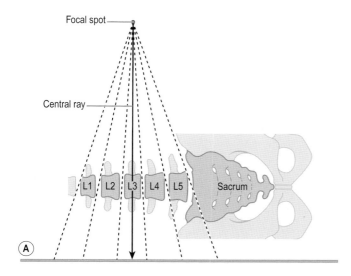

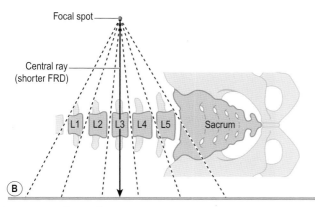

Figure 13.3 Effects of varying FRDs on joint space demonstration. This is a diagrammatic representation of the lumbar vertebrae in the lateral position. (A) shows the position, which uses a longer FRD than in (B). Notice how the obliquity of the rays at the periphery (L5/S1 and T12/L1) increase with the shorter FRD and increase the chances of vertebral overlap on the image. L3 is unaffected as it lies below the central ray.

Exposure factors

A kVp high enough to allow penetration and visualisation of the L5/S1 joint space, as well as to demonstrate the lumbar vertebrae, should be used. EU guidelines suggest 80–95 kVp.[18]

Criteria for assessing image quality

- T12 to S1, spinous processes and soft tissues anterior to vertebral bodies are demonstrated on the image
- Posterior, superior and inferior borders of each vertebral body should be superimposed
- Posterior ribs and superior surfaces of the sacral alae should be superimposed
- Joint spaces between each vertebra should be clearly demonstrated.
- Sharp image demonstrating soft tissue structures anterior to the vertebral bodies in contrast to detail of bony cortex and trabeculae; bone seen in contrast with intervertebral joint spaces between T12 and L1 down to L5/S1. Spinous processes of lumbar vertebrae visualised

Common errors	Possible reasons
The posterior condyles of the vertebral bodies are not superimposed	Rotation of the patient – MSP not parallel to the table-top. Adjust the hips and/or shoulders so that they are superimposed
Disc spaces are not clearly demonstrated – the superior and inferior surfaces of the vertebral bodies are not superimposed	The long axis of the vertebral column is not parallel to the table-top (tilt). See notes in positioning section for methods which may be used to correct or compensate
	Is there a degree of scoliosis which may be affecting joint space demonstration?
Pale (low density) over L5/S1 region, rest of lumbar spine well demonstrated	Inadequate kVp selected

Modification of technique for trauma

Clearly it is important not to move the patient if trauma is indicated; consequently, it is necessary for the lateral view to be obtained using a horizontal beam.

Lateral lumbosacral junction (LSJ)

(Figs 13.4A,B, 13.5A,B)

The LSJ or L5/S1 projection is normally only required if the joint space is not adequately demonstrated on the lateral projection (i.e. if there is overlap of the vertebral body of L5 onto S1, or if there is insufficient penetration to demonstrate the joint space or bony detail of S1), to enable assessment of the intervertebral height. Under no circumstances should this projection be undertaken 'routinely', without first having assessed the lateral projection for suitability.

It is unnecessary for the joint space to be 'perfectly' demonstrated: some superimposition of the superior surfaces of S1 and the inferior surfaces of L5 is acceptable. A clear disc space with no superimposition of the vertebral bodies is the ideal result and is what we should be looking to achieve; however, the radiation dose burden of this examination needs to be considered. In order to avoid undertaking a lateral L5/S1 projection in addition to the lateral lumbar, assessment of disc space height can often be made on a less than perfect image, as shown in Figure 13.4B, which shows the lower end of the lumbar vertebrae as they might appear on a lateral lumbar spine image. As long as the four surface edges can be identified then an assessment of joint space is possible, and an additional view of the LSJ is *not* required. These measurements can only be made when the lateral lumbar spine image shows adequate penetration and exposure that provides good detail of the bony trabeculae of the first sacral segment.

IR is usually horizontal; an antiscatter grid is employed
Erect weightbearing horizontal beam technique may be used.[6]

Positioning

- The patient is placed on to their side as for the lateral projection position, i.e. with the MSP parallel to the X-ray table and the vertebral bodies parallel with the table
- An imaginary line adjoining the PSISs will demonstrate the plane of the L5/S1 joint space. If not superimposed, the beam should be angled to coincide with this line

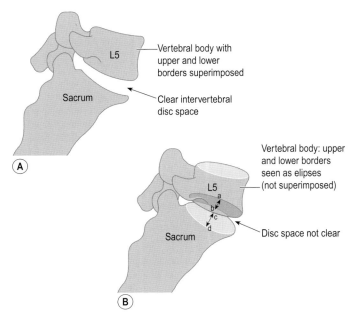

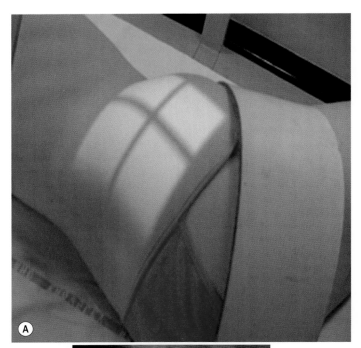

Figure 13.4 'Tilted' lateral lumbar image: assessment of joint space. (A) 'Perfect' – L5/S1 showing disc space as seen in (B); (B) acceptable – because disc height can be assessed as indicated, by measuring a–b and c–d.

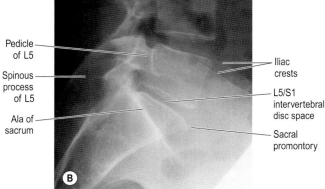

Figure 13.5 Lateral lumbosacral junction.

Beam direction and FRD

A vertical central ray, coincident with the L5/S1 joint space (vertical alignment of PSISs). Beam angulation may be required to ensure the central ray is directed through the joint space, which should be assessed by viewing:

1. The AP projection to see if there is a lateral tilt of the lower lumbar spine and/or the joint space at the LSJ. The AP projection *must* be available for assessment before attempting the lateral L5/S1 projection
2. The position of the PSISs when lying in the lateral position. They should be vertically aligned in order to justify use of a vertical central ray. Deviation from this position will mean that the central ray must be angled to coincide with the angle made by the PSISs
3. The lateral lumbar spine image. The radiographer may have used a vertical, caudally or cranially angled central ray for the lateral lumbar projection and the appearance of the lateral L5/S1 area on the lateral lumbar spine can be used as a reference point for assessment of the central ray. Modification of the central ray for this projection can be summarised thus:
   – If the lateral lumbar image undertaken with a vertical central ray shows a good L5/S1 joint space (but is underexposed or under-penetrated), angle approximately 5–7° caudally when the beam is centred over the LSJ
   – If the lateral lumbar image undertaken with a caudally angled central ray shows a good L5/S1 joint space (but is underexposed or under-penetrated), add more caudal angulation before centring the beam over the LSJ
   – If the lateral lumbar image undertaken with a cranially angled central ray shows a good L5/S1 joint space (but is underexposed or under-penetrated), use a vertical beam centred over the LSJ

   – If the lateral lumbar image undertaken with a vertical central ray shows a poor L5/S1 joint space it is most likely that a vertical central ray will be required for the lateral L5/S1 projection unless the AP projection and the PSISs show the opposite is required

100–150 cm FRD

Again, consider using the longer FRD to compensate for long ORD.

Centring point

Through the lumbosacral junction, which lies anterior to the spinous process of L5

This is most readily located as shown in Figure 13.6. An imaginary triangle is drawn between the readily palpable anterior superior iliac spine (ASIS), PSIS and apex of the iliac crest. The L5/S1 junction lies in the centre of this triangle.

Collimation

Body of L5, first sacral segment, spinous processes

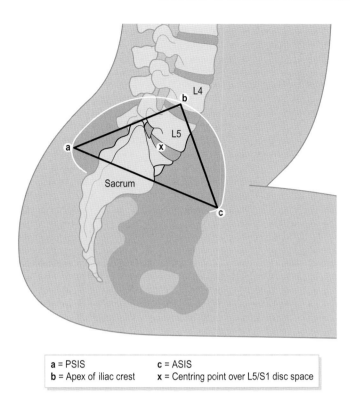

a = PSIS	c = ASIS
b = Apex of iliac crest	x = Centring point over L5/S1 disc space

Figure 13.6 Location of centring point for lateral L5/S1 projection. 'a', 'b' and 'c' show the landmarks which make the triangle around the centring point. The triangle is not necessarily equilateral or isosceles, but this is still an effective way to centre accurately.

Criteria for assessing image quality

- Bodies of L5 and S1, spinous processes and soft tissues anterior to vertebral bodies are demonstrated on the image
- Posterior, superior and inferior borders of L5 and S1 should be superimposed
- L5/S1 joint space should be clearly demonstrated (but see Fig. 13.4)
- Ala of sacrum superimposed*
- Sharp image demonstrating soft tissue structures anterior to the vertebral bodies in contrast to detail of bony cortex and trabeculae, joint space and spinous process of L5

*Use of the term 'ala' refers to the oblique white lines noted on the lateral projection, which have previously been described as ileopectineal lines, basis ossis sacri or pelvic lines.[19] The lines, whatever their correct name, do lie coincident with the sloped and expanding ala of the sacrum as they join with the pelvis at the sacroiliac joints. It is felt therefore that the use of the term 'ala' is simple and less confusing.

Common errors	Possible reasons
Both sides of ala of sacrum not superimposed; posterior parts of L5 do not appear superimposed	Rotation of the patient. MSP not parallel to the table-top (rotated) – adjust the hips and shoulders so that they are superimposed
Disc spaces are not clearly demonstrated – the superior and inferior surfaces of the vertebral bodies are not superimposed	Incorrect choice of beam angulation or The long axis of the vertebral column is not parallel to the table-top

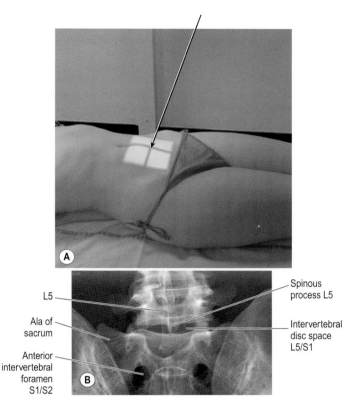

Figure 13.7 AP LSJ. (B) Notice how the appearances of L5 and its spinous process and L5/S1 joint space change from the AP lumbar spine image (Fig. 13.1B) to this, the AP L5/S1 image. This is because (1) the oblique rays in the AP lumbar image are caudal and the lumbar curve tilts the body of L5 forwards over the joint space; (2) the beam is angled opposite to this (cranially) for the AP L5/S1 projection, coinciding with the disc space.

AP L5/S1 junction (Fig. 13.7A,B)

Because of the orientation of the lumbar curve, L5 tilts in opposition to the oblique rays of the X-ray beam; thus the L5/S1 joint space is not well demonstrated on the standard AP projection. The AP L5/S1 projection is rarely used but may be used for additional evaluation in relevant clinical circumstances,[20] which is most commonly requested for specialist orthopaedic assessment.

IR is horizontal; an antiscatter grid is employed

Positioning

The patient is positioned as for an AP lumbar spine projection

Beam direction and FRD

Initially vertical, with a cranial angle of 10–20°, according to the patient's lumbar lordosis, which tends to be more extreme in the female adult.[21] The lateral projection should be viewed before assessing the angulation required

Centring point

In the midline, level with the ASISs; this may vary slightly according to cranial angle used

Collimation

L4/L5 junction, L5, transverse processes, L5/S1 junction

Criteria for assessing image quality

- L4/L5 junction, L5, transverse processes, and L5/S1 junction are demonstrated
- L4/L5 and L5/S1 joint space shown clearly
- Spinous process of L5 centralised over vertebral body
- Sharp image showing contrast between bony trabeculae of vertebral bodies and the joint spaces between

Common error	Possible reason
Poor joint space visualisation	Inaccurate angle selection

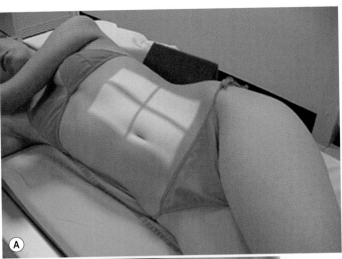

OBLIQUE LUMBAR SPINE

Oblique projections may be undertaken with the patient prone or supine. Posterior oblique projections are usually used and demonstrate the side closest to the IR. Anterior obliques could be used and would demonstrate the side furthest from the receptor, raising the side under examination and centring over the third lumbar vertebra. Oblique projections demonstrate the apophyseal joints, laminae, pedicles and pars interarticularis. They are used in particular to demonstrate defects in the pars interarticularis which may result in spondylolisthesis. Both obliques are undertaken, for comparison.

Traditionally, posterior obliques were used most extensively, in order to reduce the ORD and therefore minimise magnification unsharpness. Unfortunately, the lumbar curve lies in opposition to the oblique rays, which gradually increase in obliquity towards each end of the lumbar vertebrae, increasing the longitudinal obliquity of all but L3 on the image. Use of the anterior oblique approach would bring the lumbar curve into a position which more closely follows the pattern of central and oblique rays, reducing the longitudinal obliquity of L1, L2, L4 and L5. Although ORD would be increased for this projection, anterior abdominal tissue is compressed; this allows for reduction in scatter and a reduction in exposure factors may be considered if tissue compression is significant. However, patients with back pain or limited movement are likely to find the semi-prone position difficult, and for this reason the posterior obliques are described in more detail.

MRI is the investigation of choice in the symptomatic patient; however, non-specific abnormalities are commonly detected even in asymptomatic patients, so careful thought must be given to the appropriateness of imaging.[22]

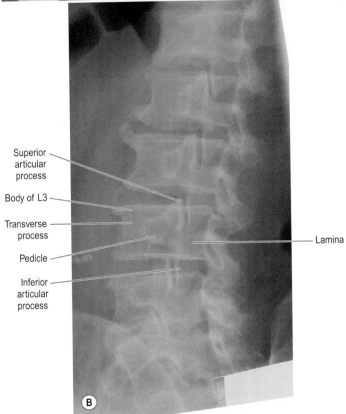

Figure 13.8 Posterior oblique lumbar spine.

Posterior obliques (Fig. 13.8A,B)

IR is horizontal; an antiscatter grid is employed

Positioning

- The patient lies supine, their MSP coincident with and perpendicular to the midline of the table
- The arm on the side under examination is raised onto the pillow, for comfort and ease of positioning
- The patient is rotated 45° *towards* the side under examination
- Radiolucent pads are placed under the trunk and raised shoulder for support. The arm on the unaffected side must be clear of the area under examination

Beam direction and FRD

Vertical

or the beam is angled with a cranial or caudal tilt of between 10° and 15° *if the patient presents with a marked lordosis*. The degree of angle used is dependent upon the degree of lordosis and the direction of angle relates to which vertebrae are under examination (e.g. caudal angle for L1 and L2, cranial for L4 and L5)

100 cm FRD

Centring point

Over the raised side of the trunk at the level of the lower costal margin (level of L3), in the midclavicular line

Collimation

T12/L1 junction, L5/S1 junction, bodies and transverse processes of lumbar vertebrae

Criteria for assessing image quality

- T12/L1 junction, L5/S1 junction, bodies and transverse processes of lumbar vertebrae are demonstrated
- 'Scottie dog' appearance seen within the associated vertebral body, with a dog's nose seen touching the edge of the vertebral body and the back of the dog's front leg coincident with the middle of the vertebral body. Structures correspond to the dog as follows:
  - Nose = transverse process
  - Eye = pedicle
  - Ear = superior articular process
  - Body = lamina
  - Neck = pars interarticularis
  - Front leg = inferior articular process
    Please note that the position of the dog in relationship to its associated vertebral body will vary slightly in a longitudinal direction, according to the relationship of the vertebral body and its distance from the central ray. It is suggested that L3 is used to assess positional accuracy, as it lies most perpendicular to the central ray
- Sharp image showing soft tissue in contrast with bone and 'Scottie dog' in contrast with the bony trabeculae of the associated vertebral body

Common errors	Possible reasons
Dog's nose is elongated and most of it lies outside the vertebral body outline	Inadequate rotation
Dog's nose squashed and lies well within vertebral body outline	Excessive rotation

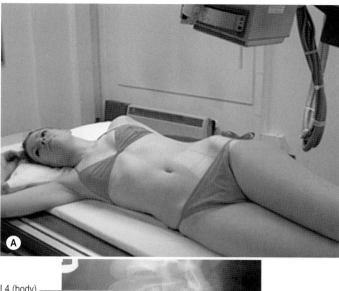
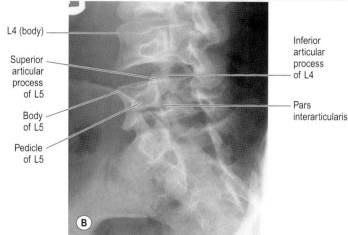

L4 (body)

Superior articular process of L5

Body of L5

Pedicle of L5

Inferior articular process of L4

Pars interarticularis

Figure 13.9 Posterior oblique L5. Compare the pars interarticularis on this image to that of L3 on Figure 13.8B. The neck of the Scottie dog in Figure 13.8B is intact, whereas here there appears to be a dark line or collar, which is suggestive of spondylolisthesis.

Posterior oblique L5 (Fig. 13.9A,B)

For this projection, positioning is as for the posterior oblique lumbar vertebrae, with the following adjustments because of the position of the vertebral body and its extreme tilt at the end of the lumbar lordosis. Anterior obliques may also be considered, with the direction of beam angulation in opposition to that used for posterior obliques and the centring point adapted to lie over the PSIS of the raised side.

Beam direction and FRD

Initially vertical, angled 10–20° cranially. The IR is displaced until coincident with the primary beam
100 cm FRD

Centring point

Level with the ASIS in the midclavicular line

Collimation

L4/L5 junction, L5, S1

Criteria for assessing image quality

- L4/L5 junction, L5 and S1 are demonstrated
- 'Scottie dog' appearance seen within L5 as explained for oblique lumbar vertebrae
- Clear joint space between L4 and 5, and L5 and S1
- Sharp image showing soft tissue in contrast with bone and 'Scottie dog' in contrast with the bony trabeculae of L5. Bone seen in contrast with joint spaces

Erect laterals in flexion and extension

Flexion and extension views may be used to demonstrate the range of movement within the lumbar spine. With the development of erect scanning by Fonar, it is now possible to perform this examination by MRI.[23,24]

IR is vertical; an antiscatter grid is employed

Positioning

- The patient is in the erect lateral position, either seated or standing. The MSP is parallel to the erect bucky, usually with the left side in contact with it
- For the flexion projection the patient bends forward, flexing the spine as far forward as possible, arms extended forward, holding a fixed support or their legs to aid immobilisation
- For the extension projection the patient leans backwards, extending the spine as far as possible; again, immobilisation devices can be provided

Central ray, FRD, centring point

Central ray horizontal, at 90° to the long axis of the spine. The rest of the technique is as for the lateral projection

SACROILIAC JOINTS

The sacroiliac joints (SIJs) are difficult to assess on AP projections of the lumbar spine or pelvis, owing to the oblique nature of the joints. The sacral angle, which lies in opposition to the oblique rays at the periphery of the X-ray beam, causes foreshortening of the joints on the AP lumbar projection. On the AP pelvis projection, the sacral and sacroiliac joint angle is far greater than the obliquity of X-rays around the central ray. The joints travel from the back of the sacrum and pelvis in an anterolateral direction (approximately 15°), again crossing the oblique rays in any AP position, rather than lying coincidentally with them. Therefore it is necessary to use a technique that considers the effects normal anatomy has on the demonstration of these joints.

Many years ago it was believed that the joints were demonstrated with a prone patient position and very short FRD; the short FRD was suggested in order to provide maximum angulation of oblique rays around the central ray and pass more accurately through the joints. This was combined with the prone position, which placed the sacral angle in a more suitable orientation. Unfortunately, although a prone position is often recommended to reduce the dose to the gonads, this method significantly increases the skin dose and is not likely to provide noticeable improvement of joint visualisation; it has been estimated that an unobtainable and unfeasible FRD of 18 cm would be required in order to provide obliquity of rays that will coincide with the 15° angles of the joints.[25] A prone projection at 100 cm FRD, with the caudal angle selected to pass through the sacral angle at 90°, is therefore recommended if a single projection is required. Alternatively, individual posterior oblique projections of each joint will demonstrate the joints most effectively, but will require the patient to be exposed to ionising radiation twice (although close collimation will reduce the associated risks of exposure to ionising radiation).

Prone SIJs (Fig. 13.10A,B)

IR is horizontal; an antiscatter grid is employed

Positioning

- The patient lies prone, arms placed on the pillow and head turned to the side for comfort
- The MSP is perpendicular to the table-top and positioned to lie coincident with the long axis of the table

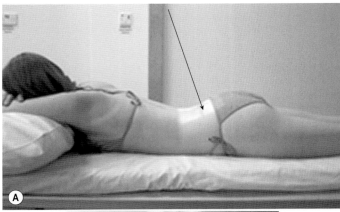

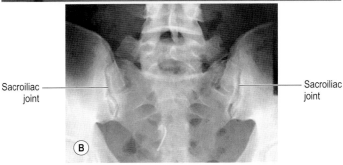

Sacroiliac joint — — Sacroiliac joint

Figure 13.10 Prone SIJs.

Beam direction and FRD

A vertical central ray is angled caudally until at 90° to the long axis of the sacrum
100 cm FRD

Centring

Midway between the PSISs

Collimation

SIJs, L5/S1 joint

Criteria for assessing image quality

- SIJs and L5/S1 joint are demonstrated
- Symmetry of sacrum and SIJs
- Sharp image demonstrating the trabecular pattern of sacrum and ilium and lower density of the SIJs in contrast with the sacrum and ilium

Posterior oblique SIJs (Fig. 13.11A,B)

Both joints are examined for comparison.
  IR is horizontal; an antiscatter grid is employed

Positioning

- The patient lies supine, with the MSP initially coincident with the long axis of the table
- The side under examination is raised 15° and a radiolucent pad placed under the raised side for immobilisation
- The arm on the lowered side is placed on the pillow for comfort and the leg on the same side flexed at the knee to aid stability
- A sheet of lead rubber is applied to the lower pelvis region, below the level of the SIJs

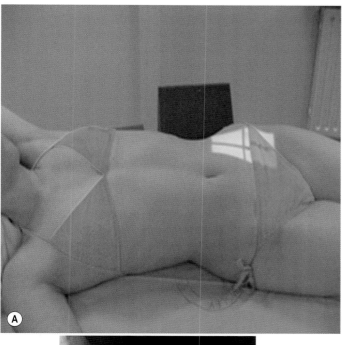

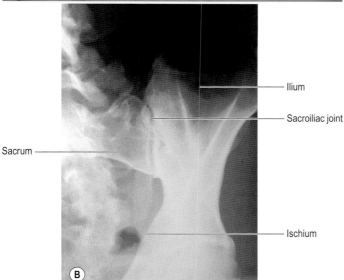

Ilium

Sacroiliac joint

Sacrum

Ischium

Figure 13.11 Posterior oblique SIJs.

Beam direction and FRD

1. Vertical *or*
2. Angled 10–15° cranially, to compensate for the sacral angle

The second option can, in some cases, project the image of the ischium over the inferior aspect of the SIJ. This is more likely in males, due to the shallower pelvis.

Centring

1. 2.5 cm medial to the ASIS on the raised side
2. 2.5 cm medial to and below the ASIS on the raised side

Collimation

SIJ on the raised side

Criteria for assessing image quality

- SIJ is demonstrated
- SIJ is shown clear of iliac crest and ASIS
- Joint space seen clearly
- Sharp image showing bony trabeculae of sacrum and ilium and the lower density joint in contrast with sacrum and ilium

Common errors	Possible reasons
Joint space overlaps	Because the joint surfaces are not flat, some irregularity of the joint will be noted. Total loss of joint space is due to inaccurate obliquity. There may be indistinct or lost joint space in cases of degenerative diseases, such as ankylosing spondylitis
Ilium superimposed over joint	Too much obliquity

OTHER IMAGING MODALITIES AND THE LUMBAR SPINE

As previously stated, MRI is generally recognised as the most appropriate modality for lumbar spine imaging in many circumstances.[1,4,22] Cost and availability are factors that will still predispose some departments to the continued use of plain radiography; the significant radiation dose burden must, however, always be considered for justification of this procedure.[15] New techniques are in development, such as erect MRI scanning, enabling a wide variety of examinations to be performed.[24]

Computed tomography (CT) has been advocated for demonstration of pars interarticularis abnormalities which lead to spondylolisthesis,[26] but its role in imaging the intervertebral disc should now be limited to patients unable to undergo MRI. CT also has a role in significant trauma where modern multislice scanners can use multiplanar and 3D bony reconstruction techniques.

REFERENCES

1. van den Bosch M, et al. Evidence against the use of lumbar spine radiography for low back pain. Clinical Radiology 2004;59(1):69–76.
2. Royal College of Radiologists Working Party. Making the best use of clinical radiology services: referral guidelines for doctors. 6th ed. London: Royal College of Radiologists; 2007.
3. Kendrick D, et al. Radiography of the lumbar spine in primary care patients with low back pain: randomised controlled trial. British Medical Journal 2001;322: 400–5.
4. Miller P, et al. Cost-effectiveness of lumbar spine radiography in primary care patients with low back pain. Spine 2002;27(20): 2291–7.

5. Editor's choice. Challenges to orthodoxy? British Medical Journal 2001;322(7283):0.

6. Wood A. Imaging the spine: Why take it lying down? Synergy 2003;Dec:16–9.

7. McQuillen Martensen K. Radiographic image analysis. Philadelphia: WB Saunders; 2010.

8. Whitley A, et al. Special procedures in diagnostic imaging. Oxford: Butterworth Heinemann; 1991.

9. Murrie VL, et al. Supportive cushions produce no practical reduction in lumbar lordosis. British Journal of Radiology 2002;75:536–8.

10. Downing N. Does flexion of the knees and hips reduce lumbar lordosis during AP lumbar spine examinations? Proceedings of UK Radiological Congress 2005; p. 97.

11. Colleran C. PA lumbar spines; a future concept. Radiography Today 1994;60(681): 17–20.

12. Mitchell F, et al. Scattered radiation and the lumbar spine. Radiography Today 1991;57(645):12–4.

13. Thomas A. Imaging the lateral thoracic spine. Synergy 2003;Apr:10–3.

14. Hart D, et al. Estimation of effective dose in radiology from entrance surface dose and dose area product measurements. NRPB 262 Chilton 1994.

15. Nicholson R, et al. Awareness by radiology staff of the difference in radiation risk from two opposing lateral lumbar spine examinations. British Journal of Radiology 1999;72:221.

16. Hart D, et al. Coefficients for estimating effective doses from paediatric x-ray examinations. NRPB 279 Chilton 1996.

17. Chapple C, et al. Awareness by radiology staff of the difference in radiation risk from two opposing lateral lumbar spine examinations. British Journal of Radiology 2000;73:568.

18. European Guidelines on Quality Criteria for Diagnostic Radiographic Images. EUR 16260 Luxembourg Office for Official Publications of the European Communities; 1997.

19. Wong-Chung J, et al. Two parallel linear densities on lateral radiographs of the lumbosacral spine: neither ileopectineal lines nor basis ossis sacri. British Journal of Radiology 1997;70:58–61.

20. ACR Practice guideline for the performance of spine radiography in children and adults. ACR; 2002.

21. Murrie VL, et al. Lumbar lordosis measurement: a study in patients with and without low back pain. Clinical Anatomy 2001;14:298.

22. ACR Appropriateness criteria. Acute low back pain: radiculopathy. ACR; 1996.

23. Jinkins J, et al. Upright, weight-bearing, dynamic-kinetic magnetic resonance imaging of the spine – review of the first clinical results. Journal of Hong Kong College of Radiology 2003;6:55–74.

24. www.fonar.com.

25. Unett EM, Royle AJ. Radiographic techniques and image evaluation. London: Chapman and Hall; 1997.

26. Mayor P. Invited review: spondylolysis: current imaging and management. Proceedings of UK Radiological Congress 2003. British Journal of Radiology 2003;76(Suppl):35.

| Chapter | **14** |

Sacrum and coccyx

Elizabeth Carver

SACRUM

Trauma relating to the sacrum may well be associated with other injury to the pelvic ring and imaging of the pelvis is likely to be required in addition to examination of the sacrum. In cases of severe trauma it is inadvisable to undertake a lateral projection of the sacral area in the position described in this section; a horizontal beam approach would be the method of choice. However, as serious pelvis trauma will probably be assessed by initial pelvis images which will be supplemented by computed tomography (CT) examination, a lateral sacrum image is unlikely to be required.

The sacrum may be a site for metastatic spread of malignancy and plain images of the region would demonstrate such lesions if the secondary tumour has eroded at least 40% of the bone. Magnetic resonance imaging (MRI) is most appropriate for assessing bone metastases.[1] Today it is rare to find radiography requested for assessment of this area, and there is no longer specific reference to assessment of the sacrum in current Royal College of Radiologists (RCR) guidelines in the UK.

The lumbar curve varies with each individual patient and causes variation in the angles created between the sacrum and lumbar vertebrae. As a result it is suggested that the cranial angulation required to strike the sacrum at 90° in the anteroposterior (AP) position will vary from 10° to 25°, according to the individual patient's build. The most efficient strategy for making a decision on appropriate angulation is to undertake the lateral projection initially and use it to assess the required angle before proceeding with the AP projection. This also applies to the coccyx.

If the examination request outlines that information on the coccyx is required, the lateral projection of the coccyx can be included on the lateral sacrum projection, to reduce the number of exposures. For this reason, the coccyx is also referred to in the description of the lateral projection.

For all projections of the sacrum and coccyx, the image receptor (IR) is horizontal and antiscatter grid is used

Lateral sacrum (Fig. 14.1A,B)

Positioning

- The patient lies on their side, with hips and knees flexed to maintain stability and the feet placed together to prevent the patient from rolling forwards or backwards. The arms are flexed at the elbow and raised to rest on the pillows for comfort and to clear them from the area of interest
- Lead rubber is applied over the raised side, diagonally from anterior superior iliac spine (ASIS) to the femoral head, to cover the anterior portion of the pelvis and to protect the gonads
- The palm of the radiographer's hand is used to palpate the posterior aspect of the sacrum and ensure that its transverse axis is perpendicular to the table-top
- The long axis of the sacrum is parallel to the table-top; this should be checked with the area at the radiographer's eye level for accuracy. If patient build affects the relationship of the sacrum to the table-top, a compensating cranial or caudal central ray can be used (see beam direction, below)

Beam direction and focus receptor distance (FRD)

Vertical, directed at 90° to the long axis of the sacrum once this has been assessed
100 cm FRD

Centring

Midway between the posterior superior iliac spines (PSISs) and sacrococcygeal junction

As the coccyx is more difficult to palpate than the sacrum, the level of its first segment may be difficult to locate. An alternative method to palpation uses the relationship of sacrococcygeal junction, which lies approximately level with the midpoint of the upper border of the symphysis pubis; palpation of the symphysis pubis anteriorly will allow the radiographer to estimate the level of the first coccygeal segment posteriorly.

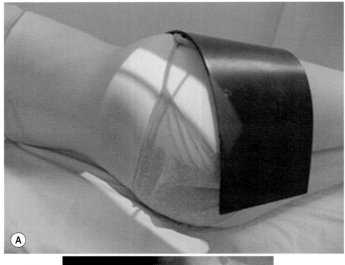

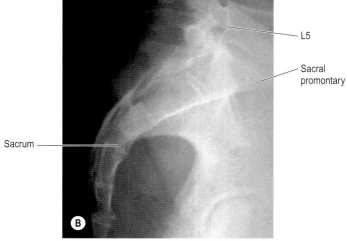

Figure 14.1 Lateral sacrum.

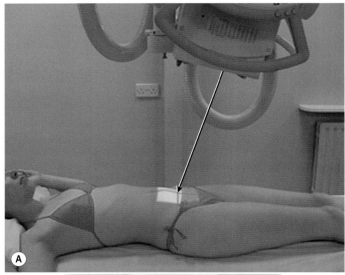

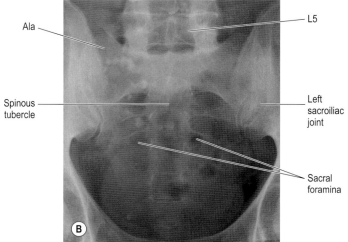

Figure 14.2 AP sacrum.

Collimation

Lumbosacral junction, sacral promontory, soft tissues overlying the sacrum posteriorly, coccyx

Criteria for assessing image quality

- Lumbosacral junction, sacral promontory, soft tissues overlying the sacrum posteriorly and coccyx are demonstrated. Omission of the coccyx from the field may be acceptable if demonstration of the coccyx is not required specifically for the examination
- Joint space at the lumbosacral junction is demonstrated
- Ala of sacrum superimposed*
- Sharp image demonstrating bony trabeculae. Adequate penetration to demonstrate detail of sacrum and less dense coccyx on the one image

*Use of the term 'ala' refers to the oblique white lines noted on the lateral projection, which have previously been called ileopectineal lines, basis ossis sacri or pelvic lines.[2] The lines, whatever their correct name is deemed to be, do lie coincidentally with the sloped and expanding ala of the sacrum as they join with the pelvis at the sacro-iliac joints. It is therefore felt that use of the term 'ala' is simple and less confusing.

Common errors	Possible reasons
Non-superimposition of ala	Rotation
Sacrum demonstrated but detail of coccyx less so, or not seen *If information relating to the coccyx is not required for the examination, repeat examination should not be attempted*	1. kVp may not be correct to demonstrate the range of densities encountered over sacrum and coccyx
	2. A combination of the higher exposure factors and increased scatter associated with larger patients may have affected image contrast and quality. This is not necessarily considered a radiographer error; close collimation will reduce scatter but will not eliminate it

AP sacrum (Fig. 14.2A,B)

Positioning

- The patient is supine with arms abducted from the trunk
- The median sagittal plane (MSP) is coincident with the long axis of the table
- For male patients, lead rubber or lead gonad protection is applied below the symphysis pubis
- ASISs are equidistant from the table-top

Beam direction and FRD

The lateral sacrum projection is examined to assess the angle of the sacrum

Initially, the central ray is vertical, angled 10–25° cranially until 90° to the long axis of the sacrum

Centring

In the midline, midway between the level of the ASISs and the upper border of symphysis pubis

The IR must coincide with the emerging central ray, and to ensure that the collimated area lies within it.

Collimation

Lumbosacral joint space, sacrococcygeal junction, sacroiliac joints

Criteria for assessing image quality

- Lumbosacral joint space, sacrococcygeal junction and sacroiliac joints are demonstrated
- Symphysis pubis is superimposed over coccyx
- Symmetry of sacral foraminae
- Sharp image demonstrating bony detail of spinous tubercles in contrast with the body of the sacrum and all bony detail of the sacrum in contrast with the soft tissues of the pelvic cavity

Common errors	Possible reasons
Asymmetry of sacral foramina	Rotation about the MSP
Symphysis pubis superimposed over lower sacral segments	Angle of beam is too great
Foreshortened sacrum	Inadequate angle used
Ala of sacrum seen but sacral segments 2–4 superimposed; fifth segment seen	Angle selected is in wrong direction (caudal)

COCCYX

Under older RCR guidelines, trauma to the coccyx and coccidynia were not routine indicators for radiographic examination of the coccyx since confirmation of effects on the coccyx does not alter patient management.[3] Current RCR guidelines say that X-ray examination of the coccyx in trauma should only be undertaken in 'special circumstances', but do not identify the circumstances that would be considered special. They also state that the variations in 'normal' appearances of the human coccyx can make radiological assessment difficult.[4]

However, although guidelines rule it out, the most frequently encountered problems associated with the coccyx are extreme pain and trauma and these may necessitate radiographic examination.

Lateral coccyx (Fig. 14.3A,B)

Positioning

- The patient lies on their side and is positioned as for the lateral sacrum and coccyx projection
- A lead rubber sheet is applied diagonally from ASIS to the femoral head

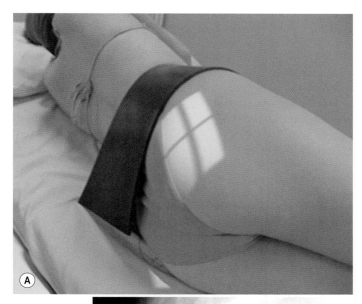

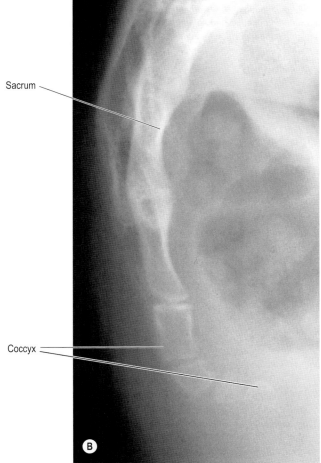

Sacrum

Coccyx

Figure 14.3 Lateral coccyx.

Beam direction and FRD

Vertical, directed at 90° to the long axis of the sacrum and coccyx
100 cm FRD

Centring

At the base of the sacrum, level with the midpoint of the symphysis pubis

Collimation

Coccyx, sacrococcygeal junction

Criteria for assessing image quality

- Coccyx and sacrococcygeal junction are demonstrated
- Sharp image demonstrating separate coccygeal segments in contrast to the surrounding soft tissues

Common error	Possible reason
Inadequate contrast to distinctly demonstrate coccyx in contrast to soft tissues of buttocks	Usually due to patient build and implications of associated scatter (see errors section under AP coccyx)

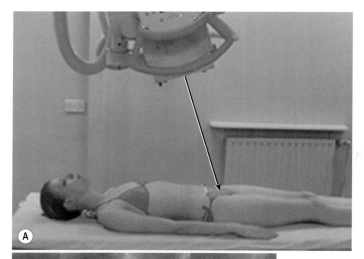

AP coccyx (Fig. 14.4A,B)

Positioning

- The patient is supine as for the AP sacrum projection
- For male patients, lead rubber or lead gonad protection is applied below the symphysis pubis, to protect the gonads

Beam direction and FRD

The lateral coccyx or sacrum and coccyx projection is examined to assess the angle of the coccyx

Initially the central ray is vertical, angled approximately 15° to 20° caudally until 90° to the long axis of the coccygeal segments.
100 cm FRD

Centring

In the midline, midway between the level of the ASISs and the upper border of symphysis pubis

The IR must coincide with the emerging central ray, and to ensure that the collimated area lies within it.

Collimation

Sacrococcygeal junction, all coccygeal segments

Criteria for assessing image quality

- Sacrococcygeal junction and all coccygeal segments are demonstrated
- Symphysis pubis is cleared from the coccyx
- Foreshortened sacrum
- Sharp image demonstrating coccygeal segments in contrast with the soft tissues of the pelvic cavity

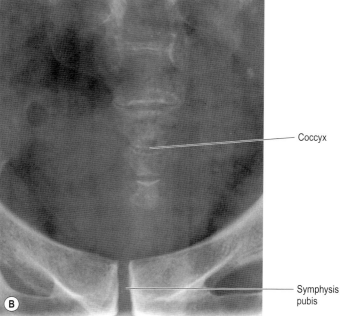

Figure 14.4 AP coccyx.

Common errors	Possible reasons
Poor contrast between coccyx and soft tissues or coccyx not demonstrated	1. Although the coccyx itself is not particularly dense, the pelvic area in the larger patient is an area of relatively large body thickness. Increased scatter associated with larger patients may thus have affected image contrast and quality. This is not necessarily considered a radiographer error and may be unavoidable in some cases
	2. Faecal matter and bowel gas may also overlie the area and mask the low-density structure of the coccyx
Coccygeal segments superimposed over the sacrum	Excessive angle used
Sacrum not foreshortened; coccygeal segments foreshortened or superimposed	Angle selected is in wrong direction (cranial)

REFERENCES

1. RCR Working Party. Making the best use of clinical radiology services: referral guidelines. 6th ed. London: The Royal College of Radiologists; 2007.

2. Wong-Chung J, et al. Two parallel linear densities on lateral radiographs of the lumbosacral spine: neither ileopectineal lines nor basis ossis sacri. British Journal of Radiology 1997;70:58–61.

3. Royal College of Radiologists Working Party. Making the best use of a department of clinical radiology: guidelines for doctors. 5th ed. London: Royal College Of Radiologists; 2003.

4. Royal College of Radiologists Working Party. Making the best use of a department of clinical radiology: guidelines for doctors. 6th ed. London: Royal College Of Radiologists; 2007.

Chapter 15

Thoracic skeleton

Elizabeth Carver

The bones of the thorax consist of the ribs and sternum, but radiographic examination of the area also involves demonstration of the sternoclavicular (SC) joints. Referrals for radiography of the ribs have declined, especially in cases of trauma. Although painful, rib fractures are treated conservatively unless displacement causes fracture fragments to penetrate the soft issue of the thorax and induce pneumothorax or haemothorax. Evidence of these conditions is definitely required via radiographic examination, but the posteroanterior (PA) chest projection is considered to be the most appropriate means for demonstration of these appearances,[1] as the most important aspect of diagnosis is that of assessing the effect injury may have had on thoracic contents. The PA chest film is also very likely to demonstrate the fractured rib and fragments causing a pneumothorax, haemothorax or evidence of visceral damage.[2,3] Ribs positioned below the diaphragm on the PA image are those that are less likely to penetrate the pleura, thus reducing or eradicating the need for separate X-ray examination of these. The PA chest image also shows ribs 1–6 reasonably well in their entirety, but not ribs 7–12.

Metastatic deposits may be demonstrated by X-ray but are better located via scintigraphy; however, as metastases in the rib may lead to pathological fracture it may be necessary to undertake plain radiography. In addition to fractures and metastasis, other rib lesions seen on plain radiography include fibrous dysplasia, aneurysmal bone cysts, myeloma and granuloma,[4] but it is questionable whether X-ray would be the method of choice to demonstrate them.

OBLIQUE RIBS

The oblique projection is designed to turn the lateral portions of the ribs away from their profiled position as seen on the PA chest radiograph. Of course, this means that other aspects of the ribs will not be well demonstrated on the oblique projection. For this reason, oblique ribs projections must always be accompanied by a PA chest radiograph.

It is more than obvious that exposures should be made on arrested respiration, but the phase varies according to the ribs under examination owing to the position of the diaphragm in relation to individual rib height. Because the diaphragm effectively splits the area covered by ribs into two different densities, this has implications for adequate demonstration of ribs on the radiograph. As a result, exposure for oblique projections of the upper ribs (1–6) is made on arrested inspiration to facilitate their demonstration over the air-filled lung tissue, and ribs 7–12 on expiration to demonstrate them over abdominal tissue below the diaphragm.

In addition to the phase of respiration, angulation can be used to maximise the number of ribs shown above or below the diaphragm. Caudal angulation will project the image of the diaphragm lower in the case of the upper ribs, as can cranial angulation to project it higher and maximise the number of lower ribs shown below the diaphragm.

Posterior oblique for upper ribs (Fig. 15.1A,B)

Image receptor (IR) is vertical for projections of the ribs unless otherwise stated; antiscatter grid is often required for lower ribs.

Positioning

- A lead rubber apron is applied to the patient's waist
- The patient stands with their back to the IR and faces the X-ray tube; the side under examination is positioned with the lateral borders of ribs 1–6 well within the IR border
- The arm on the side under investigation is raised and the forearm rested on the head; this will clear the arm from the area of interest
- The patient is rotated 30–45° towards the side under examination; the thorax on the side of interest rests against the IR

Beam direction and focus receptor distance (FRD)

Beam is initially horizontal, with 12° caudal angulation
100 cm FRD

Centring

Two-thirds of the way down the line adjoining sternal notch and xiphisternum

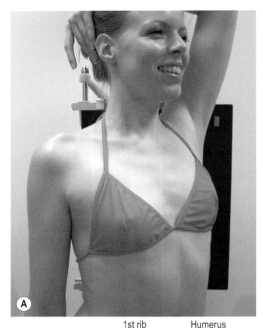

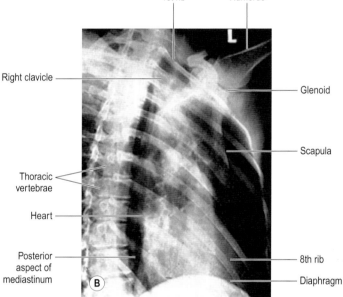

Figure 15.1 Posterior oblique – upper ribs.
(B) Reproduced with permission from Bryan GJ. Skeletal anatomy. 3rd ed. Edinburgh: Churchill Livingstone; 1996 and Gunn C. Bones and joints. 4th ed. Edinburgh: Churchill Livingstone, 2002.

IR displacement may be required to ensure that the area of interest lies within its boundaries

Collimation

C7 to T12, lateral margins of ribs on affected side, midclavicular line on the opposite side

It is not necessary for this projection to be undertaken erect, but it is described thus as it is more comfortable for the patient who has painful ribs, as their weight does not lie on their injured thoracic ribcage. Supine oblique positioning can still be adopted for patients who cannot sit or stand erect.

Traditionally the upper rib oblique projection has been described using antiscatter grid,[5,6] but as ribs 1–6 lie superior to the diaphragm in a low-density area, direct exposure is possible without an antiscatter device. This allows reduction in exposure factors and therefore affords less radiation dose to the patient. In the case of larger patients it is possible that provision of adequate contrast may be compromised by an increase in tissue density. This, coupled with the higher density over the mediastinum, may require the use of a grid.

> Expose on arrested inspiration

Criteria for assessing image quality

- The entire length of ribs 1–6 are demonstrated above diaphragm
- Arm is cleared from thorax
- Heart shadow may overlie medial aspect of sixth rib in the case of right-sided ribs, or most of the sixth rib in the case of left-sided ribs
- Oblique appearance of thoracic vertebrae
- Image of anterior ribs moved laterally in comparison to their position as seen on the PA chest image
- Sharp image demonstrating ribs in contrast to air-filled lung tissue and viscera of the mediastinum and heart

Common errors	Possible reasons
High-contrast image which does not demonstrate ribs in contrast to viscera and heart	kVp selected is too low. It will be necessary to compensate for kVp increase by reducing mAs proportionally to avoid over-blackening over the lung area
Over-blackened image generally	If automatic exposure chamber used, the central ray and chamber selected may be lying over the dense mediastinum
Pale shadow overlying lateral ribs	Arm not cleared from area
Lower ribs (4–6) pale and shown below diaphragm	Exposed on expiration

Posterior oblique for lower ribs (Fig. 15.2A,B)

Positioning

- A lead rubber apron is applied to the patient's waist
- The patient stands with their back to the IR and faces the X-ray tube; the side under examination is positioned with the lateral borders of ribs 7–12 well within the IR boundaries
- The arm on the side under investigation is raised and the forearm rested on the head; this will clear the arm from the area of interest
- The patient is rotated 30–45° towards the side under examination; the thorax on the side of interest rests against the IR

Beam direction and FRD

Central ray is initially horizontal, with 12° cranial angulation
100 cm FRD

Centring

Midway between the lower costal margin and xiphisternum

IR displacement may be required to ensure that the area of interest lies within its boundaries.

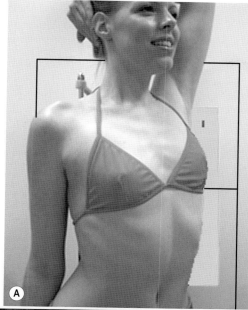

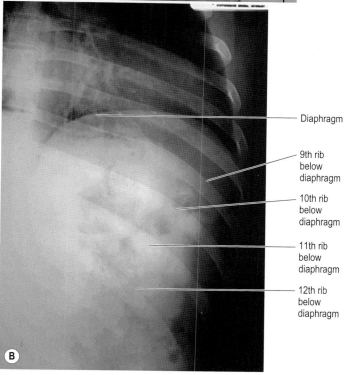

Figure 15.2 Posterior oblique – lower ribs.

Labels on Figure 15.2:
- Diaphragm
- 9th rib below diaphragm
- 10th rib below diaphragm
- 11th rib below diaphragm
- 12th rib below diaphragm

Collimation

2.5 cm below lower costal margin to midway between the sternal notch and xiphisternum, lateral margins of ribs on the affected side, midclavicular line on the opposite side

> Expose on arrested expiration

Note that the oblique for lower ribs has been described as for the upper ribs, with the patient erect. This is in contrast to other texts,[6]

which suggest this projection be undertaken with the patient in a supine oblique position. The erect position has been used here simply for reasons of patient comfort.

Criteria for assessing image quality

- The entire length of ribs 7–12 demonstrated below the diaphragm; ribs 7 and 8 are frequently shown above the diaphragm but, since the heart shadow tends to overlie these ribs in the oblique position, contrast over these ribs is usually similar to those seen below the diaphragm
- Arm cleared from thorax
- Oblique appearance of thoracic vertebrae
- Ribs appear less curved than in a PA or anteroposterior (AP) image
- Sharp image demonstrating ribs in contrast to abdominal and heart tissue

Common errors	Possible reasons
Pale shadow overlying lateral ribs	Arm not cleared from area
Ribs 7–8 dark and shown above diaphragm	Exposed on inspiration; more likely to affect the right side than the left due to there being less heart tissue superimposed over the ribs on this side

STERNUM

The mechanism for injury to the sternum is most likely to be that of a crush injury, as in a road traffic accident when the steering wheel impacts upon the driver's chest. The lateral projection is recommended for patients with sternal injury[2] and can be undertaken with the patient seated or supine on a trolley.

Lateral sternum (Fig. 15.3A,B)

IR is vertical; an antiscatter grid may be required for larger patients

Positioning

- A lead rubber apron is applied to the patient's waist
- The patient stands or sits erect with the lateral aspect of their chest placed in contact with the IR. If standing, their feet are separated for stability
- The height of the IR is adjusted to coincide with the sternum
- The median sagittal plane (MSP) is parallel to the IR
- The arms are raised above the head to clear from the area of interest as for the chest lateral; the chin is raised *or*
- The shoulders are pulled back (this may be difficult for some patients)

Beam direction and FRD

Horizontal, at 90° to the IR
100 cm FRD

Centring

Midway between the sternal notch and xiphisternum

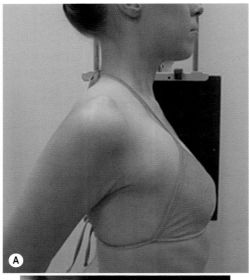

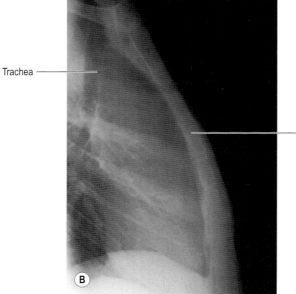

Trachea

Sternum

Figure 15.3 Lateral sternum.

Collimation

SC joints, manubrium, sternal body and xiphisternum, soft tissues of anterior sternal area, retrosternal lung tissue

Rotation of the light beam diaphragm housing to coincide with the long axis of the sternum will maximise efficiency of collimation to the field.

Expose on arrested respiration

Arrested respiration avoids movement unsharpness on the image, which is the primary function of the manoeuvre. However, arrested inspiration will serve to press the sternum further forward, which is especially beneficial when the arms are pulled backwards rather than raised.

Criteria for assessing image quality

- SC joints, manubrium, sternal body and xiphisternum, soft tissues of anterior sternal area, retrosternal lung tissue are demonstrated
- Arms are cleared from the area of interest
- SC joints are superimposed
- Sharp image demonstrating bony trabeculae in contrast with anterior soft tissues and retrosternal lung tissue

Common errors	Possible reasons
Pale density over upper sternum and SC joints	Arms not cleared from field
White sternum with no bony detail evident	kVp too low
Lower aspect of sternum not included on image	During inspiration the patient may lean back or elevate the lower chest during the manoeuvre, moving the lower sternum outside the field of collimation or off the receptor completely. Care should be taken to observe the patient during the manoeuvre

Anterior oblique sternum (Fig. 15.4A,B)

This projection is not recommended for trauma cases as it involves a prone position if the patient cannot stand, and in any case it provides no valuable additional information to the lateral. However, it has been recommended for demonstration of inflammatory conditions.[5]

The oblique position clears the sternum from the vertebral column; some texts describe a right anterior oblique,[5,7] but consideration must be given to the fact that the majority of the heart shadow lies over to the left. For this reason, the left anterior oblique is described here, where the right side is moved away from the IR to position the sternum over the right lung. The right atrium of the heart will also move to the right, but this forms a significantly lower proportion of heart tissue than that which would be projected if a right anterior oblique were performed.

The projection can be undertaken erect or prone and therefore IR orientation will depend on which is selected; antiscatter grid is often required.

Positioning

- A lead rubber apron is applied to the back of the patient's waist
- The patient lies prone *or* stands facing the IR
- The IR position should be checked to ensure the sternum lies within its boundary
- The patient is rotated 45° towards the right, into the left anterior oblique position; the right arm is raised onto the pillow if semi-prone, or on the top of the IR if erect. A 45° radiolucent pad will assist in accurate positioning for both methods, with the added advantage of immobilisation for the semi-prone position. For the semi-prone patient the knee on the raised side is flexed and used as additional immobilisation
- The sternum should lie coincident with the long axis of the IR
- A PA anatomical marker is usually used for this projection

Expose on gentle respiration, using low mA and long time selection
This will blur the rib shadows on the image.

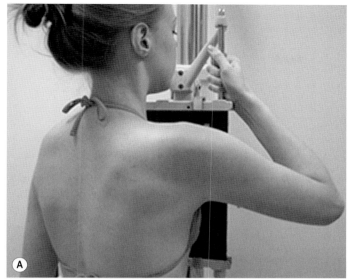

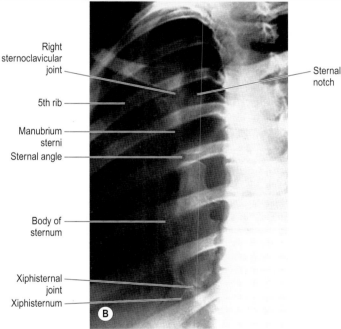

Figure 15.4 (A) Anterior oblique sternum; (B) oblique sternum.
(B) Reproduced with permission from Bryan GJ. Skeletal anatomy. 3rd ed.
Edinburgh: Churchill Livingstone; 1996 and Gunn C. 4th ed. Bones and
joints. Edinburgh: Churchill Livingstone; 2002.

Beam direction and FRD

Perpendicular to the IR
100 cm FRD

Centring

To the centre of the IR, over the raised side of the thorax

Collimation

The sternum, SC joints

Criteria for assessing image quality

- Sternum and SC joints are demonstrated
- Sternum and SC joints are clear of the vertebral column, and superimposed over the right lung
- Sharp image of the sternum in contrast with the soft tissues of the lung. Blurred rib shadows

Common error	Possible reason
Sternum partially overlying vertebral column and mediastinum	Inadequate obliquity. This most frequently occurs in the semi-prone position, when the 45° pads used to assess rotation (and aid immobilisation) are not pushed far enough under the thorax. Use of these pads to achieve a 45° rotation can be more effective if the patient lies in a lateral position initially, with the thin edge of the sponge wedge placed closely against the lowered side. The patient then lowers their right side down onto the pad, rather than raising this side from the prone position
	The weight of the patient can also compress the pad sufficiently to affect angle of obliquity. Use of two pads or one long pad placed under the thorax may prove more effective

STERNOCLAVICULAR JOINTS

The SC joints are examined for evidence of subluxation of the joints.[5]

PA sternoclavicular joints (Fig. 15.5A,B)

IR is vertical; antiscatter grid is not required

Positioning

- A lead rubber apron is applied to the back of the patient's waist
- The patient stands facing the IR
- The feet are separated for stability
- The MSP is perpendicular to the IR, assessed by ensuring that the medial ends of the clavicles are equidistant from the IR
- A PA anatomical marker is usually used for this projection

Expose on arrested respiration

Beam direction and FRD

Horizontal, 90° to the IR
100 cm FRD

Centring

Over the middle of the body of T2 and to emerge through the sternal notch

Collimation

Both SC joints

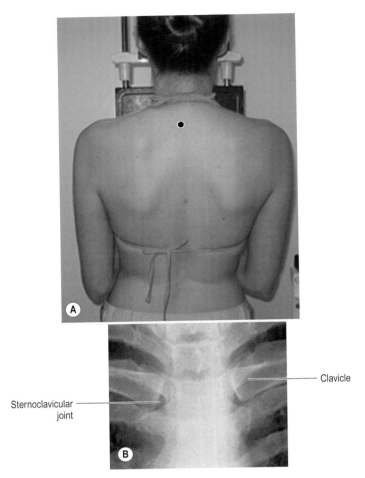

Figure 15.5 PA SC joints.

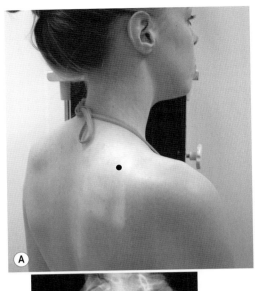

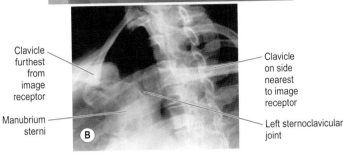

Figure 15.6 (A) Anterior oblique SC joints; (B) oblique SC joints.

Criteria for assessing image quality

- Both SC joints are demonstrated
- Medial ends of the clavicle are equidistant from the spinous processes of the thoracic vertebrae
- Sharp image demonstrating joints either side of the vertebral column in contrast to the vertebrae, medial ends of the posterior ribs, soft tissue of the lungs and sternum

Common error	Possible reason
Medial ends of clavicle not equidistant about the vertebral column; one joint only demonstrated	MSP not perpendicular to IR; the medial end of clavicle furthest from the vertebrae corresponds to the side rotated away from the IR

Oblique SC joints (Fig. 15.6A,B)

Both joints are examined for comparison.
   IR is vertical

Positioning

- A lead rubber apron is applied to the back of the patient's waist
- The patient stands facing the IR
- *To demonstrate the left SC joint* the patient is rotated 45° towards the right, into the left anterior oblique position

- *To demonstrate the right SC joint* the patient is rotated 45° towards the left, into the right anterior oblique position
- The feet are separated for stability
- A PA anatomical marker is usually used for this projection. To avoid confusion, the PA anatomical marker should indicate the side of the joint under examination *and* be placed over to the relevant side on the IR

Expose on arrested respiration

Beam direction and FRD

Vertical, 90° to the IR
100 cm FRD

Centring

Level with T2, over the side of the thorax furthest from the IR, to emerge through the sternal notch

Collimation

Both SC joints

Criteria for assessing image quality

- Both SC joints are demonstrated
- Sharp image demonstrating joint under examination contrast with clavicle and sternum

For the left joint

- Both joints are cleared from the vertebral column and shown overlying the lung apex on the right
- The right joint is shown with the medial end of the clavicle overlying the joint
- The left joint space is demonstrated as open

For the right joint

- Both joints are cleared from the vertebral column and shown overlying the lung apex on the left
- The left joint is shown with the medial end of the clavicle overlying the joint
- The right joint space is demonstrated as open

Common error	Possible reason
One or both joints are not seen clear of the vertebral column	Inadequate obliquity. A 45° pad assists in assessing angle of rotation more accurately

Anterior obliques have also been described with significantly less rotation – as little as 10° – the reason for this being that there will be clearance of the spine with minimum distortion of the joint.[8] However, it is noted from resulting images that this obliquity does not adequately clear the joint from the relatively high density of the upper mediastinum.

REFERENCES

1. Carver E, Carver B, editors. Medical imaging: techniques, reflection and evaluation. Edinburgh: Churchill Livingstone; 2006.
2. Royal College of Radiologists Working Party. Making the best use of a department of clinical radiology: guidelines for doctors. 5th ed. London: Royal College Of Radiologists; 2003.
3. Nicholson DA, Driscoll PA. ABC of emergency radiology. Cambridge: BMJ Publishing; 1995.
4. Helms CA. Fundamentals of skeletal radiology. 2nd ed. Philadelphia: WB Saunders; 1995.
5. Bontrager K, Lampignano JP. Textbook of radiographic positioning and related anatomy. 6th ed. St Louis: Mosby; 2005.
6. Whitley AS, et al. Clark's positioning in radiography. 12th ed. London: Hodder Arnold; 2005.
7. Sutherland R. Pocketbook of radiographic positioning. 2nd ed. Edinburgh: Churchill Livingstone; 2003.
8. Long BW, Rafaert JA. Orthopaedic radiography. Philadelphia: WB Saunders; 1995.

Chapter 16

Principles of radiography of the head

Elizabeth Carver

INTRODUCTION

Radiography of the head is commonly termed 'skull radiography', but because the word 'skull' refers to the cranial vault and its bones, 'skull radiography' would technically exclude the facial bones, some paranasal sinuses, mandible and temporomandibular joints.

From the mid 1980s onwards there has been a reduction in the number of requests for plain radiography of the head, as computed tomography (CT) and magnetic resonance imaging (MRI) in particular have provided more detailed and useful information (but plain radiography of the facial bones is still regularly requested). These imaging methods now provide information that is either unlikely to be provided by plain radiographic images or is only likely to be demonstrated by it in the later stages of disease processes. There has also been a reduction in the number of projections advocated per examination over the years, in order to reduce radiation dose to patients. Bearing in mind the superiority of MRI and CT, current guidelines do not recommend plain radiography of the cranial vault, even in cases of trauma, unless CT is not available at the time of examination; the exception to this is in cases of non-accidental injury in children.[1]

Despite the drop in numbers of requests and projections undertaken, chapters on the head will include a full range of descriptions of projections in order to provide information for regions where CT and MRI are less accessible or inaccessible; in addition, there will still be occasions when two cranial vault projections are required in the trauma situation. Where relevant, a discussion on the suitability of plain radiography versus specialised techniques will be presented throughout the section as each area is covered.

A LOGICAL APPROACH TO TECHNIQUE

Historically, texts on radiography have presented radiographers and students with information that has included up to approximately 50 projections.[2,3] This has proved daunting for radiographers in training, to say the least, and it is possible that the decline in frequency of use of plain radiography of the head is likely to exacerbate this.

However, if radiography of the head is approached logically it is realised that all projections are based upon a very few basic head positions, or projections, which require modification and variation by use of angulation and differing centring points. Collimation will also vary, according to the area of interest for each projection. With reference to centring points, it will appear that there are as many of these as there are projections. However, on examination of radiographs, it becomes clear that centring points used are logically selected as being in the middle of the area of interest; so it is recommended that, if in doubt, simply ensure the area of interest lies centrally in the collimated field. Realistically, the radiographer need only quote specific centring points when disseminating information to others.

Familiarity with the bony features of the skull and face, and their radiographic appearances, is vital when assessing radiographs for quality. The most important structures for recognition are:

- Orbits and the bones forming the orbits
- Bones of the vault and sutures
- Maxilla
- Sphenoid, including lesser and greater wings, sphenoid sinus, sella turcica and pterygoid processes/plates
- Petrous portion of temporal bone and its ridge
- Zygomae and arches
- Features of the mandible, temporomandibular joints
- Paranasal sinuses
- Nasal septum
- External and internal auditory meati
- Foramen magnum and atlanto-occipital joints.

Description of basic projections relies heavily on the use of planes, baselines and surface markings, and the radiographer must be similarly familiar with these (Figs 16.1, 16.2).

Surface markings, planes and baselines

(Figs 16.1, 16.2)

Glabella

The glabella is situated in the midline of the forehead just above the level of the superior orbital margins; it lies over the frontal sinuses.

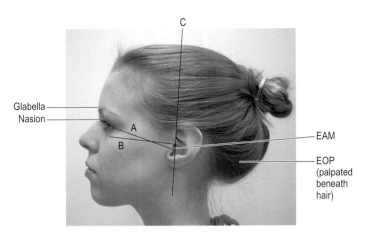

A. Orbitomeatal baseline (OMBL)
B. Anthropological baseline
C. Auricular line

Figure 16.1 Surface markings, planes and baselines – 1.

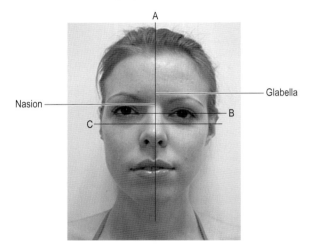

A. MSP
B. Interpupillary line
C. Infraorbital line

Figure 16.2 Surface markings, planes and baselines – 2.

External occipital protuberance (EOP)

The EOP is palpable and situated in the midline, inferiorly, over the occiput.

External auditory meatus (EAM)

The EAM is the hole surrounded by the pinna of the ear.

Nasion

The nasion is situated below the glabella, and is a depression between the orbits and above the nasal bone.

Coronal plane

The coronal place is coincident with the coronal suture and separates the body into anterior and posterior halves.

Infraorbital line

The infraorbital line connects the inferior orbital margins and lies parallel to the interpupillary line.

Interpupillary line

The interpupillary line is a horizontal line connecting the pupils of the eyes.

Median sagittal plane (MSP)

The MSP is a vertical plane in the midline of the head, separating the left and right sides.

Orbitomeatal baseline (OMBL)

The OMBL is an imaginary line extending from the outer canthus of the eye to the middle of the EAM. It is used in conventional radiography techniques of the head.

BASIC POSITIONS OF THE HEAD

In this book the names of projections are always given as a representation of the direction of the beam, so that this gives the radiographer information on the initial patient position. This is in preference to a system that uses names for some projections which reflect the original describer of the projection (for example Towne's, Waters') but gives little or no information on the position. When such a name is very commonly used in everyday practice, the alternative will be given in brackets.

Occipitofrontal (OF) (Fig. 16.3A,B)

This is a posteroanterior (PA) position, with the forehead in contact with the image receptor (IR) and the OMBL at 90° to it. It is easiest to achieve with the patient seated erect. Traditionally it is referred to as a 'PA skull' position, but as the occipitomental (OM) position is also PA this does not describe the true position of the head for the OF.

With an OF projection, beam angulation will affect the position of the ridge of the petrous portion of the temporal bone: caudal angulation lowering it in relation to the orbits and cranial angulation raising it. The effects of caudal angulation can be compared using Figures 16.4A, B and C. These positions rely on accurate positioning of the OMBL at 90° to the IR and accurate angle selection. The effects of errors on the appearance of the petrous ridge in the OF position are outlined below.

Common errors – OF projections	Possible reasons
Petrous ridge appears higher within the orbits than required, or appears above superior orbital margins	OMBL not 90° to the IR, chin down too far. Caudal tube angle selected, if used, is less than required for projection. Direction of angle incorrect
Petrous ridge appears lower within the orbits than required, or appears below inferior orbital margins	OMBL not 90° to IR, chin raised slightly. Caudal tube angle selected, if used, is more than required for projection

Symmetry of the structures on either side of the head is a requirement of all AP or PA radiographs of the head. Rotation of the head, away from the position with the MSP perpendicular to the IR, will affect this symmetry. The most obvious identifiable appearance suggestive of rotation is increased distance of the lateral orbital border from the lateral outer table of the vault on one side compared to the other

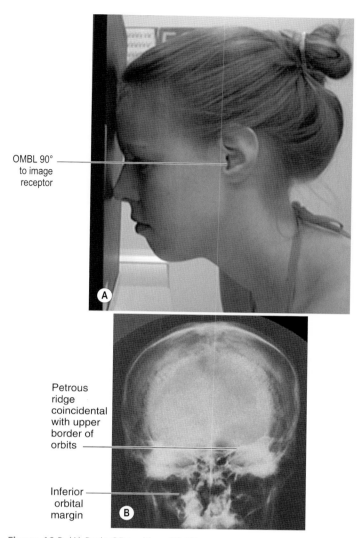

OMBL 90° to image receptor

Petrous ridge coincidental with upper border of orbits

Inferior orbital margin

Figure 16.3 (A) Basic OF position; (B) OF.

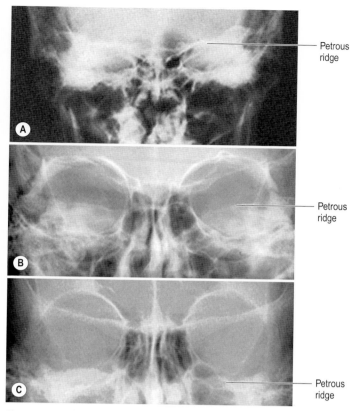

Petrous ridge

Petrous ridge

Petrous ridge

Figure 16.4 Effects of caudal angulation on petrous ridge in the OF position: (A) no angle; (B) 10° angle; (C) 20° angle.

It has been noted that it is common practice for radiographers to initially ask the patient to place their nose and forehead in contact with the IR and that nose size will affect OMBL relationship if this method is used.[4] For this reason it is advocated that the patient is asked to only place their forehead against the IR, with the radiographer adjusting OMBL position as necessary.

Fronto-occipital (FO) (Fig. 16.5)

This is an anteroposterior (AP) position, with the occiput in contact with the IR and OMBL at 90° to it. It can be undertaken erect or supine and is most often used in cases of trauma when patient condition is not suitable for an OF projection; if this is the case any caudal angulation normally given in conjunction with the OF position is directed *cranially rather than caudally*. It is used when radiographers avoid PA projections of the head because of potential difficulty in achieving and maintaining the correct position. Caudal angulation may also be applied in the FO position routinely, as for the FO 30° half axial (Towne's) projection (see Ch. 17 on the cranial vault.)

The appearance of the FO projection, with no tube angulation, should be identical to those for the OF, with the exception of relative orbital size. In the FO position the lateral orbital borders will appear

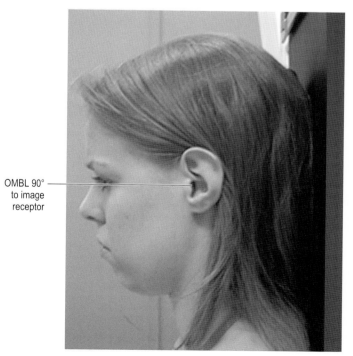

OMBL 90° to image receptor

Figure 16.5 Basic FO position.

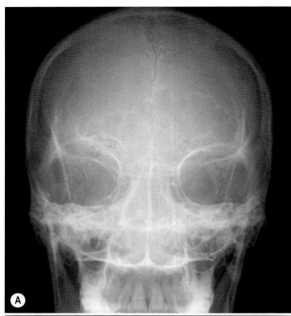

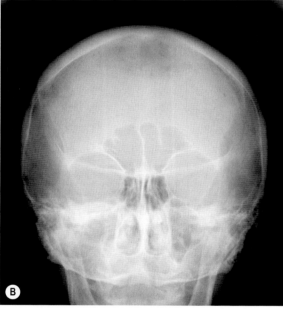

Figure 16.6 Appearances of FO and OF radiographs: (A) FO angled 20° cranially, showing lateral orbital margins further from the lateral skull margins than in (B) OF angled 20° caudally.

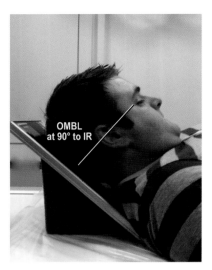

Figure 16.7 Cassette supported for supine patient.

above the orbital outlines, and becoming increasingly 'v' shaped as the angle increases. More specific guidelines on FO projectional errors are given in Chapter 17.

Positioning the OMBL at 90° to the IR can be difficult in this AP position, especially in the patient who is of stocky build or is kyphotic. If sitting erect, the patient will find it easier to press the occipital area against the IR, and achieve the correct relationship of OMBL to it, if the chair they use is placed slightly forward of the receptor unit. Leaning back towards the unit initially until their shoulders come into contact with it, they are then asked to push the back of their neck against the unit, flexing their neck until the occipital area is also in contact. It has been noted that this method is more effective than asking the patient to simply put the back of their head against the IR while dropping the chin, as the back of the head generally lies at the top of the occiput rather than in its centre.[4]

Positioning of the OMBL is more difficult for the supine patient, and it is worthy of note that most trauma patients requiring skull images will present supine on a trolley; use of a non-opaque pad under the head may help facilitate the position but is not considered ideal, as the increase in object–receptor distance (ORD) causes magnification unsharpness which increases in severity towards the vertex of the skull. For the non-neck-injured patient it is preferable to use a support under an IR with stationary grid, positioned directly under the patient's head and at 90° to the OMBL (Fig. 16.7). Other solutions and suggestions will also be considered in Chapter 17 on the cranial vault.

Occipitomental (OM) (Fig. 16.8A,B)

This is a PA position, with the chin raised and in contact with the IR. The relationship of the OMBL to the IR varies and is usually between 30° and 45° from the perpendicular, according to the requirements of the examination. With the OMBL at 30° the nose is close to, or even in contact with, the IR, but this does vary according to shape of the nose; the chin is well elevated if a 45° relationship to the IR is required, and in this position the nose is very unlikely to be in contact with it.

As for the OF and FO projections, the location of the petrous ridge on the image is also used to assess accuracy of positioning for the OM. The required level for most OM projections requires the petrous ridge to be seen at either the midpoint or the lower border of the maxillary

very close to, or even superimposed over, the lateral outer table of the vault. The OF projection will show the lateral orbital borders well within the outer margins of the vault (Fig. 16.6A,B). Clearly this is due to the difference in magnification of the orbits, as they lie close to the IR in the OF position and further away in the FO position; the distance of the lateral aspects of the vault from the IR will be similar for both and magnification of the area will also be similar.

Errors in positioning have the same effects as those for the OF projection, OMBL position affecting the position of the petrous ridge and rotation affecting symmetry. A raised chin in the FO position will have the same effect as the same action in the OF position, which is that of lowering the petrous ridge, whereas a dropped chin will raise it. The FO with caudal angulation will show the petrous ridges rising

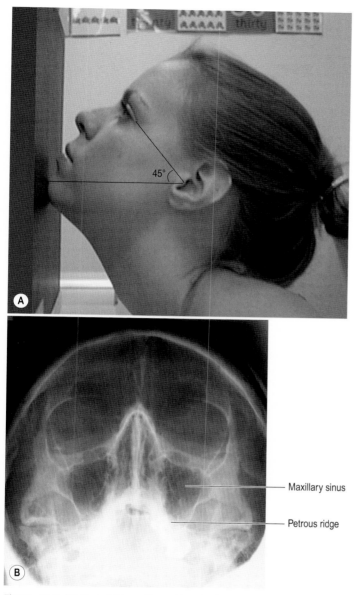

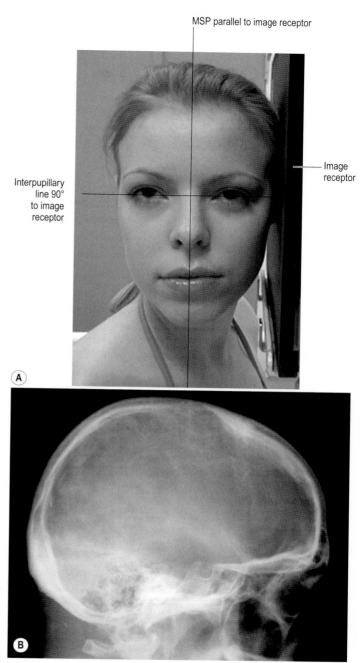

Figure 16.8 (A) Basic OM position: chin raised 45°; (B) OM 45°.

sinuses. Caudal angulation will further lower the position of the petrous ridge on this projection.

With further reference to the assessment of projectional accuracy using the petrous ridge, as for the OF and FO positions: a higher position of the ridge than that required indicates that the chin is inadequately elevated. If the ridge is lower than required the chin is over-elevated. Again, evidence of rotation is assessed by symmetry of the facial structures, especially the distance of the lateral orbital margins and rami of the mandible from the lateral aspect of the vault.

Lateral (Fig. 16.9A,B)

This is a familiar position, with the MSP parallel to the IR. Angulation can be used for some lateral oblique projections, such as those for mandible or temporomandibular joints. Both tilt and rotation of the head will affect the appearance of the lateral projection. This

Figure 16.9 (A) Basic lateral position; (B) lateral.

projection can be undertaken with the patient seated or prone but it can be difficult for them to achieve the required position; if undertaken erect, turning the patient's head into position while maintaining the MSP parallel to the IR may be more easily achieved with the chair placed very close to the IR and the patient's vertebral column vertically positioned. If a patient leans forward towards the unit there is more likelihood of tilt. Another solution lies in the use of a cassette-type IR with grid in an erect holder, or supported vertically against the side of the supine patient's head (which is elevated on a radiolucent pad), enabling the patient to be positioned with their whole MSP (head and body) parallel to the IR. This reduces the difficulty associated with turning the head and obtaining an accurate position.

Submentovertical (SMV) (Fig. 16.10A,B)

The vertex of the skull is placed in contact with the IR for this projection, facilitated by the patient initially sitting facing the X-ray tube and extending the neck and head backwards. The OMBL is parallel to the IR. The projection is not in common use as the information it provides is minimal and even inadequate compared to that given by CT and MRI. The projection can be quite difficult for some patients to achieve and maintain, especially as pressure on the vertex of the skull can be quite painful.

Table-top/trolley or erect technique?

Although radiographic examination of the skull can be undertaken erect or supine, erect positioning is easier for the patient for most positions, especially PA positions. As already mentioned, lateral projections can be difficult to achieve when the patient is erect with their head turned, but a supine horizontal projection, with the whole of the body's MSP parallel to the IR, is easier for the patient. As this method usually uses a stationary grid, this could similarly be employed using an erect IR support with the patient seated. The patient's shoulder fits comfortably under the support, without the patient needing to turn their head. A lateral with the patient prone can be very difficult and, in any case, any prone position is out of the question for the injured patient. Achieving the perpendicular relationship of the OMBL for the FO projection is also quite difficult for the supine patient. Because of this, the method selected for descriptions of radiography of the head (conventional method) is the erect technique. Modifications for the supine patient can be found in Chapter 25.

SUMMARY

There is a small range of basic projections (OF, FO, lateral, OM, SMV) upon which radiography of the head is based, and this range can be seen to be simplified when it is remembered that:

- the OF and FO projections are simply the reverse of each other
- the lateral projection is a familiar concept and therefore not a difficult one
- the SMV projection is little used
- erect positioning is often easier to achieve.

Chapters (17–20) give the relevant projections for specific areas of the head and these are described in more detail, showing use of these basic projections with modifications in angles used, centring points and collimation requirements.

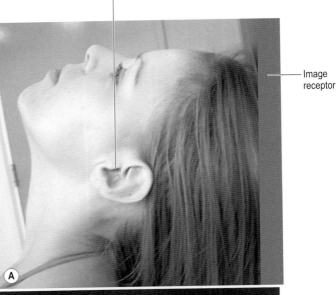

OMBL parallel to image receptor

Image receptor

(A)

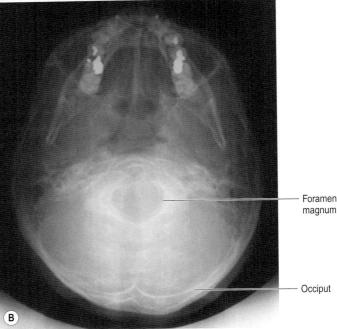

Foramen magnum

Occiput

(B)

Figure 16.10 (A) Basic SMV position; (B) SMV.

REFERENCES

1. RCR Working Party. Making the best use of clinical radiology services: referral guidelines. 6th ed. London: The Royal College of Radiologists; 2007.
2. Bontrager K, Lampignano JP. Textbook of radiographic positioning and related anatomy. 7th ed. St Louis: Mosby; 2010.
3. Whitley AS, et al. Clark's positioning in radiography. 12th ed. London: Hodder Arnold; 2005.
4. Unett EM, Royle AJ. Radiographic techniques and image evaluation. London: Chapman and Hall; 1997.

Chapter | **17** |

Cranial vault

Barry Carver

Skull radiography has been in decline for many years. It is still in limited use for the investigation of some metabolic and bone disorders, and as part of the skeletal survey protocol for cases of suspected non-accidental injury (NAI). In cases of trauma, even where still used, fewer projections are recommended for a number of years – two rather than the 'traditional' three being advised.[1]

Why is this? The easy answer appears to be radiation protection – minimisation of dose.

In 1978 Eyes and Evans, in a study of 504 patients in two Liverpool teaching hospitals, found a very low yield of positive findings on plain skull radiographs, suggesting that they were of limited value in the management of patients with head injury.[2] Both earlier and later studies in the USA agreed with these findings, the yield of fractures varying but with a low of 2.7% in agreement with the above UK study.[3–5]

Head injuries are the cause of around 700 000 hospital attendances each year in England and Wales.[6] Imaging of the head injury patient is directed at detecting the nature of the underlying pathology; once this is accomplished the brain can be protected against greater damage. Optimal imaging is dependent on the nature of the injury, with evaluation of the brain normally being of paramount importance. The advent of computed tomography (CT) has had a massive impact on the diagnosis and treatment of traumatic head injury, allowing rapid non-invasive identification of both diffuse injury and surgically treatable lesions.

It should be noted that cervical spine injury is relatively common in comatose patients with head injury,[7] hence it is important to exclude such an injury prior to mobilisation, the minimum examination being a high quality lateral examination C1–C7.

When the Royal College of Radiologists (RCR) guidelines were first produced, one purpose was to eliminate unnecessary skull radiographs, and they have been successful in reducing the number of skull images being performed. The current RCR guidelines[6] adopt the Canadian CT head rule[8] eliminating the need for radiography of the skull in trauma, except for where CT is unavailable, or in the case of NAI in children.

RCR guidance has been added to in the UK by guidance issued by the National Institute for Health and Clinical Excellence (NICE).[9] Application of the Canadian Head CT Rule has been shown to be effective in the management of patients with minor head trauma, significantly reducing the amount of scans required in this group, but patients in the high- and medium-risk groups require CT.[8]

Given its ability to demonstrate bony detail as well as much greater detail of the underlying soft tissues within the cranial vault, CT is the investigation of choice in an increasing number of circumstances. Thus the use of skull radiography, particularly in trauma, has diminished greatly, but its use is not yet obsolete: indeed, in some countries skull radiography remains in widespread use.[10] Consequently, it is still necessary for the radiographer to be competent in X-ray examination of the cranial vault.

Projections for the cranial vault may be undertaken erect, or with the patient supine or prone. The technique described here uses erect positioning, and the table-top or trolley technique must be modified by remembering that erect anteroposterior (AP) becomes supine, and erect posteroanterior (PA) becomes prone, etc. For the *injured patient*, no projections are undertaken prone, and occipitofrontal (OF) projections must be adjusted to become fronto-occipital (FO), with any cranial or caudal angulations directed in the opposite direction to those given for OF projection. For example, if an OF 20° with caudal angle is required, the FO uses a 20° cranial angle in order to reproduce the required appearances on the image.

OF cranium (Fig.17.1A,B)

Image receptor (IR) is vertical; an antiscatter grid is employed

Positioning

- The patient is seated facing the IR, their forehead in contact with it
- The orbitomeatal baseline (OMBL) and median sagittal plane (MSP) are perpendicular to the IR. The MSP position can be checked by ensuring that the distances between both external auditory meati (EAMs) and the IR are equidistant

Beam direction and focus receptor distance (FRD)

There are a range of beam directions used, which affect the position of the petrous ridge on the image produced (see Ch. 16); *20° caudal angulation* clears the ridge to the lowest border of the orbits and this

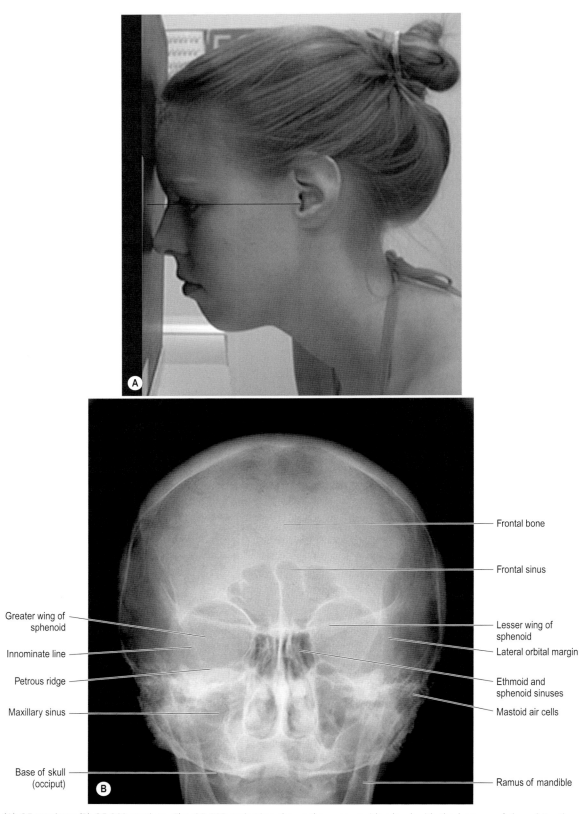

Figure 17.1 (A) OF cranium; (B) OF 20° cranium. The OF 20° projection shows the petrous ridge level with the bottom of the orbits, thus projecting as much of the cranial vault as possible above the maxilla and petrous portion of temporal bone.

angulation is probably that used most frequently, since it maximises the amount of vault shown above the maxilla

Centring

In the midline of the occiput, to emerge through the glabella

Owing to angulation, it is necessary to ensure that the collimated field lies within the IR boundaries.

Collimation

Vertex of vault, inferior border of occiput, lateral margins of vault

When a patient presents on a trolley, after a head injury, or when they cannot turn face-down for a table-top technique, the FO projection (described later) is used and adapted by using a 20° cranial angle. Centring is over the glabella.

Criteria for assessing image quality

* Vertex of vault, inferior border of occiput, and the lateral margins of vault are demonstrated
* Superior border of petrous ridge shown level with superior orbital margins, if no angle is used. For techniques using beam angulation, the petrous ridge should appear halfway down the orbits for 10° caudal angle and at the bottom of the orbits for 20° angle
* Lateral borders of orbits equidistant from lateral borders of skull
* Sharp image showing the dense petrous ridge in contrast with the orbits and occiput, frontal bone in contrast with the adjacent air-filled sinuses

Common errors	Possible reasons
Petrous ridge is seen above required level in relationship to orbits	Inadequate angle selected or OMBL used is incorrectly positioned (chin down too far)
Petrous ridge is seen below required level in relationship to orbits	Angle selected is too great or OMBL used is incorrectly positioned (chin not down enough)
Distance between lateral orbital margins is not equal	Rotation of the head; the orbit demonstrating the shortest distance between its lateral border and the lateral aspect of the vault coincides with the side towards which the head is rotated

FO 30° cranium (Fig.17.2A,B)

This projection is also referred to as the *Towne's* or *half axial* projection and may also be produced as an OF with a 30° cranial angle. The OF approach is seldom used in conventional skull techniques as the projection is mostly used to show the occiput, which is positioned closest to the IR in the FO position. However, the OF position is easier to achieve if the patient is seated erect, and the risks associated with radiation dose to eye lens and thyroid are less severe.

IR is vertical; an antiscatter grid is employed

Positioning

* The patient sits erect facing the X-ray tube
* The OMBL and MSP are perpendicular to the IR. The MSP position can be checked by checking that the distances between the EAMs and the IR are equidistant. Avoid using facial structures such as eyebrows to assess symmetry of the position, as such soft tissue structures generally are not symmetrical in their position
* For notes on how to overcome difficulties when positioning the OMBL for the FO in conventional technique, see Chapter 16.

Beam direction and FRD

Initially horizontal, then angled 30° caudally

Centring

Traditional centring is often described as being approximately 5 cm above the glabella, but this has been found to cause unnecessary irradiation of the neck and thyroid.[11] Radiographers will be familiar with the instruction to 'centre at the hairline', but unfortunately, not only do hairlines vary in their position, they are also non-existent in many males. Alternatively the central ray can be directed to a point above the glabella, ensuring that its path travels through the foramen magnum (found approximately midway between the EAM and mastoid process from the lateral perspective). Changing the centring point and central ray angle can have the effect of reducing dose to the thyroid.[12]

1. The horizontal beam is collimated to the size of the vault and angled 25° caudally
2. The beam is re-centred over the vault to include it in the collimated field; further longitudinal collimation may be possible at this point. It will be noted that the centring point is higher than when using the 30° angle

Collimation for conventional FO 30° projection

Occiput, parietal bones, foramen magnum, petrous temporal bone, lateral aspects of vault

Owing to angulation, it is necessary to ensure that the collimated field lies within the IR boundaries.

OF with 30° cranial angulation ('reverse Towne's')

IR is vertical; an antiscatter grid is employed

Positioning

* The patient is seated facing the IR, their forehead in contact with it
* The OMBL is perpendicular to the IR as for other OF projections
* The MSP is perpendicular to the IR

Beam direction and FRD

Initially horizontal, then angled 30° cranially
100 cm FRD

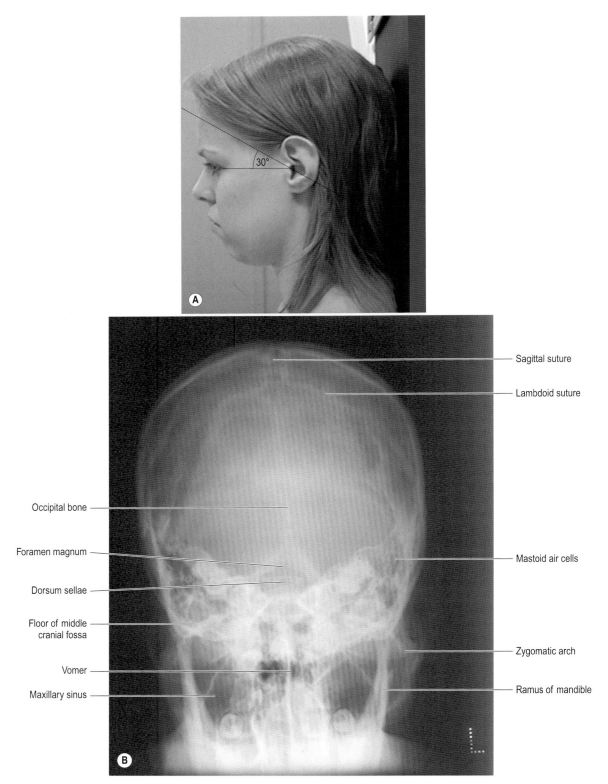

Sagittal suture

Lambdoid suture

Occipital bone

Foramen magnum

Dorsum sellae

Floor of middle
cranial fossa

Mastoid air cells

Vomer

Zygomatic arch

Maxillary sinus

Ramus of mandible

Figure 17.2 FO 30°.

Centring

Below the EOP to emerge above the glabella. The beam should pass through the foramen magnum (found approximately midway between the EAM and mastoid process from the lateral perspective)

The IR will require cranial displacement to ensure its centre coincides with the central ray.

Collimation

Occiput, parietal bones, foramen magnum, petrous temporal bone, lateral aspects of vault

Criteria for assessing image quality

- Occiput, parietal bones, foramen magnum, petrous temporal bone and lateral aspect of vault are shown
- Foramen magnum is demonstrated with dorsum sellae seen centrally within its borders
- Petrous ridge is seen as a shallow 'v' either side of the foramen magnum
- Sharp image showing dorsum sellae in contrast with the less dense foramen magnum; bones of the vault in contrast with the petrous portion of temporal bone

Common errors	Possible reasons
Foramen magnum appears short or is not evident. Dorsum sellae may be visible above the portion of the foramen magnum that is seen	Angle selected is inadequate or OMBL is positioned incorrectly (chin not down enough)
Large foramen magnum seen but curve of the posterior arch of C1 is seen in its lower third, rather than the anvil-shaped dorsum sellae	Angle selected is too great or OMBL is not positioned correctly (chin down too far)
Dorsum sellae not seen centrally in foramen magnum and petrous portions of temporal bone are asymmetrical	Rotated head; direction of rotation coincides with the direction of shift of the sella within the foramen

Lateral cranium (Fig.17.3A,B)

IR is vertical; an antiscatter grid is employed

Positioning

- The patient is seated, facing the erect IR
- The head is turned through 90°, away from the side of interest, and the side of the head is placed in contact with the IR
- The MSP is parallel to the IR

Beam direction and FRD

Horizontal, at 90° to the IR (must also be 90° to the MSP)
100 cm FRD

Centring

Midway between the glabella and external occipital protuberance

Collimation

Vertex of skull, occiput, frontal bone

Criteria for assessing image quality

- Vertex of skull, occiput and frontal bone are demonstrated
- There is superimposition of the floor of the anterior cranial fossa, superimposition of the outlines of the sphenoid and pituitary fossa; superimposition of the inner table of occiput; superimposition of the inner table of frontal bone; superimposition of the petrous portions of temporal bone
- Sharp image demonstrating bony detail of the vault in contrast with the less dense sutures, mastoid air cells and air-filled sphenoid sinus. The petrous portions of temporal should appear slightly underpenetrated in comparison to the temporal bones and the EAMs should be identified within the dense area of the petrous portions of temporal

Many structures are identified for superimposition in the lateral skull projection and not all are included in the list of image criteria above. Those not listed here include temporomandibular joints, angles of mandible and orbital outlines.

In the real world of clinical practice, experience has shown that these paired structures are almost never *all* superimposed on one lateral image. The main reason for this is the varying distance of these structures from the central ray, accompanied by the distance between the structures themselves; this serves to project the outline of the structure nearer the central ray away from the outline of the other structure in the pair.

For example, consider the lateral orbital outlines, which, on the average male adult, lie around 6 cm away from the centring point: at an FRD of 100 cm this would create obliquity of the ray passing through the lateral orbit. This obliquity can be assessed mathematically to be around 3.5°, which is enough to displace the image of the orbital outline furthest from the IR. Other structures, such as angle of mandible furthest from the IR, are even more remote from the central ray.

Common errors	Possible reasons
Vertical aspects of structures not superimposed and appear *side by side*. These include: anterior clinoids, posterior clinoids, anterior aspect of sphenoid sinus, lateral orbital margins, temporomandibular joints, petrous ridges	MSP not perpendicular to the IR; rotation of the head
Horizontal aspects of structures not superimposed and appear *one above the other*. These include: floor of the anterior cranial fossa, anterior clinoids, posterior clinoids, floor of sphenoid sinus, floor of the pituitary fossa, orbital outlines, temporomandibular joints, petrous ridges	MSP not perpendicular to the IR; tilt of the head *Note that the image produced may demonstrate both tilt and rotation*

Frequently the pituitary fossa is used as the main focus for assessment of position but it must be noted that a seriously tilted lateral may show a single pituitary fossa outline, suggesting good positioning. Severe tilt will displace one side of the fossa and lower its outline sufficiently so as to mask its outline with inferiorly positioned structures; this leaves one side of the fossa appearing to be a beautifully superimposed image of the full pituitary fossa. It is therefore recommended that the pituitary fossa is only used for position assessment in conjunction with at least one other pair of structures, for the lateral skull image.

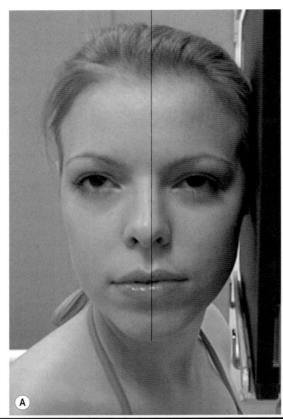

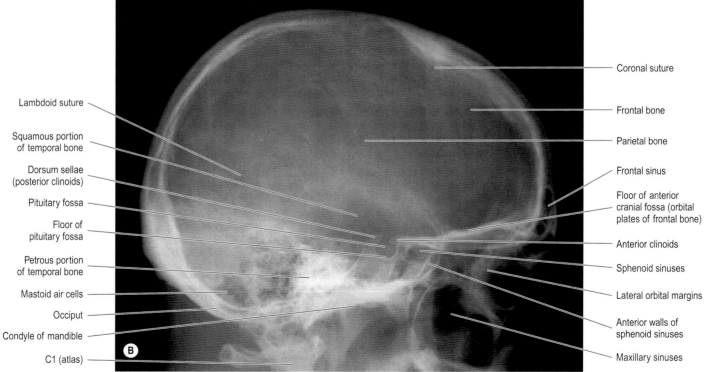

Lambdoid suture

Squamous portion
of temporal bone

Dorsum sellae
(posterior clinoids)

Pituitary fossa

Floor of
pituitary fossa

Petrous portion
of temporal bone

Mastoid air cells

Occiput

Condyle of mandible

C1 (atlas)

Coronal suture

Frontal bone

Parietal bone

Frontal sinus

Floor of anterior
cranial fossa (orbital
plates of frontal bone)

Anterior clinoids

Sphenoid sinuses

Lateral orbital margins

Anterior walls of
sphenoid sinuses

Maxillary sinuses

Figure 17.3 Lateral cranium.

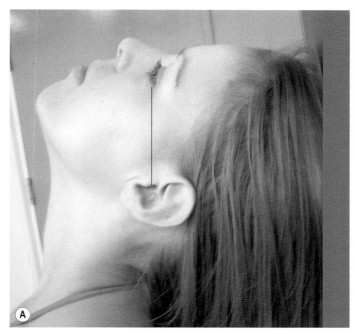

Figure 17.4 (A) SMV.

Submentovertical (SMV) cranium (Fig.17.4A,B)

IR is vertical; an antiscatter grid is employed

This projection is not possible as part of table-top technique unless equipment is available that can support the patient's trunk and legs above the table-top and allow extension of the neck to bring the vertex of the head in contact with the table-top.

Positioning

- A chair or stool is placed in front of the erect unit and pulled approximately 30 cm from it. If using a chair, its back should be perpendicular to the IR, rather than parallel with it. Brakes must be applied if the stool or chair has wheels
- The patient is seated with their back to the IR
- The patient is asked to lean back and extend their neck; the radiographer should support their shoulders gently but should avoid taking the patient's full weight
- The patient is asked to place the vertex of their head in contact with the IR
- MSP of the head is perpendicular to the IR and the OMBL parallel to it

Beam direction and FRD

Horizontal, then angled 5° cranially
100 cm FRD

Centring

Midway between the angles of the mandible

Collimation

Frontal bone, occiput, parietal bones

Maintenance of the required SMV position is very difficult for patients and their body weight is borne by the vertex of the skull; this is actually quite painful and can leave the patient feeling quite nauseous. The radiographer must position the patient confidently and efficiently, to ensure that their patient experiences minimum discomfort.

Criteria for assessing image quality

- Frontal bone, occiput and parietal bones are demonstrated
- Circular image of the odontoid process seen under the anterior rim of the foramen magnum
- Body of the mandible passes through the centre of the maxillary sinuses; symphysis menti is seen just inside the frontal bone
- Angles of the mandible are superimposed over corresponding temporomandibular joints
- Sagittal suture is seen centrally and bisects the foramen magnum; the cervical vertebrae are superimposed centrally down the MSP
- Symmetry of bilateral structures of the skull

Common errors	Possible reasons
Body of the mandible below maxillary sinuses; odontoid process seen more elongated, similar to its appearance on the AP C1–C2 projection; symphysis menti seen through the sphenoid or ethmoid sinuses; angles of the mandible below temporomandibular joints	OMBL not parallel to the IR; inadequate chin elevation
Asymmetry of anatomical structures	MSP not perpendicular to the IR (tilt of the head)

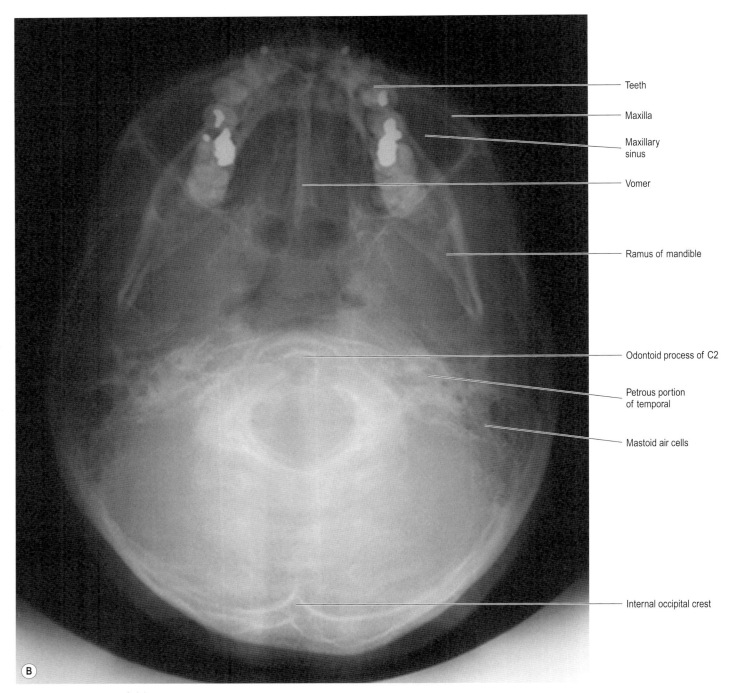

Teeth

Maxilla

Maxillary
sinus

Vomer

Ramus of mandible

Odontoid process of C2

Petrous portion
of temporal

Mastoid air cells

Internal occipital crest

Figure 17.4, Continued (B) SMV.

REFERENCES

1. McGlinchey I, et al. Comparison of two or three radiographic views in the diagnosis of skull fractures. Clinical Radiology 1998;53:215–17.

2. Eyes B, Evans A. Post-traumatic skull radiographs. Time for a reappraisal. Lancet 1978;2(8080):85–6.

3. Balasubramaniam S, et al. Efficacy of skull radiography. American Journal of Surgery 1981;142:366.

4. Strong I, et al. Head injuries in accident and emergency departments at Scottish hospitals. Injury 1978;10:154.

5. St John EG. The role of the emergency skull roentgenogram in head trauma. American Journal of Roentgenology 1968;76:315.

6. Royal College of Radiologists Working Party. Making the best use of a department of clinical radiology: guidelines for doctors. 6th ed. London: Royal College Of Radiologists; 2007.

7. Zimmerman R. Head injury. In: Taveras J, Ferrucci J, editors. Radiology on CD-ROM: Diagnosis, imaging, intervention. Philadelphia: Lippincott Williams and Wilkins; 2001;3, Ch 37.

8. Steill I, et al. The Canadian CT head rule for patients with minor head injury. Lancet 2001;357:1391–1396.

9. NICE. Head injury – triage, assessment, investigation and early management of head injury in infants, children and adults. Clinical Guideline 56. London: Nice; 2007.

10. Brell M, Ibanez J. Minor head injury management in Spain: a multicentre national survey. Neurocirugia 2001;12(2):105-24.

11. Laudicina P. Head trauma. Seminars in Radiologic Technology 2000;8(1): 7–11.

12. Denton B. Improving plain radiography of the skull: The half axial projection re-described. Synergy 1998;Aug:9–11.

Chapter | **18** |

Facial bones

Elizabeth Carver

The most frequent reason for radiological examination of the facial bones is trauma to the region; plain radiographic imaging of the area remains a popular and appropriate method of initial assessment in the acute setting, providing information relatively quickly and with a relatively low radiation dose compared to computed tomography (CT), the other imaging method best suited for providing information on bony injury to the area. Low-dose CT is considered a suitable method for demonstration and assessment of orbital fractures, as plain radiographic images can sometimes be inconclusive and may not give the 3D information needed before treatment of fractures. For many years it has been suggested that plain radiography may only be useful in cases showing clinical signs that clearly suggest surgical intervention,[1] but current guidelines still show that plain radiography has a place in the assessment of facial and orbital injury.[2] Magnetic resonance imaging (MRI) may also be considered, but as scans are undertaken supine, the teardrop effect of the herniating orbital tissue may not be as well demonstrated as in the prone CT scan with coronal sections. CT will provide better bony definition on the images.

CT may also be required to provide information in trauma cases when plain images in the general facial bones survey are inconclusive or are difficult to produce to a high enough standard; this is often due to difficulties associated with patient condition in severe trauma when excessive oedema may reduce image contrast.

The facial bones can be demonstrated by a general plain radiographic survey that includes the maxilla, mandible, orbits, nasal bones and zygomae. However, provision of specific information on some of these areas requires alternative or additional projections so that a diagnosis can be made. The mandible and zygomae both require individual examination in case of injury, and plain radiography is the initial examination method of choice for these areas. In non-trauma-related indications the mandible may require CT examination to assess the progress of dental implants.

The temporomandibular joints (TMJs) can also be imaged by plain radiography, which will provide information on condylar dislocation and loss of joint space. MRI will give more useful information regarding the joint itself and, since internal disruption is the most commonly encountered problem in the joint, MRI is most suitable. Arthrography will provide dynamic information regarding the joint.

Injury to the nasal bones is not considered a reason for routine radiographic examination, but clinical specialists (e.g. for ear, nose and throat, and maxillofacial follow-up) may consider special nasal bones projections to be useful.[2] This would be the case when assessing fragment displacement and septal deviation.

Although a significant number of patients presenting with facial trauma will attend on a trolley, patients also frequently arrive as a 'walk-in' case and can be examined erect at a skull unit or erect bucky. Erect examination with a horizontal beam is essential for some projections where it is necessary to demonstrate air–fluid levels, and must be attempted whenever possible. This is particularly relevant in the case of blow-out fractures of the orbital floor, where fluid level in the maxillary sinus is used as an indicator of this type of injury.

Similarly to requirements for imaging the cranium, the severely injured patient will present on a trolley and any occipitomental (OM) projections must be modified to a mento-occipital position, with angle direction opposite to that for OM. Laterals can be undertaken with the image receptor (IR) supported vertically at the side of the face. A description of a modified projection for zygomatic arches on the trolley-bound patient is also given. Facial examinations in the emergency situation are also covered in the A&E chapter of this book (Chapter 25).

The choice of projections for facial bones appears to vary according to referring clinical or individual hospital protocol, but rarely includes the lateral facial bones projection. It is common to find that at least two OM projections are used, with tube angle or no angle, and there have been studies in the past to investigate whether a single projection can be used;[3,4] the most likely projection that can be suggested for this is referred to as the OM 30° in related articles, but it is necessary to ask whether this means that the orbitomeatal baseline (OMBL) lies at 30° to the IR and using a central ray perpendicular to the IR, or if a true OM with OMBL at 45° is used with a caudal tube angle of 30°. Fortunately, one article does include an image that shows the petrous ridge clearly level with the middle of the maxillary sinuses, indicating that the projection required an OMBL at 30° to the IR but with no tube angle.[3] This position is familiar as the routine OM for orbits,[5] which is collimated to include only the orbital outlines and maxillary sinuses for that area; clearly, if this projection is used for full facial bones assessment then all facial bones must be included in the primary beam. Investigation of the idea of one 'ideal' projection for facial bones assessment has involved consideration of articles and textbooks relating to radiographic positioning or recommendation of projections in facial trauma, and has yielded some additional interesting results that give rise to some very pertinent points when discussing imaging and referral.

All radiographers use eponymous terms for a few projections, for example Towne's projection of the skull, Judet's views of the acetabulum and Garth's projection of the shoulder. Unfortunately, this makes the actual technique used less memorable than the name. In the last 30 years UK textbooks have aimed to use nomenclature that indicates the actual position for the projection, rather than the name of the projection's designer, with addition of the eponymous title next to the descriptive title. Unfortunately this is not necessarily the case internationally, and eponymous titles are frequently used, leading to a varying range of projection names which are then incorporated into journal articles, potentially creating confusion or even misinterpretation. A search for a list of all eponymously named projections showed that there are approximately 200 in existence,[6] although many are supplementary specialist projections that have been largely superseded by additional imaging modalities. Of this long list, only 17 appeared to be familiar in the UK.

An example of variation in nomenclature when discussing radiography of the facial bones can be centred around the OM projection and therefore has particular relevance to this chapter. In the UK OM tends to refer to a position with the OMBL at 45°, to ensure that the petrous ridge is cleared from the bases of the maxillary sinuses;[5,7,8] in the US the same projection is named PA axial, transoral, Waters' or even parietocanthal projection.[9,10] Position descriptors for this same projection also vary, with UK texts indicating an OMBL angle of 45°[5,6,8] and US texts stating 37°,[9,10] yet all who provide image evaluation criteria insist that their position will see the petrous ridge in the same place, just clear of the lower borders of the maxillary sinuses. One point to raise is that, although it is fairly easy to judge a 45° OMBL to IR angle, can anyone actually claim to accurately judge 37°? US authors do use an alternative way to ensure their positioning is accurate, by referring to alignment of the meatomental line (MML) at 90° to the IR.[9] The MML is the line joining the external auditory meatus and the chin, and it is not clear whether it can be relied on as accurate in patients with developmental deformities of the mandible, such as mandibular prognathism.

It is also noted that the way the relationship of OMBL to IR is described can also vary, with texts giving the suggested OMBL angle either related to the IR[5,7] or related to the perpendicular.[9] This is very confusing, even for experienced authors in radiography, but probably almost impossible for students to understand.

Even articles written in the UK cause confusion: another article exploring the concept of a single view assessment in trauma investigates the potential of either 'the OM 15° and OM 30° view' but does not make it clear what the actual positioning for the projections entails (again, is the OMBL at 45° for each, with caudal angle, or does the angle refer to the OMBL position?). Study of the article reveals that the OM 15° is referred to thus:

The occipitomental film with a 15° tilt (OM 15°) was considered to be the most useful view because it projects the orbital floor separate from the petrous ridge and displays the zygomatic arches.[11]

Unfortunately this means little in the search for an explanation of the actual projection details, since the tilt referred to is not explained as either tube angle or OMBL angle. Clearance of the petrous ridge to below the inferior orbital margins is seen in any OM projection with more than 20° chin lift (i.e. when the OMBL starts at 90° to the IR and the chin is raised so that the OMBL is moved through 20°), and so information on the petrous ridge in the quote above does not help clarify the situation. There is no positional information provided for the OM 30° projection in the article.

A word of warning: ensure you know the correct relationship of baselines and IR before proceeding. In addition, much work has been written by maxillofacial surgeons on appropriate projections in facial trauma; in the absence of extensive *radiographic* experience on their part, how can we expect these articles to be consistent in their meaning for everyone?

GENERAL SURVEY OF FACIAL BONES

Requests that define the desired examination as 'facial bones' require a general OM and (sometimes) lateral survey of the area. OM projections are based on a position with the OMBL at 45°, using a range of caudal beam angles. More than one OM projection may be included in the survey, and two examples are shown of the 45° OM: without angulation in Figure 18.1B and with 30° caudal angulation in Figure 18.1C. Although discussion in the previous section shows that a 30° elevation of the OMBL from a perpendicular relationship to the IR has been suggested as a standalone projection for survey of facial bones,[3] it does not appear to be universally adopted as such at present.

The IR is vertical for all projections of facial bones, orbits and nose unless the patient presents supine on a trolley; antiscatter grid is required, with the exception of lateral nasal bones.

OM facial bones – basic projection
(Fig. 18.1A,B,C)

Positioning

* The patient is seated, facing the IR
* The chin is placed in contact with the midline of the IR and the chin position is adjusted until the OMBL has been raised 45° from the horizontal
* The median sagittal plane (MSP) is perpendicular to the IR, which is assessed by checking that the external auditory meati (EAMs) or lateral orbital margins are equidistant from it

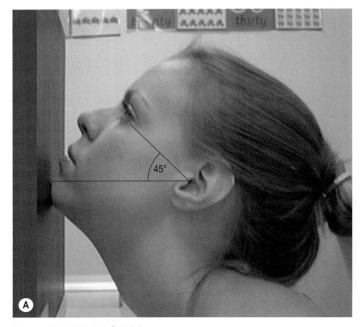

Figure 18.1 (A) OM facial bones.

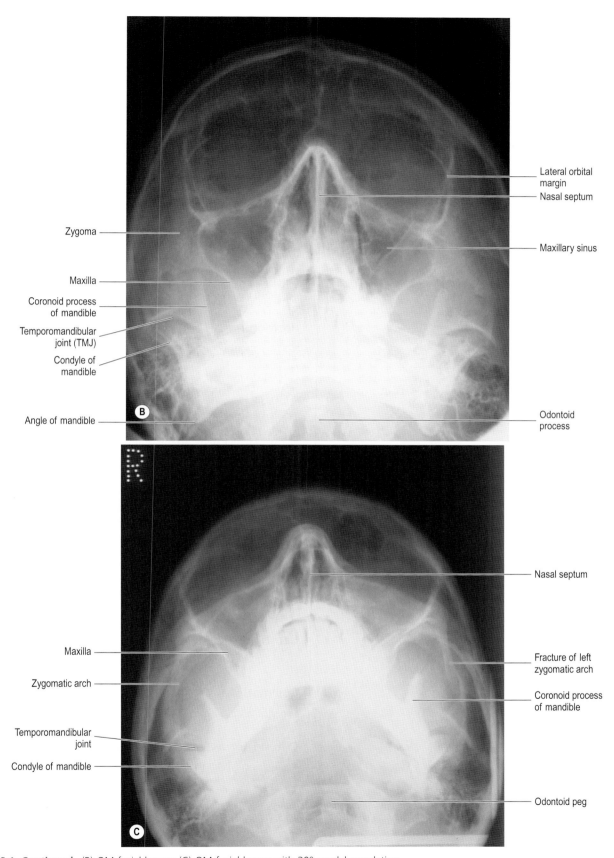

Lateral orbital margin

Nasal septum

Maxillary sinus

Zygoma

Maxilla

Coronoid process of mandible

Temporomandibular joint (TMJ)

Condyle of mandible

Angle of mandible

Odontoid process

Maxilla

Nasal septum

Zygomatic arch

Fracture of left zygomatic arch

Coronoid process of mandible

Temporomandibular joint

Condyle of mandible

Odontoid peg

Figure 18.1, Continued. (B) OM facial bones; (C) OM facial bones with 30° caudal angulation.

Beam direction and focus receptor distance (FRD)

1. Horizontal, at 90° to the IR and making an angle of 45° with the OMBL *or*
2. Initially horizontal, with caudal angulation applied according to requirements of the examination

100 cm FRD

Centring

Above the external occipital protuberance (EOP), to emerge half way between the level of the superior orbital margins and angles of the mandible

When using caudal angulation, the description for centring is unchanged, as the beam must always emerge through the middle of the area of interest; the point of entry for the central ray will become higher as angulation increases.

The centre of the IR must always be adjusted to ensure that the image is included within its boundaries.

Collimation

Orbits, zygomatic arches, mandible

Criteria for assessing image quality

- Orbits, zygomatic arches and mandible are demonstrated
- Symmetry of the facial bones on each side; equal distance of the lateral orbital margins from the outer table of temporal bones
- Odontoid process is visible between the angles of the mandible

Horizontal beam/0° beam angulation

- Upper border of the petrous portion of the temporal bone is level with the apices of maxillary antra
- Zygomatic arches seen as a tight 'C' and reversed tight 'C' laterally
- Sharp image demonstrating the zygomae, nasal bones, orbits and mandible in contrast to the cranial vault, and the air-filled regions of the paranasal sinuses

15–20° caudal angle

- Zygomatic arches are more gently curved and elongated than with the perpendicular (horizontal) central ray
- Petrous ridge falls below maxillary antra and is likely to be indistinguishable
- TMJs are clearly demonstrated either side of the coronoid processes of the mandible
- Exposure factors are assessed as for the horizontal beam projection

30° caudal angle

- Zygomatic arches are slightly curved and elongated, when viewed from this inferior, half-axial, perspective
- Orbits appear almost closed
- Sharp image demonstrating contrast between the inferior orbital margins, maxillary sinuses and the zygomatic arches overlying the cranial vault. The frontal bone and upper orbital area may appear over-blackened but the nasal bones are clearly seen

Common errors	Possible reasons
Asymmetry of facial structures	Rotation about MSP
Position of petrous ridge too high	Chin not raised enough. It has been noted that radiographers frequently ask patients to put their nose and chin onto the erect IR for this projection; this will only serve to raise the chin approximately 30°. It has also been noted that some imaging departments use this method with a 15° caudal angle, which only serves to clear the petrous ridge to the inferior margins of the antra; an almost identical image to the true OM 45° with horizontal beam will result, but there will be some distortion caused by application of the angle

Lateral facial bones (Fig. 18.2A,B,C)

This projection is largely considered of little or no value[3] but may still be used in some centres.

Positioning

- The patient is initially seated, facing the IR
- The trunk is brought as close as possible to the receptor unit and the patient is asked to sit with their spine as erect as possible. This helps the patient turn their head more easily into the required lateral position
- The head is turned through 90° to bring the affected side in contact with the IR
- The MSP is parallel to the IR; there should be no tilt or rotation of the head. This can be assessed by checking the midline of the cranium over the top and symmetry of the frontal bone and orbits
- Asking the patient to gently close their eyes will assist in maintenance of the position; as the radiographer leaves the receptor unit the patient will often follow this movement with their eyes and potentially affect the position of the head

Beam direction and FRD

Horizontal, at 90° to the IR
100 cm FRD

Centring

To the inferior border of the zygoma

Collimation

Superior orbital margins, symphysis menti, TMJs, nasal bones

Criteria for assessing image quality

- Superior orbital margins, symphysis menti, TMJs and nasal bones are demonstrated
- Superimposition of the malar processes of maxilla, orbital outlines and TMJs
- Sharp image demonstrating the malar processes of maxilla in contrast to the air-filled maxillary sinuses, and the orbits in contrast to other bones of the face. The mandible is seen in contrast to the soft tissues of the face. Nasal bones are over-penetrated

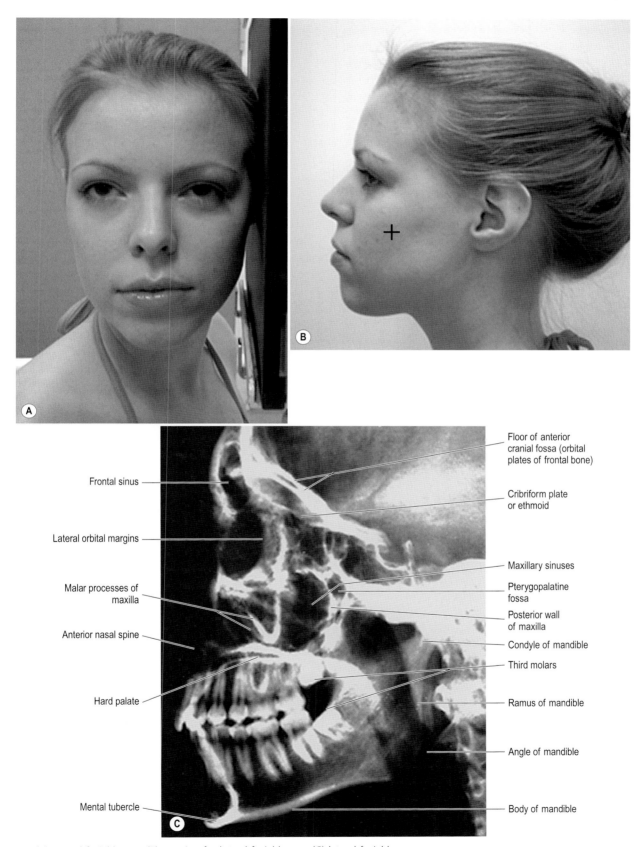

Figure 18.2 (A) Lateral facial bones; (B) centring for lateral facial bones; (C) lateral facial bones.
(C) Reproduced with permission from Bryan GJ. Skeletal anatomy. 3rd ed. Edinburgh: Churchill Livingstone; 1996 and Gunn C. Bones and joints. 4th ed. Edinburgh: Churchill Livingstone; 2002.

Common errors	Possible reasons
Non-superimposition of the floor of the anterior cranial fossa; malar processes seen as one above the other; orbital outlines seen as one above the other	MSP tilted, usually with the upper part of the head tilted towards the IR. If a patient cannot comply with the required position, a compensating caudal angle can be used to reduce the effects of the tilt
Lateral orbital margins seen side by side and not superimposed; malar processes seen displaced in a horizontal direction	Head is rotated; this is often encouraged when the patient 'slumps' in their chair rather than sitting with their spine erect, as described in 'positioning' for this projection

ORBITS

The orbits are examined for trauma or the presence and position of intraocular foreign bodies (IOFB). IOFB assessment may be made after penetrating injury or prior to MRI scanning as a safety measure to exclude the presence of ferrous material in the eye.

A horizontal beam should be used wherever possible, as air–fluid levels in the maxillary sinuses can be an indicator of orbital floor fracture. Air in the top portion of the maxillary antrum will also serve to provide contrast with any soft tissue teardrop appearance of a herniating inferior rectus muscle down through the fractured orbital floor. Clearly the OM orbital projection cannot be undertaken erect with a horizontal beam on a seriously injured patient: at the very least a lateral with horizontal beam can be attempted while this type of patient is supine.

OM orbits/OM 30° ('modified occipitomental'[7]) (Fig. 18.3A,B)

The orbital floor is not well demonstrated on the true 45° OM and this projection will show blow-out fractures more reliably than the true OM.

Positioning

- The patient is seated, facing the IR
- The chin is placed in contact with the midline of the IR and the chin position is adjusted until the OMBL has been raised 30° from the horizontal
- The MSP is perpendicular to the IR, which is assessed by checking that the EAMs or lateral orbital margins are equidistant from the IR

Beam direction and FRD

Horizontal, at 90° to the IR
100 cm FRD

Centring

Above the EOP, to emerge level with the middle of the orbits

Collimation

Orbits, maxillary sinuses

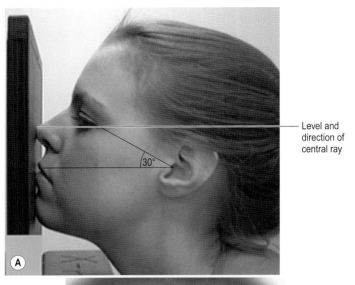

Level and direction of central ray

30°

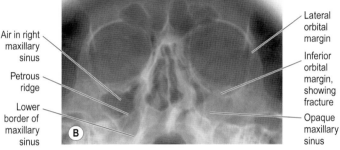

Air in right maxillary sinus

Petrous ridge

Lower border of maxillary sinus

Lateral orbital margin

Inferior orbital margin, showing fracture

Opaque maxillary sinus

Figure 18.3 OM orbits.

Criteria for assessing image quality

- Orbits and maxillary sinuses are demonstrated
- Orbital margins are equidistant from the outer table of the temporal bones
- Petrous ridge seen halfway to two-thirds down the maxillary sinuses
- Sharp image demonstrating contrast between the orbital outlines, the cranial vault, air-filled frontal and maxillary sinuses. Fine detail of the orbital floor is seen at the top of the maxillary sinuses

Common errors	Possible reasons
Asymmetry of facial structures	Rotation about MSP
Petrous ridge level with inferior orbital margins or within orbital outline	Chin not raised enough
Petrous ridge in the lower half of the antrum, or even at its lower margin	Chin elevated too high. This will have a detrimental effect upon the ability of reporting personnel to diagnose blow-out fractures of the orbital floor, which is not well demonstrated on projections with the chin elevated more than 30°

This 'modified' OM projection is suggested as ideal for a single facial bones projection;[3] to adjust this projection and utilise for positioning is the same as for full facial bones assessment the area of interest should include mandible, TMJs and orbits. The central ray will be in the midline, to emerge level with the lower borders of the zygomae.

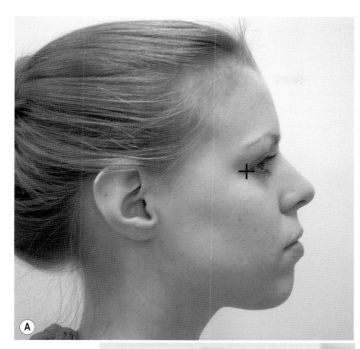

Floor of anterior
cranial fossa
(orbital plates
of frontal bone)

Lateral orbital
margins

Inferior orbital
margins

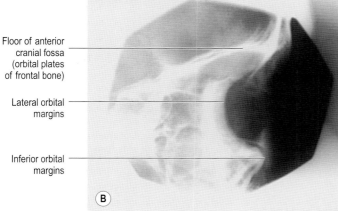

Figure 18.4 (A) Centring for lateral orbits; (B) lateral orbits.

Lateral orbits (Fig. 18.4A,B)

Positioning

- The patient is initially seated, facing the IR and positioned with their head turned as for a lateral facial bones projection

Beam direction and FRD

Horizontal, at 90° to the IR
100 cm FRD

Centring

Over the outer canthus of the eye

Collimation

All orbital outlines, maxillary sinuses

Criteria for assessing image quality

- Orbits and maxillary sinuses are demonstrated
- Orbital outlines are superimposed
- Sharp image demonstrating orbital outlines in contrast to the air-filled maxillary sinuses and ethmoid sinuses

Common errors	Possible reasons
Orbital plates of frontal bone not superimposed	MSP tilted
Lateral orbital margins not superimposed	Head is rotated

NASAL BONES

The IR is vertical for all projections of the nose.

OM nasal bones (Fig. 18.5A,B)

Positioning

- The patient is seated, facing the IR and positioned as for OM facial bones

Beam direction and FRD

Horizontal, at 90° to the IR
100 cm FRD

Centring

Above the EOP, to emerge through the centre of the nasal bone

Collimation

Nasal bone, anterior nasal spine

Criteria for assessing image quality

- Nasal bone and septum are demonstrated; there is evidence of frontal and maxillary sinuses superiorly and laterally
- Petrous ridge is evident as level with inferior maxillary antra
- Sharp image demonstrating the nasal septum centrally and the nasal bones laterally, in contrast with the air-filled ethmoid sinuses

Lateral nasal bones (Fig. 18.6A,B)

Positioning

The patient is initially seated, facing the IR and positioned as for a lateral facial bones projection

Beam direction and FRD

Horizontal, at 90° to the IR
100 cm FRD

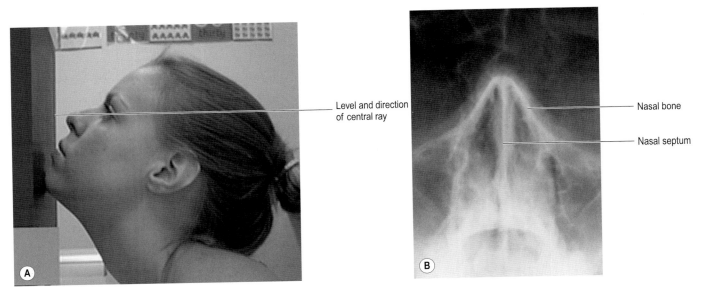

Level and direction of central ray

Nasal bone

Nasal septum

Figure 18.5 OM nasal bones.

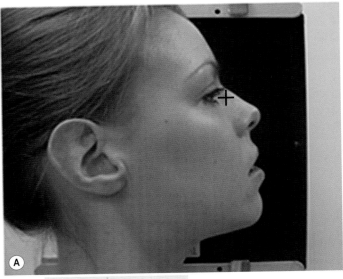

Nasal bone

Soft tissue of nose

Anterior nasal spine

Figure 18.6 Lateral nasal bones.

Centring

Over the nasal bone

Collimation

Nasal bone, anterior nasal spine, soft tissue of the nose

Criteria for assessing image quality

- Nasal bone, anterior nasal spine and soft tissue of the nose are demonstrated
- Sharp image demonstrating bony detail of the nasal bone and anterior nasal spine, in contrast to the soft tissues of the nose and air-filled sinuses

MANDIBLE

The structure of the mandible makes it difficult to image accurately using the usual approach of obtaining two images at 90° to each other. As a result several projections are available for demonstration of this bone, none of which demonstrate it adequately in its entirety:

1. The PA mandible projection, which shows the rami relatively well but causes foreshortening over the body
2. The lateral, which superimposes both sides of the mandible
3. The lateral oblique, which clears the body on the side under examination from the opposite side but foreshortens the ramus. Both lateral obliques are undertaken in any one case, as the mandible is a recognised site for contrecoup fractures

A combination of all, or any, of these projections is used to provide information on the mandible as a whole.

Alternatively, orthopantomography (OPT) can be used to demonstrate the mandible. This is a method that clearly requires specialised equipment, which is not always available. Some units are unsuitable for patients in wheelchairs and the image does have some unsharpness. The main benefit of this method is its ability to demonstrate the whole mandible and TMJs on one image, but it still may not be easy to see fractures; other projections may be required as supplements.[12]

The IR is vertical for projections of the mandible

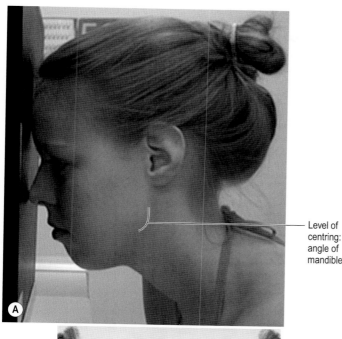

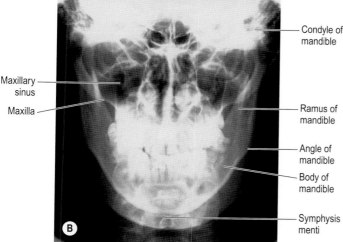

Figure 18.7 PA mandible.

Level of centring: angle of mandible

Condyle of mandible

Maxillary sinus

Maxilla

Ramus of mandible

Angle of mandible

Body of mandible

Symphysis menti

PA mandible (Fig. 18.7A,B)

Positioning

Note that, although this is described as a PA projection, the patient's head is actually positioned as for an occipitofrontal (OF) projection; because the beam will not travel through the occiput or frontal bone the projection cannot actually be named as OF.

- The patient is seated, facing the IR
- The forehead is placed in contact with the midline of the IR and the chin position is adjusted until the OMBL is perpendicular to it
- The MSP is perpendicular to the IR, which is assessed by checking that the EAMs or lateral orbital margins are equidistant from it

Beam direction and FRD

Horizontal, at 90° to the IR
100 cm FRD

Centring

In the midline of the neck, midway between the angles of the mandible

Collimation

TMJs, angles of mandible, symphysis menti

Criteria for assessing image quality

- TMJs, angles of the mandible and symphysis menti are demonstrated
- Petrous ridge is level with the top of the orbits
- Condyles are superimposed over the inferior aspect of the petrous bones laterally
- Symmetry of the mandible either side of the face and neck
- Mandible is seen as a 'U' shape
- Sharp image demonstrating the entire mandible in contrast to the soft tissues of the face and neck, and the bones of the cervical vertebrae

Common error	Possible reason
Pale area where the mandible overlies cervical vertebrae, but contrast over rami is good	kVp too low to penetrate the area over the cervical vertebrae; mAs may need to be reduced if kVp increased

Lateral mandible (Fig. 18.8A,B)

Positioning

- The patient is seated, facing the IR
- The head is turned through 90° to place the affected side in contact with the IR
- The chin is raised very slightly to reduce the density of the soft tissues of the throat which lie over the body of the mandible
- The MSP* is parallel to the IR, which is assessed by checking that the angles of the mandible are in alignment or superimposed

*Using the MSP of the head may not be appropriate for the lateral projection as the mandible may not lie in continuous alignment with the skull. It is suggested that, for this projection, the mandible should be considered to have an MSP that runs vertically down its midline and midway between the angles.

Beam direction and FRD

Horizontal, at 90° to the IR
100 cm FRD

Centring

Over the angle of the mandible

Collimation

TMJs, angles of mandible, symphysis menti

Criteria for assessing image quality

- TMJs, angles of mandible and symphysis menti demonstrated
- Condyles superimposed over each other; angles of mandible superimposed
- Mandible clear of the cervical vertebrae
- Sharp image demonstrating the entire mandible in contrast to the soft tissues of the neck and mouth

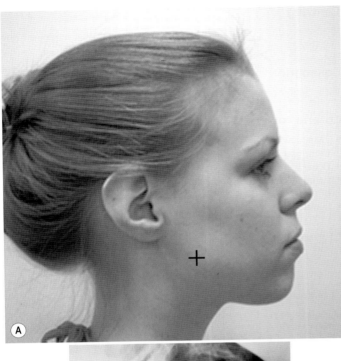

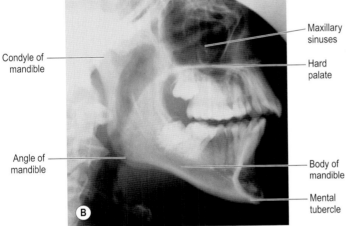

Figure 18.8 (A) Lateral mandible – centring; (B) lateral mandible.

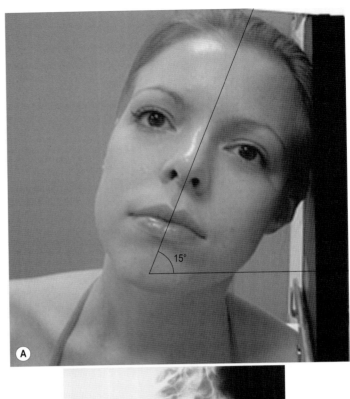

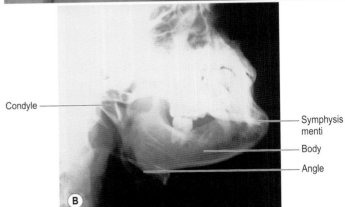

Figure 18.9 Lateral oblique mandible.

Common error	Possible reason
Non-superimposition of required structures	It is tempting to use the upper facial structures to assess the lateral position of the patient; see comments at end of the positioning section
	There may be some magnification of the side furthest from the IR on patients with wider mandibles, which will effectively take its outline outside that of the opposite side; this cannot be considered as radiographer error. Consider increasing FRD to compensate

Lateral oblique mandible (Fig. 18.9A,B)

Both obliques are undertaken in order to demonstrate the whole mandible.

Positioning

- The patient is seated alongside the IR with the side under examination nearest to it
- The chin is raised very slightly, to reduce the density of the soft tissues of the throat which lie over the body of the mandible
- The MSP is initially parallel to the IR and the head then tilted towards it until the MSP is approximately 15° to it. Care must be taken not to rotate the head during the manoeuvre
- The chin is elevated as far as possible to clear the condyle from the neck

Beam direction and FRD

Initially horizontal, then directed 10° cranially
100 cm FRD

Centring

Midway between the angles of the mandible

Collimation

TMJ and angle of mandible on the side under examination, symphysis menti

Once collimation is complete, the IR position may require adjustment until the radiation field lies within the boundaries. The outline of the soft tissues overlying the mandible should be shown as a shadow within the light beam (and within the borders of the IR).

Unfortunately the combination of angle and obliquity for this oblique method does distort and foreshorten the ramus in particular. The body of the mandible is not in contact with the IR, and this has implications for magnification and unsharpness of the body and lower portion of the ramus.

Because the lateral oblique position of the mandible itself will foreshorten the ramus of the mandible, an alternative method is to use a true lateral position of the head, with an increased cranial angle. For this the patient has been described as prone, with the head turned into the lateral position and a cranial beam angle of 25°.[13] Supine with the head turned laterally has also been described, with a 35° central ray.[14] However, a prone lateral position often proves difficult for the patient, especially if injured. The supine lateral head position can be equally difficult but the patient's trunk can be obliqued to improve the situation; for both these supine and prone positions there is the potential for increased ORD, which affects magnification of the image, although this could be improved by supporting the IR on a pad on the table-top.[13] An increase in FRD will also reduce magnification.

Use of a 25° cranial angle in conjunction with a true lateral (seated patient position) requires the tube head to be in a relatively low position and the beam is frequently attenuated by the shoulder in larger patients; an attempt to clear the shoulder can be made by posterior rotation of the shoulder nearest the tube, but this often causes rotation of the head. The shoulder can often lie within the primary beam and be superimposed over the mandible, even with the prone lateral position.

The oblique position with cranial angulation can be deemed a general survey of the mandible and modifications have also been described which will provide more specific information of different aspects of the mandible.[9]

30° rotation towards the side under examination will demonstrate the body more adequately.

45° rotation demonstrates the symphysis menti.

It is also claimed that a rotation of 15° will give a general survey of the mandible, but surely this rotation will cause the condyle to overlie the neck on the image?

Criteria for assessing image quality

- TMJs, angles of the mandible and symphysis menti are demonstrated
- TMJ, condyle, ramus and body on the side under examination are cleared from the cervical vertebrae
- Sharp image demonstrating the entire mandible in contrast to the soft tissues of the neck and mouth

Common errors	Possible reasons
Condyle on the side under examination not cleared from the cervical vertebrae	Chin too low *or* forehead is rotated towards the IR

OPT for mandible

Please refer to Chapter 22 for this examination.

TMJs

Lateral oblique (Fig. 18.10A,B)

In the lateral position the TMJs are superimposed and an oblique central ray is used to clear the image of one TMJ to reveal the other. Both sides are examined for comparison and images taken with mouth open and then closed. An erect technique is more comfortable for the patient than using a table technique.

IR is vertical; an antiscatter grid is employed

Positioning

- The patient is initially seated, facing the IR and is then positioned as for the lateral facial bones; the TMJ under examination is in contact with the IR
- The MSP is parallel to the IR; there should be no tilt or rotation of the head. This can be assessed by checking that the interpupillary line is perpendicular to the IR
- A legend is applied to the IR to indicate whether the mouth is open or closed

Beam direction and FRD

Initially horizontal, then angled 25° caudally
100 cm FRD

Centring

Above the TMJ remote from the IR, with the beam emerging through the TMJ under examination

The TMJ is palpable anterior to the tragus of the ear. If the patient is asked to open their mouth the radiographer's finger will feel a depression over the mandibular fossa as the mouth opens, as the mandibular condyle moves forwards from the mandibular fossa.

Collimation

TMJ, condyle of mandible

Criteria for assessing image quality

- TMJ and condyle of mandible are demonstrated
- Other TMJ is clear from the area of interest
- TMJ under examination anterior to EAM
- Indication of whether the mouth is open or closed is clearly seen on the image
- Sharp image demonstrating the mandibular fossa in contrast to the temporal bone and condyle of mandible

Common errors	Possible reasons
Mastoid air cells of unaffected side overlying TMJ	MSP rotated, face turning towards IR
TMJ or ramus of mandible closest to tube not cleared from TMJ under examination	1. Inadequate angle used *or* 2. Head is tilted with its vertex towards the IR, which effectively reduces the effects of angulation

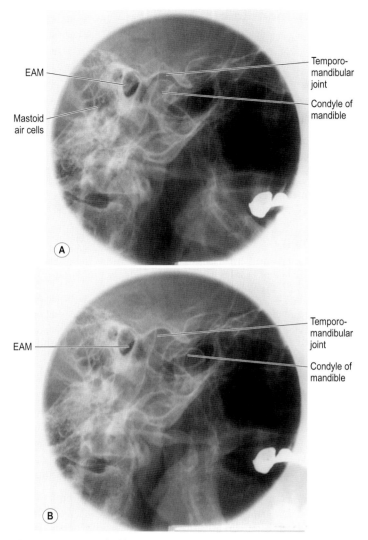

Figure 18.10 Lateral oblique TMJs: (A) mouth closed, (B) mouth open.

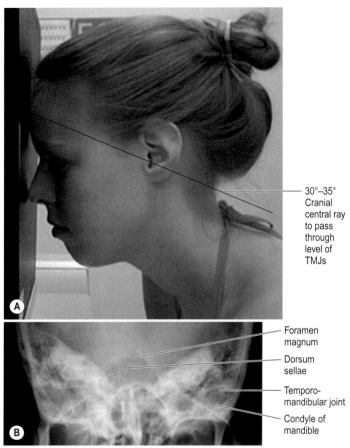

Figure 18.11 TMJs – OF 30–35°.

OF 30–35° TMJs (Fig. 18.11A,B)

IR is vertical; an antiscatter grid is employed

Positioning

- The patient is seated, facing the IR
- The forehead is placed in contact with the midline of the IR and the chin position adjusted until the OMBL is perpendicular to it, as for the basic OF position
- The IR may require displacement after accurate tube centring to ensure that the area of interest is included in its boundary
- The MSP is perpendicular to the IR, assessed by checking that the EAMs or lateral orbital margins are equidistant from it

Beam direction and FRD

Initially horizontal, with 30–35° cranial angulation
The specific angle has not been suggested here as it does appear that there is some variation in practice.[7,8] *Selection of optimum exposure factors will ensure that the joints will be well demonstrated, regardless of a 5° difference in angle.*
100 cm FRD

Centring

In the midline of the neck, to travel through the TMJs

Collimation

TMJs

Exposure is made with the mouth open, and a legend should be applied to indicate this

Most texts describe the fronto-occipital (FO) projection rather than the OF,[5,6,8,9] but, as outlined in Chapter 16, the OF position is easier for the patient, especially if they can sit in an erect position. The OF position will also help reduce dose absorbed by the lenses of the eyes and the thyroid, although the close collimation required for TMJs does ensure that dose is minimised, even in the FO position. It is unlikely that the joints will lie significantly closer to the IR on either the OF or the FO projections, therefore image sharpness should be similar on both.

FO 30–35° TMJs

IR is vertical; an antiscatter grid is used (supine technique may be used, but the FO position is difficult to achieve with the patient supine)

This projection is essentially the same position as the 30° FO projection (Towne's) used for the cranial vault, with collimation to the area of interest and alteration of height of centring.

Positioning

- The patient is seated, with their back to the IR
- The back of the occiput is placed in contact with the midline of the IR and the chin position is adjusted until the OMBL is at 90° to it
- The MSP is perpendicular to the IR, which is assessed by checking that the EAMs or lateral orbital margins are equidistant from it
- It will be necessary to adjust the height of the IR after centring

Beam direction and FRD

A horizontal central ray is angled 30–35° caudally
100 cm FRD

Centring

In the midline above the glabella, with the beam travelling through the TMJs and then the lower occiput.

Collimation

Mastoid bones, TMJs, condyles of mandible, upper rami of mandible

Criteria for assessing image quality

- Mastoid bones, TMJs, condyles of mandible and upper rami of mandible are demonstrated
- Symmetry of the petrous portion of the temporal bones on either side of the foramen magnum; the condyles of mandible are an equal distance from the lateral portions of the skull
- Dorsum sellae seen within the foramen magnum; arch of C1 may be demonstrated if a 35° angle has been used
- Sharp image demonstrating contrast between the TMJs and the denser petrous temporal and mastoids

Common errors	Possible reasons
Asymmetry of petrous temporal bones around the foramen magnum	Rotation about MSP
Pale image over the TMJ	Inadequate penetration

Orthopantomography (OPT)

As in the case of the mandible, the TMJs are seen on the OPT examination of the mandible (see Ch. 22) but the joints are shown closed in the conventional mouth position. Open-mouth exposure should also be made in order to demonstrate the joint adequately. This is a difficult manoeuvre for patients with dislocation, and examination with the TMJ open and closed may not be possible using the OPT technique.

ZYGOMATIC ARCHES

The zygomatic arches are demonstrated reasonably well in contrast to the cranium on the OM facial bones projections, but they can be shown in profile over the soft tissues of the cheeks in the FO 30° projection.

FO 30° zygomatic arches (Fig. 18.12A,B)

As mentioned for the TMJ examination in this position, a technique with the patient supine may be used but is not recommended unless absolutely necessary (for example when the patient is injured seriously enough to present supine on a trolley).

An alternative OF projection is not described, as the zygomatic arches must show some magnification in order to demonstrate them laterally at either side of the cranial vault. To undertake an OF projection would minimise magnification of the arches since they lie closer to the IR in this position; the posterior half of the vault will be magnified and potentially overlie part, or all, of the zygomatic arches.

The IR is vertical

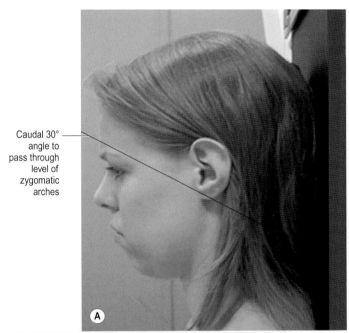

Caudal 30° angle to pass through level of zygomatic arches

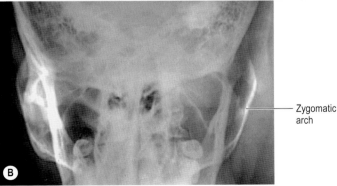

Zygomatic arch

Figure 18.12 (A) FO 30° zygomatic arches; (B) OF 30° zygomatic arches. *(B) Reproduced with permission from Ballinger PW, Frank ED. Merrill's atlas of radiographic positioning and radiologic procedures. 10th ed. St Louis: Mosby; 2003.*

Positioning

- The patient is seated with their back to the IR and positioned initially as for the FO 30° TMJ projection
- It will be necessary to adjust the height of the IR after centring, to ensure the area of interest lies within its borders

Beam direction and FRD

A horizontal central ray is angled 30° caudally
100 cm FRD

Centring

In the midline above the glabella, with the beam travelling through the zygomatic arches

Collimation

Mastoid bones, zygomatic arches, zygomae, upper rami of mandible

Exposure factors

Exposure factors must be set significantly lower than for other FO 30° projections of the cranial vault, mastoids and TMJs. This is because of the low density of the arches and the fact that no grid is necessary for the examination.

Modified submentovertical (SMV) zygomatic arches for the injured patient

(Fig. 18.13)

Note that this projection can only be used with a cassette-type IR.

Positioning

- The patient lies supine on the table or trolley; it may be necessary to place a pillow under the patient's shoulders to elevate the area of interest
- The neck is flexed back as far as possible and the IR placed vertically in contact with the top of the head, its long axis resting on the table-top
- The IR position is adjusted (angled) until parallel to the long axes of the zygomatic arches , then supported in this position by pads and sandbags
- The MSP is perpendicular to the IR and coincident with its midline

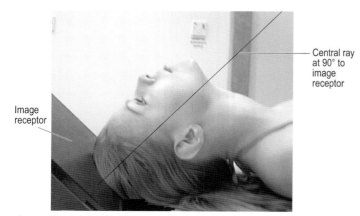

Figure 18.13 Modified SMV zygomatic arches.

Beam direction and FRD

The beam should be perpendicular to the IR and zygomatic arches

FRD 120 cm, or slightly more for patients with a large abdomen, which may lie in the way of the tube head at shorter FRD

Centring

In the midline, to travel through the midpoint of the zygomatic arches

Collimation

As for the FO 30° projection

Criteria for assessing image quality – FO 30°

- Mastoid bones, zygomatic arches, zygomae and upper rami of mandible are demonstrated
- Symmetry of the petrous portion of the temporal bones on either side of the foramen magnum
- Dorsum sellae seen within the foramen magnum
- Sharp image demonstrating contrast between the low density zygomatic arch and the soft tissues of the face

Common errors – FO 30°	Possible reasons
Asymmetry of petrous temporal bones around the foramen magnum	Rotation about MSP
Dark image with poor contrast	Quite obviously, selection of mAs and kVp is too high. Density of the arch is frequently overestimated and it should be remembered that this density is less than that of a phalanx. There is an air gap between the zygomatic arch and the IR which will need consideration when selecting exposure factors

Essentially the FO 30° projection uses a tangential approach to demonstrate the zygomatic arches; other methods that employ the tangential approach have also been described as:

1. An SMV projection with the beam centred under the chin at the level of the midpoint of the zygomatic arches. Collimation includes both sides
2. An SMV with a 15° tilt of the head (the vertex turned away from the side under examination) and centring over the apex of the arch. Each side is exposed in turn[7]

Use of the SMV may prove difficult for the patient, especially those who present supine on a trolley. Maintenance of the position is also difficult for the patient. A more comfortable position is used in the modified SMV.

Criteria for assessing image quality (SMV)

As for the FO 30° projection

REFERENCES

1. Bhattaychara J, et al. The role of plain radiography in the management of suspected orbital blow-out fractures. British Journal of Radiology 1997;70: 29–33.

2. RCR Working Party. Making the best use of clinical radiology services: referral guidelines. 6th ed. London: The Royal College of Radiologists; 2007.

3. Pogrel M, et al. Efficacy of a single occipitomental radiograph to screen for midfacial fractures. Journal of Oral and Maxillofacial Surgery 2000;58(1):24–6.

4. Goh S, Low B. Radiologic screening for midfacial fractures: a single 30 degree occipitomental is enough. Journal of Trauma 2002 Apr;24(4):688–92.

5. Carver E, Carver B, editors. Medical imaging: techniques, reflection and evaluation. Edinburgh: Churchill Livingstone; 2006.

6. http://www.e-radiography.net/names/named_views.htm#A.

7. Swallow, et al. Clark's positioning in radiography. 12th ed. London: Hodder Arnold; 2005.

8. Unett E, Royle A. Radiographic techniques and image evaluation. London: Nelson Thornes; 1997.

9. Bontrager K, Lampignano JP. Textbook of radiographic positioning and related anatomy. 7th ed. St Louis: Mosby; 2010.

10. McQuillen-Martenson K. Radiographic image analysis. 3rd ed. St Louis: Saunders; 2010.

11. Sidebottom AJ, Sissons G. Radiographic screening for midfacial fracture in A & E. BJR 1999;72:523–4.

12. Scally P. Medical imaging. Oxford: Oxford University Press; 1999.

13. Frank E, et al. Merrill's atlas of radiographic positioning and procedures. 12th ed. St Louis: Mosby; 2011.

14. Eisenberg R, et al. Radiographic positioning. 2nd ed. Boston: Little Brown and Company; 1995.

Chapter 19

Paranasal sinuses

Elizabeth Carver

X-ray examination of the sinuses is rarely undertaken in the 21st century as acute symptoms should be diagnosed and treated clinically, with computed tomography (CT) and magnetic resonance imaging (MRI) superseding plain radiography as imaging techniques, but only when treatment has proved 'ineffective' (or if malignancy is suspected).[1] The projections must be undertaken erect, with horizontal beam, to demonstrate any fluid levels that might be present in the sinuses.

For all projections of the sinuses and postnasal space the image receptor (IR) is vertical

Occipitomental (OM) sinuses (Fig. 19.1A,B)

Positioning

- The patient is seated, facing the IR
- The chin is placed in contact with the midline of the IR and the chin position is adjusted until the orbitomeatal baseline (OMBL) has been raised 45° from the horizontal
- The median sagittal plane (MSP) is perpendicular to the IR, which is assessed by checking that the external auditory meatuses (EAMs) or lateral orbital margins are equidistant from it

Beam direction and focus receptor distance (FRD)

Horizontal, at 90° to the IR and making an angle of 45° with the OMBL
100 cm FRD

Centring

Above the external occipital protuberance (EOP), to emerge at the level of the inferior orbital margins

Collimation

Frontal sinuses (the upper borders of these sinuses vary with each individual and a specific border description cannot be given), maxillary sinuses

Criteria for assessing image quality

- All paranasal sinuses are demonstrated
- Symmetry of facial bones on each side; equal distance of lateral orbital margins from outer table of temporal bones
- Upper border of the petrous portion of the temporal bone is level with the apex of the maxillary antra
- Images of premolars and molars are medial to, and clear of, the medial aspects of the maxillary sinuses
- Zygomatic arches are seen as a tight 'C' and reversed tight 'C' laterally
- Sharp image demonstrating the air-filled regions of the paranasal sinuses in contrast with the bones of the skull

Common errors	Possible reasons
Asymmetry of the facial structures	Rotation about MSP
Position of the petrous ridge is too high; it is seen through the maxillary sinuses	Chin is not raised enough. (see further notes in Ch. 18, OM facial bones)
Petrous ridge is below the maxillary sinuses; image of crowns of premolars overlying the medial aspects of the maxillary sinuses. The frontal sinuses are foreshortened and may appear over-dark	Chin is raised too high
or Position appears acceptable; frontal sinuses are over-darkened	Collimation might not be tight enough around the area of interest, thus scatter may blacken the upper anterior aspect of the frontal bone

Lateral (Fig. 19.2A,B)

It is not likely that this projection will add useful information to the OM, as the two sides of the head are superimposed. Its inclusion in this text has therefore been discontinued.

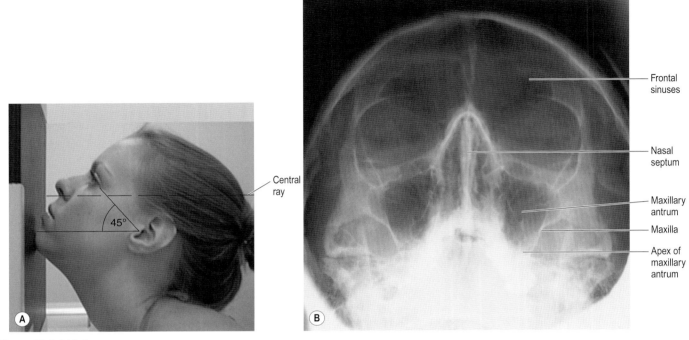

Central ray

Frontal sinuses

Nasal septum

Maxillary antrum

Maxilla

Apex of maxillary antrum

45°

A

B

Figure 19.1 OM sinuses.

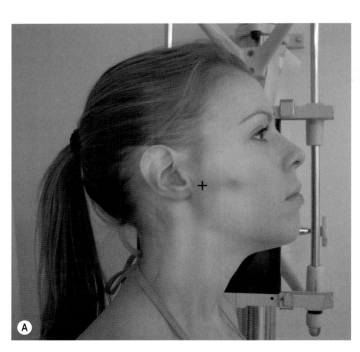

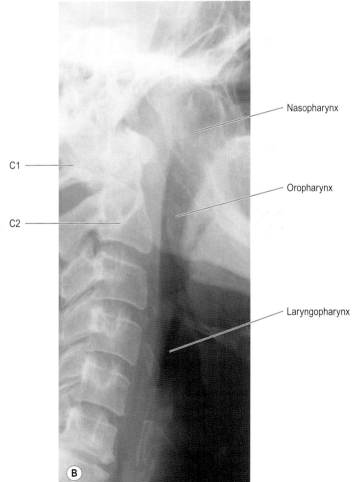

C1

C2

Nasopharynx

Oropharynx

Laryngopharynx

A

B

Figure 19.2 Lateral postnasal space.

Lateral postnasal space

UK guidelines no longer suggest X-ray examination of this area, but some anecdotal comment suggests that this may still be used for children who snore or have difficulty breathing through their nose.

Positioning

- The patient stands or sits with the side of their head next to the IR and their MSP parallel to it
- The MSP is parallel to the IR; there should be no tilt or rotation of the head. This can be assessed by checking the midline of the cranium over the top and symmetry of the frontal bone and orbits
- The chin is raised slightly, to reduce the density of the soft tissues of the throat and clear as much of the mandible as possible from the air-filled regions

Beam direction and FRD

Horizontal, at 90° to the IR
100 cm FRD

Centring

Below the midpoint of the OMBL, half way between the level of the temporomandibular joint (TMJ) and angle of the mandible

Collimation

Angle of the mandible and 3 cm anterior to this, TMJ, pharynx and down to the level of the thyroid cartilage

Criteria for assessing image quality

- Postnasal space, the posterior wall of the maxillary sinuses, the TMJ and thyroid cartilage are demonstrated
- Clear joint spaces are shown between the cervical vertebrae
- Sharp image demonstrating the darker air-filled pharynx in contrast with the soft tissues of the surrounding area and the mandible. Cervical vertebrae appear pale and low in contrast

Occipitofrontal (OF) maxillary and anterior ethmoid sinuses (Fig. 19.3A,B)

Positioning

- The patient is seated, facing the IR
- The forehead is placed in contact with the IR and the chin position is adjusted until the OMBL is at 90° to it
- The MSP is perpendicular to the IR, which is assessed by checking that the EAMs or lateral orbital margins are equidistant from it

Beam direction and FRD

Horizontal, at 90° to the IR
100 cm FRD

Centring

In the midline of the occiput, to emerge at the level of the inferior orbital margins

Collimation

Frontal sinuses (the upper border of these sinuses vary with each individual and a specific border description cannot be given), maxillary sinuses

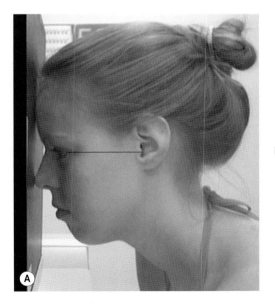

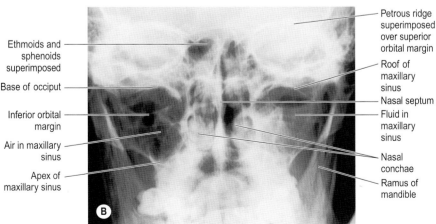

Ethmoids and sphenoids superimposed
Base of occiput
Inferior orbital margin
Air in maxillary sinus
Apex of maxillary sinus

Petrous ridge superimposed over superior orbital margin
Roof of maxillary sinus
Nasal septum
Fluid in maxillary sinus
Nasal conchae
Ramus of mandible

Figure 19.3 OF maxillary and anterior ethmoid sinuses.

Criteria for assessing image quality

- All paranasal sinuses are demonstrated
- Equal distance of the lateral orbital margins from the outer table of the temporal bones on each side
- Upper border of the petrous portion of the temporal bone is level with the superior orbital margins
- Sharp image demonstrating the air-filled regions of the paranasal sinuses in contrast with the bones of the skull. The petrous portion of the temporal appears under-penetrated

Common errors	Possible reasons
Distance of the lateral orbital margins from the lateral borders of skull differs on each side	Rotation about MSP
Position of the petrous ridge is too high; it is seen above the superior orbital margins	OMBL is not perpendicular to the IR; chin is too far down
Petrous ridge is too low; it is seen within the outline of the orbits	OMBL is not perpendicular to the IR; the chin is raised slightly
Maxillary sinuses are over-blackened with poor contrast between the air-filled sinuses and maxilla. Petrous temporal shows good contrast and detail	Over-penetration. The maxilla itself is not a particularly dense bone and this is often overlooked

OF (10°) frontal sinuses (Fig. 19.4A,B)

In the OF projection for maxillary and anterior ethmoid sinuses the frontal sinuses are foreshortened, whereas in the OM projection they are magnified and distorted. For a more accurate representation of these sinuses, the OMBL is raised to bring the vertical axis of the frontal sinus into a position where it is more parallel to the IR. 10° caudal angulation will achieve the required effect, but a horizontal beam is advised in order to demonstrate fluid levels more accurately.

IR is vertical

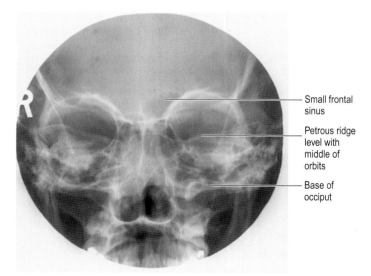

— Small frontal sinus

— Petrous ridge level with middle of orbits

— Base of occiput

Figure 19.4 Frontal sinuses.

Positioning

- The patient is positioned initially as for the OF maxillary sinuses projection
- The chin is raised 10° and a radiolucent pad placed between the forehead and IR for immobilisation

Beam direction and FRD

Horizontal, at 90° to the IR

If the chin is to be elevated 10° then a guide must be used to assess this accurately; it is arguable whether the human eye can estimate a small angle such as 10° accurately. Use of a 10° radiolucent pad for immobilisation would be appropriate. Alternatively a large protractor, or a large piece of clear plastic marked with angles, can be placed against the OMBL

100 cm FRD

Centring

In the midline of the occiput, to emerge through the nasion

Collimation

Frontal, ethmoid, sphenoid sinuses

Criteria for assessing image quality

- Frontal, ethmoid and sphenoid sinuses are demonstrated
- Symmetry of structures around the midline
- Upper border of the petrous portion of the temporal bone half way down the orbits
- Sharp image demonstrating the air-filled frontal and ethmoid sinuses in contrast with the frontal and ethmoid bones

OF ethmoid and sphenoid sinuses (Fig. 19.5)

Positioning

- As for the frontal sinuses, these sinuses can be seen on an *OF projection*, this time with *the chin lowered until the OMBL moves through 10°*

Beam direction, centring and collimation

As for the OF for frontal and anterior ethmoid sinuses

Criteria for assessing image quality

- Ethmoid and sphenoid sinuses are demonstrated
- Symmetry of structures around the midline
- Upper border of the petrous portion of the temporal bone is shown above the superior orbital margins; the petrous ridges start to elevate obliquely towards the outer table of the vault, rather than appearing horizontal
- Sphenoid and ethmoid sinuses seen in the midline, slightly above the orbits and between the petrous portions of the temporal bones
- Sharp image demonstrating the air-filled ethmoid and sphenoid sinuses in contrast with the bones of the vault and petrous portions of the temporal bones

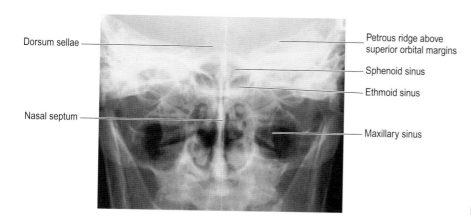

Dorsum sellae

Petrous ridge above
superior orbital margins

Sphenoid sinus

Ethmoid sinus

Nasal septum

Maxillary sinus

Figure 19.5 OF sphenoid and ethmoids.

REFERENCE

1. Royal College of Radiologists Working
   party. Making the best use of a department
   of clinical radiology: guidelines for doctors.
   6th ed. London: Royal College Of
   Radiologists; 2007.

Chapter | 20 |

Specialised projections of the skull

Elizabeth Carver

In the 21st century, the majority of hospitals in the Western world have access to specialised imaging modalities. Of these, computed tomography (CT) and magnetic resonance imaging (MRI) have largely replaced plain radiography in the diagnosis of diseases which were originally only assessed with plain radiography. Unfortunately, plain radiography frequently only provides information when disease is very advanced; CT provides more detailed and high-quality information, and MRI has the advantage of providing information on neurological and other soft tissues (with no patient dose from ionising radiation) before any bony effects are seen.

Information on plain radiography is still provided in this book, as support for radiographers working in areas with limited or no access to MRI and CT.

SELLA TURCICA (PITUITARY FOSSA)

To clarify the use of terms in this chapter, the name 'pituitary fossa' refers to the depression within the sella turcica in which lies the pituitary gland. The sella turcica itself forms the top of the central portion of the sphenoid bone, lying over the sphenoid sinus in the midline.

An enlarged and eroded sella can be a sign of a pituitary tumour or raised intracranial pressure, but this appearance is an effect of long-term disease.

For all projections of the sella turcica image receptor (IR) is vertical; an antiscatter grid is employed

Lateral sella turcica (Fig. 20.1A,B)

Positioning

- The patient is initially seated facing the IR
- The trunk is brought as close as possible to the receptor unit and the patient is asked to sit with their spine as erect as possible. This helps the patient turn their head more easily into the required lateral position
- The head is turned through 90° to bring the side of the head in contact with the IR
- The median sagittal plane (MSP) is parallel to the IR; there should be no tilt or rotation of the head. This can be assessed by checking the midline of the cranium over the top and symmetry of the frontal bone and orbits

Beam direction and focus receptor distance (FRD)

Horizontal, at 90° to the IR
100 cm FRD

Centring

Midway between the posterior tubercle of the first cervical vertebra and the glabella *or* 2.5 cm anterior to the external auditory meatus (EAM), along the orbitomeatal baseline (OMBL), and 2.5 cm above this point

The second centring point will have variable efficacy due to variations in the skull size of the individual patient.

Collimation

Sphenoid bone from lesser wing (anterior clinoid processes) anteriorly and posterior clinoids posteriorly

Criteria for assessing image quality

- Anterior and posterior clinoid processes, sella turcica, sphenoid sinus and dorsum sellae are demonstrated
- Superimposition of both sides of the floor of pituitary fossa and floor of the anterior cranial fossa
- Anterior clinoid processes are superimposed
- Posterior clinoid processes are superimposed
- Sharp image demonstrating outline of the clinoids and pituitary fossa in contrast with the temporal bones and sphenoid sinus

Common errors	Possible reasons
Both pairs of clinoid processes over-lapped, seen one above the other	Tilted skull
Both pairs of clinoid processes overlapped, seen side by side	Rotated skull
'Double' floor of sella turcica; two lines over floor area	Tilted skull or floor is eroded on one side by tumour

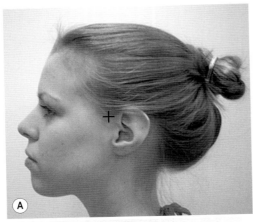

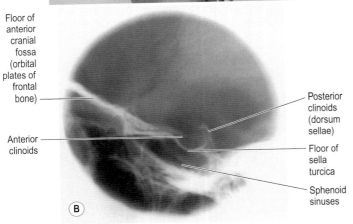

Floor of anterior cranial fossa (orbital plates of frontal bone)

Anterior clinoids

Posterior clinoids (dorsum sellae)

Floor of sella turcica

Sphenoid sinuses

Figure 20.1 Lateral sella turcica.

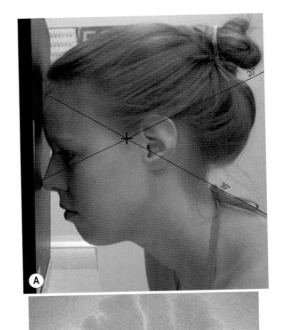

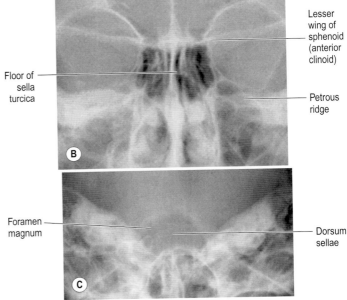

Lesser wing of sphenoid (anterior clinoid)

Floor of sella turcica

Petrous ridge

Foramen magnum

Dorsum sellae

Figure 20.2 (A) OF sella turcica; (B) OF 20° sella turcica; (C) OF 30° sella turcica.

Occipitofrontal (OF) sella turcica (Fig. 20.2A,B,C)

The OF 20° projection will demonstrate the floor of the sella turcica, seen as asymmetry of the floor if the floor is eroded on one side. The OF 30° projection has limited value, demonstrating the dorsum sellae through the foramen magnum; the dorsum will appear as low density if it is eroded.

IR is erect

Positioning

- The patient is seated facing the bucky, their forehead in contact with it
- The OMBL and MSP are perpendicular to the IR

Beam direction and FRD

(a) Initially horizontal, a *20° caudal* angle will demonstrate the floor of the pituitary fossa through the ethmoid and sphenoid sinuses
(b) A *30° cranial* angle will demonstrate the dorsum sellae through the foramen magnum
100 cm FRD

Centring

(a) With *20° caudal* angle: Above the external occipital protuberance (EOP) to emerge through the nasion
(b) With *30° caudal* angle: Below the EOP, on the neck, to emerge through the glabella

Collimation

OF 20°: Lesser wing of sphenoid, sphenoid and ethmoid sinuses
OF 30°: Ethmoid sinus, foramen magnum

Criteria for assessing image quality

OF 20°

- Lesser wing of the sphenoid, sphenoid and ethmoid sinuses are demonstrated
- Medial aspects of the superior border of petrous ridge are shown superimposed on the inferior orbital margin
- Lesser wing of sphenoid seen medially and symmetrically across the upper portion of the orbits
- Medial borders of the orbits are equidistant from nasal septum
- Floor of pituitary fossa is seen as a horizontal line across the ethmoid sinuses. In cases of erosion of the floor of the fossa, this line may deviate from horizontal orientation
- Sharp image showing the fine line indicating the floor of the pituitary fossa in contrast with the air-filled ethmoid sinus

OF 30°

- Foramen magnum is demonstrated
- Dorsum sellae is seen in the centre of the foramen magnum
- Sharp image showing dorsum sellae in contrast with the less dense foramen magnum

Common errors – OF 20°	Possible reasons
Petrous ridge seen above the level of the inferior orbital margins	Inadequate angle selected or OMBL is incorrectly positioned (chin down too far)
Petrous ridge seen below the level of the inferior orbital margins	Angle selected is too great or OMBL is incorrectly positioned (chin not far enough down)

Common errors – OF 30°	Possible reasons
Foramen magnum appears short or is not evident. Dorsum sellae may be visible above the portion of the foramen magnum that is seen	Angle selected is inadequate or OMBL is positioned incorrectly (chin not far enough down)
Large foramen magnum seen but curve of the posterior arch of C1 is seen in its lower third, rather than the anvil shape of dorsum sellae	Angle selected is too great or OMBL is not positioned correctly (chin too far down)

MASTOIDS

Lateral oblique mastoids (Fig. 20.3A,B)

Positioning for this projection is identical to that for lateral oblique temporomandibular joints (TMJs), although the centring point differs. The pinna of the ear must also be cleared from the mastoid area. Both sides are examined for comparison.

IR is vertical; an antiscatter grid is employed

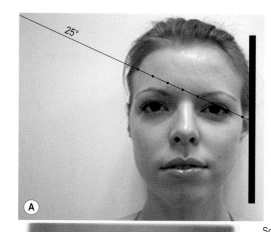
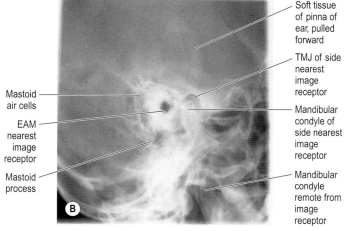

Figure 20.3 Lateral oblique mastoids.

Labels: Soft tissue of pinna of ear, pulled forward; TMJ of side nearest image receptor; Mandibular condyle of side nearest image receptor; Mandibular condyle remote from image receptor; Mastoid air cells; EAM nearest image receptor; Mastoid process

Positioning

- The patient is initially seated, facing the IR
- The trunk is brought as close as possible to the receptor unit and the patient is asked to sit with their spine as erect as possible. This helps the patient turn their head more easily into the required lateral position
- The head is turned through 90° to bring the mastoid on the side under examination over the IR. The location of this bone can be detected by palpating the mastoid process, which lies inferiorly and posteriorly to the EAM
- The pinna of the ear on the side nearest the IR is then gently pulled forward and the head rests against the IR to keep the pinna forward. This clears the image of the pinna from the area of interest
- The MSP is parallel to the IR; there should be no tilt or rotation of the head. This can be assessed by checking the midline of the cranium over the top, symmetry of the frontal bone and orbits, and that the interpupillary line is perpendicular to the IR
- Asking the patient to close their eyes will assist in maintenance of the position; as the radiographer leaves the receptor unit, a patient will often follow this movement with their eyes and potentially affect the position of the head

Beam direction and FRD

Initially horizontal, angled 25° caudally
100 cm FRD

Centring

Above the mastoid process on the side remote from the IR, to emerge over the mastoid process on the side nearest the IR

Collimation

EAM, mastoid process, air cells behind the pinna of the ear

Criteria for assessing image quality

- EAM and air-filled mastoid are demonstrated posterior to the EAM
- Condyle of mandible and mastoid air cells of the opposite side are projected clear from those under examination
- Soft tissue of ear is seen as folded forward and cleared from the mastoid
- Air cells of the mastoids are seen in contrast to bone; bony detail of the mastoid bone is demonstrated

Common errors	Possible reasons
Mastoid closest to tube not cleared from mastoid under examination	1. Inadequate angle used or
	2. Head is tilted with its vertex towards the IR, which effectively reduces the effects of angulation
TMJ of opposite side not cleared from mastoid	Inadequate angle, or tilt as above or the head is rotated with the face away from the IR

Profile of mastoid process (Fig. 20.4A,B)

Both sides are examined for comparison.
   IR is vertical

Positioning

- The patient is initially positioned as for an FO projection.
- The head is rotated approximately 30° away from the side under examination, until the process is in profile and cleared from ramus of the mandible

Beam direction and FRD

Initially horizontal, angled 25° caudally
100 cm FRD

Centring

Over the mastoid process under examination (nearest the IR)

Collimation

Mastoid air cells, mastoid process

Criteria for assessing image quality

- Mastoid and mastoid process are demonstrated
- Mastoid process is cleared from the mandible and zygoma
- Mastoid bone is seen in contrast to air-filled cells and soft tissues of the neck

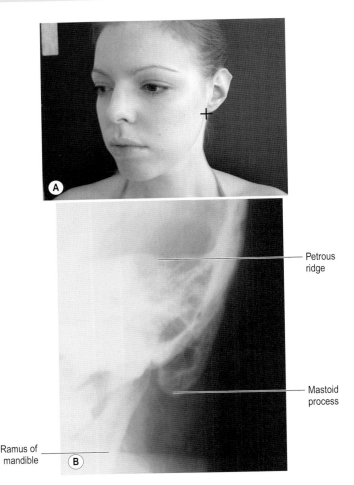

Figure 20.4 Profile of mastoid process.

Common errors	Possible reasons
Mandible and/or zygoma overlying mastoid process	Inadequate obliquity
Occiput overlies mastoid process	Excessive obliquity

OF 30° mastoids (Fig. 20.5A,B)

IR is vertical; an antiscatter grid is employed

Positioning

- The patient is seated facing the bucky, their forehead in contact with it
- The OMBL and MSP are perpendicular to the IR

Beam direction and FRD

Initially horizontal, angled 30° cranially
100 cm FRD

Centring

In the midline of the neck, to travel through the mastoid processes
   It may be necessary to further displace the IR, to ensure the area of interest lies within its borders.

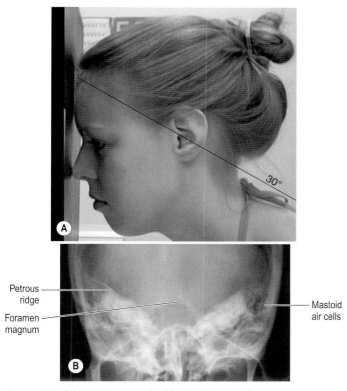

Figure 20.5 (A) OF 30° mastoids; (B) OF 30° mastoids.

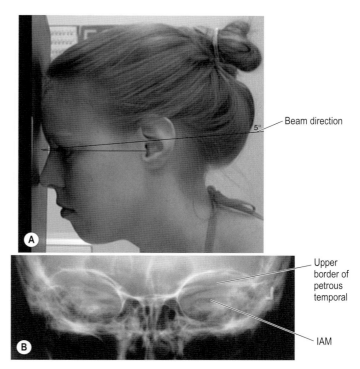

Figure 20.6 OF 5° IAMs.

Collimation

Temporal bones, mastoid processes

Criteria for assessing image quality

- Air-filled mastoid bones are demonstrated on the lateral portions of the temporal bones
- Dorsum sellae and posterior clinoid processes are projected through the centre of the foramen magnum
- Petrous temporals seen as a slight 'v' shape about the foramen magnum
- Symmetry of the petrous portions of the temporal around the midline
- Sharp image demonstrating the air-filled mastoids in contrast to the denser bones of the vault

Common errors	Possible reasons
Foramen magnum appears short or is not evident. Dorsum sellae may be visible above the portion of the foramen magnum that is seen	Angle selected is inadequate or OMBL is incorrectly positioned (chin not far enough down)
Large foramen magnum seen but curve of the posterior arch of C1 is seen in its lower third, rather than the anvil shape of dorsum sellae	Angle selected is too great or OMBL is incorrectly positioned (chin too far down)

TEMPORAL BONE: PETROUS PORTION FOR INTERNAL AUDITORY MEATUS (IAM)

OF 5° IAMs (Fig. 20.6A,B)

IR is vertical; an antiscatter grid is employed

Positioning

- The patient is seated facing the bucky, their forehead in contact with it
- The OMBL and MSP are perpendicular to the IR
- The nasion is coincident with the middle of the IR

Beam direction and FRD

Initially horizontal, angled 5° caudally
100 cm FRD

A central ray perpendicular to the IR has previously been described[1] for this projection, but as the petrous ridge lies coincident with the upper border of the orbits, location of the IAM can be difficult. Use of the 5° caudal angle brings the ridge just below the upper border of the orbits; this acts as a distinguishable landmark, below which lies the low-density channel for the IAM (Fig. 20.6B).

Centring

Above the EOP to emerge through the nasion

Collimation

Superior orbits and base of skull (occiput)

Criteria for assessing image quality

- Superior orbits and base of skull (occiput) are demonstrated
- Petrous ridge is seen just below the superior margins
- Symmetry of structures is seen through the orbits; semicircular canals seen at the outer limits of the IAMs can be assessed as to their equidistance from the lateral orbital outlines
- Sharp image demonstrating contrast of the petrous portions of temporal bones with the outline of the orbits and the less dense IAMs lying within the petrous portion

Common errors	Possible reasons
Petrous ridge seen above required level in orbits	Inadequate angle selected *or* OMBL is incorrectly positioned (chin too far down)
Petrous ridge seen below required level in orbits	Angle selected is too great *or* OMBL is incorrectly positioned (chin not far enough down)

Anterior oblique (OF oblique) IAMs

(Fig. 20.7A,B)

This projection is also known as *Stenver's projection*.[1] It aims to place the petrous portion of the temporal bone parallel to the IR while using the cranial angle to clear the image of the petrous bone above the zygomatic arch and over the flatter, less detailed image of the temporal and parietal bones. The obliquity of the petrous portion of the temporal bones for the Stenver's position is given as approximately 45° but variations according to build have been highlighted as ranging from 40° in the dolicocephalic head (long narrow vault as seen from above), through 47° in the mesocephalic ('average') and as much as 54° in the brachycephalic (short and broad vault when seen from above).[2]

IR is vertical; an antiscatter grid is used

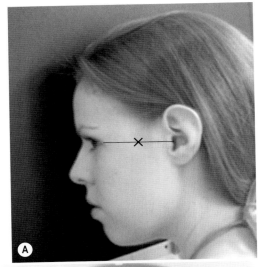

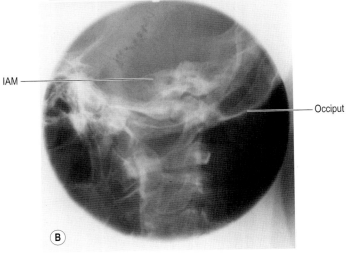

IAM

Occiput

Figure 20.7 AO (OF oblique) IAMs.

Positioning

- The patient is initially positioned in an OF position
- The head is rotated 45° away from the side under examination

Beam direction and FRD

Initially horizontal, angled 12° cranially
100 cm FRD

Centring

Midway between the EOP and the EAM remote from the IR, to emerge midway between the EAM nearest the IR and outer canthus of the eye. It may be necessary to displace the IR to ensure the area of interest lies within its borders.

Collimation

Temporal bone under examination

Criteria for assessing image quality

- Orbits, base of occiput and petrous portion of the temporal bone are demonstrated
- Mastoid air cells of the side under examination projected shown laterally in relation to semicircular canals
- Image of the curve of the occipital outline (of the side not under examination) travels through the mastoid air cells
- Lines representing the right and left sides of the base of the skull are horizontal and at the same level
- IAM, semicircular canals and vestibule of the ear are seen below the arcuate eminence, above the head of mandible
- Sharp image demonstrating the dense petrous portion of temporal in contrast to the IAM, semicircular canals and the vestibule

Common error	Possible reason
Short meatus	Incorrect rotation; this will show the internal occipital crest crossing the meatus or semicircular canals

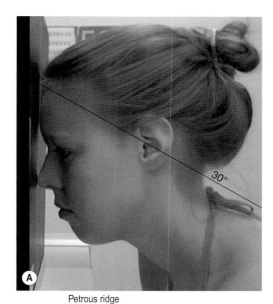

Petrous ridge

IAM | Foramen magnum | Semicircular canal

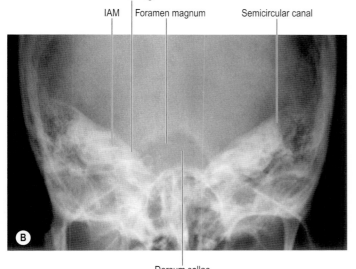

Dorsum sellae

Figure 20.8 OF 30° petrous temporal.

OF 30° petrous temporal (Fig. 20.8A,B)

IR is vertical; an antiscatter grid is employed

Positioning

* The patient is seated facing the bucky, their forehead in contact with it
* The OMBL and MSP are perpendicular to the IR

Beam direction and FRD

Initially horizontal, angled 30° cranially
100 cm FRD

Centring

In the midline of the neck, to travel through the level of the EAMs. It may be necessary to displace the IR to ensure the area of interest lies within its borders.

Collimation

Temporal bones to include petrous portion

Criteria for assessing image quality

* Temporal bones, including petrous portions, are demonstrated
* Dorsum sellae and posterior clinoid processes are projected through the centre of the foramen magnum
* Petrous temporals are seen as a slight 'v' shape about the foramen magnum
* Symmetry of petrous portions of temporal around the foramen magnum
* Sharp image with dense petrous portions of temporals seen in contrast to the less dense acoustic meati and the occiput

Common errors	Possible reasons
Foramen magnum appears short or is not evident. Dorsum sellae may be visible above the portion of the foramen magnum that is seen	Angle selected is inadequate *or* OMBL is incorrectly positioned (chin not far enough down)
Large foramen magnum seen but curve of the posterior arch of C1 is seen in its lower third, rather than the anvil shape of dorsum sellae	Angle selected is too great *or* OMBL is incorrectly positioned (chin too far down)

OPTIC FORAMEN

Occipitomental (OM) oblique/anterior oblique (AO) optic foramen

(Fig. 20.9A,B)

Both optic foramina are examined for comparison.
    IR is vertical; an antiscatter grid is employed

Positioning

* The patient is seated, facing the IR
* The chin is placed in contact with the IR
* The chin position is adjusted until the OMBL has been raised 30°; the head is then rotated through 30°, away from the eye under examination

Beam direction and FRD

Horizontal, at 90° to the IR
100 cm FRD

Centring

Behind and above the mastoid process nearest the X-ray tube, to emerge through the middle of the orbit under examination

Collimation

Bony outline of the orbit under examination

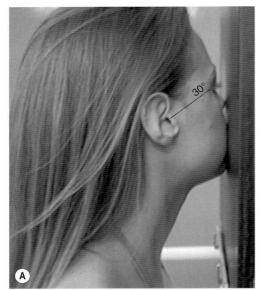

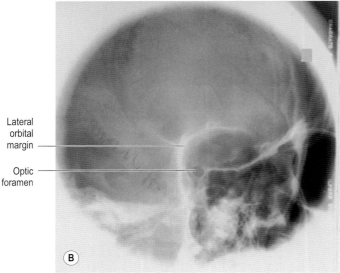

Lateral
orbital
margin

Optic
foramen

Figure 20.9 AO optic foramen.

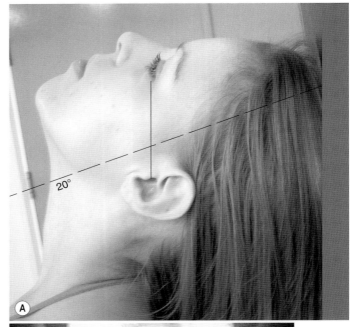

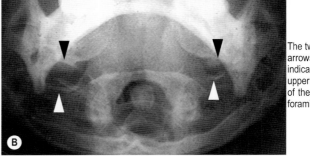

The two black arrows indicate the upper aspect of the jugular foramina

Figure 20.10 (A) SMV jugular foramina; (B) SMV 20° jugular foramina. *(B) Reproduced with permission from Ballinger PW, Frank ED. Merrill's atlas of radiographic positioning and radiologic procedures. 10th ed. St Louis: Mosby; 2003.*

Criteria for assessing image quality

- Outline of orbit is demonstrated in full
- Optic foramen seen as a low-density circle within the orbit, level with its midpoint and nearer the lateral margin of the orbit
- Sharp image demonstrating the low-density foramen in contrast to the bones forming the orbit and the overlying bones of the vault

Common errors	Possible reasons
Lateral orbital margin obscuring part, or all, of the foramen	Head is rotated too far
Inferior orbital margin obscuring part, or all, of the foramen	Chin is raised too far
Foramen appears elliptical and is located nearer to the medial aspect of the orbit than is required	Inadequate rotation
Foramen appears to be cylindrical and is located in the upper half of the orbit	Inadequate raising of the chin

JUGULAR FORAMINA

Submentovertical (SMV) 20° jugular foramina (Fig. 20.10A,B)

IR is vertical; an antiscatter grid is employed

Positioning

- A seat is placed midway between the X-ray tube and the erect bucky; the patient sits on the stool, facing the X-ray tube
- The patient leans back gently onto the radiographer's arm and flexes their neck and back until the vertex of their head can be placed in contact with the bucky

Beam direction and FRD

20° cranially
100 cm FRD
It may be necessary to displace the IR to ensure the area of interest lies within its borders.

Centring

Midway between the angles of the mandible

Collimation

Angles of mandible, symphysis menti, foramen magnum

Criteria for assessing image quality

- Angles of the mandible, symphysis menti and foramen magnum are demonstrated
- Odontoid process of C2 is demonstrated, through the upper half of the foramen magnum
- Mandible is raised clear of the jugular foramina and superimposed as an arch over the petrous temporal bones
- Both jugular foramina are demonstrated symmetrically on either side of the midline, midway between the edge of the foramen magnum and angle of mandible
- Sharp image demonstrating dense bone of the skull base, in contrast with the jugular foramina

Common errors	Possible reasons
Mandible overlying foramina	Chin is not elevated enough
Mandible is clear but foramina not clear	Chin is elevated too much

REFERENCES

1. Swallow RA, et al. Clark's positioning in radiography. 11th ed. London: Heinemann; 1986.

2. Eisenberg R, et al. Radiographic positioning. 2nd ed. Boston: Little, Brown; 1995.

Chapter 21

Dental radiography

Elizabeth Carver

Dental radiography is still a widespread imaging technique required by dentists and oral surgeons in dental surgeries and hospitals. Intraoral techniques in particular are low dose in relation to examinations undertaken elsewhere in the body, but this does not mean that dose should be considered irrelevant in examinations of the teeth and mouth.

DOSE REDUCTION AND RADIATION PROTECTION

As long ago as 1994 in the UK, the National Radiological Protection Board (NRPB) issued guidelines stating that there was no justification for the routine use of lead rubber aprons.[1] In practice, the artefacts caused by incorrect placement of lead rubber aprons during orthopantomography (OPT) were considered to be a common cause of repeat radiographs, thereby doubling the radiation dose received by the patient. At this stage the NRPB also concluded that dental radiography posed no risk to women at any stage during pregnancy; however, as the use of lead rubber does not actually increase the dose to patients, it could be suggested that its use for any intraoral or cephalometry technique may be of 'psychological' benefit to the patient. This may be especially appropriate in the case of the patient who is aware of the risks associated with ionising radiation but who is not reassured by the radiographer's explanation that there is no likelihood of danger when undergoing dental radiographic examinations. Since the 1994 NRPB document there have been key documents issued regarding guidelines and regulations on the use of radiation for medical exposure, each referring less specifically to the use of lead rubber for dental examinations but emphasising the responsibility of the radiographer to reduce the radiation dose wherever possible.[2-4] In view of this, and the previous comments on the 'psychological' benefits to the patient, it may be more appropriate to offer all patients lead rubber aprons for intraoral and cephalometric examinations.

DIFFICULTIES IN PROVIDING ACCURACY OF DENTAL ASSESSMENT

The teeth themselves provide the radiographer with problems of accurate imaging, owing to the nature of their various shapes. This, added to their positions within the alveolar ridges of the maxilla and the mandible, their arched arrangement in the mouth and the varying positions of the teeth in each individual, shows that the implications for accurate representation of dentition are complex.

TERMINOLOGY ASSOCIATED WITH DENTAL RADIOGRAPHY

Dental techniques require an understanding of some terms that are not encountered in radiography of the rest of the body; these are outlined in Table 21.1.

TECHNIQUES USED IN DENTAL RADIOGRAPHY

Intraoral techniques

Bitewings: Demonstrate the crowns and interproximal surfaces of the teeth.
Periapicals: Demonstrate the whole tooth.
Occlusals: Demonstrate a range of structures and aspects of the mouth, including the hard palate, incisors and canines, unerupted canines, confirmation of position of unerupted canines, premolars, submandibular salivary glands and ducts and the symphysis menti.

Table 21.1 Dental terminology

Buccal/labial (Fig. 21.1)	The (outer) aspect of the teeth that lies between the teeth and the cheeks or lips
Lingual/palatal (Fig. 21.1)	The (inner) aspect of the teeth that lies between the teeth and the tongue
Distal (Fig. 21.2)	The direction of the dental arch towards the molars, posteriorly and outwards away from the MSP. Used to describe beam shift, tube shift or angulation
Mesial (Fig. 21.2)	The direction of the dental arch towards the incisors, anteriorly and inwards towards the MSP. Used to describe beam shift, tube shift or angulation and is in the opposite direction to distal movement
Alatragal line (Fig. 21.3)	An imaginary line from the tragus of the ear to the middle of the ala of the nose (the flare of soft tissue around the nostril)
Occlusal plane (upper) (Fig. 21.3)	The line of the biting surfaces of the upper teeth. When the mouth is closed this is deemed to be the occlusal plane rather than the upper occlusal plane. The line lies parallel to the anthropological baseline and the alatragal line. It lies approximately 4 cm below the alatragal line
Occlusal plane (lower)	*With the mouth open*, this line lies parallel to, and approximately 2 cm below the line which lies between the tragus of the ear and the outer canthus of the mouth. Because all radiography of the teeth should be undertaken with the mouth closed around an IR holder or occlusal film, this plane is not actually used in this text and is therefore not illustrated
Medial sagittal plane (MSP) (Fig. 21.4)	Plane running vertically down the middle of the face, separating the left and right sides

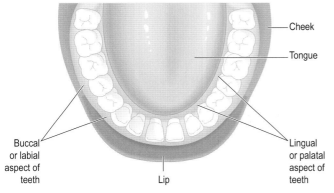

Figure 21.1 Buccal/labial, lingual/palatal aspects of the teeth.

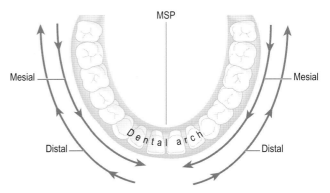

Figure 21.2 Distal and mesial.

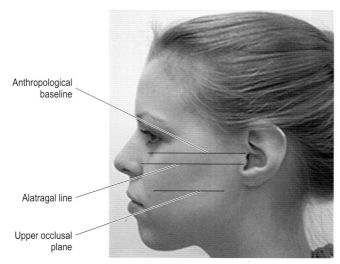

Figure 21.3 Reference lines used in dental radiography.

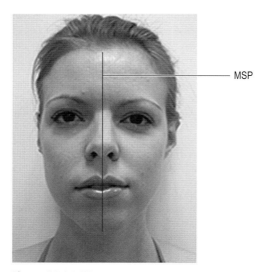

Figure 21.4 MSP.

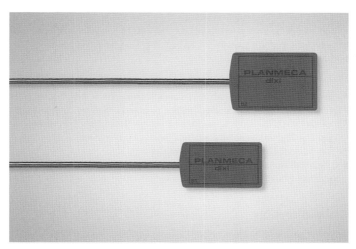

Figure 21.5 Digital dental image receptors.
Reproduced with permission from Xograph Imaging Systems.

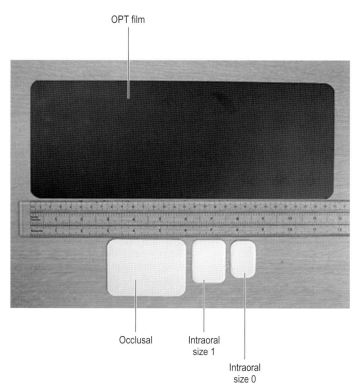

Figure 21.6 Dental film sizes.

Extraoral techniques

Orthopantomography (OPT or OPG)/dental panoramic tomography (DPT): Demonstrates the whole mouth, including dentition, mandible, maxillary sinuses and temporomandibular (TMJ) joints. This technique is covered in Chapter 22.
Lateral cephalometry: Mainly used to assess the extent of malocclusions and facial deformities prior to and post surgery. This technique is covered in Chapter 22.

RECORDING AND DISPLAYING THE IMAGE

Since the first edition of this book there has been an increase in use of digital imaging for dental examinations, but there still exists a proportion of film-based radiography in dental units; this is likely to continue to decrease as dental surgeries replace ageing equipment. It is therefore still necessary to give direction on the use of film and display of film images.

Digital dental units use small image receptors (IRs) which are connected to the digital unit (Fig. 21.5) and these are similar in size to films used in dental radiography.

Receptor sizes (Fig. 21.6)

A range of film/receptor sizes are available: *size 0* is the smallest and is used in periapical examinations for children and adults with small mouths. *Size 1* is also used in periapical examinations, usually for adults, and also for parallax technique. *Occlusal* receptors are larger than size 0 and 1, as they are designed to cover a larger area of dentition. Intraoral techniques do not use a film/screen system as the area under examination is of low density and exposure factors used are relatively low, so that intensifying screens are not necessary even in the non-digitised situation.

Cassettes and film used in OPT are usually of a specific size designed solely for this examination, approximately 14–15 × 30 cm. They are used in conjunction with intensifying screens used, as the area under examination is significantly denser than individual teeth. Lateral cephalometry film is 18 × 24 cm or similar. Digital units for both OPT and cephalometry incorporate the IR into the X-ray unit.

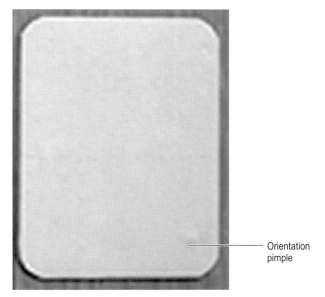

Figure 21.7 Orientation pimple.

Receptor orientation

A consistent method must be used to orientate the film in the mouth, since it is impossible to tell whether teeth are from the left or right side, from the mandible or the maxilla. The most familiar method was to use the orientation 'pimple' when using film; this is a tiny but palpable raised lump on the tube side of the film (Fig. 21.7). The pimple is always positioned towards the crowns of the teeth in periapical and occlusal examinations. For bitewings the pimple is usually orientated towards the roots of the upper teeth. Digital IRs are always used with the lead leaving the edge of the receptor, which is outside the mouth, and identification must be annotated onto the resulting image at the postprocessing stage.

Displaying film images

Films are usually mounted with patient and tooth/projection identification in clear holders or stapled to clear film or translucent mounting medium. The 'pimple' must face outwards, towards the viewing radiographer. Left and right teeth are also clearly indicated. Before the widespread use of OPT for whole-mouth examinations, whole-mouth periapical images were displayed in the format of the mouth itself.[5]

Intraoral techniques: bitewings

These demonstrate the crowns, interproximal surfaces and gingival margins of the premolars and molars. Bitewing film is available, which is a small dental film with a centralised flap of paper on the tube side of the film. Film/IR size is equivalent to size 1. The patient's teeth bite on the flap in order to immobilise and maintain position (Fig. 21.8A).

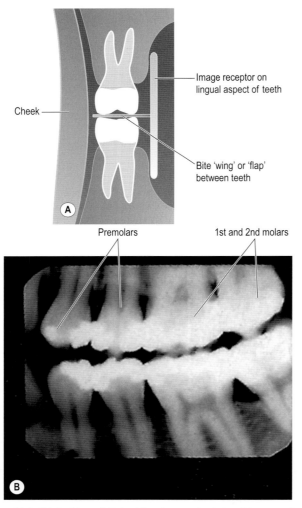

Figure 21.8 (A) Position of IR for bitewings and relationship to teeth; (B) bitewing image.
(B) Reproduced with permission from Whaites E. Essentials of dental radiography and radiology. 3rd ed. Edinburgh: Churchill Livingstone; 2002.

Bitewing holders are also available: these are a disposable device into which the film is inserted; a plastic flap at 90° to the film is placed between the patient's teeth.

Positioning

- The patient is seated with their neck leaning on a support
- A bitewing film or bitewing holder is placed with its tube side in contact with the lingual surface of the teeth under examination and the flap between the occlusal surfaces of the teeth
- The patient closes their teeth over the flap
- The median sagittal plane (MSP) is vertical and the upper occlusal plane horizontal

Beam direction

Initially horizontal, then angled 5° caudally

Centring

To the middle of the IR, over the occlusal plane

Include

Crowns of the teeth under examination and alveolar crests

Criteria for assessing image quality

- Crowns of the teeth and alveolar crests are demonstrated
- No evidence of elongation or foreshortening of teeth
- No overlap of adjacent teeth
- Slight separation of occlusal surfaces of teeth
- Sharp image demonstrating enamel in contrast with pulp cavity and the alveolar crests

Common errors	Possible reasons
Foreshortening of the teeth	Poor beam selection or the IR has slipped away from the lingual surface of the teeth
Overlap of the crowns at their interproximal surfaces	Beam not at 90° in the mesiodistal direction

Intraoral techniques: periapicals

Periapical examinations are generally used to demonstrate individual or small groups of teeth. Before the introduction of OPT/OPG or DPT the whole of the mouth was examined in this way, with images mounted to represent the layout of the dentition.[5] OPT examination has almost exclusively superseded this approach.

As already mentioned in the introduction to this section, the structure and position of teeth cause problems for the radiographer when attempting to provide high-quality images of the area. Ideally the radiographer places any body part so that its long axis is parallel to the IR and the X-ray beam is 90° to the body part and the IR.

More specifically, the most significant problems can be identified as:

1. The teeth are surrounded at their neck and root by the bones of the maxilla or mandible, which are themselves surrounded by the gum. This reduces the proportion of the tooth that can

be placed in close contact with the IR. When added to the arched construction of the hard palate, positioning of the IR parallel to the tooth becomes problematic. The teeth themselves are arranged in a variation of angles in the mouth, the incisors being at a much greater angle than the molars.

2. The size of the patient's mouth will affect the possibility of positioning the IR, since a narrow dental arch may not accommodate the IR.

3. Overlapping teeth when the dentition is overcrowded will mean that it is impossible to provide images of some teeth without some superimposition.

Two techniques are available for periapicals: *bisecting angle* and *paralleling*. Each aims to reduce the effects of the obliquity of the teeth and the problems outlined in the introduction to this section. There are advantages and disadvantages associated with each method, which will be discussed after descriptions of the techniques.

Periapicals: bisecting angle technique

It is already acknowledged that an angle will be made between the long axis of the IR and the long axis of a tooth if the IR is placed on the labial aspect of the tooth and gum surrounding the root. Rather than directing the beam at 90° to either the tooth or the IR, for this technique the beam is aimed 90° to the bisector of the angle made by the tooth and IR – in other words, a compromise is reached (Fig. 21.9).

For this method, the angle of the individual patient's teeth must be estimated before commencing the examination. Although texts and dental radiography units list suggested beam angulation for this technique,[5,6] human dentition varies widely and each patient must be assessed individually. Visual examination of the dentition in a mesio-distal direction will give the radiographer an idea of beam direction in order to ensure that it will pass through the teeth at 90° and avoid overlap of the crowns at their interproximal surfaces. When assessing the angle of the long axis of the tooth in premolars, the centre of the crown must be assessed rather than the longest (labially positioned)

cusp, which is usually curved and does not give an accurate indication of the tooth as a whole.

If film is used, a size 0 or 1 dental film is selected for this examination. The film should always be used with the 'pimple' facing outwards towards the X-ray tube and orientated towards the crowns of the teeth under examination. When film is used, a bisecting angle holder (Figs 21.10, 21.11, 21.12A) must always be used, as using the patient's finger for support is not acceptable.

Positioning

- The patient is seated with their neck supported
- The IR has its tube side in contact with the lingual aspect of the crowns of the teeth. The IR is vertically aligned for incisors and canines and transversely for premolars and molars
- The tooth under examination is centred to the IR, or the midpoint of the range of teeth intended for inclusion is centralised
- The patient closes their teeth over the holder for incisors and canines, and closes their lips over the holder for the other teeth, to immobilise the IR and maintain its position
- The head is adjusted until the MSP is vertical and the occlusal plane is horizontal

Beam direction

Initially horizontal, then adjusted until at 90° to the bisector of the angle formed between the long axis of the tooth and the long axis of the IR *and* 90° to the IR mesiodistally

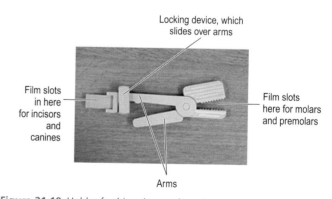

Figure 21.10 Holder for bisecting angle technique.

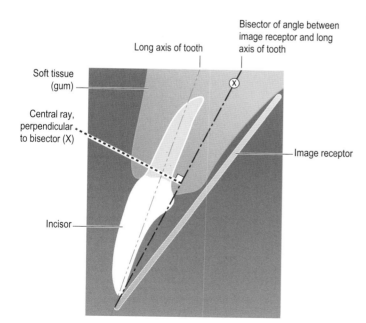

Figure 21.9 The bisecting angle.

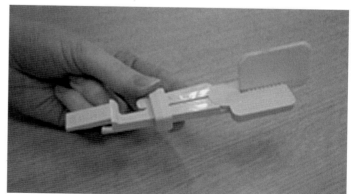

Figure 21.11 Bisecting angle holder – film in holder for molars and premolars.

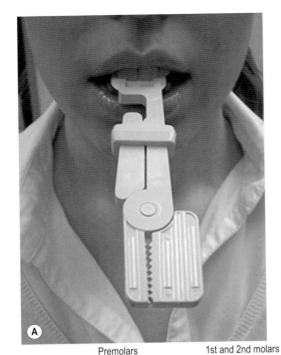

Premolars 1st and 2nd molars

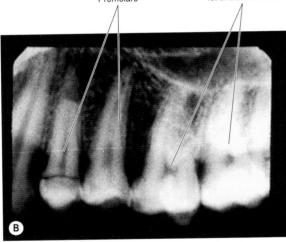

Figure 21.12 (A) Bisecting angle holder – film in position for incisors; (B) bisecting angle periapical.
(B) Reproduced with permission from Whaites E. Essentials of dental radiography and radiology. 3rd ed. Edinburgh: Churchill Livingstone; 2002.

Centring

Over the buccal surfaces of the teeth, to the centre of the film

A guide for *approximate* angles for 'normally positioned' teeth is given in Table 21.2.

Collimation

Crowns and roots of the teeth under examination, surrounding bone

Table 21.2 Suggested approximate angulations for bisecting angle periapical technique (the alatragal line must be horizontal for use with these angles)

Upper teeth		Lower teeth	
Incisors	55–60° caudal angle	Incisors	25–30° cranial angle
Canines	45–50° caudal angle	Canines	15–20° cranial angle
Premolars	35–40° caudal angle	Premolars	10° cranial angle
Molars	25–30° caudal angle	Molars	Horizontal beam

Criteria for assessing image quality

- Crowns, roots of the teeth and surrounding bone are demonstrated
- Minimal evidence of elongation or foreshortening* of tooth/ teeth, or overlap of adjacent teeth *if there is no overcrowding of teeth in that region*
- Sharp image showing contrast of the alveolar bone and its trabeculae, pulp cavity and enamel of the tooth/teeth

*Ideally there would be no evidence of foreshortening or elongation, but as there will always be some evidence of this owing to the arrangement of the teeth and gums, their exclusion cannot be expected.

Common errors	Possible reasons
Foreshortening of teeth; cusps of premolars and molars seen en face and crown appears 'squat'	Beam not at 90° to the bisecting angle in the craniocaudal direction
Overlap of crowns at their interproximal surfaces	Beam not at 90° in the mesiodistal direction *unless* there is actual overlap of teeth in the mouth

Periapicals: paralleling technique

(Figs 21.13, 21.14, 21.15, 21.16, 21.17A)

This technique also attempts to tackle the problems associated with producing accurate images of the teeth in this difficult body area. It also makes use of holders that maintain the position of the IR parallel to the long axis of the tooth and enable accurate selection of the central ray at 90° to the IR.

Positioning

- The patient is seated with their neck supported
- The IR is placed in a paralleling holder, longitudinally for incisors and canines, transversely for premolars and molars (Figs 21.13, 21.14)
- The holder is placed in the mouth with the tube side of the IR facing the lingual surface of the teeth
- The IR is parallel to the long axes of the teeth under examination but is distant from the surface of the teeth; this may appear to be a significant distance to the radiographer, being toward the soft palate for incisors and into the opposite half of the mouth for premolars and molars
- The tooth under examination is centred to the IR, or the midpoint of the range of teeth intended for inclusion is centralised
- The patient closes their mouth over the holder to immobilise the IR and maintain its position (Figs 21.15, 21.16)

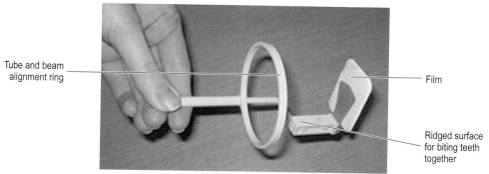

Figure 21.13 Paralleling technique holder – film (incisors and canines).

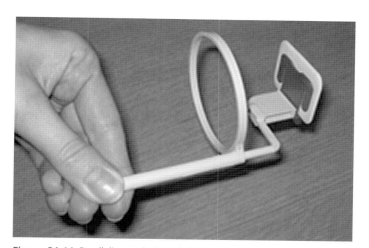

Figure 21.14 Paralleling technique holder – film (molars and premolars).

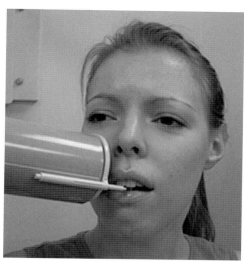

Figure 21.16 Tube aligned with paralleling holder.

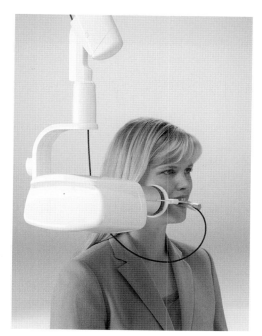

Figure 21.15 Paralleling technique – digital receptor.
Reproduced with permission from Xograph Imaging Systems.

Beam direction and centring

The beam is aligned to the centre of the indicator on the paralleling holder, in the direction indicated by the holder

Collimation

Crowns and roots of the teeth under examination, surrounding bone

Criteria for assessing image quality

This is as for the bisecting angle technique; the teeth will appear slightly larger than with the bisecting angle technique but will be less distorted

Which to use, bisecting angle or paralleling technique?

The two periapical techniques described each have advantages and disadvantages. These are briefly outlined in Table 21.3, which is intended to provide a résumé of the points that should be considered by the radiographer before selecting a suitable method. However, as these points for consideration may be likely to lead to an equivocal

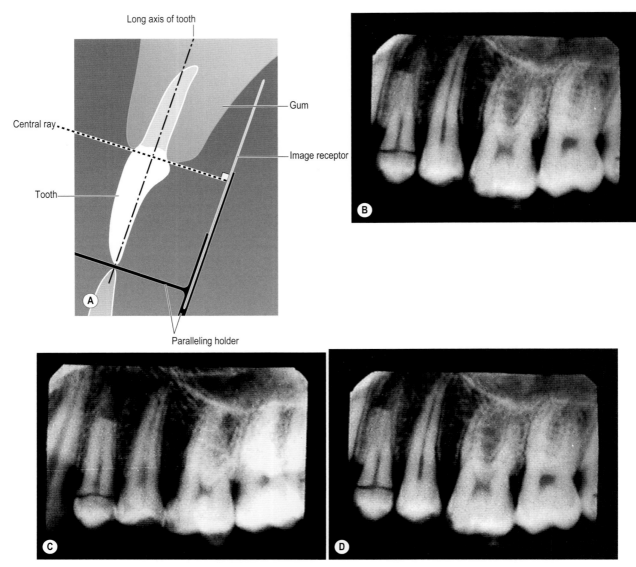

Long axis of tooth

Central ray

Tooth

Gum

Image receptor

Paralleling holder

Figure 21.17 (A) Position of IR for paralleling technique; (B) paralleling periapical. Comparison of bisecting angle and paralleling technique on periapical images: (C) bisecting angle technique, (D) paralleling technique.
(B), (C) and (D) Reproduced with permission from Whaites E. Essentials of dental radiography and radiology. 3rd ed. Edinburgh: Churchill Livingstone; 2002.

opinion, the final decision may be based solely on the availability of equipment, familiarity with one technique or preference for a particular type of film holder. Some digital units may not provide equipment that offers a choice.

Occlusals

As identified at the start of this chapter, occlusals have many uses, which are more specifically identified in Table 21.4.

There is one basic patient position used for most occlusals and this is described first, followed by the modification in position for the only exception, the submental occlusal. Relevant tube displacements and angulations are listed after the description of the basic position, alongside the area demonstrated for each (Table 21.5).

IR suitable for occlusals is selected for all these examinations.

Positioning (basic head position)

- The patient is seated with their neck leaning on a support
- The IR is in the mouth, tube side upwards for maxillary teeth and down for mandibular teeth
- The IR is pushed back as far as possible, at least to the first molars and to include the incisors
- The midline of the IR is coincident with the MSP
- The teeth are closed over the IR and the MSP is vertical
- The *occlusal plane is horizontal* for most examinations
- *Submental occlusal* (for submandibular ducts) requires extension of the neck as far as possible to bring the occlusal plane towards the vertical. The head and neck are supported in this position
- The basic position is shown in Figures 21.18A, 21.19A, 21.20A, 21.21A

Table 21.3 Advantages and disadvantages of periapical techniques – a comparison of Figs 21.9 and 21.17C,D will help illustrate these points

Bisecting angle	Paralleling
Object–receptor distance (ORD) varies along the length of the teeth, as the IR becomes more remote from crown to root; however, at no point is it as distant from the tooth as in paralleling technique. Magnification (and therefore unsharpness) increases towards the root	Relatively long ORD along the entire length of the tooth has implications for magnification and unsharpness. Also, large teeth may not fit within the periphery of the IR
Some image distortion as beam is not perpendicular to any structure	Minimum image distortion as the receptor is always parallel to the long axis of the tooth and the beam perpendicular to the IR
Selection of angle is less likely to be as accurate as for paralleling technique, since it requires estimation of the bisecting angle. Centring may also be less accurate	Use of the alignment and centring indicator on the paralleling holder ensures accuracy of beam centring and angulation
Holders are relatively small compared to the paralleling holders	Holders are more bulky for patients; however, their use is more widespread than bisecting angle holders and radiographers may prefer their use due to familiarity with the technique and equipment

Table 21.4 Occlusal projections

Projection	Demonstrates
70° maxillary occlusal (also known as standard anterior oblique maxilla)	Upper incisors, canines, hard palate
Oblique maxillary occlusal (also known as posterior oblique lateral maxilla)	Unerupted upper canines, upper premolars
Oblique mandibular occlusal (also known as posterior true mandible)	Unerupted lower canines, lower premolars
45° submandibular occlusal (also known as anterior oblique mandible)	Lower incisors, symphysis menti of mandible
Submental occlusal (also known as anterior true mandible)	Lower incisors, submandibular and sublingual ducts

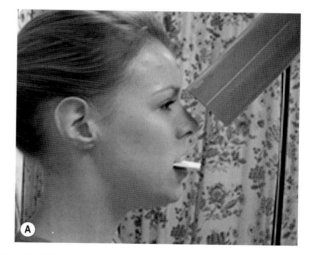

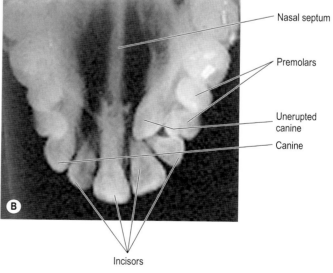

Figure 21.18 70° maxillary occlusal.

General comment on errors

Errors most commonly occur when the occlusal plane is not maintained in the correct relationship to the beam, or when the IR slips from the position prepared by the radiographer. For this reason it must be emphasised that initial patient preparation must include an explanation of the procedure to follow, reinforced by stressing the importance of immobilisation. The radiographer should also express understanding that the procedure may be uncomfortable for a short time.

Table 21.5 Beam direction and centring for occlusals

Area under examination	Projection identification	Beam direction and centring
Upper incisors, canines, hard palate	70° maxillary occlusal (Fig. 21.18A,B)	*Beam direction* 1. Initially vertical central ray; the tube head is in front of the patient's face, coincident with the MSP 2. The tube is then angled 20° towards the face, making a 20° angle with the IR *Centring* Over the nasal bone in the midline, to emerge over the middle of the IR
Unerupted upper canines, upper premolars	Oblique maxillary occlusal (Fig. 21.19A,B)	*Beam direction* 1. Initially a horizontal central ray; the tube head is at the side of the head under examination, next to the eye and perpendicular to the MSP 2. The tube is angled 65° caudally, and then angled distally 45° until at 45° to the MSP *Centring* Over the edge of the ala of the nose on the side under examination, to emerge over the middle of the IR
Unerupted lower canines, lower premolars	Oblique mandibular occlusal (Fig. 21.20A,B)	*Beam direction* 1. Initially a horizontal central ray; the tube head is at the side of the head under examination, next to the corner of the mouth and perpendicular to the MSP 2. The tube is angled 45° cranially, and then angled distally 45° until at 45° to the MSP *Centring* Under the inferior aspect of the mandible below the corner of the mouth, to emerge over the middle of the IR
Lower incisors, symphysis menti of mandible	45° submandibular occlusal (Fig. 21.21A,B)	*Beam direction* 1. Initially a horizontal central ray; the tube head is in front of the patient's face, coincident with the MSP 2. The tube is then angled 45° cranially *Centring* Under the symphysis menti, to emerge over the middle of the IR
Lower incisors, submandibular ducts	Submental occlusal (Fig. 21.22A,B)	*Beam direction* Initially horizontal, central ray is angled cranially until 90° to the occlusal plane *Centring* Under the symphysis menti to emerge over the middle of the IR

Criteria for assessing image quality – occlusals

70° maxillary occlusal	Anterior arch of the maxillary teeth back to the first molars are demonstrated. Incisors and canines are foreshortened; premolars and molars are demonstrated axially. Symmetry of the maxillary arch
Oblique maxillary occlusal	Full length of incisors, canines and premolars including alveolar bone surrounding roots is demonstrated (on the side under examination). Incisors, canines and premolars are elongated (on the side under examination). Dental arch on the side under examination appears flattened. Superimposition of teeth on the side that is not under examination
Oblique mandibular occlusal	Canines and premolars of the side under examination are demonstrated. Mandibular arch on the side under examination appears flattened. Superimposition of teeth on the side that is not under examination
45° submandibular occlusal	Symphysis menti and mandibular arch back to first molars are demonstrated. Foreshortening of lower incisors. Superimposition of the teeth over the mandible
All projections except submental occlusal	Sharp image demonstrating detail of the teeth under examination and their roots, in contrast to alveolar bone, pulp cavity and enamel
Submental occlusal	Mandibular arch from incisors to first molars is demonstrated. Mandibular arch is demonstrated axially (i.e. from below); incisors and canines are foreshortened. Medial aspect of distal premolars overlying lingual aspect of the mandible. Sharp image demonstrating the soft tissues of the floor of the mouth in contrast with the mandible

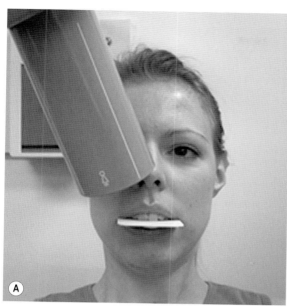

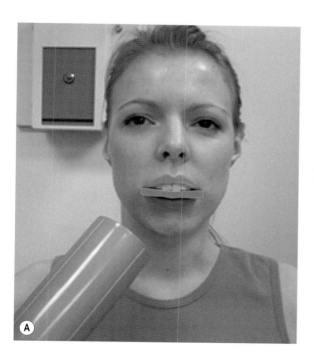

Maxillary sinus

Incisors

Canine

Molars   Premolars

Figure 21.19 Oblique maxillary occlusal.

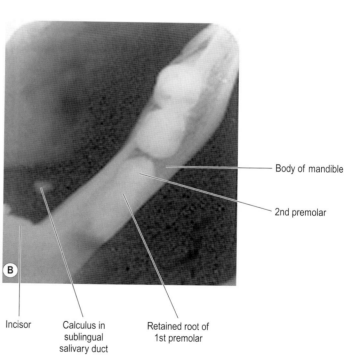

Body of mandible

2nd premolar

Incisor   Calculus in   Retained root of
           sublingual   1st premolar
           salivary duct

Figure 21.20 Oblique mandibular occlusal.

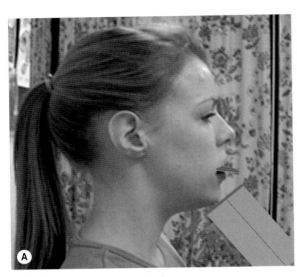

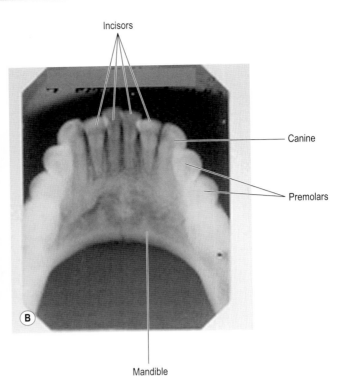

Figure 21.21 45° submandibular occlusal.

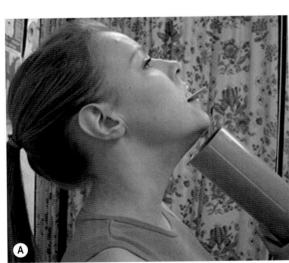

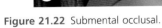

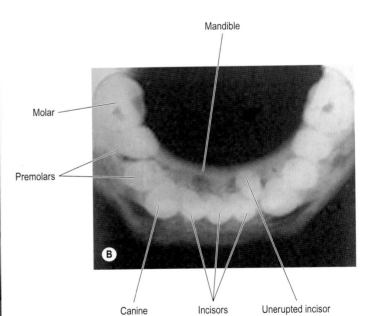

Figure 21.22 Submental occlusal.

LOCATION OF POSITION OF UNERUPTED CANINES ('PARALLAX' PROJECTION)

It is sometimes necessary to produce images that provide information in addition to that provided by occlusal projections. Specifically, these may be required to help identify the position of an unerupted canine in relation to other anteriorly placed teeth in an anterior or posterior direction. The method is only recommended for the area from the incisors to the first premolars.

An initial orthopantomograph may initially be required to show the orientation of the unerupted tooth, as they can sometimes be found lying horizontally and high within the maxilla. The principle of so-called parallax projections is to take two intraoral images, using tube shift (angulation) between the two images, to provide slightly varying images which allow the position of the unerupted tooth to be assessed. An occlusal or periapical approach can be used and, although periapical images are likely to be easier to interpret, occlusals will prove beneficial in demonstrating the high, horizontally positioned canine.

Once tooth orientation has been ascertained, the next stage of the examination is based on two separate bisecting angle or occlusal examinations.

Bisecting angle approach for parallax

The first examination uses a basic bisecting angle technique and the second employs bisecting angle technique plus tube shift to project the more anteriorly placed teeth (or tooth) laterally compared to the initial image (Fig 21.23). In other words, a labially positioned unerupted canine will move further in the direction of angle (towards the MSP) than the erupted teeth on the second image; a palatally positioned unerupted canine will appear to shift away from the direction of angle (away from the MSP).

Positioning

- The patient is seated with their neck supported
- The IR has its tube side in contact with the lingual aspect of the crowns of the teeth. The IR is vertically aligned for incisors and canines and transversely for premolars and molars
- The tooth under examination is centred to the IR, or the midpoint of the range of teeth intended for inclusion is centralised
- The patient closes their mouth over the holder to immobilise the IR and maintain its position
- The head is adjusted until the MSP is vertical and the occlusal plane is horizontal

Beam direction and FFD

First image: initially horizontal, which is then adjusted until at 90° to the bisector of the angle formed between the long axis of the tooth and the long axis of the IR
Second image: from the angle and direction selected for the first image, the tube is shifted 25–30° in a distal direction (to form a mesially directed angle of 25–30° to the beam used for the first image)

Centring

Over the buccal surfaces of the teeth to the centre of the receptor; for the second image, the IR is displaced slightly in a mesial direction to ensure its centre is coincident with the central ray

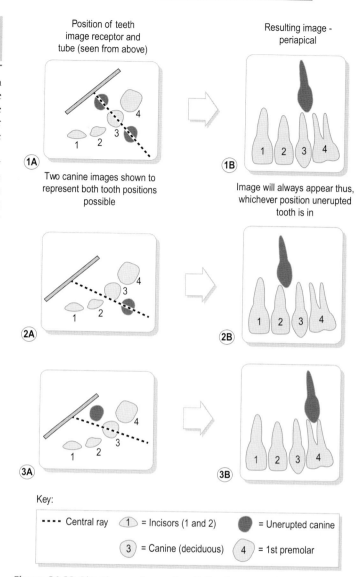

Position of teeth image receptor and tube (seen from above)

Resulting image - periapical

Two canine images shown to represent both tooth positions possible

Image will always appear thus, whichever position unerupted tooth is in

Key:

---- Central ray   1 = Incisors (1 and 2)   ● = Unerupted canine

3 = Canine (deciduous)   4 = 1st premolar

Figure 21.23 Bisecting angle parallax. Shift of unerupted canine related to its position: the left hand column (A) shows position of teeth, IR and tube (seen from above); the right hand column (B) shows the resulting periapical image. (*1A*) shows the (left) teeth from above, with unerupted canines anteriorly or posteriorly positioned (either way will give the periapical appearance seen in (*1B*). An erupted canine tooth is included in this illustration and this would be a deciduous tooth; however, a deciduous canine tooth may not be present in all cases. (*2A*) shows the teeth from above, with an anteriorly positioned unerupted canine. The beam angulation created by tube shift will move this unerupted tooth further mesially (as in image *2B*) than the erupted canine, making it appear nearer to the second incisor than on the original periapical seen in (*1A*). (*3A*) shows the teeth from above, with a posteriorly positioned unerupted canine. The beam angulation created by tube shift will move the erupted teeth further mesially (as in *3B*) than the unerupted canine, making the unerupted canine appear nearer to the first premolar than on the original periapical seen in (*1A*).

The main purpose of the two exposure tube shift/angulation technique is to use geometric principles in order to ascertain the position of the unerupted tooth. This applies to both periapical and occlusal approaches.

Occlusal technique for parallax

If the occlusal method is used, tube shift is undertaken on the second exposure, as in the periapical method. The occlusal approach may be advisable if the unerupted tooth has a horizontal orientation and lies high in relation to the erupted teeth, and some authors recommend only this method for position location.[7] The tube movement can be either horizontal (distal tube head movement to form a mesial angle) or vertical (creating a more caudal angle) in relation to the first exposure.[7]

If horizontal tube shift is used a labially positioned unerupted canine will move further in the direction of angle (towards the midline) than the erupted teeth on the second image; a palatally positioned unerupted canine will appear to shift away from the direction of angle (away from the midline). If a vertical tube shift is used for the second exposure, a labially positioned unerupted canine will appear to shift down over or towards the erupted teeth, and a palatally positioned unerupted canine will show the erupted tooth to fall even lower compared to their position on the first image (opening up any space between them and the unerupted tooth above).

Identification of images and location of position of the unerupted tooth

Although it is essential that procedures for correct identification and image orientation are followed for all dental and other imaging procedures, parallax images need special attention to detail. It is vital that each image produced for the parallax examination is identified as to whether it is the initial image or the second image with tube shift. Only with accurate identification can the position of the unerupted tooth be assessed. Images should be displayed side by side in order to assess the relative positions of the teeth.

REFERENCES

1. Royal College of Radiologists NRPB. Guidelines on radiology standards for primary dental care. Documents of the NRPB 5; 3 Didcot: NRPB; 1994.

2. European Commission. European Guidelines on Quality Criteria for Diagnostic Radiographic Images. Office for Official Publications of the European Communities. Brussels: 1996.

3. Statutory Instrument 1999 No. 3232. The Ionising Radiations Regulations 1999. London: HMSO; 1999.

4. The Ionising Radiation (Medical Exposure) Regulations 2006. London: HMSO; 2006.

5. Swallow RA, et al. Clark's positioning in radiography. 12th ed. Oxford: Hodder Arnold; 2005.

6. Unett EM, Royle AJ. Radiographic techniques and image evaluation. London: Chapman and Hall; 1997.

7. Whaites E. Essentials of dental radiography and radiology. 3rd ed. Edinburgh: Churchill Livingstone; 2002.

Chapter | 22 |

Orthopantomography and cephalometry

Elizabeth Carver

ORTHOPANTOMOGRAPHY (OPT OR OPG) OR DENTAL PANORAMIC TOMOGRAPHY (DPT)

This technique requires the use of a specialised OPT unit (Fig. 22.1A,B), the tomographic principle being that which is used to produce the image of the full mouth and its dentition. The moving tube effectively blurs out the shadow of overlying structures by placing the dental arch in the axis of the tomographic movement. Structures not lying within this axis are effectively blurred, and so their detail does not overlie the image of the teeth and mandible. However, the area of interest does show some element of unsharpness compared to radiographic images of other body parts when a non-moving tube is used.

The technique opens out the image of the dental arch to appear in a linear arrangement on the final image. It has long been employed in the dental setting and has largely replaced full mouth periapical examinations. As mentioned in Chapter 18, the OPT examination can be used to demonstrate the temporomandibular joints and mandible.

The tomographic movement of the unit attempts to follow the dental arch, which it keeps within the tomographic axis of the beam as it travels around the patient's face. Because of this, accurate positioning aims to place the dental arch within this axis and horizontally to follow the plane of tube movement. Positioning also aims to keep unwanted structures such as the cervical vertebrae clear from the tomographic axis.

Some tomographic units use a system of slit light beams that are aligned with the incisors, median sagittal plane (MSP), anthropological baseline or alatragal line. Lights are also used to assess the patient's position in an anteroposterior (AP) direction; these vertical slit beams are seen as superimposed when the patient is in the optimum plane but are separated if the patient is too far forward or not forward enough. Since all these light arrangements are used in varying ways for each manufacturer, it is difficult to describe the use of each different system. Suffice to say, use of these light systems will ensure that the patient is actually in the position as described in the positioning section below. It can often be difficult to align the baselines with the

lights on the OPT unit once they are switched on. Visually assessing the baselines *before* switching the lights on often helps, and the radiographer uses the lights to check height and positioning accuracy afterwards.

The X-ray beam leaves the tube housing via a slit collimator and the thin beam moves around the dental arch and across the image receptor (IR); this arrangement reduces the inevitable penumbra that would be caused by a wider beam. However, some penumbral effect is unavoidable.

The tomographic movement travels around the head with a horizontal beam, in opposition to traditional tomographic units that move over the supine patient and use a beam which is initially vertical and moves longitudinally or in a circular, elliptical or helical course.

Owing to the nature of this horizontal movement the use of the OPT unit may be distracting for the patient during exposure. Advance preparation must include demonstration of tube movement for the patient, using the 'test' setting. The unit is then returned to the start position.

If used, an OPT cassette is inserted into the erect cassette holder on the unit. Digital equipment incorporates the receptor into the unit and OPT/DPT is selected on the unit.

Positioning (Fig. 22.2)

- A disposable bite rod is inserted into the chin rest, or a disposable plastic cover is applied to the permanent bite rod
- The patient is seated or standing with their chin resting on the chin support and in the correct position to facilitate the dental arch being placed in the correct tomographic plane (with the anthropological baseline and alatragal line horizontal and the head far enough forward, often indicated by slit light indicators as designed by the manufacturer)
- The patient bites with their incisors in the groove on the bite rod, to effect separation of teeth on the image
- The MSP is vertical and perpendicular to the bite rod. The height of the unit is adjusted until the occlusal plane is horizontal (assessed by checking that the alatragal line or anthropological baseline are horizontal)

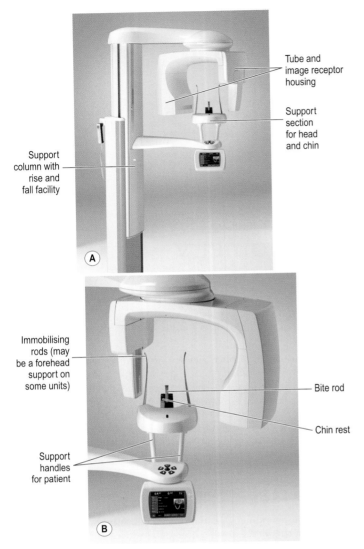

Figure 22.1 OPT unit.
Reproduced with permission from Xograph Imaging Systems.

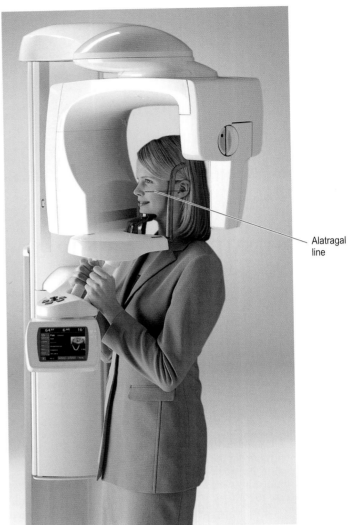

Figure 22.2 Patient positioned in OPT unit. The patient's MSP is vertical and there must be no rotation. The alatragal line is horizontal, as indicated by the black line on the model. Note how the patient has stepped forward to bring the cervical vertebrae into the correct position. *Reproduced with permission from Xograph Imaging Systems.*

- The patient holds onto the support handles and is asked to step forward slightly to bring the cervical spine vertical. If seated, their chair is pulled forward by the radiographer. Throughout this manoeuvre the head must not tilt or rotate and the chin must not lift or drop
- The head clamp is applied for immobilisation
- The patient is asked to close their lips and press their tongue forwards against the teeth and the roof of the mouth for the duration of the exposure
- Exposure is made after a reminder to the patient to keep still during tube movement

Criteria for assessing image quality (Fig. 22.3)

- All of the mandible, including symphysis menti inferiorly and condyles superiorly, is demonstrated. The hard palate and lower part of the maxillary sinuses are demonstrated
- Dentition is demonstrated in a horizontal line
- Bite rod is shown between upper and lower central incisors with separation of occlusal surfaces of all teeth

- All teeth are seen relatively sharply
- Slightly blurred shadow of the anterior aspect of the neck structures is superimposed over images of the incisors; sharper image of bodies of the cervical vertebrae seen at both lateral edges of the image, cleared from the area of interest
- Mandible outline is continuous and not 'stepped'

Common errors	Possible reasons
Step appears in the image, particularly noticeable over the mandibular outline	Patient may have moved chin during exposure
Part of the image is blurred whereas the rest appears sharp	Patient movement at some point during exposure, but not throughout exposure

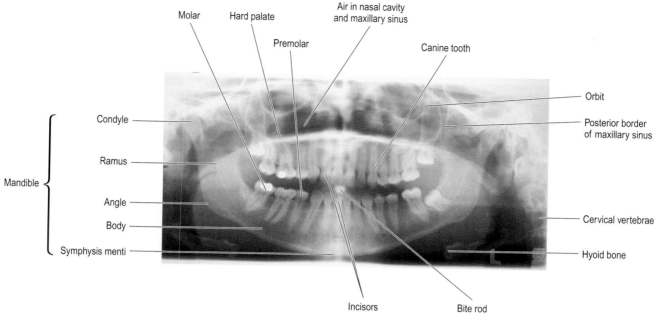

Figure 22.3 OPT/DPT image.

Dentition layout not seen as horizontal, mouth appears to smile; mandibular incisors may be blurred and slightly magnified	Occlusal plane not horizontal; chin is lowered slightly
Dentition layout not seen as horizontal, mouth appears upturned (sulking); maxillary incisors may be slightly blurred and magnified	Occlusal plane not horizontal; chin is raised slightly
Dentition layout not seen as horizontal, appears tilted. Unsharp posterior teeth	MSP not vertical
Middle section of the mandible not seen sharply, outer sections appear more sharp. Unsharp posterior teeth	MSP rotated
Very narrow incisors; cervical vertebrae may be seen centrally	Patient's chin too far forward into the unit
Broad, unsharp incisors; these are sometimes likened to 'piano keys'	Patient's chin not far enough into the unit
Sharper image of cervical vertebrae superimposed over the incisors (some OPT units may produce some cervical shadowing as normal)	Patient's head too far forward in the unit and the cervical vertebrae are further towards the panoramic axis. Patient may not have stepped forward to reduce the cervical curve; the middle vertebrae may protrude into the axis[1]
Dark band seen across the roots and upper aspect of crowns of upper teeth	Tongue not depressed against roof of mouth during exposure; lips may not be closed

CEPHALOMETRY

Prior to maxillofacial surgery and orthodontic treatment it is usually necessary to examine the relationship of the soft tissues of the face to facial bones and teeth. After treatment further assessment is made and it is therefore essential that all images in the series are comparable. To ensure that this is the case, specialised equipment is used to produce consistent images.

The unit can be independent or form part of a unit which has dual function for OPT and lateral cephalometric applications; Fig. 22.1 shows a unit which incorporates the cephalometry function into an OPT unit, and Figure 22.4 focuses on the cephalometry section of that unit. In any case the cephalometry part of the unit usually includes:

1. Fixed focus receptor distance (FRD) (minimum 150 cm to minimise magnification and geometric unsharpness). If the object film distance (OFD) can be altered in a unit, the distance of the median sagittal plane (MSP) from the IR must be registered to allow accurate assessment; measurement facility may be found on the nasion support (see point 3, below).
2. Head clamps with ear plugs. These are inserted into the external auditory meati (EAMs) to ensure accurate and consistent positioning.
3. Nasion support, which slides in an anteroposterior (AP) direction in relation to the patient. This ensures that different sized heads can be immobilised in the unit. They also slide along a measured scale, and measurements from this scale are used in units with automatic filter positioning, to ensure that the filter lies in a position that is accurate for each patient.
4. A filter which is used to compensate for the range in density from facial soft tissue to facial bones. This filter can be permanently situated in the tube head (both free-standing and OPT units) or, in older equipment, an aluminium wedge is attached to the light beam diaphragm. The latest equipment uses a digital IR.

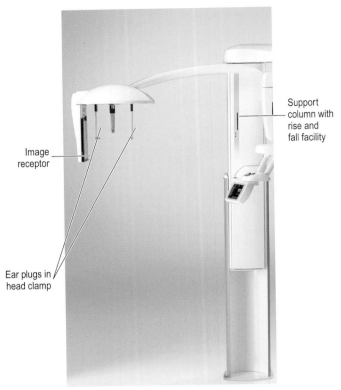

Figure 22.4 Cephalometry unit.
Reproduced with permission from Xograph Imaging Systems.

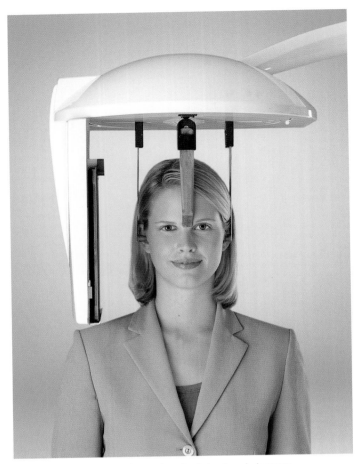

Figure 22.5 Positioning the patient for lateral cephalometry.

If used, a 24 × 30 cm cassette is placed longitudinally in the erect cassette holder on the unit. For digital units, the cephalometry option is selected on the unit.

Positioning (Fig. 22.5, Fig. 22.6)

- The patient is erect with their MSP parallel to the cassette
- The height of the unit is adjusted until the earplugs can be placed in the EAMs
- The occlusal plane is horizontal
- The nasion support is positioned in contact with the nasion
- If not permanently situated within the tube housing, the wedge filter is inserted over the light beam diaphragm with its thicker end aligned over the soft tissues of the face
- The patient is asked to close their back teeth and relax the lips; this is maintained during exposure

Beam direction

Horizontal, at 90° to the IR; this is fixed for most units

Centring

Over the earplugs and the middle of the IR; this is fixed for most units

Collimation

Fixed collimation is usually found in most units and includes soft tissue outlines of the forehead, face/nose and mandible

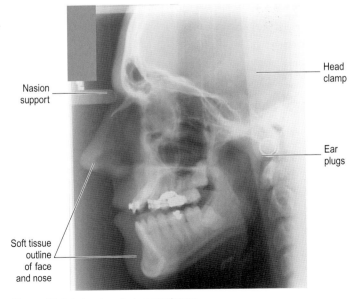

Figure 22.6 Lateral cephalometry image.

Criteria for assessing image quality

- Soft tissue outline of face including forehead, nose, lips and chin are demonstrated
- Whole of mandible and ear plugs are demonstrated
- Superimposition of both the ear plugs and of the right and left facial structures
- Anthropological baseline is horizontal
- Sharp image demonstrating detail of the facial bones *and* soft tissues of the face

Common errors	Possible reasons
Soft tissues of the face too dark	Filter not applied, or not selected on the unit
Denser soft tissues below the chin in comparison with the other soft tissues of the face	Anthropological baseline not horizontal; the chin is down and increases the density of the soft tissues under the mandible

Projection is usually acceptable on lateral cephalogram images, since the use of the ear plugs ensures accuracy. If the ear plugs are not inserted fully this is likely to impinge upon positioning of the MSP

REFERENCE

1. Iannucci Haring J, Jansen Lind L. Radiographic interpretation for the dental hygienist. Philadelphia: Saunders; 1993.

Section | 3 |

Chest and abdomen

Chapter 23

Chest and thoracic contents

Elizabeth Carver

Plain radiographic examination of the chest, in particular the postero-anterior (PA) projection, is considered to be the most commonly performed examination in the imaging department and is still used every day. Current guidelines suggest chest X-ray is useful in the following cases:

- Acute chest pain
- Suspected aortic dissection
- Suspected pulmonary embolism
- Suspected pericarditis/pericardial effusion, myocarditis, heart failure
- Chronic angina (stable)
- Suspected heart valve disease
- Congenital heart disease
- Pneumonia
- Pleural effusion
- Haemoptysis
- Insertion or removal of devices in the very sick[1]

Despite the reduction in referrals resulting from efforts to cut the numbers of unnecessary medical irradiations,[2,3] it can be seen that there is still a wide range of referral reasons that are considered valid. Plain radiography of the chest was used more extensively in the 20th century than today and is no longer justified in the following cases:

- Non-cardiac related chest pain
- Preoperative assessment ('routine', in patients who are not considered at risk from administration of anaesthetic)
- Screening medicals (with exception of high risk immigrants and those who need employment-specific imaging; RCR guidelines give an example of this as 'deep sea divers')
- Upper respiratory tract infection

Although anecdotal evidence shows that chest radiography has certainly been discontinued from the non-recommended list above, an internet search during the writing of this text did show that there is evidence that some hospital protocols still include recommendation for 'routine' chest radiography in some cases.[4]

Common findings on the chest image

Common findings on the chest image include abscess; atelectasis; bullae; calcifications; cardiomegaly; consolidation; emphysema; empyema; fibrosis; haemothorax; hiatus hernia; hilar enlargement or displacement; mastectomy; mediastinal enlargement (including lymph node enlargement); metastasis; neoplasm; pleural effusion; pleural plaques; pneumonectomy; pneumonia; pneumoperitoneum; pneumothorax; pulmonary oedema; raised diaphragm/s; rib fractures; thyroid goitre; tracheal shift; vertebral collapse.

Note that this is not a list of indications for referral for chest radiography; it is a résumé of commonly encountered appearances.

THE PA CHEST PROJECTION AND COMMENTS ON ITS IMPLEMENTATION

The PA chest projection is the primary method for demonstration of the thoracic contents. It is universally acknowledged that the gold standard for demonstrating the chest is to execute it with the patient in the erect, PA position. Reasons for this are straightforward and logical.

Erect

1. Undertaking the projection in the erect position allows for demonstration of unnaturally located fluid, which finds its natural level within the thoracic cavity and is well demonstrated as more dense in appearance than the air-filled lung tissue. In the supine position this pleural fluid will lie posteriorly in a layer which will show as an increased density over the hemithorax in which it lies; this density may overlie other pathology.[5] Wherever possible radiographers should undertake chest radiography erect; in the case of the infirm patient an erect sitting projection is a suitable alternative and this can be achieved using a stool or, preferably, a commercially built chair designed for stability and versatility. These chairs have wheels for manoeuvrability, wheel locks for stability, and removable back and arms for versatility. A PA erect chest can therefore be undertaken with the chair back removed but chair arms in place (Fig. 23.1A,B,C,D). For patients who must remain in a wheelchair, on a trolley or bed, an erect anteroposterior (AP) projection can be undertaken.

2. Inspiratory effort is more effective when the thorax is in the erect position.

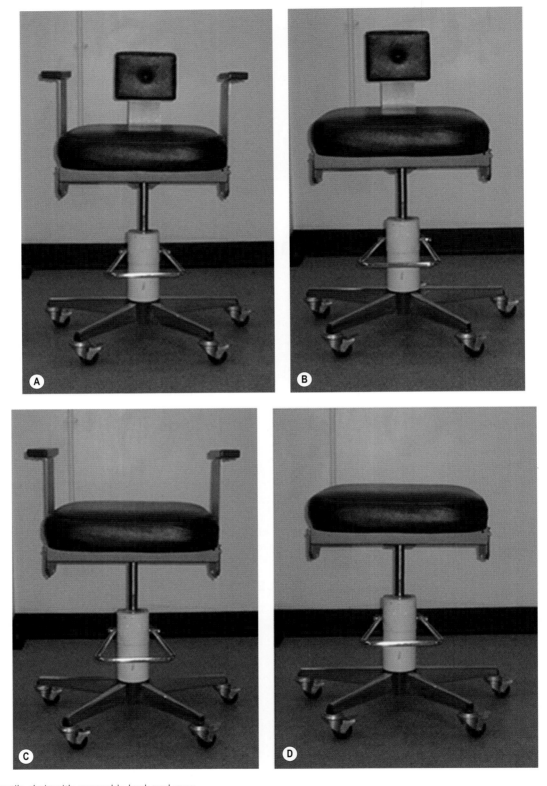

Figure 23.1 Versatile chair with removable back and arms.

PA

1. The PA projection allows forward tilt of the thorax to elevate the lung apices above the clavicles. Tuberculosis (TB) frequently manifests itself in the lung apex, thereby indicating the importance of clearing this area from the image of the clavicles (although a lordotic projection will clear the clavicles entirely above the apices, allowing visualisation of the lung apex without superimposition of the clavicles over the lower apical portion). Numbers of reported cases of TB in the 21st century are relatively insignificant in the UK compared to the 17th, 18th and 19th centuries and the first half of the 20th century, but it is by no means non-existent; after a period of increase the *incidence rate* per thousand (global population) levelled off in the period around 2005, but actual numbers increased because of population increase.[6] In the UK, numbers of recorded TB cases fell to their lowest level in 1987, reaching the low plateau of 5000–6000 cases per year for some years afterwards; the first signs of a very slight increase were noted around 1997,[7] increasing until 2009 but then falling again in 2010.[8]

   In addition to revealing the lung apices, forward tilt also avoids a lordotic appearance of the image; lordosis affects the accuracy of cardiothoracic ratio (CT ratio) assessment for cardiomegaly.

2. The chin can be supported clear of the apices by its position resting upon the upper border of the image receptor (IR).

3. As the heart lies anteriorly within the thorax (Fig. 23.2) the degree of magnification of this organ is minimised in the PA position; again, in assessment of the CT ratio, minimal magnification is preferred.

4. In an adult woman, compression of breast tissue against the IR will reduce body thickness and ensure the lowest exposure factor settings can be used.

5. It is acknowledged that the use of PA projections reduces the dose to anteriorly positioned radiosensitive organs, owing to the higher average beam energy after travelling through the posterior portions of the chest (thereby producing less absorption in these anterior organs). The sternum and female breasts lie within the field of primary radiation and will also benefit from reduction of dose in the PA position.

6. Obliquity of the X-ray beam at the periphery of the thorax will assist projection of the scapulae away from the area of the lung fields. The angle of this obliquity is likely to vary, as the distance of the scapulae from the central ray will differ according to the width of the chest, but it is likely that this angle will be quite small, even in the patient who has a wide chest. Examples of such angles of obliquity of the beam at 2 m focus receptor distance (FRD), at different points around the beam centre (when using a central ray at 90° to the IR) and using geometric calculations, are given as approximate figures in the following table (figures are given to the nearest decimal point).

Distance from centring point (cm)	Angle of oblique rays at this point (2 m FRD)
12	3.4°
17	4.8°
21.5	6.2°

Comments on exposure technique selection

In order to image the lung tissue adequately in contrast to air within the thorax, for the most part of the 20th century exposure factors with a fairly low kVp were traditionally selected for chest radiography. These were usually in the range of 60–75 kVp and accompanied by values of 6–12 mAs. However, structures overlying dense areas such as the heart failed to be demonstrated owing to the low penetration of the beam. EC guidelines in 1996 not only stressed the importance of using a high-energy beam in order to penetrate such areas, but also emphasised the reduction of absorbed dose by using high kVp techniques, namely 125 kVp.[9] These high kVp techniques may well require the use of an antiscatter grid or bucky, and use of automatic exposure devices (AEDs) is recommended in the 1996 EC guidelines, selecting the right chamber.

Positioning choices for the PA projection

There have been relatively few published comments in the past regarding actual positioning techniques (although there has been reasonably frequent comment on exposure factor techniques, radiation protection and dedicated chest radiology systems).

Historically, and internationally, descriptions for PA chest techniques have included a confusing range of centring points (T4–T7), suggestions for caudal angulation or use of the horizontal beam. This range of techniques should be questioned, especially as consistency of approach is desirable when aiming to provide a quality-led service.

Direction of central ray

It appears that, internationally, beam angulation is not in widespread use and the UK appears to be the area most likely to use it.[10] Caudal angulation has been suggested as inappropriate as the (minimal) obliquity of the beam used is actually likely to reduce the amount of posterior inferior lung tissue demonstrated above the diaphragm on the image (this is despite the common belief that its use 'opens out the lung fields' or maximises the amount of lung tissue seen above the diaphragm).[11] The effectiveness of small angles has also been challenged.[12] In addition, caudal angulation takes the beam direction towards the abdomen, thereby potentially increasing radiation dose to this region. To summarise, the use of caudal angulation does not offer improvements in image quality, may reduce the amount of lung tissue seen above the diaphragm, and potentially adds to the radiation burden for abdomen and gonads; it is can therefore be considered pointless.

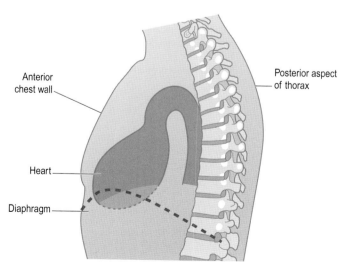

Figure 23.2 Heart in relationship to anterior chest wall.

Centring point

As indicated, suggestions for centring have varied from T4 to T7,[13-16] with the middle of the IR, chest or thorax also mentioned in some texts.[15-17] In some cases more than one suggestion is given. So which is most appropriate? An additional question is: do texts specifying a vertebral level mean the body *or* the spinous process of that which is indicated? This is an important point when it is remembered that the body of a thoracic vertebra lies level with the spinous process of the one above it. It is also important that a suggested centring point be located as a palpable surface marking, so in this chapter spinous process will be referred to.

One suggestion for accurate assessment of the centring point involves using a ruler to measure the radiographer's hand span in order to help locate a centring point (given in centimetres and inches from T1) for use on the 'average' male and 'average' female,[18] but how can this be standardised or accurate when the assessment (and opinion) of 'average' is likely to vary from radiographer to radiographer, and any set measurement in centimetres or inches varies in its distance down each individual spine from a given point?

Centring points are most effective when simply in the centre of the area of interest, whether or not tube angle is used, and this should similarly apply to the chest region. Considering the issue of using a sensible centring point for the chest, the previous edition of this book suggested a move from traditional centring points as high as T6 (which lies only one-third of the distance from apices to costophrenic angles) after research showed that this point almost never lies in the middle of the area of interest: indeed, study of PA chest images has shown that the vertebral body that most frequently lies level with the midpoint of the lungs is the body of T8 (spinous process of T7).[19]

Yet the reality of actually visualising this centring level accurately, and at a distance of 2 m, can also be questioned, despite accurate palpation at the skin surface. Of course, a mark can be made at the appropriate level on the patient's gown after palpation, but realistically, only female patients undergo chest radiography in an examination gown. Would marking of the skin on a male patient be ethical? Probably not. Alternatively, a removable sticker could be applied to the back of male patients, but this may also not be acceptable to every individual.

In support of the question regarding the ability to accurately select a centring point at 2 m, it has been found that radiographers frequently believe that they use a specific centring point for PA projection of the chest but in reality ensure that the area of interest lies centrally over the IR. They then centre to the middle of the IR and the area of interest.[20] This provides a well-centred image and suggests that radiographers are accurate at centring appropriately at 2 m, but not at selecting the point they believe they use. For this reason the description of technique and centring point in this book reflects a combination of this second method and selection of a specific centring point.

PA chest projection (Fig. 23.3A,B,C)

IR is vertical

Positioning

- A lead rubber apron is applied to the patient's waist
- The anterior aspect of the chest is placed in contact with the IR
- The height of the IR is adjusted until the whole of the thorax is included in its perimeter. The beam is collimated to the patient's thorax
- The patient's feet are separated slightly, for stability
- The patient leans forward and the chin is raised slightly and rests against the IR, or upon its upper border if a cassette type IR is used

- The median sagittal plane (MSP) is perpendicular to the IR; this is checked by ensuring the sternoclavicular joints are equidistant from the IR. The MSP is coincident with the long axis of the IR
- The elbows are flexed and the backs of the hands are placed on the sides of the waist, resting on the lateral aspects of the iliac crests. The elbows are then gently pressed forward towards the IR, to clear the scapulae from the lung fields on the image. Ensure that the hands are actually on the *lateral* aspect of the waist, as this maximises forward movement of the shoulders; positioning of the hands on the posterior aspect significantly reduces the range of forward movement
- A PA marker is most frequently used, on the relevant upper corner of the radiation field

Beam direction and FRD

Horizontal
2 m FRD

Centring

Positioning as described should ensure that centring is over the middle of the thorax, coincident with the spinous process of T7 (body of T8)

Collimation

First thoracic vertebra, first rib, lateral margins of ribs 2–10, costophrenic angles

---

Expose on arrested inspiration; maximum effort required

Before exposure the radiographer should check that the shoulders are not raised during the inspiratory effort, or that the arms and shoulders have not relaxed backwards. The time lapse between initially pressing the arms forward during positioning and exposure may seem relatively short, yet patients frequently, and usually imperceptibly, relax their arms enough to superimpose at least some scapular outline over the upper lung fields during this short time.

Criteria for assessing image quality

- First thoracic vertebra and first rib, lateral rib margins and costophrenic angles are demonstrated. The costophrenic angles must be demonstrated above the collimated field
- 3–5 cm of apical tissue is projected above the clavicles
- Posterior aspects of the ribs are slightly inclined from the thoracic spine down towards their lateral borders
- Anterior aspects of the ribs are inclined more steeply than the posterior aspects, from their lateral borders down towards the midline
- Medial ends of the clavicles are equidistant from the midline of the thoracic vertebrae
- Scapulae are cleared from the lung fields
- Six anterior or nine posterior ribs are demonstrated above the diaphragms
- Sharp image demonstrating the vascular pattern of the lungs to the periphery in contrast with the air-filled lung tissue and dense structures of the hila and mediastinum (heart, aorta). Trachea and proximal bronchi should be visible, as should the retrocardiac lung and mediastinum. The thoracic vertebrae (intervertebral disc spaces) should be evident through the cardiac image. Diaphragms and costophrenic angles should be clearly seen. These exposure factor criteria relate to high kVp technique as outlined by EC 96 regulations.[3] For images produced with kVp lower than 85–90, penetration is assessed by checking that the spinous process of T4 is adequately seen in the midline as in

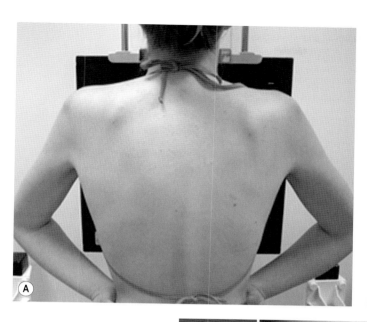

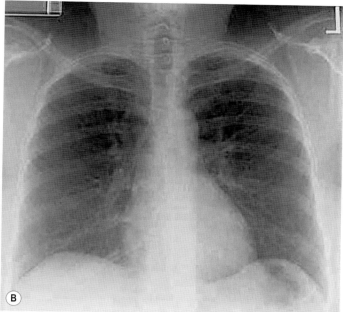

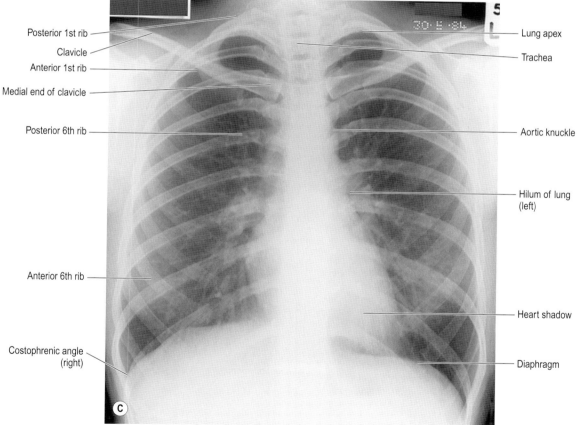

Posterior 1st rib

Clavicle

Anterior 1st rib

Medial end of clavicle

Posterior 6th rib

Anterior 6th rib

Costophrenic angle (right)

Lung apex

Trachea

Aortic knuckle

Hilum of lung (left)

Heart shadow

Diaphragm

Figure 23.3 (A) PA chest; (B) PA chest using high kVp; (C) PA chest using lower kVp.

Figure 23.3C. (Note that the patient positioning in Fig. 23.3C is superior to that in Fig. 23.3B.)

Adherence to quality standards outlined above is particularly important in the PA chest radiograph:

- *Poor inspiratory effort, lordosis and rotation* will all affect the accuracy of CT ratio assessment. *Rotation* will also cause hilar markings to appear more prominent on one side of the thorax and potentially mimic the suggestion of pathology. Density in each lung will appear to be different in the rotated patient. A rotated position will also cause the mediastinum to appear widened and the trachea to appear shifted laterally.[5,21]

- It is vital to include *all* the outline of the whole of the costophrenic angle on each side, as a significant volume of 100 mL of pleural effusion may be present before blunting of the costophrenic angle will be demonstrated.[5] This is related to the fact that the diaphragm level sits lower on the posterior aspect of the thorax in relation to its anterior portion. Pleural fluid can collect in this lower posterior portion before it is actually demonstrated in the anterior portion and on the PA erect chest radiograph, when it is seen to cause blunting of the costophrenic angle as its earliest appearance.[21] Although the lateral radiograph is more sensitive than the PA when demonstrating pleural effusions, most often a good-quality PA is the first indication that the lateral will be necessary.[21] It is therefore essential that the PA image includes the whole costophrenic angle to ensure that the earliest radiographic signs of pleural effusion can be noted as soon as possible.

Common errors	Possible reasons
Medially positioned soft tissue shadow, between and/or overlying the apices	Chin not raised adequately
Apices inadequately cleared above the clavicles; posterior and anterior aspects of the ribs flattened	Patient is lordotic, i.e. not leaning forward towards the IR
Medial ends of the clavicles not seen at an equal distance from the thoracic vertebrae	Patient is rotated. The medial end of the clavicle furthest from the vertebrae corresponds to the side rotated away from the IR. Any evidence of scoliosis? If the patient has scoliosis, it may not be possible to ensure the clavicles lie equidistant from the midline[22]
Scapulae overlying upper, lateral aspects of lung fields	Elbows and shoulders not pushed forward adequately, or patient has relaxed their arm position Patients with limited shoulder movement may not find it possible to fully comply with the required action; try extending the patient's arms in forward abduction, with internal rotation at the shoulder
Fewer than six anterior ribs or nine posterior ribs are demonstrated above the diaphragms	*Miscounted ribs*; check again. The first and second ribs cross over superiorly on the image and can sometimes be erroneously counted as one, rather than two. A tip when checking rib numbers is to assume that the posterior aspects of the first and second ribs appear to cross over, like a kiss on a birthday card – so always 'count the kiss' first and remember that the kiss = ribs one and two. Counting the thoracic vertebrae is another method that can be used to identify posterior ribs and confirm rib number
	Poor inspiratory effort. Obese patients or patients with dyspnoea may find improvement difficult
	Any evidence or history suggestive of infective or cardiac disease, lobar collapse, lobectomy, subphrenic abscess, phrenic nerve paralysis or upper abdominal mass? These are likely to affect diaphragm height and improvement may not be possible

AP erect chest (Figs 23.4, 23.5)

The AP erect chest is undertaken when a patient is too ill or frail to stand or sit PA erect.

IR is vertical

Positioning

- A patient who can sit on a chair sits with their back to the IR (Fig. 23.4)
- For a patient who presents on a trolley or bed the IR is (a) brought to the back of the patient (digital plate technique), (b) placed in the erect holder or (c) supported by a large 45° pad which rests on the raised back of a trolley or bed (Fig. 23.5)
- The posterior aspect of the chest is placed in contact with the IR
- The height of the IR is adjusted until the whole of the thorax is included in its perimeter. Ensuring that the first thoracic vertebra is below the upper border of the receptor will ensure that the lung apices are included at the top of the image
- The patient sits, supported with their back against the IR
- A lead rubber apron is applied to the patient's waist
- The beam is collimated to the patient's thorax and its upper border positioned level with the upper border of T1
- A small radiolucent pad is placed behind the shoulders to reproduce the slight elevation of the lung apices above the clavicles achieved in the PA position. The chin is raised slightly and the MSP is coincident with the long axis of the IR
- The MSP is perpendicular to the IR; this is checked by ensuring the sternoclavicular joints are equidistant from the receptor

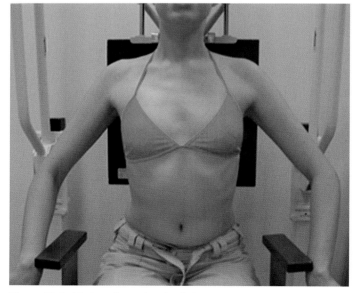

Figure 23.4 AP chest for patient in chair.

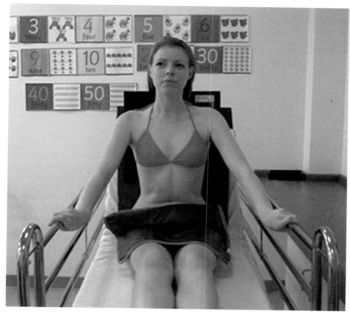

Figure 23.5 AP chest for patient on trolley.

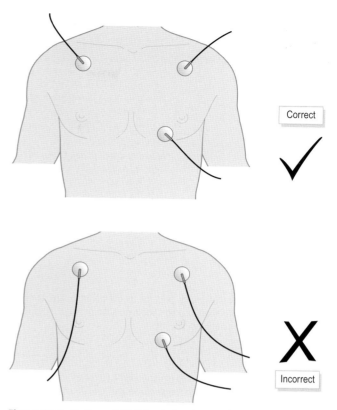

Figure 23.6 Position of ECG leads for chest radiography.

- For the patient who is sitting on a chair, the elbows are flexed and the backs of the hands are placed on the sides of the waist, resting on the lateral aspects of the iliac crests. The elbows are then gently pressed forward towards the IR, to clear the scapulae from the lung fields on the image. This is exactly the same action as that required for the PA projection. Some patients in bed or on a trolley may also be able to achieve this position
- For patients unable to clear the scapulae by the above method, the arms are abducted and, if possible, rotated internally at the shoulders until the thumbs are directed to the floor. Resting the forearms on the trolley or bed sides, while maintaining some internal rotation, is an effective method of achieving and maintaining this position (Fig. 23.5)
- An AP marker is used, within the relevant upper corner of the radiation field
- If the patient has electrocardiogram (ECG) leads attached to their chest, or is using an oxygen mask, care must be taken to clear these artefacts from the field. ECG leads should leave the chest area by the 'shortest route' if they cannot be temporarily detached (Fig. 23.6)
- An 'erect AP' legend is applied next to the anatomical marker

Beam direction and FRD

Horizontal
2 m FRD

A caudal angle may be used to reduce the effect of lordosis if the patient (unavoidably) is leaning back. The angle should be selected by assessing the degree of recumbence, although approximately 5° has been suggested.[18] Use of such an angle should be carefully considered, as significant deviation from the use of a horizontal beam may affect demonstration of fluid in the chest cavity.

Centring

To the middle of the thorax (approximately midway between the sternal angle and xiphisternum)

Collimation

First thoracic vertebra, first rib, lateral margins of ribs, costophrenic angles

Expose on arrested inspiration; maximum effort required

Criteria for assessing image quality

Criteria are identical to those for the PA projection, but it should be remembered that elevation of the apices above the clavicles may be less successful than on a PA image, despite use of the radiolucent pad suggested in the positioning description. It is likely that there will still be some lordosis, as it is tempting for the infirm patient to lean back, using the IR for support. This is potentially made worse when the patient attempts good inspiratory effort. Elevation of the chin is often difficult for the infirm patient and is made more difficult if the thorax is tilted slightly forward by the radiolucent pad. Forward tilt will also cause some magnification of the upper thorax.

Lordosis is more likely to occur in bed- or trolley-bound patients, where the IR is supported by a sponge and the patient's legs extend forward, increasing the tendency of the thorax to lean back. The possibility of lordosis increases further when pillows are substituted for the pad. The potential risk of lordosis in the AP position does not validate approval of its presence on the image, and maximum effort should be made to avoid its incidence.

Common errors (see also errors outlined under PA projection)	Possible reasons
Lordosis	Patient using IR as support for their back. If lordosis cannot be improved, a compensating caudal angle may be effective in reducing the effect
Soft tissue shadow over lower lung fields	Abdominal tissue may be superimposed; usually seen in lordotic patients on a trolley or bed. It is especially prevalent in patients who have a large abdomen

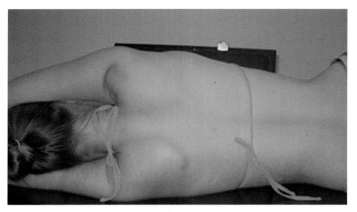

Figure 23.7 Lateral decubitus PA chest.

Supine AP chest

This is undertaken on the very sick patient, most often in the mobile situation. Two people are required to facilitate safe manual handling while positioning the patient on the IR.

Positioning

- The patient's trunk is elevated from the bed or trolley and the IR is placed underneath the chest, to include the whole of the thorax within its boundaries
- MSP is perpendicular to the IR and coincident with its long axis
- A lead rubber apron is applied over the abdomen, below the diaphragm
- The chin is raised slightly
- The arms are abducted and, if possible, rotated internally at the shoulders
- An AP marker is used, on the relevant upper corner of the radiation field
- A 'supine AP' legend is applied next to the anatomical marker
- Artefacts should be moved as described for the AP erect projection

Beam direction and FRD

Vertical; however, a caudal angle of 5° will reduce the appearance of lordosis on the image
FRD as high as possible – up to a maximum of 2 m; FRD can be maximised by lowering the bed

Centring

To the middle of the thorax, as for erect AP chest

Collimation

First thoracic vertebra, first rib, lateral margins of ribs 2–10, costophrenic angles

Expose on arrested inspiration; maximum effort required

For patients on a ventilator it may be necessary to ask for suitably designated staff to facilitate suspension of respiration by controlling the ventilator.

Consideration for radiation protection – mobile radiography

Although some patients will be examined in the supine position on a trolley in the imaging department, the majority of supine chest examinations are undertaken as mobile examinations on the ward or A&E recovery, i.e. in a radiation supervised area rather than a controlled area. Therefore, the radiographer's responsibility regarding radiation exposure is of paramount importance, particularly regarding protection of personnel and other patients in the vicinity.

Criteria for assessing image quality

Criteria are identical to those for the PA and AP projections, with the risk of lordosis similar to that for the AP projection. Suspension of adequate inspiration is likely to be more difficult in the case of the unconscious patient who is breathing independently, therefore a maximum attempt to achieve an adequately inspired, sharp image must be made.

Unfortunately it is often not possible to achieve the optimum FRD of 2 m for the supine projection, owing to equipment or environment restrictions. This will cause magnification that is greater than for examinations undertaken at 2 m FRD. With the additional consideration of the fact that the heart is already magnified in the AP position, assessment of CT ratio is further compromised. The mediastinum will also appear enlarged.

Lateral decubitus PA chest (Fig. 23.7)

This projection should be used when it is vital that a horizontal beam is used to demonstrate pleural effusions; ultrasound can also be used to confirm or exclude this condition.[5] Occasionally small pneumothoraces require demonstration using this method.[16]

IR is vertical

Positioning

- The patient lies on a radiolucent pad: (a) *on their affected side*, to allow for the settlement of pleural fluid in the lateral portion of the lung or (b) *on their unaffected side* to allow the demonstration of air in the pleural cavity. The knees are flexed for comfort and stability and the arms raised to clear them from the area of interest and primary beam

- The IR is placed vertically, its long axis parallel to the long axis of the table-top, trolley or bed
- The anterior aspect of the chest is placed in contact with the IR and the position is adjusted until the whole of the thorax is included in its perimeter, with the first thoracic vertebra included. The MSP is coincident with the longitudinal axis of the receptor
- A lead rubber apron is applied to the patient's waist
- The chin is raised slightly to clear it from the lung apices. The MSP is perpendicular to the IR; this is checked by ensuring the sternoclavicular joints are equidistant from the IR
- A PA marker is applied

Beam direction and FRD

Horizontal
2 m FRD

Centring

To the middle of the thorax, over the spinous process of T7 (body of T8)

Collimation

First thoracic vertebra, first rib, lateral margins of ribs 2–10, costo-phrenic angles

Criteria for assessing image quality

Criteria follow those for the PA erect chest. However, if the suspected pathologies outlined as reasons for use of this projection are found, it may not be necessary to repeat the examination in the case of rotation, poor inspiration, poor scapular clearance or lordosis. The most important criterion for this projection is the inclusion of the whole area of interest, especially the lateral border of the hemithorax related to the pathology in question.

Lateral chest (Fig. 23.8A,B)

Unless there is known pathology related to a particular side of the chest, the PA projection should be examined to determine the pathology site before taking the decision to use this projection. Decision on the appropriate lateral is made on the basis that the side with the most significant pathological feature is selected for positioning closest to the IR. Use of the lateral projection has declined since the late 1980s with the increased use of computed tomography (CT).

Under no circumstances should a lateral projection be undertaken as 'routine' or without relevant clinical reason.

As for the PA chest, EC guidelines also recommend use of antiscatter grid in conjunction with 125 kVp exposure technique and use of AED,[9] although this is not currently widespread in practice. Commonly, a grid is only used for larger patients and kVp is often lower than 125.

Positioning

IR is vertical
- A lead rubber apron is applied to the patient's waist
- The arms are raised and the lateral aspect of the chest is placed in contact with the IR
- The height of the IR is adjusted so the thorax lies within its perimeter and the beam is collimated to include the whole of the thorax
- The feet are slightly separated for stability
- The elbows are flexed and the hands clasped at the back of the head; the humeri are adducted medially until parallel. Upper arm tissue and humeri must be cleared from as much of the apices and upper lungs as possible
- A slight forwards tilt of the trunk will bring the thorax into a vertical position
- The MSP is parallel to the IR

Patients who cannot comply with the positioning described above can be examined with modifications listed below.

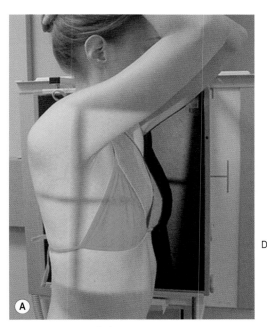

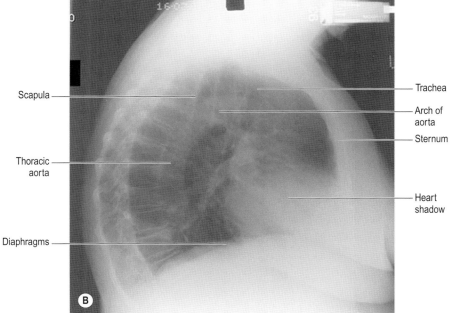

Scapula —
Thoracic aorta —
Diaphragms —

Trachea
Arch of aorta
Sternum
Heart shadow

Figure 23.8 Lateral chest.

Difficulty	Modification or adaptation
Patient cannot maintain position of raised arms, cannot raise arms or cannot flex elbows comfortably	Patient holds vertical structure with raised hands. Commonly a drip stand is used for this
Patient cannot stand	Projection can be undertaken using a stool or chair (Fig. 23.9)
Patient needs support at their back (if sitting)	A radiolucent pad can be placed behind the patient's back as in Figure 23.10

Beam direction and FRD

Horizontal
2 m FRD

Centring

Midway between the sternum and posterior ribs anteroposteriorly, level with a point midway between the sternal angle and the xiphisternum

Collimation

Shoulder, sternum, spinous processes of thoracic vertebrae, posterior and anterior costophrenic angles

Criteria for assessing image quality

- Shoulder, sternum, spinous processes of thoracic vertebrae, posterior and anterior costophrenic angles are demonstrated
- Shoulder and soft tissue of upper arms overlying lung apices only
- Condyles on posterior aspect of thoracic vertebrae are superimposed; posterior aspects of ribs are superimposed
- Intervertebral joint spaces are clear
- Image of left diaphragm seen slightly above right
- T11 is demonstrated above the posterior diaphragm
- Sharp image demonstrating lung markings in contrast with the heart, aorta, air-filled trachea and ribs. The sternum, posterior heart border, diaphragms, anterior and posterior costophrenic angles and thoracic vertebrae should also be demonstrated

Common errors	Possible reasons
Non-superimposition of condyles of vertebral bodies; non-superimposition of posterior aspects of ribs	Rotation; MSP not parallel to IR
Intervertebral joint spaces not cleared	Patient tilt; MSP not parallel to IR *or* patient has scoliosis. The PA chest image will confirm this
Pale shadow over upper lungs	Unavoidable at extreme upper lung area (apices); soft tissue shadow lower than this is almost certainly due to the upper arms dropping from their required position. Take care not to confuse the appearance with pathology

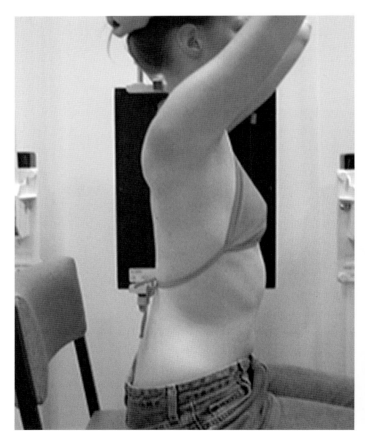

Figure 23.9 Lateral chest in chair.

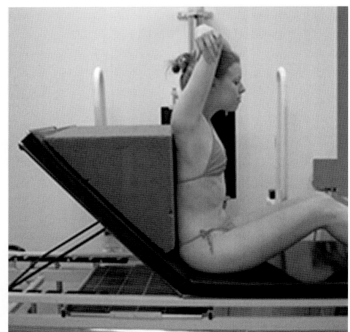

Figure 23.10 Lateral chest on trolley.

LUNG APICES

As with the lateral projection, modern imaging methods have largely superseded the use of apical projections, but it may be a low radiation dose approach to use apical projections to clarify whether a suspicious appearance needs further investigation.

Suspected lesions in the lung apex may well be seen above the clavicle on a PA chest image, but there is some risk that the clavicle itself will overlie some appearances. The lung apex can be cleared from the clavicle in one of the following ways:

1. With the patient initially AP or PA, the thorax is tilted in extreme lordosis to elevate the clavicles above the lung apices. A horizontal beam is used (Figs 23.11A,B, 23.12)
2. With the patient initially PA, a horizontal beam is angled 30° caudally to project the lung apices below the clavicles (Fig. 23.13)
3. With the patient initially AP, a horizontal beam is angled 30° cranially to project the clavicles above the lung apices. An appropriate method to clear the clavicles from the apices should be chosen after consideration of imaging principles and dose implications

Method 1 (lordotic AP or PA with horizontal beam)

The horizontal beam image has less distortion than methods using angulation, but the AP position has implications for increased dose to the thyroid, eye lens, breast and sternum compared to the PA position. In the AP position the patient can lean back onto the IR for support, but unless there are suitable structures for the patient to hold on to, the PA method can be unstable. In the AP position the apical region is closer to the IR, whereas there is increased lung-apex-to-film distance in the PA position, which has implications for magnification unsharpness of the area. An air gap will also exist, requiring some increase in exposure. However, the air gap will have the effect of some reduction in scatter and hence improved image quality.

Method 2 (PA position with 30° caudal angulation)

The benefits of the PA position are as those for method 1 but the 30° angulation will cause some image distortion.

Method 3 (AP position with 30° cranial angulation)

Disadvantages of using the AP position are as those outlined in method 1, but in addition to this the angulation will cause some image distortion, as in method 2. Because the angle is directed cranially, the dose to the lenses of the eyes and thyroid will be greater than with AP method 1.

This method will be more acceptable to patients who cannot comply with requirements for sitting or standing in a PA position, as for the routine chest PA projection. It can be used in the supine position, with a vertical central ray directed 30° cranially.

A lordotic projection can also be used to demonstrate right middle lobe collapse, using the PA position described in method 1, and inclusion of all thoracic anatomy as for the routine PA chest projection, centring at the level of T8.

Apparent lesions adequately seen above the clavicle on the PA projection can be demonstrated in a different plane by using a lordotic apical projection, since information on lung apices cannot be gleaned from a lateral chest image. Beam angulation will provide a more distorted image and is therefore of limited value. The current recommendation for investigation of suspicious lesions in this region is to use CT, whenever readily available.

Exposure factors

As the apices are not overshadowed by dense structures such as the mediastinum, in apical projections it is not necessary to use a high kVp technique or antiscatter grid. A lower kVp will help reduce scatter and increase contrast quality. The projections should be well collimated, which will reduce dose and therefore also ensure optimum contrast by assisting with scatter reduction.

Lung apices: AP lordotic (Fig. 23.11A,B)

IR is erect

Positioning

- A lead rubber apron is applied to the anterior aspect of the patient's waist
- The patient initially sits erect in the AP position, with their seat approximately 25–35 cm from the IR. Distance varies according to patient height: taller patients will need to sit further away than shorter patients
- The patient leans back to rest the backs of their shoulders upon the IR; the clavicle should lie horizontally level with the C7/T1 region
- The IR is adjusted until the area of interest lies within its boundaries
- The MSP is perpendicular to the IR
- The sternoclavicular joints are equidistant from the IR
- Scapular clearance is required as for the PA chest projection
- An AP marker is used

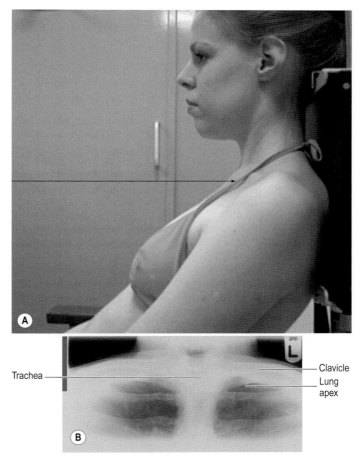

Trachea —

Clavicle
Lung apex

Figure 23.11 AP lung apices with lordosis.

Beam direction and FRD

Horizontal

2 m FRD

Note that magnification reduction is not as great an issue as in the full PA chest projection, since the CT ratio is not relevant to the projection. Therefore it is not inappropriate to use a shorter FRD.

Centring

Over the sternal angle

A visual check that the shadow of the upper border of the soft tissue above the shoulder and clavicle lies within the light beam field and within IR boundaries will ensure that the tops of the lung apices are included.

Collimation

Upper border of T1, clavicles, lung apices, lateral borders of ribs 1–5, fifth thoracic vertebra

Lung apices: PA lordotic (Fig. 23.12)

IR vertical

Positioning

- A lead rubber apron is applied to the posterior aspect of the patient's waist
- The patient initially sits erect in the PA position, with their seat directly in front of the IR
- The patient leans back, away from the IR, until their clavicles lie horizontally level with the C7/T1 region
- The patient holds onto the unit, bucky housing or handles for stability
- The sternoclavicular joints are equidistant from the IR
- Scapular clearance is required
- A PA marker is used

Beam direction and FRD

Horizontal

2 m FRD

In contrast to the AP method, this distance is essential in order to reduce magnification and unsharpness.

Centring

Over the midline of the patient, to emerge through the sternal angle

Collimation

Upper border of T1, clavicles, lung apices, lateral borders of ribs 1–5, fifth thoracic vertebra

For both the PA and AP lordotic projections of the apices, a visual check that the shadow of the upper border of the soft tissue above the shoulder and clavicle lies within the light beam field will ensure that the tops of the lung apices are included.

Lung apices: PA with 30° caudal angulation

(Fig. 23.13)

Most dedicated digital chest units have a fixed central ray which is perpendicular to the IR; this method, and the AP with cranial angulation, is therefore unsuitable for use with this type of unit.

IR is erect

Positioning

- A lead rubber apron is applied to the posterior aspect of the patient's waist
- The patient sits erect in the PA position
- The sternoclavicular joints are equidistant from the IR
- Scapular clearance is required
- A PA marker is used

Beam direction and FRD

Initially horizontal, which is then directed 30° caudally

2 m FRD

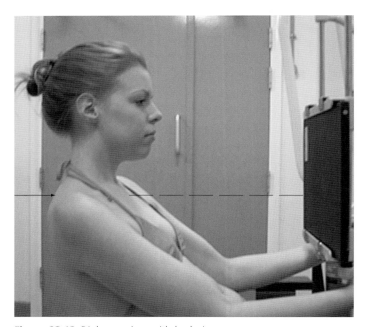

Figure 23.12 PA lung apices with lordosis.

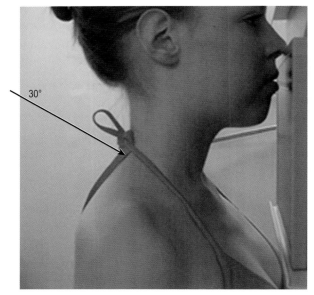

Figure 23.13 PA lung apices with 30° caudal angulation.

Centring

Over the vertebral column, to emerge at the sternal notch

Collimation

Upper border of T1, clavicles, lung apices, lateral borders of ribs 1–5, fifth thoracic vertebra

A visual check that the shadow of the upper border of the soft tissue above the shoulder and the clavicle lies within the light beam field will ensure that the tops of the lung apices are included.

Lung apices: AP with 30° cranial angulation

(Fig. 23.14)

IR is vertical

Positioning

- A lead rubber apron is applied to the anterior aspect of the patient's waist
- The patient sits erect in the AP position
- The sternoclavicular joints are equidistant from the IR
- Scapular clearance is required
- An AP marker is used

Beam direction and FRD

Initially horizontal, which is then directed 30° cranially
1 m FRD

Centring

To the sternal angle

Collimation

Upper border of T1, clavicles, lung apices, lateral borders of ribs 1–5, 5th thoracic vertebra

A visual check that the shadow of the upper border of the soft tissue above the shoulder and clavicle lies within the light beam field will ensure that the tops of the lung apices are included.

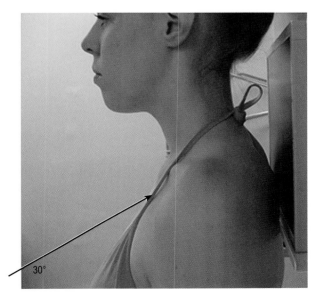

Figure 23.14 AP lung apices with 30° cranial angulation.

All methods

Expose on arrested inspiration

Common errors	Possible reasons
Overall image density low	Insufficient exposure given; the projection requires an increase from that used for the PA projection as the beam travels through an increased thickness due to lordosis or beam angulation. If PA lordotic method used, has the increased air gap been considered?
One lung apex more dense than the other	Rotation
Clavicles overlying lung apices	Lordosis or beam angle is insufficient

Criteria for assessing image quality

- Upper border of T1, clavicles, lung apices, lateral borders of ribs 1–5 and fifth thoracic vertebra are demonstrated on the image
- Clavicles cleared above the tops of the lung apices
- Flattened appearance of the ribs
- Medial ends of clavicles equidistant from the midline of the thoracic vertebrae
- Scapulae cleared from the lung fields

OBLIQUE PROJECTIONS OF THE CHEST

Prior to the widespread use of CT, oblique projections of the chest were valuable for demonstrating the estimated 40% of lung tissue obscured by dense structures in the chest.[23] In addition, oblique projections can be used to demonstrate the mediastinum, heart and great vessels, trachea, hila and pleural plaques evident in cases of mesothelioma.

45° anterior oblique chest (RAO, LAO)

(Fig. 23.15A,B,C,D)

IR is vertical for all oblique projections of the chest

Positioning

- A horizontal beam is collimated to the size of the patient's thorax, with the patient standing with the front of their chest in contact with the receptor
- A lead rubber apron is applied to the patient's waist
- The IR height is adjusted until the area of interest lies within its boundaries
- From a PA position, the patient rotates 45° to the left for the RAO or 45° to the right for the LAO projection
- The feet are slightly separated for stability
- The arms are raised at the sides of the head and then flexed at the elbows; the forearms are then rested across the top of the head. This clears the arms from the field
- Without leaning forward, the patient is immobilised by resting the shoulder nearest the IR against the IR
- A PA marker is most frequently used on the upper aspect of the IR. The RAO should bear a right marker and the LAO a left marker, which should always lie above the side nearest the IR

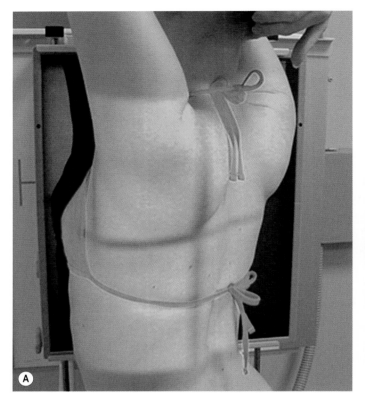
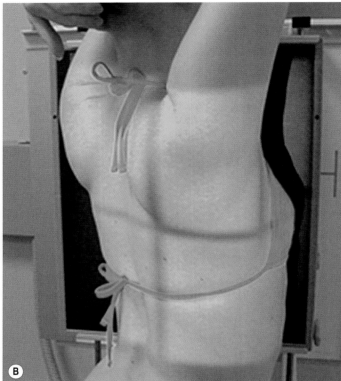
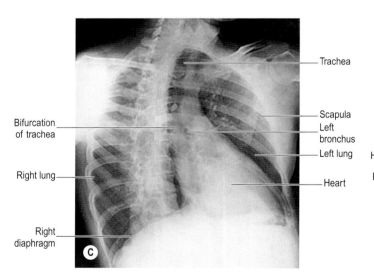
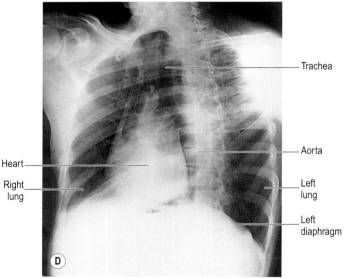

Figure 23.15 (A) RAO chest; (B) LAO chest; (C) RAO chest; (D) LAO chest.
(C) and (D) Reproduced with permission from Ballinger PW, Frank ED. Merrill's atlas of radiographic positioning and radiologic procedures. 10th ed. St Louis: Mosby; 2003.

Beam direction and FRD

Horizontal
2 m FRD

Centring

To the middle of the IR, at the level of the spinous process of T7 (body of T8), midway between the vertebral column and the lateral borders of ribs on the side furthest from the IR

Collimation

First thoracic vertebra, first rib, lateral margins of ribs 2–10, costophrenic angles

Criteria for assessing image quality

- First thoracic vertebra and first rib, all rib outlines and diaphragms are demonstrated
- Arms are cleared from the lung fields

- Vertebral column shown closer to the lateral border of the thorax on the side positioned nearest the IR
- Heart shown in its entirety over the vertebral column and side positioned furthest from the IR
- Seven anterior ribs are demonstrated above the diaphragms. These should be counted on the side positioned nearest to the IR
- Sharp image demonstrating the dense mediastinal structures in contrast with air-filled lungs

Common errors	Possible reasons
Heart shadow slightly overlapping onto side nearest IR	Less than 45° rotation on the thorax
Appearance of space between heart shadow and vertebral column on side furthest from IR	More than 45° rotation on the thorax

Other anterior oblique chest positions

The 45° obliques described are probably the most useful obliques today, as they are most appropriate for a general oblique survey of the chest and adequate for demonstrating pleural plaques when ongoing assessment may not require CT at every stage. Other obliques are suggested for demonstration of more specific structures:

1. Trachea, great vessels and cardiac outline will best be seen with a greater angle of rotation (60°) on the RAO projection.[15,18] The structures are seen well clear of the vertebral column, as is the descending aorta.
2. Bifurcation of the trachea and arch of aorta can be demonstrated by using a 70° rotation on the LAO projection.[15] Structures are seen cleared from the vertebral column but the descending aorta is seen to overlie it.

THORACIC INLET

The trachea can appear deviated or compressed on plain radiographic images, owing to tumour or thyroid goitre. It can also deviate from the midline towards the side of lobar collapse on AP or PA projections. Rotation when positioning the patient will cause apparent deviation of the trachea from the midline. In the 21st century, the area covered by the thoracic inlet is largely examined by MRI, CT or radionuclide imaging (RNI) studies.

IR is erect for all projections of the thoracic inlet

PA thoracic inlet (Fig. 23.16A,B)

Positioning

- A lead rubber apron is applied to the patient's waist
- The patient faces the IR; the feet are slightly separated for stability
- The MSP is coincident with, and perpendicular to, the long axis of the IR
- The chin is raised until the occiput and mandible are superimposed, to maximise the amount of upper trachea demonstrated on the image
- A PA marker is most frequently used, on the upper aspect of the IR

Beam direction and FRD

Horizontal
100 cm FRD

Centring

Through T2 to emerge through the sternal notch

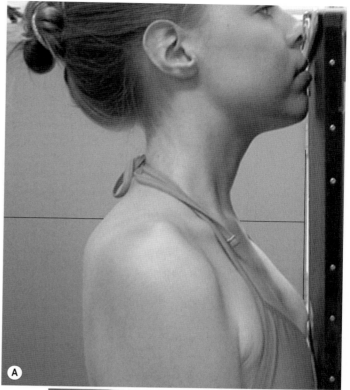

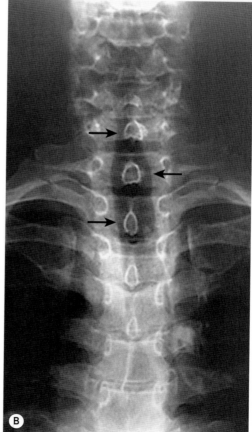

Figure 23.16 PA thoracic inlet. (B) The arrows outline the lateral margins of the air-filled trachea.
(B) Reproduced with permission from Ballinger PW, Frank ED. Merrill's atlas of radiographic positioning and radiologic procedures. 10th ed. St Louis: Mosby; 2003.

Expose on arrested inspiration or Valsalva manoeuvre

The Valsalva manoeuvre is forced exhalation against a closed upper airway, i.e. not actually exhaling but forcing air from the lungs into a closed mouth and nasal passage. It has been likened to the bearing down action of defaecation. The action serves to fill the trachea with air in order to provide a contrast with the soft tissues surrounding it.

Use of the Valsalva manoeuvre has traditionally been advocated for use with projections of the thoracic inlet, but this action may be difficult while the patient is being asked to maintain a particular position. It must therefore be suggested that the Valsalva manoeuvre is exercised with caution in the patient who is standing erect. It must also be considered that, since the trachea is a structure that does not naturally rest with closed walls, like the oesophagus, it will in fact always contain air even if the patient's lungs are not in an inspirational phase. So, for lower thoracic inlet demonstration, is the Valsalva maneouvre actually necessary?

Collimation

C4–T6 longitudinally, lateral soft tissue outlines of the neck

Criteria for assessing image quality

- Trachea down to its bifurcation and lateral soft tissue outlines of the neck are demonstrated
- Spinous processes of vertebrae and the trachea are demonstrated down the centre of the vertebral bodies and medial ends of clavicles equidistant from the spinous process
- Mandible and occiput are superimposed
- Sharp image demonstrating air-filled trachea in contrast to the soft tissue of neck and vertebral column

Common errors	Possible reasons
Symmetrical dense white shadow of occiput obscuring upper trachea	Chin raised too high
Symmetrical shadow of mandible obscuring upper trachea	Chin not raised enough
Asymmetrical shadow of occiput and/or mandible superimposed over upper neck	Head is rotated. If appearances are accompanied by rotation of the trunk (see next comments below) the whole of the MSP is incorrectly positioned
Trachea not centralised over vertebral column	MSP not perpendicular to IR or some deviation may be due to external common compression (for example in cases of thyroid enlargement). This, of course, is not due to radiographer error

Lateral upper respiratory tract and thoracic inlet (Fig. 23.17A,B)

Positioning

- A lead rubber apron is applied to the patient's waist
- The patient stands erect with their MSP parallel to the IR; the feet are slightly separated for stability. This projection may be undertaken with the patient sitting
- The chin is raised until the mandible is cleared as far as possible from the upper trachea
- The shoulders are relaxed downwards to clear them from the inlet into the thorax

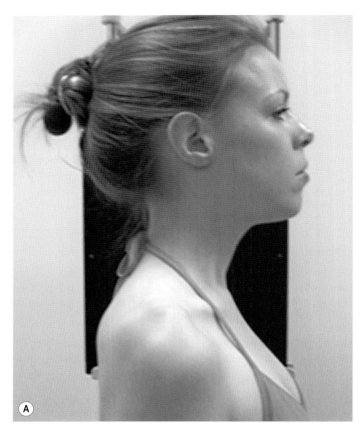
(A)

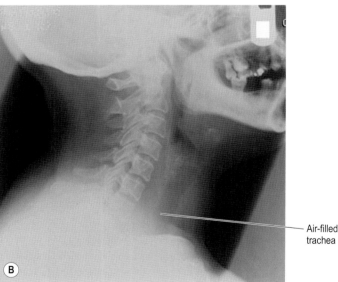
(B)
Air-filled trachea

Figure 23.17 Lateral upper respiratory tract.

Beam direction and FRD

Horizontal

200 cm FRD

This is an increase from the 100 cm used for the PA projection. It aims to reduce magnification of the trachea, which lies further from the IR owing to the shoulder's position against the IR

Centring

To the middle of the neck, at the level of the thyroid eminence

Collimation

Nasopharynx and down to include medial end of clavicle, anterior soft tissue outline, vertebral bodies of cervical vertebrae, T1

Good collimation, avoiding irradiation of the orbits, can be improved by slightly rotating the light beam diaphragm so that its long axis follows the angle of the neck.

Expose on arrested inspiration

Criteria for assessing image quality

- Nasopharynx, oropharynx, upper trachea, medial end of clavicle and anterior aspect of soft tissues of neck are demonstrated
- Mandible is elevated to clear it from as much of the trachea as possible (but there will still be some superimposition)
- Sharp image demonstrating air-filled trachea in contrast to the soft tissue of the neck. The vertebral column will be underpenetrated

Common error	Possible reason
Soft tissue shadow obscuring clavicle and trachea	Poor patient posture during exposure (shoulders not relaxed). This may be a problem with kyphosed patients

Lateral lower trachea and thoracic inlet

(Fig. 23.18A,B,C)

A grid may be used for this technique

Positioning

- A lead rubber apron is applied to the patient's waist
- The patient stands erect with their MSP parallel to the IR; the feet are slightly separated for stability. This projection may be undertaken with the patient sitting
- The arms are extended and raised either side of the head, until vertical. The chin is raised to further effect this manoeuvre, which aims to clear the humeral heads from the retrosternal area of the trachea

The method described for clearance of humeral heads from the area of interest is contrary to those previously described,[15] where the hands are clasped behind the back and the shoulders pulled back (Fig. 23.18B). This method is difficult for many patients, particularly those with degenerative disease of the joints and some who are overweight. The method using raised arms has previously been suggested as an alternative for patients with stiff shoulders[14] and is a viable first choice owing to its easy implementation. It must be remembered, however, that failure to raise the chin adequately and bring the arms vertical will limit the effectiveness of the manoeuvre.

Beam direction and FRD

Horizontal
200 cm FRD

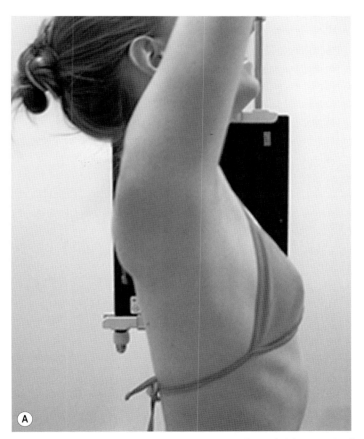
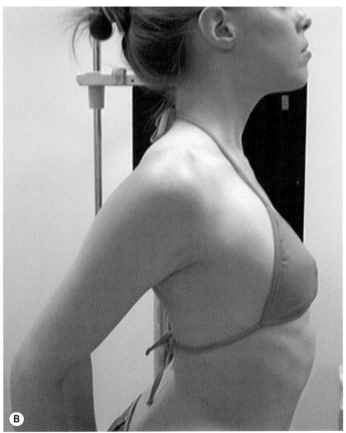

Figure 23.18 Lateral lower trachea and thoracic inlet with (A) arms raised and (B) arms pulled back.

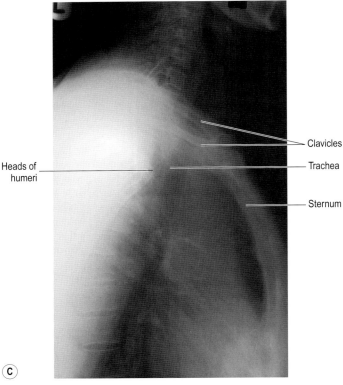

Heads of humeri

Clavicles

Trachea

Sternum

(C)

Figure 23.18, Continued (C) Lateral lower trachea and thoracic inlet.

As for the lateral of the upper region, this FRD is selected to counteract magnification caused by increased object–receptor distance (ORD).

Centring

Below the sternal notch, at the level of the sternal angle

Collimation

Thyroid eminence and carina of trachea, soft tissue anterior to trachea in neck and thorax, bodies of cervical vertebrae, lung tissue posteriorly

It is important that the whole of the trachea is demonstrated by the combination of the two lateral projections described for the trachea and thoracic inlet. As a result, the crossover area, which is that of the inlet of the trachea into the thorax level with the sternal notch, must be seen adequately on both images. Because two exposures are made this has implications for dose to the patient; it is possible to undertake one projection of the whole area, using a high kVp technique and centring at the level of C6–C7 while collimating to include the whole of the trachea.[18]

Expose on arrested inspiration

Criteria for assessing image quality

- Trachea from above the sternal notch down to its bifurcation, manubrium sterni, lung tissue anterior and posterior to the trachea are demonstrated
- Soft tissue of shoulders and heads of humeri are cleared from the trachea
- Sharp image demonstrating air-filled trachea in contrast to the lung tissue, clavicle and manubrium

Common error	Possible reason
Density overlying trachea on image	Arms and shoulders inadequately raised or not pulled back

REFERENCES

1. RCR Working Party. Making the best use of a clinical radiology services: guidelines for referrers. 6th ed. London: The Royal College of Radiologists; 2007.
2. The Ionising Radiation (Medical Exposure) Regulations 2006. London: HMSO; 2006.
3. Radiation Protection 118. Referral Guidelines for Imaging. Luxembourg: European Commission; 2000.
4. https://audit.rcplondon.ac.uk/fbh/files/a%20to%20z.pdf.
5. Scally P. Medical imaging. Oxford: Oxford University Press; 1999.
6. World Health Organization factsheet on TB. http://www.who.int/mediacentre/news/releases/2007/pr08/en/index.html.
7. World Health Organization Report. Global tuberculosis control. Geneva: WHO; 2003.
8. Pedrazzoli D, et al. Tuberculosis in the UK: Annual report on tuberculosis surveillance in the UK. Health Protection Agency; 2011. Available at: www.hpa.org.uk.
9. European Commission. European guidelines on quality criteria for diagnostic radiographic images. Brussels: Office for Official Publications of the European Communities; 1996.
10. Sjovall A. (*Correspondence*) PA chest films. British Journal of Radiology 1982;55:168.
11. Smith RF. (*Correspondence*). Radiography 1982;April:80.
12. Dimmick R. (*Correspondence*). Radiography 1981;March:79.
13. Clark KC. Positioning in radiography. 4th to 10th ed. London: Heinemann; 1945–79.
14. Unett EM, Royle AJ. 1997. Radiographic techniques and image evaluation. London: Chapman and Hall; 1997.
15. Swallow RA, et al. Clark's positioning in radiography. 11th ed. London: Heinemann; 1986.
16. Ballinger PW, Frank ED. Merrill's atlas of radiographic positioning and radiologic procedures. 10th ed. St Louis: Mosby; 2003.
17. Watkins P. A practical guide to chest imaging. Edinburgh: Churchill Livingstone; 1984.

18. Bontrager K, Lampignano JP. Textbook of radiographic positioning and related anatomy. 7th ed. St Louis: Mosby; 2010.

19. Unett E, Carver B. The chest X-ray: centring points and central rays – can we stop confusing our students and ourselves? Synergy 2001;Nov:14–7.

20. Unett E, Carver B. The chest X-ray: centring points and central rays – can we stop confusing our students and ourselves? Synergy 2001;Dec:8–9.

21. Meholic A, et al. Fundamentals of chest radiology. Philadelphia: WB Saunders; 1996.

22. McQuillen Martensen K. Radiographic Image analysis. 3rd ed. Philadelphia: WB Saunders; 2010.

23. Chotas H, Ravin C. Chest radiography: estimated lung volume and projected area obscured by the heart, mediastinum and diaphragm. Radiology 1994;193:403–4.

Chapter 24

Abdomen

Elizabeth Carver

Plain radiography of the abdomen is often used for assessment of gross anatomical deviation, such as displacement of organs in the case of abdominal tumours or obstruction of the alimentary tract. Information on the urinary system can be provided by the plain abdominal image, preceding other imaging procedures, also providing information on gross anatomical deviation within the urinary system. The appearance of radio-opaque calculi will be demonstrated on the image but urography, ultrasound, radionuclide imaging or computed tomography (CT) will be required to provide information on renal function, site of urinary obstruction or extent of obstruction. The role of these imaging methods in genitourinary investigations is considered in Chapter 31.

Supine abdomen (Fig. 24.1)

Image receptor (IR) is horizontal, used with antiscatter grid

Positioning

- The patient is supine with the arms slightly abducted from the trunk
- The median sagittal plane (MSP) is coincident with the long axis of the table and the centre of the bucky
- Lead rubber or lead gonad protection is applied, below the symphysis pubis, to male gonads
- Anterior superior iliac spines (ASISs) are equidistant from the table-top
  - The iliac crests are level with the middle of the IR, *or*
  - Using the calibrated markings on the light beam diaphragm, collimate to the IR boundary: ensure that the lower edge of collimation lies below the lower border of the symphysis pubis
- Because of magnification, owing to the significant distance from the symphysis pubis to the IR, the symphysis pubis should lie well above the lower boundary of the IR
- Central ray and the middle of IR should be accurately aligned

Beam direction and focus receptor distance (FRD)

Vertical, at 90° to the IR
100–120 cm FRD, selected to ensure magnification is at its minimum and include the maximum amount of abdominal tissue on the image

Centring

Positioning for (a) over a point in the midline of the abdomen, level with the iliac crests
  Note that this point refers to the actual *highest point of the crests at the back*, rather than the lower level palpated on the lateral aspect of the abdomen.
Positioning for (b) is to the centre of the IR
  The midline of the abdomen, or MSP, can be identified by palpating the middle of the upper border of the symphysis pubis and the xiphisternum. The line joining these surface markings will represent the position of the MSP.

Collimation

Symphysis pubis, as much upper abdomen as possible, lateral soft tissue outlines

Comments on centring, collimation and area of interest

It has been stated that the 11th thoracic vertebra should be included in the collimated field as it lies above the renal outlines and at the tip of the right lower lobe of liver and spleen.[1] It is noted that in most adults this would not usually allow for the inclusion of all the upper abdominal contents; however, with the exception of examination of the upper gastrointestinal tract, ultrasound is the most appropriate imaging modality for the upper abdomen. This would negate the necessity for the inclusion of abdominal tissue immediately below the diaphragm. When the supine abdomen position is used to demonstrate the kidneys, ureter and bladder, and additional abdominal information is not required, lateral collimation can be made to the ASIS on each side to more effectively reduce radiation dose.

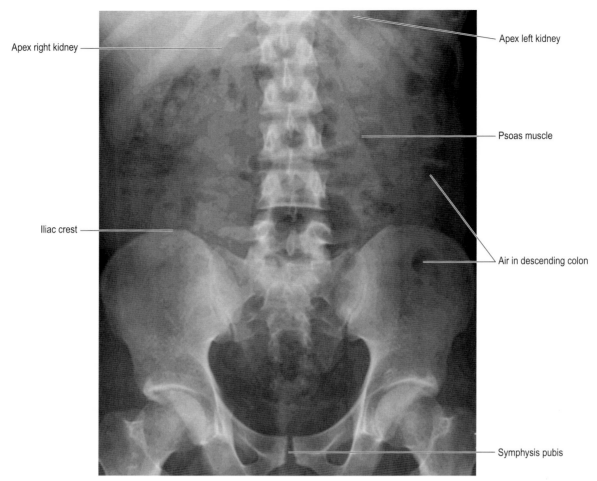

Apex right kidney

Apex left kidney

Psoas muscle

Iliac crest

Air in descending colon

Symphysis pubis

Figure 24.1 Supine abdomen.

Traditionally a specific centring point has been given when describing the anteroposterior (AP) supine abdomen. This has usually been stated as level with the iliac crests in the midline, as in centring (a), above.[2] Unfortunately, the continuing trend for an increase in average height, noted especially in Europe and the Western world and estimated to be increasing by between 10 and 30 mm per decade,[3] affects the amount of body tissue that can now realistically be included on the image. Although the iliac crests do appear midway between the diaphragm and symphysis pubis on the image, centring point (a) will only be useful in smaller patients, i.e. those whose abdominal tissue will actually 'fit' within the maximum receptor length. Selection of the centring point/positioning method will therefore depend upon the radiographer's assessment of the patient's size.

An additional complication occurs with larger patients, whose adipose tissue will cause further elevation of the symphysis pubis above the table-top; this increases the effect of magnification, potentially adding to the risk of the image of the symphysis being projected below the lower border of the IR. Using the suggested method (b) of centring will reduce the risk of projecting the symphysis pubis off the lower end of the image in these cases.

Compensation for magnification may be made by increasing the FRD,[4] but this may still not be effective enough for very tall patients. Unfortunately, in these cases it may be necessary to undertake an additional projection of the upper abdomen if it is essential to include this area in the examination. Indeed, it has been suggested that the hypersthenic patient requires two, separately centred, abdomen images.[5] This does seem somewhat excessive and would result in a higher radiation dose to the patient than undertaking an additional, well-collimated, upper abdomen projection.

With regard to the increase in average height of a population, it is a positive step that larger image receptors are becoming increasingly available. Unfortunately, not all manufacturers currently offer the 35 × 47 cm IR as an option; hopefully this will change in the future.

Expose on arrested respiration during exposure

Clearly, exposure must be made on arrested respiration to reduce the risk of movement unsharpness on the image, caused by the shift of abdominal organs during diaphragmatic movement. There is a range of recommendations regarding the phase of respiration to suspend,[1,6] and questions regarding the most appropriate choice arise from this. Suspension of respiration after exhalation cannot be excluded as it facilitates lower density of abdominal tissue, necessitating the selection of lower exposure factors and hence reducing dose compared to exposure in the opposite phase of respiration.

Unfortunately, when this issue is considered alongside that of the tall patient, as discussed above, it can be argued that exhalation will exacerbate the problems of including all the required area on the image.

Therefore, the concept of exposure on arrested inspiration to compress abdominal contents into an apparently shorter area may become more acceptable, as it reduces the area covered by the abdominal contents (i.e. the area from the diaphragm to the symphysis pubis), increasing the chance of a single exposure examination. This is clearly an opportunity for the reflective practitioner to base their decision on practice using a benefit-versus-risk approach.

Criteria for assessing image quality

- Symphysis pubis, as much of the upper abdomen as possible, and lateral soft tissue outlines of the abdomen are included on image
- Spinous processes of vertebrae seen coincident with the midline of the image and centralised and aligned down the middle of the vertebral bodies
- Symmetry of the iliac crests
- Sharp image demonstrating soft tissue in contrast with bowel gas and bony structures

Note that scoliosis will affect the symmetry of the vertebral column and position of the vertebrae coincident with the long axis of the film. It is distinguishable from rotation due to position error by the distinct lateral curve of the column and potential variation of rotation down its length.[1] If inclusion of the relevant body area on the image is acceptable, a repeat should not be considered. In the case of positional rotation it must be remembered that correction will be possible and will improve accuracy in the appearance of organ position within the abdominal cavity.

Common errors	Possible reasons
Symphysis pubis is not included on the image	Inaccurate centring/positioning or tall patient? Centring point at the level of the iliac crests may have been used. Try centring method (b)
Upper abdomen is not included; symphysis pubis is well above the lower edge of the film	May have been centred using the lateral borders of iliac crest rather than the highest point at the back
Vertebral column is not coincident with the midline of the film	Xiphisternum to symphysis line is inaccurately positioned or scoliotic patient
Spinous processes are not demonstrated in the midline of the vertebral bodies	MSP is not perpendicular to the table-top; palpate ASIS to ensure it is equidistant from the table or the patient is scoliosed

Erect abdomen

Validity of use of this projection

The erect abdomen has traditionally been requested to diagnose/exclude obstruction of the bowel, alimentary perforation or the effects of stab injury. The erect position allows air to rise above fluid levels in the obstructed bowel where the inferior level of the air shadow appears flat, or under the right diaphragm in cases of perforation. Towards the close of the 20th century the validity of requests for the erect abdomen examination began to be questioned, as it was recognised that other projections demonstrate appearances suggestive of obstruction or perforation. More specifically, in the case of the supine acute abdomen, these appearances are:[7]

- *Sentinel loop sign*: an isolated loop of distended bowel indicates the effects of inflammatory processes such as appendicitis or pancreatitis, causing ileus
- *Dilated small bowel loops*: indicate small bowel obstruction. Loops are centrally sited and there is absence of faecal matter; eventually the distal bowel becomes airless as it collapses, but the stomach may still contain air. Air in the distended small bowel may appear as a ladder or stack of coins
- *Dilated colon*: points to obstruction. Dilation of the colon with air is noted, up to the site of obstruction. The bowel is much distended, with distended haustra, and the appearances are notable around the edges of the abdomen, rather than the more centralised loops as in the case of obstructed small bowel
- *Volvulus*: obstruction appears as a distended portion of looped bowel. The obstruction is caused by the closed ends of the loop, which may have a 'coffee bean' appearance.

As the right diaphragm lies at a higher level than the left, in cases of perforation gas or air in the peritoneal cavity will rise to lie under the right diaphragm. The appearance is that of a dark line under the diaphragm, often following its curve, created by the contrast of the gas itself against the dense abdominal tissue. In addition, it should be remembered that heart and chest disease – myocardial infarction, dissecting aortic aneurysm, pneumonia and pulmonary embolism in particular – may give rise to symptoms that mimic an 'acute abdomen'.[7] Is there a need to irradiate the whole abdomen simply to demonstrate the subdiaphragmatic area? Probably not. This is largely supported by guidelines from the Royal College of Radiologists in their referral guidelines for imaging, where a supine abdomen accompanied by an erect chest examination is recommended for patients with symptoms suggestive of the acute abdomen; however, these guidelines do suggest that an erect abdomen examination may be considered if strongly suspected obstruction is not confirmed on a supine abdomen image. A lateral decubitus projection of the abdomen *is* suggested if the patient cannot be examined erect for the chest film in cases of suspected perforation;[8] this projection is described in Chapter 29. The erect chest radiograph itself should not be forgotten as a useful projection for this region: apparent upper abdominal pain can be due to lower lobe pneumonia and an erect chest radiograph will provide evidence of either, on one image and with one exposure, which uses lower exposure factors than those for an abdomen radiograph. Prior to positioning and exposure, the patient must always have been in an erect position for at least 5 minutes to allow air to rise to the highest point in the abdominal cavity.

For infirm patients, an erect projection of the chest can be attempted in the AP position with the patient sitting supported, in bed or on a trolley (Ch. 23). For some patients even this will prove difficult; in these cases a left lateral decubitus (right side raised) projection of the upper abdomen can be undertaken. This is described in Chapter 29 on the examination of the gastrointestinal tract.

Positioning

IR is vertical, used with an antiscatter grid

- The patient is sitting, or standing erect with legs separated for stability
- MSP is perpendicular to the IR and coincident with its long axis
- The middle of the IR is level with the iliac crests or its upper border should include the upper abdomen if this area is required

Beam direction and FRD

Horizontal, at 90° to the IR
FRD 100–120 cm, selected to ensure magnification is at its minimum and include the maximum amount of abdominal tissue on the image

Centring

To the centre of the IR

Collimation

As much upper abdomen as possible, lateral soft tissue outlines
The symphysis pubis need not be included as it should be included on the supine abdomen projection.

Exposure factors

Exposure factors will require an increase from the supine AP projection, to allow for increased density due to sagging of the abdominal tissue in this position.

Image quality

Image quality is assessed as for the supine abdomen, but there may be a reduction in contrast compared to the AP projection, due to increased exposure factors and abdomen sag. The symphysis pubis need not be included.

REFERENCES

1. McQuillen Martensen K. Radiographic image analysis. 3rd ed. Philadelphia: WB Saunders; 2010.
2. Eisenberg R, et al. Radiographic positioning. 2nd ed. Boston: Little Brown and Company; 1995.
3. Cole TJ. Secular trends in growth. Proceedings of the Nutrition Society 2000;59(2):317–24.
4. Gunn C. Radiographic imaging: a practical approach. 3rd ed. Edinburgh: Churchill Livingstone; 2002.
5. Bontrager K, Lampignano JP. Textbook of radiographic positioning and related anatomy. 7th ed. St Louis: Mosby; 2010.
6. Swallow RA, et al. Clark's positioning in radiography. 11th ed. London: Heinemann; 1986.
7. Nicholson DA, Driscoll PA. ABC of emergency radiology. Cambridge: BMJ Publishing; 1995.
8. RCR Working Party. Making the best use of a clinical radiology services: guidelines for referrers. 6th ed. London: The Royal College of Radiologists; 2007.

Section | 4 |

Accident and emergency

Chapter 25

Accident and emergency

Darren Wood, Elizabeth Carver

This chapter will evaluate the position of the imaging professional within the multidisciplinary team, consider the advancing role of the radiographer, and review how an understanding of injury mechanisms and pattern recognition informs the choice of projection and technique adaptation in the traumatised patient. Special considerations for techniques, in addition to choice of radiographic equipment, will also be considered for this wide field of service provision.

THE ROLE OF THE RADIOGRAPHER IN THE MULTIDISCIPLINARY TEAM

The progression of highlighting abnormalities through the use of a 'red dot' system[1] has been well documented, and by 2004 a national survey showed that 81% of hospital trusts/boards were using this aspect of role development.[2] Alongside this, the development of the advanced trauma and life support (ATLS)[3] approach to dealing with the patient with multiple injuries and the inception of the four-tier system[4] of working in the UK have advanced the position of the radiographer within the accident and emergency (A&E) multidisciplinary team. Gradual development of service provision through advanced training, to create the reporting radiographer, has further ensured the value of this team member in the A&E department.

The role of the reporting radiographer has ensured that an invaluable service can now be provided instantly in the A&E department. Acting as report writer, advanced A&E imaging practitioner, advisor to junior radiographic staff or students and other professionals in the multidisciplinary team, the reporting radiographer keys in neatly with (at a minimum) the advanced practitioner or consultant practitioner level of the 'four-tier' system of work that has evolved during the first part of the 21st century. Moving forward with this, the current recommendations are for radiographers to give an initial interpretation of their image by issuing a comment;[5] this aspect will be discussed later in this chapter.

Although the advanced practitioner may be seen as a key representative for imaging within the multidisciplinary team, it should be remembered that the radiographer has a developing responsibility to ensure they contribute fully to the trauma service. As a member of the ATLS team, the imaging practitioner must take command of their aspect of the service provided for the patient. A highly experienced team may not necessarily always provide this service and, in a stressful situation, the radiographer must control their contribution through being confident and assertive; this ensures that a good outcome is achieved while maintaining safety for patients and the wider ATLS team. In this way the radiographer becomes an advocate for all those who come into contact with ionising radiation in the resuscitation room.

It is not only in the ATLS situation that the radiographer will display the versatility to cope with the demands of the varied A&E patient presentations, across widely ranging age groups and varying requirements for adaptation of techniques. The radiographer also displays their value to the multidisciplinary team for all A&E cases in which they are involved. However, admitting a lack of knowledge or ability should not be seen as a suggestion of general inability; examples of this are most likely to lie in unusual circumstances, difficult patient presentations or difficulty with highlighting perceived abnormalities. Admission of lack of knowledge or ability, and acceptance that another more experienced or skilled member of the team may provide a better service, is the most responsible and appropriate action for this situation. This may be reflected in discussing A&E images, or requests for imaging, with the referrer or radiologist so that the best patient outcome may be achieved. Also, knowledge and its application in the form of advising alternative imaging, perhaps with a protocol-driven application of the Ionising Radiation (Medical Exposure) Regulations [IR(ME)R 2006],[6] is further evidence of the extended service provision of the radiographer within the multidisciplinary team. Indeed, acting as a gatekeeper of ionising radiation exposure to the general public is one of the more demanding roles, expected even of the newly qualified radiographer.

It is necessary that the radiography professional understands the following:

- Trauma mechanisms
- Most common injury presentations associated with trauma mechanisms
- How trauma mechanism and presentation may influence projection or technique selection
- How trauma mechanism and presentation may influence technique adaptation, in varied situations

Being able to draw on a wide experience base that has been developed through reflection upon practice (be this formalised or in an intuitive way) is another expectation of the A&E radiographer. With this in mind, it is the professional and medicolegal responsibility of radiographers to ensure that they maintain and continually develop their skills. Ensuring participation in continuing professional development (CPD) is paramount for even the most experienced, and this is reinforced by Health Professions Council (HPC) requirements that radiographers must show evidence of ongoing CPD, in order to maintain registration with HPC.

The team role of the radiographer: image interpretation

The 'red dot'[7] system has become an accepted norm for the practising radiographer and features in many undergraduate radiography courses in the UK, along with a move towards providing initial comment on images.

The radiographer's expertise in image appreciation begins with their ability to evaluate images for quality purposes, and one of the main purposes of this text is to promote a logical and systematic approach to this. During quality evaluation the radiographer will recognise pathologies or abnormalities, and so they are already effectively commenting to themselves or colleagues prior to the application of a red dot. The application of a number of basic pointers makes image review possible:

- Correct patient identifier
- Correct anatomical marker
- Correct area included (on all projections)
- Correct radiographic position
- Adequate exposure factors used (for contrast, density and sharpness)

These pointers apply to all radiographic images and relate to the structures used in this text, which are projection specific rather than broad in their application. As the image produced should be of a diagnostic standard, implementation of these checks is vital before the radiographer can comment on abnormal appearances adequately and with confidence. As for image quality assessment, there are some basic pointers to enable accurate assessment of the image for identification of any pathologies/abnormalities:

- Assess the whole area,[8] avoiding the urge to focus on the 'obvious'
- Examine the cortical outline and trabecular pattern[8,9] (follow the outline of the bone, assess for disruption)
- Look at the soft tissue[9,10] (any change may indicate a subtle fracture)
- Check radiographic lines, zones and arcs[10] (for this the radiographer needs to be aware of the basics and how to use them)
- Research any previous/recent imaging[10]

Using these basic pointers will enable radiographers to expertly analyse images so as to be able to pass comment on them; when commenting systems are introduced this is likely to lead to the issue of training, so that the comments follow a standardised format. With the aid of reporting radiographers and radiologists this should prove to be a simple issue.

The introduction of a commenting system must be logically presented to all involved, from referral to image retrieval, so that practitioner and referrer are aware that this is not a *final report* but rather the opinion of a professional within their own field; it should be used as an aid by the referrer in deciding on a final diagnosis. A system where all radiographers are expected to participate will give the referrers more confidence in that system, especially compared to the 'red dot' scheme where radiographers may have opted out of making a decision, putting the onus on to the clinician/referrer. In addition to a suitable design, the success of such a system will require continued review and audit.

It may be difficult to ascertain the medicolegal position of a commenting system unless a test case were to be presented. Even if a radiographer is not held responsible in civil proceedings, there is no reason why disciplinary or professional conduct hearings would not find the radiographer guilty of negligent conduct in situations relating to comments on anatomical appearances, if the employer has implemented a suitable framework for a commenting scheme. Vicarious liability by the employing hospital trust expects reasonable standards of care to have been exercised when supporting its employees in the execution of their duties. This includes operating within recognised protocols, working to professional standards, and also, on the part of the employer, the provision of appropriate educational support and safe working practices agreed by all participants.[11]

Similarly, radiographers who provide a reporting service, and have necessarily undergone significant postgraduate education, should offer the same standard of report; it is not acceptable to provide a lower standard of report simply because they are not radiologists.[12]

The team role of the radiographer: suitable equipment choice

Experience also plays a significant role in the activities of service provision, especially on the ancillary equipment selection front. Frequently, this type of equipment for support to the A&E imaging department is often selected without including the radiographer in the purchasing exercise. As an example, the choice of trolleys that are widely used across disciplines often results in difficulties not only for radiology staff but also for the patient and the wider team in the A&E department. In the end, a poor-quality service is often delivered because of a lack of foresight in operating as a cohesive team. Holistic care demands cooperation across boundaries seen as traditional divides; however, borders are created where they are inappropriate.[4] This is a particular problem where professions that form the minority in an area of operation are perceived as lacking in appreciation for what is best for that department area or the patient. Advocacy for the patient and service can take many different forms that are frequently not recognised.

MECHANISMS OF INJURY

A range of reasons exists as to why patients present in A&E. Certain patterns of trauma present themselves time and again, i.e. the 'common occurrences', although some injuries present after apparently minor trauma or as a result of seemingly ridiculous circumstances. Probably the most famous of all causes of injury is the 'fall onto outstretched hand' or FOOSH. Another commonly encountered trauma involves twisting of the ankle, which generates injury patterns which are linked, as force is transmitted along the whole of the leg. Certain age groups, because of their involvement in specific activities, or alternatively as a result of pathological processes influencing bone integrity, display unexpectedly severe presentations of injury following apparently innocuous trauma forces. Table 25.1 attempts to draw together injuries linked to the mechanism so that potential plain film skeletal imaging projections can be determined and expected injury patterns anticipated.

An awareness of the developmental anatomy of the skeleton is important, as injury patterns change with age. Young children may

Table 25.1 Mechanism of injury related to examination requirements

Mechanism	Part injured	Projections	Additional or alternative projections	Alternative imaging
FOOSH	Carpometacarpal joint	DP, DPO, lateral hand	Ball catcher's projection to show discreet fractures of the base of the fifth metacarpal	
	Scaphoid Distal radius (Colles' fracture)	PA wrist/scaphoid with ulnar deviation PA oblique scaphoid Lateral wrist/scaphoid PA with forearm raised 30° (see Fig. 5.24A) PA and lateral wrist	If scapholunate dissociation stress projections similar to standard scaphoid images may be needed later, as treatment effectiveness is assessed PA oblique wrist	RNI or MRI for occult scaphoid fracture MRI or US for suspected ligament damage
	Radial head	AP and lateral elbow	Specific radial head projections (see Chapter 6)	
	Glenohumeral joint	AP shoulder Axial or Y view of scapula	Modified axials as described and discussed in Chapter 7	CT, MRI or US to evaluate for Bankart lesion of glenoid labrum or rotator cuff damage
	Acromioclavicular joint	AP A/C joint		US or MRI for long standing injury – used also to evaluate rotator cuff
	Coracoid process	AP of shoulder region	Inferosuperior coracoid (AP with 20–30° cranial angle)	
Inversion at ankle	Ankle	AP and lateral ankle	30° internal oblique ankle (mortice) or external oblique ankle Stress projections for ligament integrity evaluation	US to examine ligament integrity
	Base of fifth metatarsal	DP and DPO foot		US may be used to evaluate peroneus brevis or related ligaments
	Neck of fibula	AP and lateral tibia and fibula		
Falls from a height	Calcaneum	Axial and lateral calcaneum	Standing axial (if possible) Subtalar oblique projections	CT to evaluate fracture fragments
	Ankle	AP and lateral ankle		CT to evaluate fracture fragments
	Pelvis	AP pelvis Lateral hip (if indicated – see related discussion, Chapter 10)	Judet's view of acetabulum Sacrum/sacroiliac joint	CT to evaluate fracture component relationship/3D reconstruction
	All spinal regions	AP and lateral of spinal region (see Chapter 11 for discussion on C spine)	Obliques	CT to evaluate fracture component relationship/3D reconstruction
Flexion/ extension or compression of spine	Cervical spine	Odontoid process (open mouth) AP and lateral (see Chapter 11 for discussion on C spine)	Obliques Flexion and extension laterals if neck is stable Lateral skull for ?C1 crush injury	CT and MRI to evaluate bone fracture relations and soft tissue damage respectively (see Chapter 11 for discussion on C spine)
Flexion/ extension or compression of spine	Thoracic spine	AP and lateral		CT and MRI to evaluate bone fracture relations and soft tissue damage respectively
	Lumbar spine	AP and lateral		CT and MRI to evaluate bone fracture relations and soft tissue damage respectively
Rotation forces	Knee	AP and lateral	Intercondylar notch Internal/external obliques of knee	
	Elbow	AP and lateral	Modified AP, for the elbow in flexion as described and discussed later in this chapter	CT to evaluate fracture component relationships; US to evaluate ligament damage; MRI for longer-term soft tissue damage evaluation
	All spinal regions	AP and lateral	Oblique projections of area as required to evaluate intervertebral articulations and vertebral foramina	CT to evaluate bone relations and soft tissue damage; MRI for soft tissue damage

not yet possess the skeletal components that generate adult injury characteristics, and indeed the maturity of bone may be responsible for causing variations in presentation. With their understanding of this, the radiographer can act as a resource of information for the referrer, so that an appropriate examination is embarked upon with least detriment to the child radiologically.

It is with all the above in mind, and the need to deal with the psychological aspects of the traumatised patient and accompanying relatives or friends, that the role of the radiographer is a wide-ranging one, acting as the advocate for holistic imaging management. Following recognition of the above it is appropriate to consider the more esoteric projections or adaptations to plain X-ray imaging that may be considered useful adjuncts to the trauma radiographer's range of skills.

FURTHER PROJECTIONS AND ADAPTED TECHNIQUES

Working around the patient in non-standard and trauma situations is one of the greater skills of the experienced A&E radiographer, and an understanding of how radiographic equipment or body parts may safely be moved to achieve the required positions is of major importance. As well as appreciating these subtleties, the radiographer has a further responsibility for ensuring that appropriate radiation protection methods can be achieved for the patient, staff or relatives who may have to be present in these situations. Good collimation, selection of appropriate imaging equipment and radiation protection techniques – all considered 'run of the mill' aspects of good practice – will require adaptation to ensure successful application. Clean technique approaches will also be required where open wounds present, with appropriate protection for the radiographer and supplementary considerations for equipment and the cleaning of this thereafter. Cling-film is sometimes used in the A&E department to wrap equipment, as protection against contamination from blood and other body fluids. Alternatively, plastic sheaths may be made for foam immobilisation pads or cassettes; care must be taken to ensure that these covers are kept clean and do not cause problems through artefact generation on images.

The upper limb

Common mistakes made in obtaining projections of the hand and fingers frequently occur as a result of the mistaken belief that the radiographer is being kinder to the patient by not causing excessive pain. Another example is when the radiographer attempts to obtain several finger projections in a single exposure. In both these instances it becomes immediately apparent that a less than acceptable image might be obtained, resulting in an increased risk of inaccurate diagnosis from the projection provided for radiological opinion. This lack of foresight and poor practice serves no purpose except to place the patient at risk and to lay the practitioner open to claims of negligent practice. Although hand injuries may not appear severe, the actual effects of the injury may be quite significant. By understanding this, the radiographer should realise that the highest standard of imaging possible must be achieved. This requires assertiveness (with respect to encouragement of achieving an ideal position when the patient may resist) in order to gain the best result, or adaptation of a technique to allow an image to be obtained in less than ideal circumstances. Further up the upper limb, towards the elbow and shoulder, similar demands surface to ensure that unambiguous radiographic representation of the traumatised limb or joint is achieved. Of particular concern are the supracondylar and radial head regions of the elbow,

and adequate evidence of the relatively rare, but easily missed, posteriorly dislocated shoulder is vital.

Adapted projections of the hand

Frequently the patient requiring hand radiography will present to the X-ray department on a trolley, as a result of shock after experiencing trauma and being able to see the effects of the damage inflicted upon the limb. It is possible that routine projections of the hand may be undertaken with the arm extended across onto a table or platform, but adaptation may be necessary if other injuries prevent this. At this point the radiographer must consider adapting technique to ensure a diagnostic image is produced, without the serious compromise of increased radiation dose to radiosensitive tissues. However, there are other methods of providing images of the hand, and this section identifies a range of these.

Lewis[13] identified a way to address the perceived problems of the inadequacy of hand projections by suggesting that the dorsipalmar (DP) projection is obtained with the forearm medially rotated at the elbow so that the ulnar border of the hand is lifted from the cassette surface. A 15° radiolucent foam pad is placed under this aspect of the hand to immobilise the limb and raise the medial portion of the hand (Fig. 25.1), with the remainder of the technique used following that of the DP hand described in Chapter 5.

As patients are often reluctant to flatten their hand and extend their fingers following trauma, or soft tissue swelling prevents this from happening, this small change to technique allows the interphalangeal, metacarpophalangeal and carpal joints to be displayed squarely so that a true representation of the bony relationships can be gathered. The elevation of the medial aspect of the hand also places the little finger and 5th metacarpal into a DP position, rather than the oblique position in which they lie in the routine DP hand position.

Lewis continues to make further suggestions about hand radiography that would improve visualisation of certain digits.[14] Of the thumb he makes the point that, in the normal anteroposterior (AP) and lateral projections, the thenar eminence and other structures medial to the thumb are frequently superimposed over the first metacarpophalangeal joint, preventing clear visualisation owing to imperfect

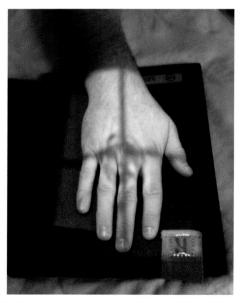

Figure 25.1 Clear joint presentation in the injured hand. Placing a 15° pad under the fifth metacarpal enhances the joint visualisation of the injured hand.

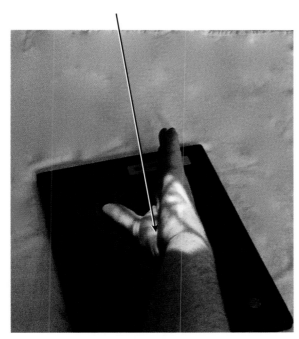

Figure 25.2 Angulation to clear the thenar eminences of the thumb. Angulation 10° cranially along the long axis of the first metacarpal ensures the thenar eminences do not superimpose and a good view of the articular surface of the metacarpal base is achieved.

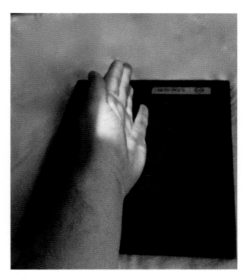

Figure 25.3 Fifth metacarpal neck projection. Slight over-rotation of the lateral hand allows visualisation of the neck of the fifth metacarpal. The thumb is further abducted before exposure.

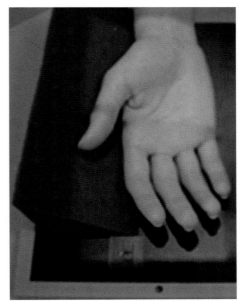

Figure 25.4 Ballcatcher's projection to show metacarpal heads tangentially.

achievement of radiographic density. He suggests, for the AP projection, that the radiographer simply angles the central X-ray beam 10–15° along the long axis of the thumb, towards the wrist, so that the soft tissue structures are projected away from the area of interest. Using this technique helps reveal the proximal joint region without juggling with exposure factors that may overexpose the distal part of the thumb while attempting to reveal the proximal aspect (Fig. 25.2). Quite frankly, the supine AP thumb technique described in Chapter 5 is probably most suitable, especially for the patient who presents on a trolley.

In a third suggestion about hand technique modifications Lewis describes another projection of the fifth metacarpal, a bone which is difficult to demonstrate owing to the anatomical relationship of the bones or soft tissues of the hand in the dorsipalmar oblique (DPO) or lateral projections.[15] He recommends further external rotation of the hand from the lateral position by an extra 5–10° so that the overlying second to fourth metacarpals no longer superimpose. The central ray is directed towards the middle of the fifth metacarpal and angled so that the ray is parallel with the thumb, which has been extended and abducted such that it does not overlie the fifth metacarpal (Fig. 25.3). Although an elongated projection is generated, almost the whole of the fifth metacarpal becomes visible.

Normally used for visualising the small joints of the fingers in the arthritic patient, the ballcatcher's[16] projection may be used to show the extent of damage in the 'fight bite' situation (Fig. 25.4). Puncture of the assailant's skin by the victim's tooth may lead to the development of osteomyelitis. Other than the clinical signs of the puncture wound or soft tissue swelling, little evidence of such an injury may be noted. However, the tangential representation of the metacarpal heads generated by this projection allows the viewer to see the indentation caused when the tooth has impacted with the metacarpal during a punching injury. The technique is described in Chapter 5, but it is not necessary to expose both hands and centring must be altered to coincide with the head of the third metacarpal, collimating to the single hand.

Adapted projections of the thumb

Injuries to the thumb are highly debilitating, as the ability to grip is compromised. Assessment of the integrity of the ulnar and radial collateral ligament at the metacarpophalangeal joint is achievable through the use of self-applied stressing forces in the posteroanterior (PA) thumb projection. This is achieved by using the index finger of the affected hand to generate adduction and abduction forces. The patient is asked to adduct the thumb by placing their index finger over the distal surface of the tip of the thumb and pulling it medially towards the finger; abduction is achieved by placing the tip of the index finger against the medial aspect of the tip of the thumb before pushing the tip of the thumb laterally, away from the index finger

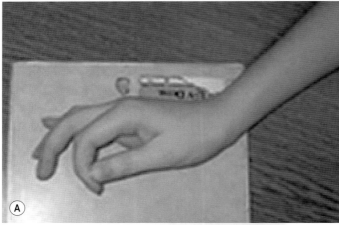

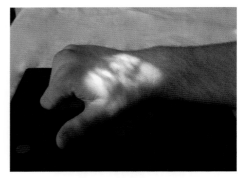

Figure 25.6 The Gedda–Billings lateral projection of the thumb. This projection gives an uninterrupted lateral perspective of the base of the first metacarpal.

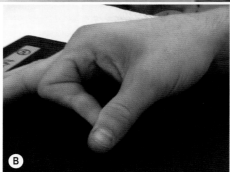

Figure 25.5 Stress projections of the thumb. (A) The stressed thumb is being pulled towards the hand by the index finger while (B) shows the opposite stressing force. These projections are used to show radial and ulnar collateral damage, respectively, around the first metacarpophalangeal joint.

(Fig. 25.5A,B). Through stressing in a horizontal direction, the ulnar and radial collateral ligaments are strained to reveal their integrity. Rupture is revealed by widening of the respective side of the metacarpophalangeal joint that is associated with the damaged ligament.

Should a true lateral projection of the base of the first metacarpal be required to reveal subtle fractures, the Gedda–Billings projection can be used.[17] Position as for the lateral thumb projection and angle the central ray 10° along the axis of the metacarpal, towards the forearm. This will free the articular surface from any superimposition over the trapezium (Fig. 25.6).

Adapted projections of the wrist and forearm

As noted with the hand, occasionally it is necessary to adapt the positioning of the patient to achieve the correct projection. One of the neatest tricks that may be used to obtain PA and lateral projections of the wrist is to encourage the patient to extend their arm and abduct it; this makes external rotation for the lateral projection easier. If the patient cannot externally rotate to a lateral position, the pronated hand and wrist can be raised onto a radiolucent pad, with the image receptor (IR) supported vertically against the medial aspect of the wrist; a horizontal beam is used lateromedially. Appropriate upper arm support may also be required with this technique. A mediolateral approach may be used if the arm cannot be abducted sufficiently to achieve the lateromedial technique, but care must be taken to avoid

irradiating the trunk unnecessarily. If it is not possible to move the forearm into a pronated position for the PA wrist projection, place the wrist in the lateral position and raise it onto a radiolucent pad with an image receptor (IR) supported vertically against the anterior aspect of the wrist, using a horizontal beam technique for the central ray. Where independent cassette-type IRs are not available and direct digital units are used, the arm and pad can be supported on a small table placed next to the vertical detector; if the patient is on a trolley then the trolley must be at 90° to the digital unit and the patient's arm fully abducted, to ensure that the trunk is not near the primary beam. An AP approach will be necessitated in this instance.

With an injury to the forearm it can be extremely difficult for the patient to assume the standard (anatomical position) attitude required for radiography. If this is the case the forearm is best treated as two separate objects for imaging, although the individual joint aspects will manifest themselves as correct radiographic presentations on the resultant images. Handling of the limb is recommended as follows (this requires shoulder movement, and the radiographer should ascertain that this is safely possible):

- At the commencement of positioning ensure the table is level with the shoulder
- Abduct the limb from the trunk at the shoulder, while encouraging the patient to extend their elbow so that the whole arm may be rested on the table-top
- Externally rotate the shoulder to bring the elbow joint into a true AP position as the arm is supinated
- Often when in this position the patient will naturally want to rest the arm, with the wrist very close to the lateral position; this will allow an AP elbow and lateral wrist projection to be obtained on one image. Clearly there will be crossover of the shaft of radius over the ulna
- After obtaining the previous image, the arm is internally rotated at the shoulder and the elbow flexed. The medial aspects of the upper arm and elbow are placed in contact with the table-top. The positions of radius and ulna in relation to the humerus do not alter. The forearm thus assumes a position that now generates lateral elbow and, through natural pronation of the hand, PA wrist projections. Again, there will be crossover over the radial and ulnar shafts
- For both positions described, centre to the mid forearm and collimate to include the whole of the lower forearm

Although this is not an anatomically correct approach, at least two views of the injured forearm at 90° to each other are obtained so that some approximation of the anatomical relationship can be gleaned (Fig. 25.7A,B).

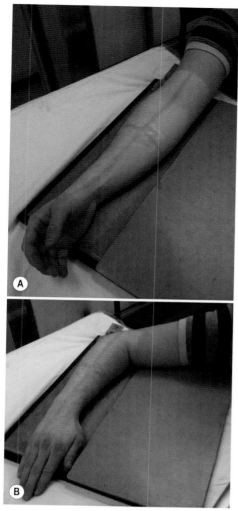

Figure 25.7 Trauma projections of the forearm. Non-standard positions of the forearm to aid the patient who is injured by obtaining projections that are (A) lateral wrist with AP elbow and (B) vice versa.

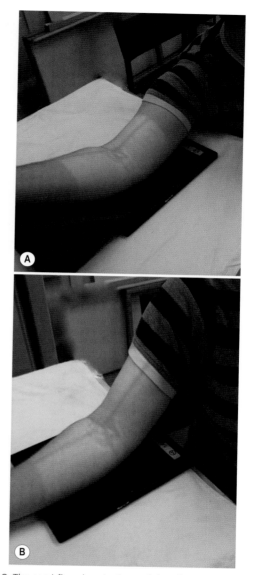

Figure 25.8 The semi-flexed projections of the elbow. Obtaining the semi-flexed elbow image from the frontal aspect as two separate projections allows the tangential viewing of the articular surfaces to be achieved thus providing a detailed examination of the injured joint.

Shoulder injury is likely to affect the ability to achieve some of the positions described above, and a horizontal beam technique (as those described for the wrist) may be required. This technique is highly valued in such limiting situations but is very dependent upon the position in which the patient's forearm and the IR can be supported. The approach must be taken from the perspective that minimal patient movement is required, and similar results can be obtained as indicated above with the least pain to the patient. However, care must be exercised with respect to achieving these projections without unnecessary exposure to primary radiation from the horizontal beam technique, as there are implications for its direction towards the trunk. Careful use of an appropriate thickness of lead rubber over the trunk, collimation, and turning the patient's head away from the X-ray tube are all essential measures that must not be ignored.

Adapted projections of the elbow and humerus

The elbow is one of the most difficult areas to examine adequately following trauma, owing to concerns about exacerbating possible neurovascular damage. Frequently the patient will present with the elbow partially flexed and will resist attempts to extend it for an AP

projection because of pain. To negotiate this problem individual images of each half of the elbow joint, i.e. proximal radius and ulna or distal humerus, should be obtained. In this way a relationship between major elbow components is noted and the articular surfaces are shown to advantage.[17] For AP images the posterior aspects of forearm and humeral portions of the elbow should be placed in contact with the IR in turn, thus allowing the radial and ulnar joint surfaces to be seen tangentially, or the trochlear/capitellar surfaces of the humerus to be displayed clearly, for each projection (Fig. 25.8A,B). A vertical central ray, or beam perpendicular to the joint portion of interest if a horizontal beam technique has to be used, is centred in turn at a point in the middle of the two articulation areas, i.e. over the proximal radioulnar joint for the proximal forearm and through the coronoid/olecranon fossa region for the distal humerus.

Patients with significant elbow injury may also present with the elbow held in full flexion as this guards against excessive pain. There is an association between this position and the likelihood of there

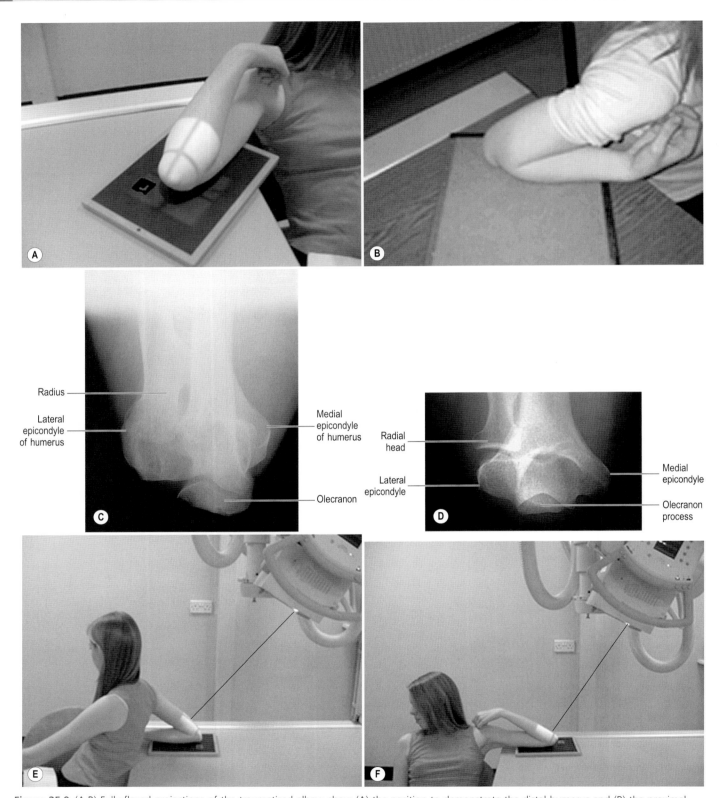

Figure 25.9 (A,B) Fully flexed projections of the traumatised elbow show (A) the position to demonstrate the distal humerus and (B) the proximal radius and ulna; (C) X-ray image of flexed elbow projection to demonstrate humerus; (D) X-ray image of flexed elbow projection to demonstrate radius and ulna; (E) elbow in flexion – upper arm in contact with receptor, with beam angulation – this projection will show proximal radius and ulna; (F) elbow in flexion – forearm in contact with IR, with beam angulation – this projection will show distal humerus.

being a fracture to the supracondylar region of the humerus, particularly in the younger patient. In these instances any attempt to extend the arm would be inappropriate, as it could cause further damage to the soft tissue structures in the area. The worst-case scenario would be permanent disability, as in Volkmann's ischaemic contracture. Instead of extending the elbow for the AP projection, take an image of the elbow with the arm still flexed but held in an AP distal humerus position, resting the posterior aspect of the upper arm on the cassette, which has been placed on the examination table. The upper arm should be positioned with the elbow level with the shoulder (Fig. 25.9A) and the vertical beam is centred midway between the humeral epicondyles. Collimate to the area of interest, but use exposure factors modified (increased) to allow for the greater thickness of the tissue overlying the elbow; higher kVp should be used to even out the range of densities that are required for demonstration. The distal radius and ulna can be similarly demonstrated in the flexed elbow by positioning the posterior aspect of the forearm in contact with the IR. This time the elbow and wrist lie in the same plane (Fig. 25.9B). Centring remains as for the projection for distal humerus, as do considerations for exposure factor selection.[18] Use of both projections may be necessary to demonstrate the elbow adequately (Figs 25.9C, D), but justification for this must be ascertained, as there are implications for radiation dose owing to the use of two exposures. It must be noted that the image of the elbow joint will not be as accurate as in the routine AP projection. However, elbow flexion *is* required for the lateral projection of the joint, and this projection is less likely to be compromised by the flexed elbow position. Positioning the arm into the correct position for the lateral is also relatively easy, thereby lessening the risk of further injury to the joint, but it must be remembered that the optimum flexion in this projection is 90° and incorrect flexion will affect fat pad appearance. Using an adapted technique to demonstrate the radial head, as described later in this chapter and in Chapter 6, is also possible with the elbow retained in a flexed position.

Still considering examination of the elbow in flexion, if the patient is unable to place the appropriate aspect of the arm in contact with the cassette (e.g. if information on radius and ulna is required, the patient is supine and cannot sit to put their forearm in contact with the IR, or if information on distal humerus is required and the posterior aspect of the upper arm carries significant abrasion), then the flexed elbow position can be modified. For proximal radius and ulna, when the posterior aspect of the forearm cannot be placed in contact with the IR, place the posterior aspect of the humerus in contact with the IR and use a beam angle perpendicular to the long axis of radius and ulna (Fig. 25.9E). For distal humerus, when it is not possible to place the posterior aspect of the upper arm in contact with the IR, place the posterior aspect of the forearm in contact with the IR and angle the central ray until it is perpendicular to the humerus (Fig. 25.9F). The centring point for each is midway between the humeral epicondyles. Note that the angle for either will vary greatly with each patient, due to variations in upper arm build, the degree of elbow flexion the patient holds the injured arm in, and the amount of abduction achievable at the shoulder.

Clearly the patient who presents on a trolley is unlikely to be able to sit next to a table for flexed elbow projections, but it is possible to reproduce them with the patient supine and the flexed joint positioned on the trolley, the arm abducted from the supine trunk (if cassette type IRs are used). In order to achieve projections fixed horizontal direct digital receptors should be used alongside the trolley and the arm abducted over the receptor. A horizontal beam technique may be necessary if the shoulder rotation needed to bring the elbow into the correct position is not possible; this would be appropriate for both AP and lateral projections. The elbow is supported on a radiolucent pad and the IR vertically positioned against the posterior aspect of the

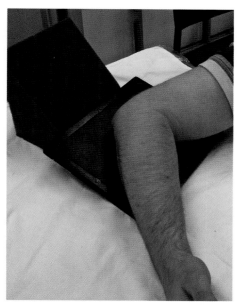

Figure 25.10 Reduced movement lateral projection of the elbow. Note the IR is supported obliquely to ensure a comfortable but accurately positioned limb. The hand and shoulder are in the same plane and the hand supported to maintain this. In this case a slight mediolateral angle will ensure that the beam is perpendicular to the IR. This projection can be used for trolley-bound patients.

humerus, as described for the modified projections of the wrist and forearm.

With more specific reference to the lateral projection for the injured elbow, obtaining a satisfactory lateral image frequently demands ingenuity in adaptation if the patient is unable to sit at the end of the table. The general rule, however, is to ensure that the elbow is supported on the IR so that the shoulder and elbow are at the same level, as in the routine lateral elbow position. This may be quite easy in a supine patient if the shoulder is mobile. However, it may not be possible to achieve this, even in a patient who is able to sit at the table, and often it is the extent of required external rotation at the shoulder that limits positioning; often the patient is limited to a position where their wrist and elbow joints lie lower than their shoulder. To reduce the effects of this, the lateral elbow projection can be modified by supporting the IR and arm with wedge-shaped pads and using a beam angle that will strike the IR at 90° (Fig. 25.10). Erect digital plate detector units are often versatile in that they can be angled to accommodate such modification. Similarly, the AP projection can be adapted so that it does not require the extent of external rotation at the shoulder. This is a horizontal beam approach where the elbow lies in a lateral position in relation to the table-top, but has the IR vertically behind its posterior aspect (Fig. 25.11). Again this may require the support of several foam immobilisation pads, and care should be taken to ensure that the arm lies parallel to the table-top.

When the patient cannot move their upper arm, but can stand or sit, a useful alternative technique for the lateral elbow projection is to position them erect PA and facing a vertical IR as if for a full lateral humerus projection. The flexed elbow, supported at the forearm by the hand of the uninjured side, should be abducted away from the body so that, viewed from the posterior aspect of the patient, the medial aspect of the elbow is visible (Fig. 25.12). This approach may also be adopted for the patient who might present on a trolley but is able to sit with their legs over the side. With the trolley placed close to the erect IR a similar result to that described may be obtained.

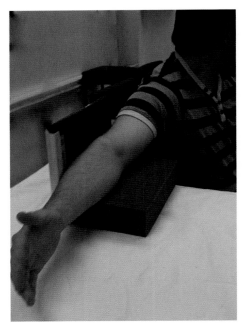

Figure 25.11 Horizontal beam AP projection of the elbow. This is used when the patient cannot externally rotate the shoulder for a routine AP, in conjunction with horizontal beam. This figure shows how the projection can be used for partially flexed elbows as well as extended elbows. The projection can be achieved for trolley-bound patients.

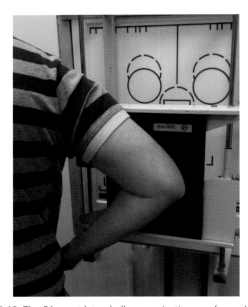

Figure 25.12 The PA erect lateral elbow projection, performed in much the same way as the lateral full length humerus.

Elbow injury that also involves the bones of the forearm is relatively common and frequently creates damage that may not be identified. Rotating the elbow externally from the true AP position so the humeral epicondyles lie at 45° relative to the IR cassette allows visualisation of the *radial head, neck and tuberosity* without superimposition of other bones (Fig. 25.13). An image of this is shown in Chapter 6 (Fig. 6.5B). The humeral capitellum will also be clearly displayed with this projection. Internal rotation of the elbow from the AP position will

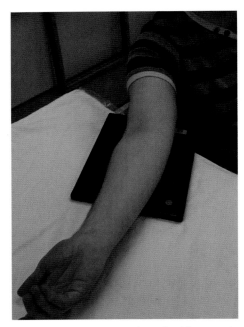

Figure 25.13 External rotation to reveal proximal forearm details. Further external rotation from the AP elbow position will allow visualisation of the radial head, neck and tuberosity.

advantageously display the coronoid of the ulna, the trochlea and an elongated medial epicondyle of the humerus (see Fig. 6.8A,B).

The radial head can also be further visualised in the lateral position by rotating from the lateral elbow position start point. Four exposures can be made with the forearm, in this lateral position, displaying maximum supination, lateral with the ulnar border of the forearm in a comfortable position, pronation of the hand and hyperpronation of the hand with the hand positioned as if attempting an AP projection of the thumb. This gradually rotates the radial head so that aspects of the proximal radial profile are displayed (see Figs 6.6A,B and 6.7A,B). Finally, the Coyle projection[19] of the radial head employs lateromedial angulation of 45° across the forearm, which is in a lateral position (Fig. 25.14A,B). This projection separates the radial head and capitellum from superimposing structures to reveal indistinct injuries that may be too subtle to detect on the normal lateral image.

Fractures of the *humerus* often appear dramatic owing to deformation of the limb, and these demand the utmost care from the imaging practitioner. In cases like this the patient is best examined erect so that the most information can be obtained using a single projection, in the same way as follow-up images would be achieved. However, if the patient presents on a trolley or has to be examined on the X-ray table, an immobilisation pad support will be necessary to obtain a true projection of the limb. Although images reveal their best information by being taken with the IR in close proximity to the limb, using an IR tray or under-trolley tray may be a desirable option to minimise movement of the arm and reduce patient discomfort. The associated projection at 90° to the first can be obtained using a combination of overlapping horizontal beam projections from the shoulder down and elbow up. Moving the arm away from the body and elevating it on supporting pads to allow clear visualisation of the limb may be necessary for these projections. The required arm positions can be achieved with (non-cassette type) fixed digital receptors in the same way as described for the forearm and elbow above. Good communication techniques and appropriate analgesia are the most helpful additions that can be offered in this setting – as in most trauma imaging approaches (Fig. 25.15A,B,C).

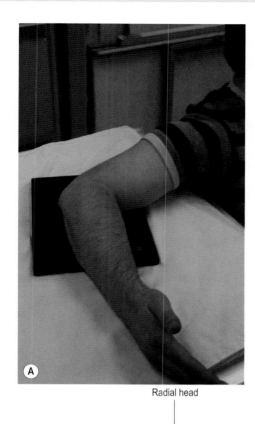

Radial head

Humerus

Ulna

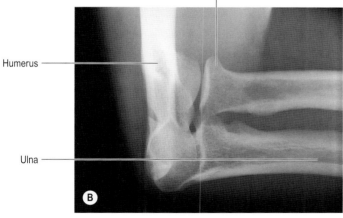

Figure 25.14 (A) Coyle radial head projection; by angling 40–45° lateromedially, this view separates the radial head from the superimposing ulna for suspected radial head/neck fractures; (B) Coyle radial head X-ray; by angling 40–45° lateromedially, this view separates the radial head from the superimposing ulna for suspected radial head/ neck fractures.

Adapted projections of the shoulder joint

The shoulder joint (specifically the glenohumeral joint) has been the source of the generation of many tailored projections to prove various injury and degenerative processes. This section will consider the supplementary projections of value following trauma.

Confusion is occasionally apparent regarding the degree of external rotation required for the AP projection of the shoulder. Ideally, appropriate clinical evaluation will result in the indication by the referrer; for example, if the *clavicle* is the injured component for which a radiological opinion is sought, this would necessitate a clavicular

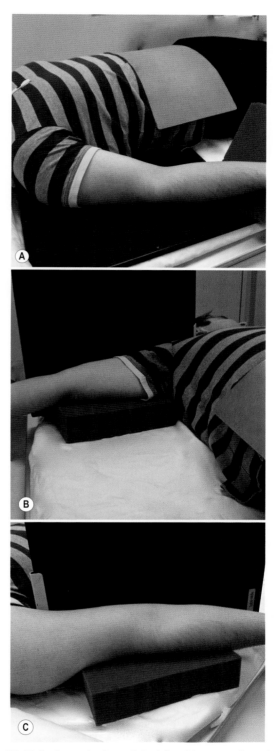

Figure 25.15 Supine projections of the injured humerus. Several options are available for obtaining images of the injured humerus with differing impacts on the patient from a movement (A,B) and potential radiation dose (C) perspective.

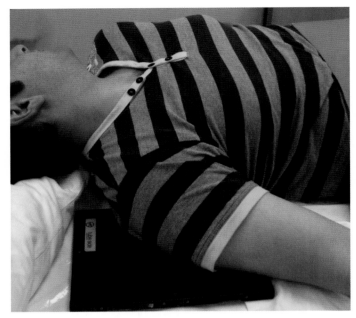

Figure 25.16 The Garth projection. The Garth projection to reveal dislocation of the glenohumeral joint. This projection produces a half axial view of the shoulder and is one option to consider where a true axial image might not be possible. It can also be undertaken sitting or standing.

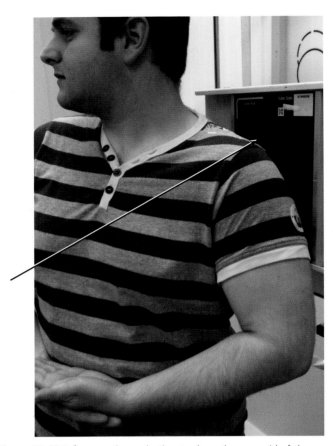

Figure 25.17 Inferosuperior projection to show the coracoid of the scapula. The coracoid projection also allows good visualisation of the acromioclavicular joint, projected clear of other shoulder structures.

Further discussion on the options for shoulder projections, including considerations for implementation in trauma situations, can be found in Chapter 7.

---

projection. Where this is not the case, and foreshortening of the clavicle is not a consideration, appropriate external rotation of the trunk to the affected side should be attempted so that the glenoid edge will be projected in profile. This will allow the viewer to scrutinise the *glenohumeral joint* effectively so that the image can be correctly evaluated for the presence of subtle dislocation or fracture characteristics. This rule also applies for patients who present in a supine position, depending of course on the potential for causing further injury by rotating the patient. The suitability of different alternatives to the axial shoulder projection must be considered before a technique is selected; discussion on this is given in Chapter 7.

The modified axial projection is one that can be used in any situation. Essentially, the projection is obtained by positioning the patient as for an AP shoulder, as seen in Chapter 7 with 30–45° caudal angulation from the original perpendicular beam direction (Fig. 7.5A,B); it is easily undertaken on the supine patient (Fig. 25.16). This can also be undertaken with 45° rotation on the trunk; this is sometimes known as the Garth projection or Garth apical oblique,[20] and is used to assess dislocation by examining the position of the humeral head relative to the glenoid of the scapula. The projection can also be undertaken erect or supine. On the resulting images for either of these angled AP projections, if the humeral head lies inferiorly to the glenoid then the dislocation is anterior, with the positions of the anatomical structures reversed for posterior dislocations, i.e. the glenoid edge is lower in relation to the humeral head. Where the patient is unable to be seated and presents on a trolley, true inferosuperior or superoinferior projections may be achieved by gently encouraging the patient to abduct the arm so that an IR can be placed in the axillary space. Alternatively, the IR is placed above the shoulder and the central ray directed from below the joint. This may be feasible, while minimising pain, as relatively small amounts of movement are required following the performance of the AP projection that complements the above.

Owing to the structure of the shoulder, the *coracoid process* has other structures superimposed over it on the image. This may be a particular problem in younger patients, where secondary ossification of the coracoid tip could mimic a fracture; this necessitates clear visualisation of this aspect of the shoulder.

If any kyphosis of the thoracic region is present, simply angle 20–30° cranially with the patient in the normal AP shoulder position (Fig. 25.17). Greater kyphosis will require greater angulation. This image can also be helpful in the evaluation of the *acromioclavicular joint*.

Adapted projections of the foot, ankle and leg

Where injuries of the *foot* are concerned radiographers frequently have to work around the patient, depending heavily at times on the versatility of the radiographic equipment. This means that, although projections are standardised or similar, the equipment must be manoeuvred into various positions, rather than moving the patient's limb. Horizontal ray techniques are often used to create a projection that is at least similar to the standard projection in the less injured patient.

When the patient presents in a *wheelchair* for foot examinations, consider placing the IR on the floor or on a small step for the patient to place the injured foot upon. In this way the frail patient does not have to be moved and a standard projection is possible. Slight extension of the ankle, required to clear the tibia and fibula from the majority of the tarsus, is also easier in this position. The *trolley-bound patient* can be examined with the leg fully extended or with the hip and knee slightly flexed. The cassette-type IR can be supported on a pad under the plantar aspect of the foot, or the fixed digital plate angled and brought into contact with the plantar aspect of the foot; it does not matter at what angle the IR and foot lie, as long as the central ray is correctly angled until it is perpendicular to the IR. In some cases it may be necessary to elevate the foot slightly by resting the back of the heel on a radiolucent pad, so that the knee and lower leg are not projected over the image. This would be most likely in the patient whose leg is fully extended. The practitioner's skills are of paramount importance here, with respect to angling the beam and accurately positioning the IR.

Working in this way indicates that the patient probably requires no more than the equivalent of the basic 'two projections at right-angles' series. That said, orthopaedic colleagues may request further projections, such as views of the *subtalar joints*. The best projections to reveal the most information on the whole region are the medial and lateral ankle obliques, where the foot is rotated respectively internally and externally from the AP ankle position to form an angle of 45° to the IR (Fig. 25.18A,B). The central ray is angled 20° cranially and directed towards the talus. Collimate to include the ankle joint, talus calcaneum and both malleoli.

Examinations for injury related to areas proximal to the ankle can usually be obtained by using a combination of routine and horizontal ray techniques. Splinting devices may be present and, where possible, these should be removed to avoid artefact generation. Should the leg be so badly injured that gross rotation of one part relative to another is displayed (e.g. shaft of tibia and fibula rotated in relation to the ankle joint), then obtain projections that ensure that at least one part of the limb is projected with its joint in the correct orientation, so that the associated portion of the injured part can be assessed relative to the part that is correctly projected. Using the lower leg as an example, this would mean AP knee and lateral ankle obtained by vertical X-ray beam; lateral knee and AP ankle obtained by horizontal ray technique.

Not all leg injuries will be as remarkable as the example above. When the patient is able to climb onto the examination table, further simple projections may be helpful in elucidating subtle injuries. Internal and external oblique projections of the ankle can be performed with the foot rotated through the axis of the ankle to form the required angle of 45° to the table-top for the respective views. The vertical central ray is centred on the ankle joint and collimated as described for the AP ankle in Chapter 8. The internal oblique will show the *distal tibiofibular joint* and *lateral malleolus* clearly, with the external oblique displaying the *medial malleolus* and *talus* to advantage. Under- and over-rotation of the ankle joint in the lateral position are also useful images to obtain from the perspective of displaying (a) the posterior tibial lip in the under-rotated lateral and (b) the posterior margin of the fibula in the over-rotated lateral.

Stress projections to reveal ligament integrity in the ankle may also be required. The inversion stress view shows the integrity of the *lateral collateral complex*, whereas the eversion stress view is helpful for showing the integrity of the *medial collateral complex*. As the referring clinician is normally responsible for the action of stressing the joint in each direction, the radiographer must control the situation by taking care to ensure any lead rubber protective devices used do not impinge on the region being imaged. One such example would be to ensure that the clinician's hands and the lead rubber gloves, worn while applying stress to the joint, do not overlie the area of interest. It is also relatively easy for the clinician to inadvertently move the

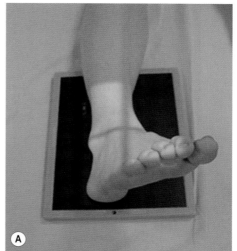

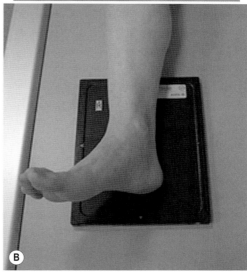

Figure 25.18 (A) The 'common' subtalar projection – the 'common' subtalar view, whereby a midpoint angle of 45° internal and external rotation of the ankle is accompanied by 20° cranial angulation of the central ray to reveal the majority of the subtalar articulation in a pair of images; (B) 45° external oblique ankle.

ankle from the AP position, which is adopted as a baseline, so that the area under examination is projected incorrectly; this would make detection of subtle injury difficult. Alternatively, some radiology departments have developed stressing devices as a variation on the Thomas wrench, which the patient may control manually, though usually this device is operated by the medical practitioner.[21] This may produce the desired result, but care is required so that the patient does not over-stress the joint and cause more injury. More likely, however, is the chance that the patient will not exert enough force on the joint to achieve a diagnostic result.

To assess the *tibiotalar* and *talofibular ligaments* of the ankle using the lateral projection, the anterior draw stress view can be attempted without the presence of the clinician; this is a variation on that described by Horsfield and Murphy.[21] The back of the heel of the patient's affected limb is rested on a wooden block that has been placed on the table- or trolley-top; the ankle joint is therefore raised above the table or trolley (Fig. 25.19). An IR is positioned on the medial aspect of the ankle and a horizontal X-ray beam is centred over the lateral malleolus. A medium-sized sandbag should be placed on

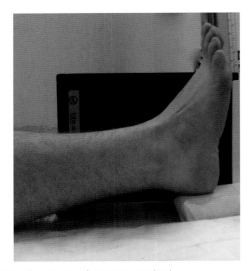

Figure 25.19 The anterior draw stress projection.

the mid-shaft of the tibia so that the ankle joint is gently stressed for approximately 1 minute before exposure. Collimation must include the whole of the ankle joint as well as at least 5 cm of the distal tibia. Be sure the malleoli are equidistant from the *block*, as for the AP position (malleoli are positioned relative to the *block* rather than to the IR). A positive response to stressing the joint shows the talus to have subluxed anteriorly, indicating damage to the ligaments indicated. Remember to remove the weight as soon as possible after exposure as this examination is often uncomfortable for the patient.

Adapted projections of the knee, thigh and hip

Knee injuries are usually best evaluated via the routine AP and horizontal ray lateral so that subtle soft tissue signs such as lipohaemarthrosis may be detected. This has added advantages in that (a) the patient need not be moved in more serious trauma situations, and (b) any radiographic evidence that may indicate an effusive collection in the suprapatellar region will not be disturbed. That said, the presence of an effusion should merely prompt the search for an underlying, more serious, bony cause.

Fractures of the *patella* are most commonly in a transverse direction, which should not be disturbed by bending the knee to achieve a lateral projection. However, the vertical fracture pattern that may not be obvious on the AP projection may require a tangential/inferosuperior skyline projection to reveal its nature. In these situations a projection with a small (around 30°) angle of flexion at the knee, the degree of flexion probably being governed by the extent of compliance attainable by the patient in conjunction with clinical history, should be attempted. Unfortunately this minimal flexion will require the central ray to be directed quite closely towards the body and head of the patient; however, this problem may be navigable by asking the patient to lie on the affected side with the slightly flexed knee resting in a lateral position close to the edge of the examination table (see patellar projections in Chapter 9). The head should be tilted back to clear the eyes as far as possible from the primary beam. In this way a grazing angle tangential to the patella is achieved which allows the patient to lean back from the track of the central ray, thereby reducing the likelihood of exposing the torso and head. Flexion must not be considered if derangement of the knee complex is suspected, or in the case of suspected tibial plateau fracture.

Femoral fractures are normally the result of significant force and are often accompanied by other injuries, so that adapted techniques are frequently required to obtain the images necessary for patient management. As with earlier examples, the use of horizontal beam techniques is vital in these situations, as is negotiating around splinting devices. The lateral is best undertaken with a horizontal beam and IR supported vertically at the side of the thigh. Lateromedial projections are favoured when it is difficult or inadvisable to raise the other leg to clear it from the femur under examination, although the lateromedial approach will involve the primary beam being directed towards the leg not under examination. AP projections can be obtained with the IR in a trolley tray, so that the limb is not moved unnecessarily. Image magnification is likely to be a problem if the IR is placed in a tray for this projection, and an increase in film receptor distance (FRD) will be required to help compensate for this. The approach to the lateral projection will mean that the IR may not extend sufficiently far along the thigh to include the injury site for evaluation in a single projection. The long femur may also not actually fit within the boundary of the IRs available (see Chapters 9 and 24, where the issue of patient length is discussed), and the only option in this instance is to obtain overlap images so that minimal movement of the patient is maintained. Also note that the femur is an area with a range of densities along its length, necessitating the use of a higher kVp non-gridded technique. To summarise these suggestions, an acceptable compromise must be reached that may result in some loss of the contrast and detail in the image but allow a single projection to be obtained, with concomitant reduction in radiation dose to the patient.

Adapted projections of the pelvis and hips

Most hip fractures are found in the elderly, but some younger patients may present with conditions such as slipped upper femoral epiphysis (SUFE), or after involvement in high-energy accidents that may have caused dislocation at the hip. Patients who have undergone total hip replacement may present with dislocation of the femoral portion owing to such simple manoeuvres as standing from a seated position in a low chair. Occasionally young athletes may present with stress injury to the neck of femur or, more rarely, a true fracture of the same region.

When the neck of femur has been fractured, two projections at right-angles are often required: a full AP pelvis, to allow full evaluation of the pelvic girdle for other injuries, and a horizontal beam lateral of the hip (although some centres accept that if an obvious fracture is seen on the AP then a further view is unnecessary; Chapter 10 provides further comment on the need for a lateral hip projection). A common error with the horizontal ray lateral projection is to allow the thigh of the unaffected side to obstruct the X-ray beam, thereby creating a soft tissue artefact. Proprietary devices are available to help the patient keep the uninjured limb suitably raised; the hip and knee are flexed until the thigh is as near vertical as possible, so that the thigh is cleared from the beam path. See Chapter 10 and Figures 10.8 and 10.9A for description of this technique, using a proprietary device to keep the thigh raised. A less expensive alternative is to use a large radiolucent foam pad, which can be positioned appropriately under the leg; this does not allow for visualisation of the centring point and must be positioned after centring and collimation have taken place.

These methods of producing a horizontal beam lateral are possible only when the patient is able to elevate the unaffected limb. An example of such a situation is when the patient has had a recent hip replacement in the uninjured hip, and there is a risk that the movements described above might cause dislocation of the unaffected side, which would be a disastrous result. When this is the case an axial oblique that will give lateral orientation information can be attempted. For this the patient remains supine with the IR initially positioned as for the horizontal beam lateral. From this position the cassette is tilted backwards 25° and supported with sandbags and foam pads. The horizontal central ray is angled 25° caudally and then rotated on the ceiling mount until the central ray is perpendicular to the IR. This tip

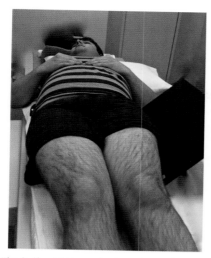

Figure 25.20 The half-axial hip projection. The half lateral/semi-axial hip projection for patients unable to elevate the opposite side to produce a horizontal ray lateral. Use of a larger IR will facilitate inclusion of the upper third of femur to provide a lateral projection of the shaft.

beam is centred over the medial aspect of the upper thigh at the level of the greater trochanter, to pass through the hip level with the femoral pulse (Fig. 25.20). Collimate the beam appropriately and select exposure factors slightly lower than those indicated for the horizontal beam lateral.

Regarding major trauma, an AP examination of the pelvis is standard in the major trauma series associated with the ATLS protocols. However, in a trauma situation there are likely to be inherent problems that will require additional care in undertaking the examination. The fractured pelvis carries serious risks associated with unstable bony components and vascular damage, requiring movement of the patient to be minimised, especially until haemodynamic stability is achieved. As a result the patient must be examined on the trauma trolley, using an IR with grid in the tray beneath the trolley. Often, accurate centring of the IR to coincide with the median sagittal plane (MSP), area of interest and central ray is difficult, as the IR is positioned under the patient by 'guess' or estimation. Patients rarely present perfectly centralised on a trolley and often lie obliquely across its central long axis. Some practitioners peer down the gap between the trolley top and the cassette tray to assess the alignment of the IR and MSP; unfortunately this is not the most accurate way of assessing the situation, as the narrowness of the gap means that the cassette and the patient cannot be seen at the same time. Where space permits, the following are useful in ensuring accurate alignment:

- Ensure the trolley is parallel to the wall of the X-ray room and the tube ceiling track
- At the head end of the trolley, find the midpoint of the trolley top or central handle (not the mattress, which is often not centralised on the trolley) and position the vertical central ray over this point
- Move the tube down the trolley towards the patient's pelvis, without any crosswise shift of the tube
- When the tube is level with the pelvis, assess the distance between the patient's MSP and the central ray; this will give a good indication of how far to displace the IR laterally if the MSP is displaced from the midline of the trolley; it may be necessary to turn the IR slightly if the patient's pelvis is lying diagonally
- Reposition the tube to lie over the midline of the pelvis and the correct centring point
- Collimate as for routine pelvis or hips AP

This tip can prove useful for any supine AP projection of the spine, abdomen or pelvis.

Less severely traumatised trolley-bound patients may also be examined on the trolley; attention to detail will ensure the correct projection is obtained and that the body part is centralised to the IR. Some imaging departments prefer to move the patient on the trolley mattress across to the examination table to ensure that a degree of imaging standardisation is achieved. However, this does expose practitioners and patients to risk of injury through manual handling.

When the resuscitation room is not being used as the examination area, other projections beyond the AP pelvis may be requested if the patient has been stabilised haemodynamically. These include:

- Judet's iliac oblique acetabulum (may be performed as a whole pelvis examination)
- Judet's obturator oblique acetabulum (may be performed as a whole pelvis examination)
- Posterior oblique of ilium
- AP pubis
- Inlet view of pelvis
- Outlet view of pelvis

Judet's projections involve 45° rotation of the patient, (a) towards the affected side to reveal the *iliac* portion of the hemipelvis and (b) away from the affected side to show the *obturator* aspects. Respectively, the projections show (a) the posterior or ilioischial column and anterior acetabular rim (when the affected side is lowered) and (b) the anterior or iliopubic column and posterior acetabular rim. When undertaken in order to show each half of the pelvis the whole hemipelvis should be included and the central ray directed to the acetabulum in both projections.[22] See Chapter 10 and Figures 10.10 and 10.11 for a full description of the obliques.

Good visualisation of the anterior portion of the iliac bone and the crest is achieved by positioning as for the iliac oblique (Chapter 10), but centring the vertical central ray over the iliac wing and remembering to collimate and adjust exposure as appropriate. A supplementary projection of the *pubis* may be helpful, especially where the syndesmosis is 'bobbly' or it is unclear as to whether or not a fracture is present. Position the patient as for the AP projection of both hips. Apply 20° cranial beam angulation for males and 30° cranial angulation for females (to allow for the differences in pelvic shape). Centre to the lower border of the symphysis pubis and collimate to include the pubic and ischial rami, ensuring that the image lies within the boundaries of the IR. The view gives an apparently elongated (although in fact more accurate) projection of the pubic and ischial rami compared to the AP pelvis, as the effects of the natural tilt of the pelvis are countered by the cranial angle, thereby preventing foreshortening.

The pelvic inlet and outlet projections provide added information for the evaluation of the degree of pelvic component movement after a fracture to the area.[23] For the *inlet* projection, position the patient as for the AP pelvis. Use a central ray angled 40° caudally, centred to the level of the ASIS, along the midline. Collimate the beam to include the whole of the pelvis and ensure that the image lies within the boundaries of the IR. This view is used to assess the degree of posterior displacement of the hemipelvis or inward/outward rotation of the anterior pelvis following trauma. The pelvic ring should be clearly demonstrated when exposure factors are selected to demonstrate the anterior and posterior structures; if this is the case, then the iliac wings are usually overexposed. For the *outlet* view, position as above but angle the central X-ray beam 40° cranially, centring the central ray to a point at the inferior border of the symphysis pubis. As with the pubic bone AP view, the effect of pelvic tilt is countered, so the view shows these unforeshortened bones clearly. Visualisation of the iliac wings is poor because of superimposition of the acetabula.[24]

Finally, *SUFE* presentation requires the use of the trauma frog lateral in conjunction with the AP pelvis projection. Starting in the position for AP pelvis, flex the knees and externally rotate the hips through approximately 40–60° and bring the soles of the feet into contact with each other. Support the legs at the knees with foam immobilising pads and sandbags. Using a vertical X-ray beam, centre at a point 1–2.5 cm proximal to the symphysis pubis (according to the size of the child) in the midline, and collimate the beam to include both hips/femoral necks. In this view the pelvis is shown as an AP projection. The proximal femora are projected laterally as for the 'turned' lateral projection; however, when visualised together this view may be called the modified Cleaves projection.[25] This may be a first attendance for this presentation so apply gonad protection carefully so that essential aspects of anatomy, particularly the heads of the femora, are not obscured.

Adapted projections of the spine

Although this section will consider the adapted projections of the spine, it should be apparent that the majority of regions of the spine require just AP and lateral projections to be obtained following trauma. In practice, computed tomography (CT) is probably used in most departments as the frontline investigation where the index of suspicion is high,[26] as clinical answers can be readily achieved and its sensitivity is far greater than that of plain radiography.[27] Although CT is used more frequently today, the following techniques are still an important adjunct and still as a frontline investigation in many circumstances following current guidelines.[26]

The cervical spine

Standard AP and lateral projections are often requested following whiplash-type injuries; the patient is frequently able to sit or stand for the lateral view as they often present 24–48 hours after the accident. A supine lateral is required for the patient who is at risk from movement, and the lateral image must always be examined before a decision on further patient management is made. The common belief is that the lateral cervical projection must take preference as the first projection undertaken in the cervical spine; this is appropriate if there is serious concern that significant neck trauma has occurred. However, if the AP cervical spine projection is required and is undertaken first *without moving the patient's neck*, would subsequently moving to the lateral projection really be considered dangerous?

The problems of shoulder shadow impingement upon the cervicothoracic region are typically similar to those encountered in the patient attending for examination of the cervical spine to evaluate degenerative changes and, as such, may be treated with similar techniques. Where more severe injuries necessitate patient presentation on a trolley, either in the imaging department or in the resuscitation room, then adaptation will be necessary to negotiate the shoulder superimposition problem. Frequently, where the patient is conscious, explaining what the radiographer is attempting to achieve enables the patient to reach down towards their feet with their arms and clear the soft tissue of the shoulders from the lower cervical vertebrae. This is especially effective if coupled with an expiration breathing technique prior to exposure.

The supine patient may be advised to use an arm folding technique, if this is considered safe; for this the arms are extended and crossed at the wrists, with the medially rotated hands clasped together (Fig. 25.21A). If the patient is in pain and holds the shoulders in spasm, or should the patient be unconscious, then different techniques are required. Some resuscitation room practitioners may advocate pulling the patient's arms by a member of the medical staff who is wearing appropriate radiation protection garments. This may seem sensible, but unfortunately there is a potential risk of further damage to either

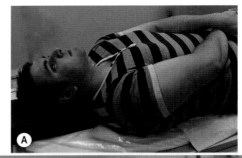

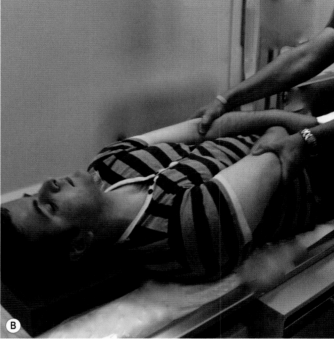

Figure 25.21 Arm folding may help reveal the cervicothoracic junction. The (A) folded and (B) pulled folded arm technique to reveal the lower cervical spine in the lateral projection.

the neck or the upper limbs. Also, personnel are frequently not strong enough to achieve sufficient movement of the shoulders, or the arms are held by the distal portions of the limb, so that laxity within the joints means the arms cannot be physically pulled sufficiently far to remove the shoulder from the projection. An alternative is to fold the patient's arms across their chest and pull from the distal humeral portion; the slight anterior abduction of the humeri more efficiently clears the soft tissue of the shoulder in an anterior direction (and away from the lower cervical vertebrae) (Fig. 25.21B).[28] Use of these shoulder clearance techniques assumes that the patient's arms are not injured and can be subjected to such forces.

When the arms are injured, possibly the best approach is to adopt a high kVp technique that will reduce contrast while ensuring that the whole lateral projection can be visualised on a single image. Many departments will immediately adopt the swimmer's position, which can be undertaken supine as well as erect, as described in Chapter 11 (Fig. 11.4A,B,C), but the validity of its use can be questioned as it necessitates significant movement of the shoulders for the neck-injured and multiply-injured patient, carries somewhat confusing information due to overlying structures, and is often low in quality due to scatter produced by area density and increased exposure factors. All these factors make interpretation more difficult; unsurprising, then, that it has been found that almost half of the swimmer's views

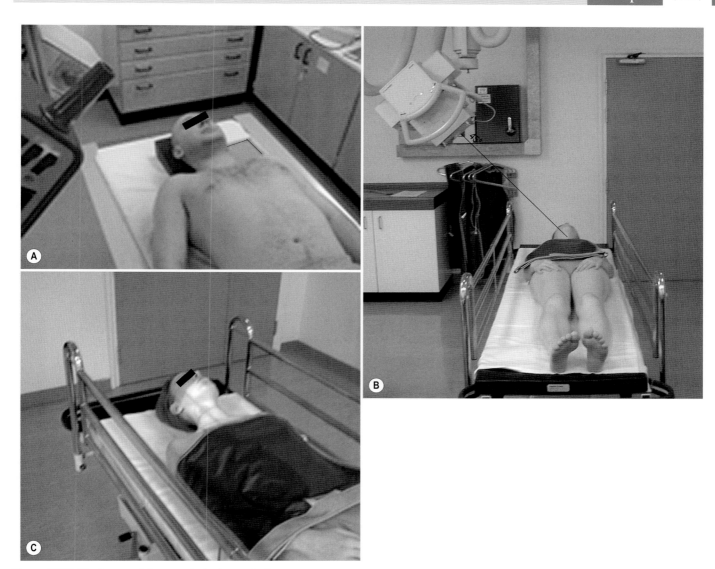

Figure 25.22 The trauma oblique cervical spine projection.

studied in one piece of research were inadequate for use as a diagnostic tool.[29] There is additional discussion on the validity of the swimmer's view in Chapter 11.

A dichotomy exists in more difficult cases with respect to how some kind of adequate projection might be obtained to reveal possible injuries to the cervical spine. Suggestions have been made regarding the performance of trauma obliques,[30,31] but unfortunately this is often met with resistance from some (usually inexperienced, non-radiologic or non-radiographic) personnel, who imply that reading the images is 'difficult'.[32,33] To produce images for the oblique cervical projection, the patient is supine on the examination table (but usually on a trolley). An IR is placed in the trolley tray or directly on the table-top next to the patient's neck. When the trolley-top method is used this may mean the IR is pushed partially under the head. This should only be done under supervision, but will not be a problem with the tray method. Angle the X-ray tube 45° in a lateromedial direction, the central ray entering the side of the neck furthest from the IR at the level of C4 (Fig. 25.22A,B,C). Both obliques are undertaken. No grid is necessary, but if one is required for a large patient ensure that the grid lines are running parallel to the direction of the central ray. This avoids grid 'cut-off'. To produce a more elongated image of the posterior spinal elements and the vertebral bodies, perform the same projection as above but with the lateromedial angulation at 60°. Although the bodies will not be projected in good relief, the posterior elements will be shown to advantage, so that injury to these regions will be revealed. In both techniques, images should be obtained from each side of the neck.

See Chapter 11 for useful additional discussion on the cervical spine and the spine in trauma.

The thoracolumbar spine

Generally speaking, most images of these regions can be obtained by appropriate use of AP vertical ray techniques with the patient on the trolley or examination table. Horizontal ray techniques allow the lateral projections to be obtained without the need to move the patient. Care is required, however, to ensure the IR is in the appropriate position without risk of injury to the patient and the projection of table or trolley-top artefacts onto the image. The latter is most problematic as objects built into the trolley or table impinge upon the posterior spinal elements.

Adapted projections of the craniofacial skeleton

Chapters 16–18 indicate techniques that were once the mainstay of craniofacial imaging in the radiology department. The trolley-top skull technique is mentioned in this chapter as it shows necessary adaptation of technique; the reality is that the likelihood of its use for the cranial vault is very low, as CT is now the imaging modality of choice.[33]

All skull and facial examinations can be achieved using the trolley-top method when embarked upon with a logical approach that uses the vital skills of understanding patient anatomy and the principles of angulation and geometry. Whereas many projections are described in this book (see Chapters 16–18) as being obtained from a PA direction to enhance radiation protection considerations, simply reversing angles through 180° allows images to be obtained from the AP perspective. Obviously, magnification will cause differences in the appearances of some projections: for example, the orbits are particularly affected by magnification. Care must also be taken where the IR has to be placed directly under the head, which is usually impossible for patients with neck injury; in these cases the IR can be placed in the IR tray under the trolley, if suitable for the technique required.

The cranial vault

As with the descriptions in earlier chapters, the ability to achieve skull projections hangs on the fact that the orbitomeatal baseline (OMBL) is perpendicular to the IR. If this is not possible, and when the patient can be safely moved, a large radiolucent support under the neck or spine can be an advantage. This is particularly useful for kyphotic individuals. Placing this wedge beneath the shoulders will aid patient comfort and encourage the head to fall naturally into a position that will place the OMBL perpendicular to the IR, which is placed directly under the skull (Fig. 25.23). The radiographer should avoid placing the IR under any support as this increases the object–receptor distance. The central ray must be angled to ensure that it forms the required angle to the OMBL. If it is still not possible to position the OMBL at 90° to the IR, compensation can be made by initially aligning the central ray with the OMBL and then adding the appropriate angle for the relevant projection before centring the beam. As a more specific example, consider a patient whose chin is raised so that the OMBL is raised 10° from the perpendicular: for a projection that requires a 20° cranial angle the central ray will initially be selected as 10° caudally to coincide with the OMBL and then angled 20° cranially from this point to achieve the correct 20° to the OMBL. On examination the beam will be 10° cranially. An alternative is to position the external auditory meatus level with the lower border of the orbit and use a vertical central ray; the petrous ridges will lie at the bottom of the orbits on the resulting image, as if a 20° cranial angle had been used in conjunction with an OMBL relationship of 90° to the IR.

The fronto-occipital (FO) 30° (Towne's) projection of the occipital region is essentially an AP projection anyway, and the OMBL is positioned by the use of pads as for other FO projections. As mentioned in Chapter 16, pads must never be placed under the head and must be placed under the IR.

Lateral projections are fairly straightforward, with the IR supported vertically at the side of the head, which is supported on a radiolucent pad (Fig. 25.24). If a neck-injured patient cannot be moved to raise the head on a pad, the IR must be positioned alongside the trolley with its lower edge well below the occiput; this will create an increased object–receptor distance and the FRD should be increased to compensate for magnification and unsharpness.

Facial bones

Facial views can almost always be obtained when the patient is compliant and can be examined in an erect sitting position; for those who are severely injured the likelihood is that CT will be the frontline investigation, although plain radiography does yield useful information in this area.

For the supine patient the occipitomental projections are replaced by AP mento-occipital positions, with the chin raised to place the OMBL either 45° or 30° from the vertical, depending on the required projection. If it is too difficult for the patient to lift the chin adequately, one solution, where presentation permits, is to place supports under the shoulders so room is made for the head to be tilted backwards to allow the OMBL to form an appropriate angle relative to the IR (Fig. 25.25A,B). The centring point is in the midline, level with the

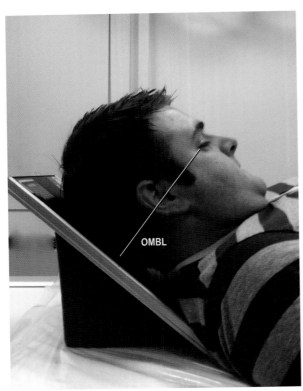

Figure 25.23 An adaptation for the FO skull. The AP table-top projection of the skull, where the patient is unable to lie flat. Note the pad lies under IR and patient, rather than under the head and on top of the IR.

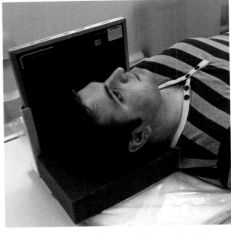

Figure 25.24 Continuing to work around the patient to generate a table-top lateral skull. The horizontal beam lateral projection of the skull with the head elevated on a radiolucent pad.

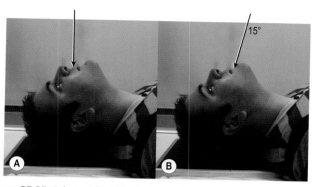

Figure 25.25 Adapted facial techniques where patient can extend the neck. Tilted head projections to show the facial bone structures as equivalent (A) OM and (B) OM 15° projections.

midpoint of the facial structures required for inclusion on the image. When this modification is not possible, an alternative has been described[33] where the head is supported on a radiolucent rectangular pad and the IR is supported vertically at the vertex of the skull. The OMBL is parallel to the IR. The X-ray tube is initially horizontal and the caudal angle is then applied according to the requirements of the projection. For this the tube has to be positioned close to the chest of the supine patient for some angulations, and this may be difficult with units having bulky tube housings. Increasing FRD with the adjustment of exposure factors will act to overcome this. Another alternative involves slight tilting of the IR in conjunction with chin adjustment (if possible) to ensure the OMBL lies parallel to the IR. This allows the tube to be used in a higher position; the initial tube position will of course change from horizontal to 90° to the IR.

SELECTION OF TRAUMA IMAGING EQUIPMENT

A&E and its associated imaging department should ideally be sited as close neighbours, if not in the same departmental area. The rooms themselves should display features that will enable them to handle the wide variation in patient presentation that spans ages from cradle to grave. X-ray rooms should be spacious, with a large 'footprint', so that enough room is available for practitioners to work around the patient in relative ease, while using X-ray equipment capable of performing the maximum range of movement possible. This is often in the face of fairly tight budgetary constraints. However, despite likely restrictions on cost, the use of a rise and fall table is a must for the range of patients who may be examined in A&E (many of the projections identified in the earlier sections necessitate this versatility), and who must be worked around to obtain the required images.

As stated earlier, ancillary equipment should be chosen to meet the demands of adaptability and ease of use,[34] and support equipment must also be robust and available either as static units in the examination room, or reliably mobile if the decision is made to share facilities. Ideally, piped gases and suction should be provided in any newly built department, and all staff should be trained in the use of this and other general equipment. Short-handedness through lack of education in a moment of demand will not carry any weight in a court of law, should litigation be instigated as a result of neglect.

Some A&E imaging departments will show signs of age owing to the degree of obsolescence of X-ray equipment in use. Initiatives such as the guidelines generated by the National Institute for Clinical Excellence (NICE)[35] for evaluation and treatment of head injuries have contributed to the death of plain film assessment in these situations.

If equipment breaks down the versatility of the experienced practitioner comes to the fore with their ability to instantly translate static techniques to mobile equipment. Therefore, patients can still expect to receive a service that, although adapted, will provide the answers needed in a traumatic situation. Advances in mobile X-ray unit technology have enabled the mobile ward service, breakdown situations in A&E or in some departments the imaging service in the resuscitation room, to move from good to excellent. Indeed, the use of mobile equipment support in the resuscitation room is seen by many to be an advantage over static units, particularly in the USA, as evidenced by television documentaries. By offering versatility and manoeuvrability, with an X-ray tube and generator that can provide almost identical qualities to those offered by static equipment, the mobile unit can be perceived as superior. Another bonus for mobile radiography is the availability of digital mobile units, with versatile IR sizes and even wireless digital IRs. Although state of the art equipment may be built into a new establishment, the anecdotal experience of the authors and others has shown that implementation of this does not always meet the demands of the service or its users. Much depends upon the activity of the hospital and how assertive staff may be in the resuscitation area. Resuscitation is for just that – for very ill patients; radiation protection issues and the impact of image quality on performing radiographic examinations in an area not fully designed for X-ray imaging makes us ask why radiography is performed in an area out of context. Even so, many radiographers appreciate the fact that their needs are being recognised by commissioning of such equipment; however, they are able to perform perfectly well when a breakdown occurs and mobile machinery has to be employed.

REFERENCES

1. Berman L, et al. Reducing errors in the accident department: a simple method using radiographers. Radiography 1986;52(603):143–4.

2. Price RC, Le Masurier SB. Longitudinal changes in extended roles in radiography: A new perspective. Radiography 2007;13(1):18–29.

3. American College of Surgeons. Advanced trauma life support student manual. 7th ed. Chicago: American College of Surgeons; 2003.

4. Department of Health. A health service of all the talents: developing the NHS workforce. London: HMSO; 2000.

5. College of Radiographers. Medical Image Interpretation & Clinical Reporting by Non-Radiologists: The Role of the Radiographer. London: College of Radiographers; 2006.

6. Health and Safety Executive. The Ionising Radiation (Medical Exposure) Regulation 20. (Statutory Instruments, 2000; no.1059). London: HMSO; 2000.

7. Society and College of Radiographers. Reporting by radiographers: a vision paper. London: SCoR; 1997.

8. Chan O. ABC of emergency radiology. 2nd ed. Oxford: Blackwell Publishing; 2007.

9. Hardy M, Snaith B. Musculoskeletal trauma: A guide to assessment and diagnosis. London: Churchill Livingstone, Elsevier; 2011.

10. Raby N, et al. Accident and emergency radiology: a survival guide. 2nd ed. London: Saunders; 2005.

11 Dimond BC. Legal aspects of radiography and radiology. Oxford: Blackwell Science; 2002.

12 Dimond BC. Red dots and radiographer's liability. Health Care Risk Report October 2000.

13 Lewis S. New angles on the radiographic examination of the hand – I. Radiography Today 1988;54(617):44–5.

14 Lewis S. New angles on the radiographic examination of the hand – II. Radiography Today 1988;54(618):29.

15 Lewis S. New angles on the radiographic examination of the hand – III. Radiography Today 1988;54(619): 47–8.

16 Eyres KS, Allen TR. Skyline view of the metacarpal head in the assessment of the human fight-bite injuries. Journal of Hand Surgery (British volume) 1993;18(1):43–4.

17 Long BW, Rafaert JA. Orthopaedic radiography. Philadelphia: WB Saunders; 1995.

18 Swallow RA, et al. Clark's positioning in radiography. 11th ed. London: Heinemann; 1986.

19 Coyle GF. Radiographing immobile trauma patients. Denver: Multi-Media Publishing; 1980.

20 Garth WP, et al. Roentgenographic demonstration of instability of the shoulder: the apical oblique projection: A technical note. Journal of Bone and Joint Surgery 1984;66A(9):1450–3.

21 Horsfield D, Murphy G. Stress views of the ankle joint in lateral ligament injury. Radiography 1985;51(595):7–11.

22 Monks J, Yeoman L. Judet's views of the acetabulum: a demonstration of their importance. Radiography Today 1989;55(628):18–21.

23 Foster LM, Barton ED. Managing pelvic fractures, part 2: physical and radiologic assessment. Journal of Critical Illness 2001;16(5):255–6, 258.

24 Hunter JC, et al. Pelvic and acetabular trauma. In: El-Khoury GY, editor. Imaging of orthopedic trauma. Radiologic Clinics of North America 1997;35(3):ix, 491–781.

25 Hardy M, Boynes S. Paediatric radiography. Oxford: Blackwell Science; 2003.

26 Royal College of Radiologists. Making the best use of a department of clinical radiology: guidelines for doctors. 6th ed. London: RCR; 2007.

27 Bailitz J, et al. CT should replace three view radiographs as the initial screening test in patients at high, moderate and low for blunt cervical spine injury: A prospective comparison. Journal of Trauma 2009;66:1605–9.

28 Carver BJ, Roche D. An alternative technique for visualisation of the C7 T1 junction in trauma. Supplement to British Journal of Radiology 2000;73:73.

29 Rethnam U, et al. The swimmer's view: does it really show what it is supposed to show? A retrospective study. BMC Medical Imaging 2008;8(2):1–4.

30 Ireland AJ, et al. Do supine oblique views provide better imaging of the cervicothoracic junction than swimmer's views? Journal of Accident & Emergency Medicine 1998;15(3):151–4.

31 Fell M. Cervical spine trauma radiographs: swimmer's and supine obliques; an exploration of current practice. Radiography 2011;17(1):33–8.

32 Daffner RH. Radiographic interpretation of cervical vertebral injuries. Topics in Emergency Medicine 1997;19(3):11–25.

33 National Institute for Clinical Excellence. Triage, assessment, investigation and early management of head injury in infants, children and adults. London: HMSO; 2003.

34 Ponsford A, Clements R. 1991 A modified view of the facial bones in the seriously injured. Radiography Today 1991;57(646):10–2.

35 Carver BJ, Unett EM. The Aintree bucky. Journal of Diagnostic Radiography and Imaging 2001;3(3):127–32.

Section |5|

Breast imaging

Chapter 26

Breast imaging

Judith Kelly, Sara Millington, Julie Burnage

INTRODUCTION AND RATIONALE

Mammography is considered to be the most commonly implemented method of imaging the breast, and, definitively, it is *radiographic* imaging of the breast. The majority of mammograms are performed by women on women, and for the purposes of this chapter it is assumed that both client and mammographer are female. It is not our intention to present a complete work on mammography and breast imaging – this is a brief introduction to a specialised field.

Although mammography is considered to be a major contributor to breast imaging, other methods of imaging the area are not ignored. A résumé of other methods is given in the chapter and ultrasound of the breast is given additional focus because of its complementary role alongside mammography.

Historically, mammography has always been performed by radiographers; however, in 2000 the Department of Health announced changes to be made to the Breast Screening Programme which meant a 40% increase in skilled staff was necessary.[1] To cope with the already critical shortage of radiographers and radiologists and the increase in demand a 'Skills Mix Project in Radiography'[2] was established and a four-tier structure was formed, the four tiers being:

- Consultant/lead practitioner
- Advanced practitioner
- Practitioner
- Assistant practitioner

Assistant practitioners work towards National Vocational Qualifications in the workplace, after which they are able to perform basic mammographic procedures under the supervision of a radiographer practitioner. Radiographers have the opportunity to undertake postgraduate training in order to advance their careers into clinical roles traditionally undertaken by radiologists, such as image reading, ultrasound, ultrasound reporting, and performing biopsies under ultrasound or stereotactic guidance.[2]

Mammography is widely used in the investigation of symptomatic breast disease and is the modality used for breast screening. The Million Women Study calculated the sensitivity and specificity of mammography by following over 120 000 women after their screening mammogram, showing sensitivity to be 86.6% and specificity 96.8%.[3]

SYMPTOMATIC MAMMOGRAPHY

Symptomatic women are usually referred by a clinician and present with a potentially significant breast problem, i.e. they have symptoms such as a palpable lump, nipple discharge and pain, or a visual change such as skin tethering or puckering.

ASYMPTOMATIC MAMMOGRAPHY

The National Health Service Breast Screening Programme (NHSBSP) invites all women aged 50–70 years who are registered with a general practitioner (GP) to attend for a routine 3-yearly mammogram. Asymptomatic women with a significant history of breast cancer are offered yearly mammograms between the ages of 40 and 49.[4] Such women may also have a mammogram if they are taking part in a research trial.

Whatever a woman's reason for attending, there will always be common anxieties. The most significant concern is likely to be the outcome or fear of positive results following the investigation, but for many women there are concerns about the procedure itself – is it painful, is it safe?

COMMUNICATION WITH WOMEN UNDERGOING MAMMOGRAPHY

As for all interactions between patient and health professional, effective communication is vital during mammography and starts before the woman even attends for her mammogram. All women should receive suitable, accurate and helpful written information prior to their appointment. This could include information about the procedure itself and, for breast screening, details about the risks and benefits, thus enabling women to make an informed decision. Any other information that may help to reduce the potential for anxiety should be incorporated, such as instructions on how to find the unit, waiting times, and other tests that may be undertaken during their visit.

The majority of women attending for a mammogram will be given a 'normal' result and therefore will be likely to meet only one member of the breast team: the mammographer. With this in mind the mammographer has a vital role in ensuring that the client receives all the information she requires and needs, and that it is imparted in a compassionate and understandable manner.

Essential communication stages:

- Before the mammogram, so that the woman knows what to expect and what is expected of her
- During the mammogram to ensure that she knows what is currently happening and to enable her to voice any concerns or indicate any discomfort she may be experiencing
- After the mammogram so that she knows when and how the results will be imparted

BREAST SCREENING

In 1957, the Commission of Chronic Illness in the United States defined screening as 'the presumptive identification of unrecognised disease … by the application of tests, examinations or other procedures which can be applied rapidly'.[5]

No screening test can be considered perfect, but the World Health Organization's International Agency for Research on Cancer (IARC) concluded that there was sufficient evidence for the efficacy of breast screening of women between 50 and 69 years.[6] Some essential considerations for a screening programme include:

- Is the disease an important health problem for the population?
- Can the population at risk be readily identified?
- Does early treatment lead to a better outcome?
- Are the benefits of screening greater than the harm caused?
- Does the screening identify the disease at a preclinical stage?
- Is treatment of the preclinical disease widely available?
- Is the screening modality acceptable to the target population?
- Is the method to be used cost effective?

In the UK mammography is currently offered every 3 years to women between the ages of 50 and 70. A pilot study currently underway may result in the age range being extended to 47–73 years.[7]

Mammography has been the screening modality used for every randomised trial that has shown a significant population reduction in breast cancer mortality.[8–11] It has a high sensitivity in the detection of breast cancers, particularly invasive carcinomas and ductal carcinoma in situ (DCIS).[3]

The use of a multidisciplinary approach when women are recalled following their initial mammogram ensures that the screening process is specific. The assessments used are further imaging, clinical examination and tissue sampling through biopsy.

Publication of the Forrest Report[5] on breast screening and the subsequent implementation of the NHSBSP revolutionised mammography in the UK. The report made numerous recommendations: projections that should be undertaken on each breast; the screening interval; interpretation of the mammograms; assessment and follow-up; and implementation of quality assurance and quality control procedures at every step of the programme. Recommendations regarding the setting up of an advisory committee and the Pritchard

Report[12] then led to guidance on quality issues. Recommendations made in the Forrest and Pritchard Reports do not pertain only to screening mammography services, as they are pertinent wherever mammography is offered, thus ensuring equity of provision for all women.

BREAST DISEASE DEMONSTRATED WITH MAMMOGRAPHY

Benign breast conditions

There are a number of benign breast conditions that may manifest on mammograms. Some examples are:

- *Benign breast change:* There is no evident disease process and changes are often brought about by hormonal variations. Conditions such as mastitis and fibroadenosis would come under this umbrella.
- *Cysts:* Cystic changes in the breast are very common and, as with most benign breast conditions, tend to be bilateral.
- *Fibroadenoma:* These are often found incidentally as they are usually too small to feel. Larger lesions occur in younger women. Fibroadenomas in postmenopausal women do not grow (except in women on hormone replacement therapy) and new lesions seldom appear.

Benign breast conditions and their mammographic appearances	
Cysts	Visualised as an increase in density usually with smooth edges
Fibroadenoma	Has no specific characteristic features but is usually smooth, rounded, well defined, and causes displacement of the surrounding tissues. When calcification occurs the lesion is said to have a 'popcorn' appearance

Breast cancer

United Kingdom breast cancer facts and statistics:[13]

- Breast cancer is the most common cancer in women
- The lifetime risk of developing cancer of the breast is 1 in 8
- 80% of breast cancers occur in postmenopausal women
- 5–10% of breast cancers are hereditary
- 90% of breast lumps are benign
- Around 300 men are diagnosed in the UK each year
- Breast cancer can be divided into two main types:
  - In situ carcinoma: this is contained within the breast ducts or lobules, although it has the potential to become invasive
  - Invasive carcinoma: this has spread from the ducts or lobules into the surrounding breast tissue. It has the potential to metastasise, via the blood or lymphatic systems, to other parts of the body and may ultimately shorten the patient's life. Invasive cancers are graded histologically from 1 to 3, according to how similar the breast cancer cells are to normal cells of the same type. The higher the grade the more different the cancer cells are from normal cells and the more rapidly they reproduce[14]

Cancer type and mammographic appearance

Cancer type	Appearance
DCIS	Microcalcifications
Invasive ductal carcinoma	Usually spiculate mass, but often has calcification and parenchymal distortion
Invasive lobular carcinoma	Similar to ductal carcinoma but microcalcification is less common

Mammography is often not able to distinguish between benign and malignant masses, which is why breast imaging services do not stop at mammography but incorporate other imaging modalities such as ultrasound and magnetic resonance imaging (MRI). However, it is possible to make some general observations from mammographic appearances:

- A spiculated mass with microcalcifications is highly suspicious and strongly indicates malignancy; any mass with distortion should be assumed to be malignant until proved otherwise
- Microcalcifications are difficult to evaluate but could represent DCIS
- Well-defined masses are likely to be benign

Dose implications for the breast undergoing mammography

It is important to remember that mammography uses radiation and therefore has the potential to induce carcinoma by the biological effects of radiation. The risk is considered to be low for the patient undergoing a single mammogram because the dose is well below the threshold for deterministic effects, and the reproductive cells are not exposed to primary radiation. Risks are highest in young women and are estimated to range from 9.1 fatal carcinomas induced per million per mGy in the 30–34-year age group, falling to 7.5 fatal carcinomas induced per million per mGy in the 45–49-year age group and 4.7 fatal carcinomas induced per million per mGy in the 60–64-year age group.[11]

For women of screening age in the UK the risk of radiation-induced breast cancer (including non-fatal tumours) is approximately 1 in 100 000 per mGy. Radiation dose for women attending the NHSBSP is taken to be on average 4.5 mGy per two-view screening examination. The risk of radiation-induced cancer for a woman attending mammographic screening (two views) by the NHSBSP is about 1 in 20 000 per visit, and it is estimated that about 170 cancers are detected by the NHSBSP for every cancer induced.[15]

Digital mammography

The NHSBSP approved the use of digital mammography for breast screening following the results of the Digital Mammographic Imaging Screening Trial (DMIST), which enrolled almost 50 000 women. Each woman in the trial underwent both film mammography and digital mammography and various factors were recorded, such as the age of the woman, density of the breast, thickness of the compressed breast, and radiation dose. Digital and film mammograms were reported separately before being compared, and it was determined that the sensitivity of film mammography was comparable to that of digital mammography in women with fatty breasts. However, in women with dense breasts the trial demonstrated significantly improved sensitivity of digital mammography over film mammography. Furthermore, the

trial revealed that the radiation dose with digital mammography was 22% less than with film mammography.[16] In 2007 the Department of Health stated that all screening units should have at least one digital mammography set by 2010.[17]

ALTERNATIVE AND COMPLEMENTARY IMAGING TECHNIQUES

Magnetic resonance mammography (MRM)

MRM is increasingly used as an adjunct to mammography and ultrasound, although it currently has disadvantages such as high cost, limited availability and several contraindications (women with pacemakers, pregnant women, those with claustrophobia and women who are unable to lie in the required prone position, which is necessary when using a breast coil). It is, however, particularly useful for:[18]

- The assessment of implant leakages
- Imaging of dense, glandular breasts
- Evaluation of indeterminate breast lesions
- Imaging of suspected multicentric or multifocal lesions
- Differentiation of recurrent breast cancer from scar tissue
- Evaluation of the response of breast cancer to treatment

Nuclear medicine

There are two main uses of nuclear medicine in breast imaging:

1. *Sentinel node biopsy.* This involves the use of technetium-labelled colloid to label the first axillary lymph node to drain the breast – the sentinel node. If this node is metastasis free then axillary clearance can be avoided. Sentinel node status is able to accurately predict axillary lymph node status in over 95% of cases.[19]
2. *Scintimammography.* This involves the use of technetium-labelled sestamibi and, used as an adjunct to mammography, is comparable to MRM in both sensitivity and specificity in the demonstration of both palpable and impalpable tumours.[18]

Ultrasound

Ultrasound of the breast has increased in recent years, owing to advances in ultrasound technology. Ultrasound is a useful adjunct but is not a standalone method for imaging the breast. It is, however, used more extensively than MRI, computed tomography (CT) and radionuclide imaging (RNI). As breast ultrasound is frequently used in conjunction with mammography, more detail on this imaging modality is included following descriptions of mammography technique.

Digital breast tomosynthesis

Some newer digital mammography sets have this function. The woman is positioned as for a normal mammogram, but with a little less compression. The tube then moves over the breast in an arc, taking a series of low-dose images as it moves. Once these images have been reconstructed (a matter of seconds) a three-dimensional image is produced which is displayed as slices throughout the breast, much like a CT scan. This is particularly useful for dense breasts as it eliminates the problem of overlapping tissue. The use of tomosynthesis as part of a breast screening programme has been trialled in the US and results so far have demonstrated that, when performed as an adjunct to digital mammography, there is a 30–40% reduction in women being recalled for assessment.[20,21] When tomosynthesis is performed without digital mammography the recall rate is reduced by 10%.[20,21] Research is currently under way at King's College Hospital in London to look into the potential of using tomosynthesis within the NHS breast screening programme.[22]

MAMMOGRAPHY TECHNIQUE

Equipment

The purchase, commissioning and quality control of suitable equipment are essential for the provision of a quality mammography service.[23] Equipment must be acceptable to both the operator and the client: it must be light and easy for the operator to use, and there must be no sharp edges in the sections of the unit that come into contact with the client. In addition, handles are necessary to help the client maintain the correct arm position for the oblique projection and for support, if necessary.

The machine consists simply of an X-ray tube connected to a breast support which houses the imaging detector on a C-shaped arm, with a moveable compression paddle between the two (Fig. 26.1).

Functional requirements

- *High-voltage generator*. The generator must supply a near DC high voltage with ripple less than 5%.
- *Kilovoltage (kVp) output*. Most modern mammography machines have automatic selection for kVp in order to optimise contrast. The generator provides a constant potential and the high voltage

applied to the tube must be from 22 to 35 kVp in increments of 1 kVp.

- *Focal spot size*. The focal spot should be as small as possible to ensure adequate resolution, for example 0.3 mm for general mammography and 0.1 mm (small focus) for magnification views.
- *Tube current (mA)*. In order to keep exposure times to a minimum (and thus reduce the likelihood of movement unsharpness) the tube current should be as high as possible. At 28 kVp the current should be at least 100 mA on large focus.
- *Grid*. A grid is essential to ensure optimum image quality; this may be incorporated within the detector on some digital systems.
- *AED*. An automatic exposure device is essential because of the wide variation in breast sizes and compositions. (As there is a need for high radiographic contrast and hence the system has low latitude, there is little scope for error in the selection of mAs.)[23]

Image recording

In line with other radiographic examinations, film/screen mammography is currently being replaced by digital mammography. The digital images are sent electronically to a computer workstation where they are post processed, before being stored in the picture archiving and communication system (PACS). From here the images can be retrieved remotely on reporting workstations and monitors throughout the hospital. The images can also be viewed in other hospitals provided a suitable network link is in place.

Digital mammography

Digital mammography has several advantages over film/screen mammography. Chemical processing is not required and there are no cassettes to change; this means that the examination time is reduced, as is the time between patients being examined. Markers are applied digitally and images can be manipulated once produced. One of the main advantages of image manipulation is its ability to magnify the image with significantly less unsharpness than that associated with macro or magnification images, sometimes required to demonstrate suspicious areas already seen on mammograms. A further benefit of digital magnification is that it does not involve an additional exposure to radiation, unlike traditional magnification views.

Viewing images

Digital mammography images can be viewed on any monitor linked to the network. However, for reporting purposes high-resolution 5 megapixel monitors are required.[24]

It is recommended that craniocaudal (CC) images are viewed 'back-to-back' with the posterior aspects of the breasts touching (Fig. 26.2A,B). Mediolateral obliques are viewed with the pectoral aspects touching (Fig. 26.3A,B). These strategies facilitate vital comparison of similar areas of each breast for each projection.

MAMMOGRAPHIC PROJECTIONS

Anatomical markers must be used on all projections undertaken and markers used in mammography usually incorporate legends, which identify the side under examination, the projection and, sometimes, the orientation of the axilla.

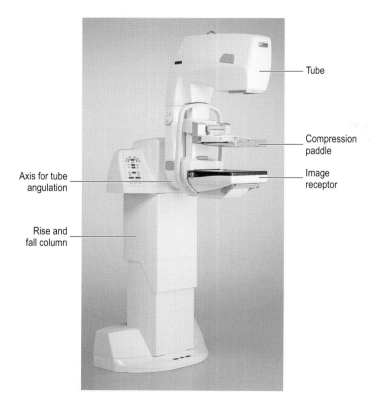

Figure 26.1 Mammography unit.
Reproduced with permission from Xograph Imaging Systems.

Tube

Compression paddle

Image receptor

Axis for tube angulation

Rise and fall column

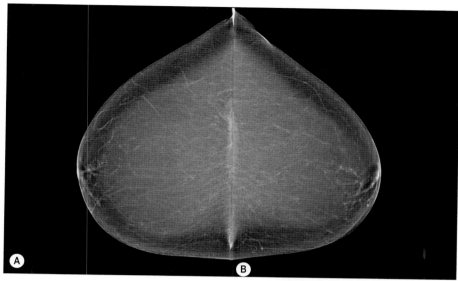

Figure 26.2 Mounting craniocaudal images for viewing. (Permission to use images by courtesy of IMS Italy).

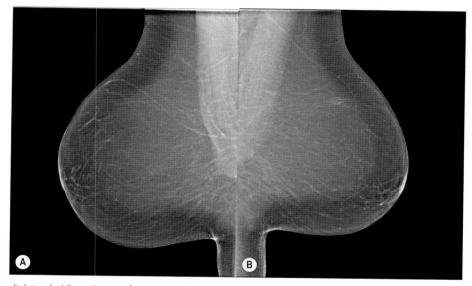

Figure 26.3 Mounting mediolateral oblique images for viewing. (Permission to use images by courtesy of IMS Italy).

Craniocaudal (CC) (Fig. 26.4A,B)

Positioning

- The mammography unit is positioned with the image receptor (IR) holder horizontal and the height adjusted to slightly above the level of the inframammary angle
- The client faces the machine, standing approximately 5–6 cm back from it
- The client's arms hang loosely by her side and her head is turned away from the side to be examined
- The breast is lifted gently up and away from the chest wall (the mammographer will use the left hand to raise the right breast and the right hand to raise the left breast)
- With the mammographer supporting the breast, the height of the unit is adjusted so that the IR holder makes contact with the breast at the inframammary fold and the breast is at approximately 90° to the chest wall

- The client is asked to lean slightly forward until her rib cage is in contact with the machine. The breast is carefully placed onto the IR holder, ensuring that no skin folds are created underneath the breast
- The client is asked to lean slightly towards the side to be examined to bring the outer quadrant of the breast into contact with the IR holder. The mammographer gently pulls the lateral aspect of the breast onto the IR holder whilst making sure that the medial aspect of the breast remains in place. It may be necessary to adjust the unit height to ensure that the inferior aspect of the breast lies horizontally on the IR holder
- The mammographer places her thumb on the medial aspect of the breast and her fingers on the superior aspect; she then pulls gently forward towards the nipple to ensure no skin folds are created, while compression is applied slowly. During this process it is advisable that the mammographer maintains gentle pressure on the client's back, to ensure the maximum amount of breast tissue is included on the image

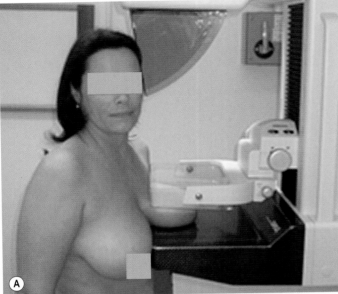

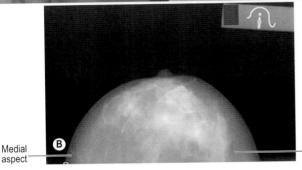

Medial aspect

Lateral aspect

Figure 26.4 (A) CC projection; (B) CC image.

Application of the correct amount of compression comes with experience, although there are guidelines concerning the amount of pressure to be used. The maximum pressure allowed in the UK is 200 N,[1] although in practice this amount is not necessary and many manufacturers limit their equipment to 160 N.

Criteria for assessing image quality

- The nipple is in profile
- The majority of the medial and lateral breast tissue (including some of the axillary tail) is included
- Pectoral muscle is at the centre of the edge of the image. However, this is only seen in approximately 30% of individuals
- An appropriate exposure has been used to provide optimum contrast between the different structures within the breast and adequate image density to demonstrate glandular tissue, muscle and fat
- Absence of artefact, including skin folds
- Absence of movement

Common errors	Possible reasons
Nipple is pointing downwards	1. IR holder may be too high – reduce height
	2. Skin on the underside of the breast may be caught at the proximal edge of the IR holder – reposition the breast by lifting it and gently pulling the underside of the breast forward
	3. Excess loose skin on the superior surface of the breast – apply tension to the skin surface, pulling it gently towards the thorax
Folds at the lateral aspect of the breast	1. There may be a pad of fat or skin above the upper outer quadrant – alter position of the arm
	2. The client may be leaning towards their medial aspect
	3. The breast may be twisted

- The light beam diaphragm can be used while compression is applied, to check that:
  - the nipple is in profile
  - all the breast is within the main beam
  - both the medial and lateral margins are included
  - there are no skin folds
  - compression of the breast is adequate*
- The client may need to hold their other breast laterally and against their body in order to avoid its inclusion on the image. Compression is a vital component in achieving good mammographic images. It is also a part of the examination that causes much concern for women. If the mammographer explains the need for compression at the start of the examination the client may be more able to tolerate any possible discomfort, knowing that better-quality images will be produced and the need for repeat examinations less likely.

*Compression of the breast greatly improves image quality by:
  - reducing the thickness of breast tissue irradiated, thereby reducing the superimposition of breast tissues and reducing the radiation dose to the breast
  - reducing geometric unsharpness
  - reducing movement unsharpness
  - improving contrast (by reducing internal X-ray beam scatter)

Mediolateral oblique (MLO) (Fig. 26.5A,B)

Positioning

- The client faces the unit with feet apart
- From the position used for the CC projection, the unit is rotated through 40–50°, with the IR holder on the side of examination; the height is adjusted to bring the upper border of the IR holder level with the axilla. It may be necessary to further adjust the height during positioning
- The client raises the arm on the side under examination and also raises her chin (thus preventing superimposition of the mandible over the breast)
- The mammographer stands next to the side not under examination and holds the lateral aspect of the breast with one hand, whilst placing the other hand on the client's back
- The client is encouraged to lean forward into the machine and, with feet still facing forward, is asked to lean laterally towards the IR holder
- The mammographer slides her hand forward from between the lateral aspect of the breast and the IR holder, gently pulling the breast forward

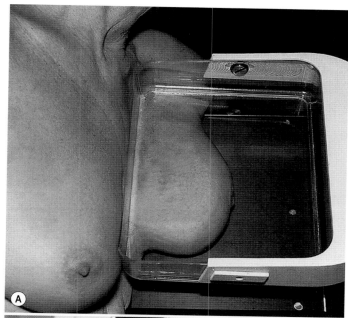

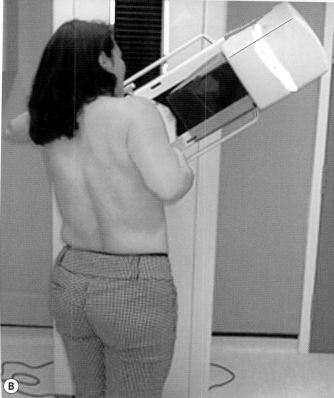

- From the side under examination, the mammographer gently pulls the client's raised arm across and behind the IR holder, so that the corner of the receptor holder sits in the axilla. The client's hand is guided to the handle of the mammography unit for support and the elbow is positioned so it hangs down comfortably behind the IR holder
- The mammographer returns to the side not under examination and, with one hand holding the superior aspect and the other hand holding the inferior aspect of the breast, the mammographer gently lifts the breast and pulls it forward. The mammographer then uses the palm of one hand to hold the breast in place, whilst using the other hand to ensure there are no creases in the inframammary angle
- The thumb of the hand holding the breast is positioned under the breast while the fingers are spread across the breast. This maintains breast position in preparation for compression
- The light beam diaphragm is used to check that:
    - the nipple is in profile
    - the inframammary angle is clearly visible and included within the boundaries
    - there are no skin folds
    - the edge of the compression plate is adjacent to the thorax from immediately below the clavicle down to the inframammary angle
- Compression is applied slowly and evenly using the foot pedal while the mammographer maintains the breast in position, gradually moving her fingers forwards towards the nipple during compression. The thumb maintains the lift of the breast until compression is complete and the breast is held in place by the compression paddle
- When imaging large breasts it is advisable to use the fingers of the opposite hand to support the inferior aspect of the breast in order to avoid straining the thumb

Criteria for assessing image quality

- The entire breast and skin surface are included
- The pectoral muscle lies at the level of the nipple and at an angle of 20–35° from the vertical
- The nipple is in profile
- The inframammary angle is clearly demonstrated
- There are no skin folds
- An appropriate exposure is used to provide optimum contrast between the different structures within the breast and adequate image density to demonstrate glandular tissue, muscle and fat
- There is absence of artefact
- There is absence of movement

Figure 26.5 (A) MLO projection; (B) MLO position demonstrating 45° angle of unit.
(A) Reproduced with permission from Lee L, et al. Fundamentals of mammography. 2nd ed. London: Churchill Livingstone; 2003.

Common errors	Possible reasons
Skin folds at axilla	IR holder may be too high
Skin folds at inframammary angle	Overlap of the breast and abdominal wall – ask the client to stick their bottom out a little and ease out any creases
Nipple is not in profile	IR holder may be too high. The client may have rotated their hips – reposition
Pectoral muscle not across the image	IR holder may be too high – adjust and reposition the shoulder

PGMI (PERFECT, GOOD, MODERATE, INADEQUATE) SYSTEM

The PGMI system was introduced in the UK in the early 1990s as a grading system and guide to performance criteria in the classification of oblique mammograms. It is still used in training centres and mammography departments as a means of evaluating mammograms. It is important to remember, however, that CC films, though not assessed by the PGMI system, must not be forgotten in performance evaluation. Indeed, many breast screening units have modified the original PGMI forms to include the criteria necessary to evaluate CC films.

As the PGMI system is subjective it is possible that individuals using it might grade the same images differently on separate occasions, and this is the main reason for questioning its validity. However, without a better system that uses both the MLO and the CC projections for training and continuing development, mammographers will continue to use PGMI.

The PGMI system: summary[23]

P = perfect

To be graded as a 'perfect' image the following must apply.

1. Whole breast imaged thus:
   - Pectoral muscle to nipple level
   - Pectoral muscle at correct angle
   - Nipple in profile
   - Inframammary angle shown under the breast
2. Correct annotations:
   - Patient identification and examination date
   - Correct anatomical markers
   - Mammographer identification
3. Correct exposure
4. Adequate compression
5. No movement unsharpness
6. Absence of skin folds
7. Symmetrical images

G = good

To be graded 'good', both oblique images must meet criteria 1–5 from the list in the Perfect section. Inadequacy in 6 and 7 can be accepted if shown in a minor degree.

M = moderate

'Moderate' images are considered acceptable for diagnostic purposes. Acceptable errors are:

- Pectoral muscle not level with the nipple or not at the correct angle but the back of the breast is adequately shown
- Nipple not in profile but the retroareolar area is well defined
- Inframammary angle is not clearly demonstrated but the breast is adequately defined
- Artefacts are present but the image is not obscured
- More severe skin folds but the breast image is not obscured – when other criteria are adequately fulfilled

I = inadequate

- If part of the breast is not imaged
- Inadequate compression: this may result in image unsharpness and reduce contrast
- Incorrect exposure
- Artefacts or skin folds that cover the image of the breast
- Inadequate or incorrect identification or annotation of anatomical markers

SUPPLEMENTARY PROJECTIONS

There are a number of additional projections that can be used to supplement the basic CC and MLO projections. They are used to gain further information when a lesion or possible lesion has been seen on the original images, and are often all that is required to clarify any uncertainty. These additional projections can also be used in situations where the client has difficulty achieving the original position, leading to an inadequate examination, for example women who are disabled, wheelchair bound, or those whose physical shape renders positioning difficult and/or painful.

Medially rotated CC projection (extended CC) (Fig. 26.6A,B)

This projection is useful to demonstrate more of the outer breast, towards the axillary tail. The equipment and the client are positioned as for the CC projection but the client then turns her feet 5–10° to the opposite side to that being examined, and is then turned further

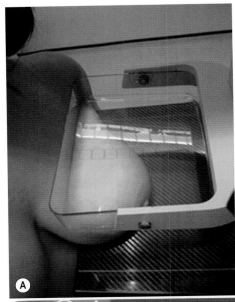

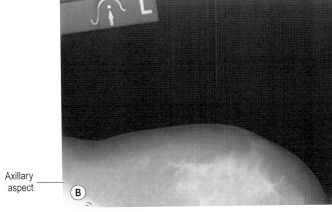

Axillary aspect

Figure 26.6 Extended CC.

to include the lateral aspect of the breast. The medial portion of the breast will not be included on the image.

This projection will demonstrate lesions in the extreme lateral portion of the breast that are seen on the MLO but not on the CC image. It can also be used for women with large breasts who require more than one image in the CC position.

Mediolateral projection (Fig. 26.7A,B)

This projection is used to assess the depth of lesions for localisation and is particularly useful after localisation. The majority of the breast tissue is demonstrated, with the exception of the axillary tail.

Positioning (left breast described)

* The IR holder is vertical
* The client faces the machine with the lateral edge of the chest wall in line with the IR holder
* The left arm is raised and the client is encouraged to hold the support handle. The breast should be in line with the centre of the IR holder
* The mammographer uses her left hand to lift the client's humerus and her right hand to lift the breast up and away from the chest wall. The client is encouraged to lean into the machine, and while keeping the nipple in profile and the inframammary angle in view the right hand is used to ease the patient's axilla onto the corner of the IR holder by carefully pulling the upper portion of the pectoral muscle forward
* The client's arm is rested on top of the machine and, while supporting the breast with the right hand and maintaining the position of the left shoulder with the left hand, the mammographer applies compression ensuring that the nipple is in profile and the inframammary angle is clearly demonstrated prior to making the exposure

Criteria for assessing image quality

* Inframammary angle is included
* Nipple is in profile
* Inferior portion of pectoral muscle is included

A *lateromedial* projection may also be undertaken if it is still necessary to demonstrate the inframammary angle. This essentially uses the opposite position of the mediolateral projection, with the client initially standing with the vertical IR holder between the breasts; the medial aspect of the breast under examination is placed against the IR holder's surface and the breast elevated, positioned and compressed similarly to the mediolateral projection (Fig. 26.8).

Localised compression views (paddle views)

These are used to demonstrate whether a lesion has clear or ill-defined borders and to demonstrate whether a lesion is merely a superimposition of tissues or indeed a genuine lesion. A small compression paddle is attached to the compression unit and this is applied over the area of the suspected lesion; it has the capacity to apply more effective and localised compression to a particular area of the breast.

Equipment requirements are:
* Fine focus
* Small localised compression paddle
* Moving grid
* Full field diaphragm

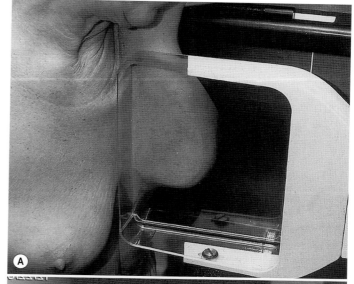

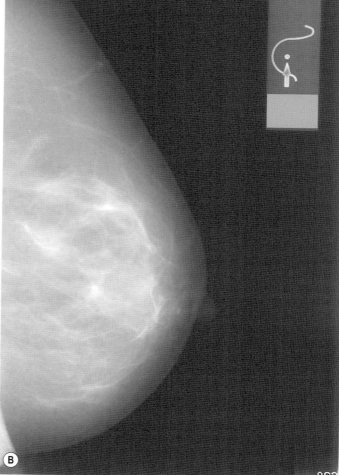

Figure 26.7 Mediolateral.
(A) Reproduced with permission from Lee L, et al. Fundamentals of mammography. 2nd ed. London: Churchill Livingstone; 2003.

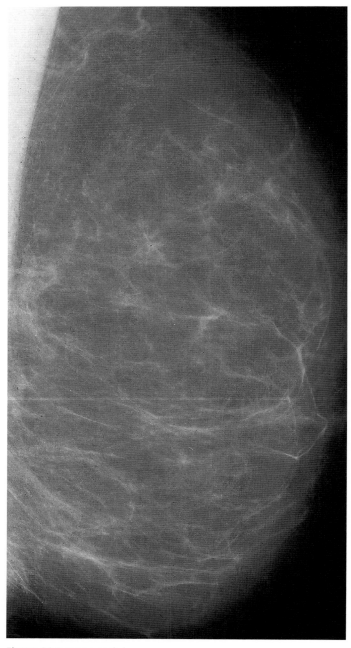

Figure 26.8 Lateromedial.
Reproduced with permission from Lee L, et al. Fundamentals of mammography. 2nd ed. London: Churchill Livingstone; 2003.

Magnification (macro) views

These are used to magnify areas of suspicion seen on mammograms, usually areas of microcalcification, which may well demonstrate their characteristics more clearly when magnified. Additional magnification views are less likely to be needed with digital equipment, as the image can be magnified digitally with excellent detail of the area in question. The benefits of this include avoidance of a second exposure to radiation, reduction of examination time and no additional discomfort for the client.

When undertaking magnification views, communication and explanation is important: if the client is aware of what is being done, why it is being done and what is required of her, she will be able to assist the mammographer more effectively.

Adaptations to equipment are required as follows:

- Fine focus
- Magnification platform
- Small localised compression paddle
- Full field diaphragm

Positioning is selected from existing images, using the projection most likely to demonstrate the suspicious appearance well; for calcifications these are CC and lateral. The breast is positioned in contact with the magnification platform rather than directly over the IR. The localised paddle is brought down over the area of suspicion.

ULTRASOUND

The use of ultrasound as an adjunct to X-ray mammography in the work-up of benign, indeterminate and suspicious breast lesions (and as a first-line imaging investigation in women under 35 with dense breasts) is now firmly embedded in breast diagnostic practice. Furthermore, ultrasound-guided interventional procedures (biopsies and localisations) have not only revolutionised the diagnostic management of impalpable and palpable breast lesions but have also resulted in very accurate preoperative diagnoses. Ultrasound-guided intervention is also recognised as preferable for sampling even clinically palpable lesions, as it is more accurate (thanks to real-time imaging) and considerably safer owing to the proximity of some breast lesions to the chest wall. Consequently, diagnostic excision (open) biopsies are now an infrequent procedure. Ultrasound is also used in initial staging of the axilla in patients with suspected breast cancer, and this facilitates the most appropriate surgical management for such cases. Any equivocal or suspicious nodes are sampled (either fine needle aspiration or core biopsy) preoperatively, and if found to contain metastatic disease an axillary clearance is performed. If no diseased nodes are found preoperatively the patient proceeds to sentinel node biopsy at the same time as surgery to remove the lesion.

As already mentioned in this chapter, magnetic resonance imaging (MRI), ultrasound and radionuclide imaging (RNI) all have a role in identifying breast disease, but the technological developments in ultrasound have meant that this modality now offers high-quality images that are most suitable for demonstrating both breast anatomy and breast pathology. With regard to the dose implications of RNI and the range of contraindications and costs of MRI, the benefits of ultrasound are clear: availability, speed of examination and equipment cost.[25] Technologies are still evolving, with add-on software applications such as *elastography* becoming increasingly available. This application allows further lesion characterisation by providing information that assesses tissue stiffness, leading to improved diagnostic confidence. However, the overall clinical benefits of such technology are yet to be fully realised and integrated into routine practice.

The use of ultrasound in the diagnosis of breast disease, both independently and as an adjunct to mammography, is well documented and there are numerous texts and articles devoted to it. This chapter aims to provide an overview of breast ultrasound rather than exploring it in great depth.

NORMAL ULTRASONIC APPEARANCES OF THE BREAST

The breast comprises a mixture of tissue components which depend on age, hormonal status, structural changes (pathological, involutional, congenital) and particular individual characteristics. In young women breast tissue generally contains very little fat (i.e. is mainly breast parenchyma) but the ageing process causes glandular tissue to be replaced by fat and connective tissue. However, this does vary, and young women with large breasts may still have considerable volumes of fatty tissue.

Observing the breast in schematic sagittal section the following anatomy is seen:

* The skin surface: this is the superficial component of the breast and, when using high-resolution probes, demonstrates a homogeneous band which is more echogenic than the underlying fatty tissue
* Subcutaneous fat
* Cooper's ligaments (the septa of connective tissue surrounding and supporting the glans from the dermis to the pectoral fascia) appear as hyperechoic, oblique lines going into the parenchyma
* Breast parenchyma (ducts and lobules)
* Interlobular fibrofatty tissue
* The deep mammary fascia
* Pectoralis major and minor muscles
* Ribs and intercostal spaces
* Pleura and lung

A young, predominantly glandular breast is variably echogenic, whereas older breasts with more adipose tissue present as hypoechoic. Breast parenchyma is therefore not homogeneous. The parenchyma is seen to be triangular in shape with the apex towards the nipple, and is visualised as a well-defined, rounded nodule of medium echogenicity.

COMMON LESIONS SEEN WITH ULTRASOUND

Cysts

Cysts are such a common finding in women between the ages of 35 and 50 years that they are virtually considered a normal variant; however, they are rare in women under 25 and over 60 years.[25] Cysts can present as single or multiple and are often bilateral.

Simple cysts generally:
* have well-defined margins
* appear as rounded or ovoid in shape
* are anechoic (no internal echoes)
* are compressible
* are seen to have a well-defined posterior wall with enhanced sound transmission
* are seen to have thin shadows at the lesion edges
* are completely encompassed by a thin echogenic capsule.

Complex cysts

A complex cyst can be defined as any cyst that does not meet the strict criteria for definition as a simple cyst (given above). They are also considered to be a common finding and the use of higher-resolution equipment probably contributes to this, owing to its ability to demonstrate small fluid particles and artefactual echoes within cysts. When characterising cystic breast lesions it is important that the operator excludes the presence of artefactual echoes within a simple cyst that can erroneously make them appear as solid lesions or complex cysts. Internal echoes can also often occur after incomplete aspiration of a simple cyst.

Benign solid lesions

The majority of benign breast tumours comprise a mixture of the three breast components: parenchyma, connective tissue and fat. The most common lesions are:

* *Fibroadenoma:* The most common benign breast tumour, affecting women between 20 and 40 years of age. They appear as a well-defined, solid lesion with smooth margins. Fibroadenomas are hypoechoic and internal echoes are usually present due to their macroscopic structure. They have an elongated shape and are not easily compressed.
* *Lipoma:* Lipomas are less echogenic than fibroadenomas, being approximately isoechoic to intramammary fat. Lesion encapsulation differentiates them from normal fatty tissue and they are more compressible than fibroadenomas.

Malignant lesions

Ultrasound is used in the diagnosis of breast cancer as an adjunct to mammography, which is the main initial diagnostic imaging tool. Carcinomas can exhibit a variety of ultrasonic characteristics and there is frequently an overlap between benign and malignant lesions (approximately 2% of carcinomas exhibit fibroadenoma-like features, i.e. smooth margins and homogeneous internal structure). However, in general malignant lesions are very variable in shape; hypoechoic; cause posterior acoustic shadowing (as they are solid); have ill-defined/irregular margins and mixed internal echoes.

Limitations of ultrasound in breast disease diagnosis

Like all imaging techniques ultrasound is very examiner dependent, and therefore experience and technique have a great effect on diagnostic accuracy. It is also equipment dependent and, as already indicated, the quality of equipment used, appropriate transducers and settings are of paramount importance in achieving optimal images. Reproducibility can often be problematic, especially following any needle intervention (if haematoma has occurred), as this can alter ultrasonic appearances for some time afterwards.

Thorough, systematic examination can be very time-consuming in large, dense breasts and visualisation of microcalcification (often an indication of DCIS) is still unreliable, even with the most up-to-date equipment.

BREAST ULTRASOUND EQUIPMENT

Adequate ultrasound examination of any organ requires the use of appropriate equipment. Performing accurate high-quality breast ultrasound requires technical specifications at the very least equal to those for any other body part, demanding excellent spatial and contrast resolution. Only high-resolution instrumentation capable of producing high-quality images should be used.[26]

The breast is a superficial structure which requires the use of high-frequency near-field imaging using real-time handheld transducers

(7.5–15 mHz) with a linear array configuration and a 'footprint' of approximately 4–7 cm. When such equipment is used many more normal structures in the breast tissue are seen, as well as appearances resulting from proliferative and fibrocystic change. A detailed knowledge of breast anatomy and pathology is therefore essential for accurate interpretation of such findings.

The use of Doppler analysis during an examination provides the sonographer with an indication of blood flow to and from a lesion, thus helping further with the formation of a differential diagnosis. Doppler modes available include colour Doppler, power Doppler and pulsed Doppler with spectral analysis. As with conventional breast ultrasound such applications require high-frequency transducers. There are a number of specific situations where there is a role for Doppler, including determination of the aggressiveness of suspicious or malignant lesions (high-grade lesions tend to have noticeably increased flow, whereas low-grade lesions have less tumour neovascularity); assessing response to tumour therapy; distinguishing fat necrosis and scarring from recurrent disease; distinguishing between inflammation and metastases where lymphadenopathy is seen.

THE ROLE OF ULTRASOUND WITH MAMMOGRAPHY

Breast ultrasound as a complementary imaging modality is most often used in the following situations:

- Evaluation of a mass already demonstrated mammographically; with an experienced sonographer ultrasound is highly sensitive in differentiating between solid and cystic lesions in the breast[25]
- To assist with needle guidance for localisation of lesions prior to surgery (see section on breast lesion localisation later in the chapter)
- To assist with needle guidance during breast interventional procedures, e.g. cyst aspirations or lesion biopsy
- Evaluation of dense breast tissue in symptomatic patients. Women most likely to have dense breasts are younger, premenopausal or on hormone replacement therapy. In the presence of dense breast tissue it is frequently difficult to distinguish mass lesions on mammograms

Wherever possible, mammograms for the patient under examination should be available to the sonographer to further aid the scan procedure, and to inform the differential diagnosis of breast problems.

SONOGRAPHY AS A STANDALONE DIAGNOSTIC TOOL

Ultrasound alone is not an appropriate means of screening women for breast cancer, and it is acknowledged that 'the use of ultrasound in population screening of asymptomatic women is associated with unacceptably high rates of both false positive and false negative outcomes'.[27] However, ultrasound is often used as the initial, and sometimes the only, imaging modality in the following situations:

- Determination of the nature of a palpable lump – solid or cystic
- Follow up for patients with recurrent cysts
- Where the level of clinical suspicion at initial assessment is low and use of radiation may raise concern, e.g. in pregnant patients
- When the patient is under 35 years of age and presents with a clinical abnormality thought to be benign. Such a patient is likely

to have dense breasts, greatly reducing the sensitivity and efficacy of mammography
- In extreme cases when a patient presenting with a clinical abnormality refuses mammographic assessment
- To ascertain the integrity of breast prostheses when rupture is clinically suspected. This method is not used in all centres and the alternative is to refer patients of this type for MRI as a first-line investigation
- In cases where compression used in mammography would be intolerable or inappropriate for the patient, e.g. in acute breast conditions such as abscess, recent trauma, and for assessment of the axilla only in cases of very advanced local disease

SUMMARY OF BREAST ULTRASOUND TECHNIQUE

- The patient is undressed from the waist up and is (usually) in the supine or supine oblique position, thereby reducing breast thickness, improving sound penetration and improving visualisation of deeper breast structures. Occasionally upper quadrant masses are better demonstrated in the erect position.
- The arm of the side under examination is extended above the head to stretch the pectoralis muscle, thereby enabling better fixation and immobilisation of the breast and ensuring good visualisation of the lower quadrants and the inframammary fold. This position also facilitates the reproducibility of clinically palpable findings.
- For optimal scanning the transducer should be held at the base, perpendicular to the skin surface, with gentle pressure applied to ensure complete contact. An angled transducer results in poor sound penetration. Compression is useful in reducing the thickness of the area to be examined and to assess changes in the shape of a lesion, e.g. flattening a cyst to confirm its nature. However, care must be taken that the pressure applied is just sufficient to maintain uniform contact with the skin surface but not so excessive that lesions are inadvertently pushed out of the scanning plane or structures are deformed within the parenchyma (the latter making them difficult to evaluate). Glandular tissue and fat are easily deformed but tumours are much firmer, exhibiting considerably less compressibility.
- The whole of the breast and its adjacent tissues are examined, from the inframammary fold to the peripheral areas of the upper quadrants, and from the anterior midaxillary line and the axillary tail to the lateral aspect of the sternum.
- Both sagittal and transverse scans are undertaken, involving overlap of scanning planes to ensure complete, systematic coverage of the breast, along with radial scanning around the areola complex. Because the lactiferous ducts converge radially toward the nipple areola from the periphery and terminate within the nipple, radial scans facilitate examination of the breast ductal structures.
- Any focal lesions demonstrated should be described along with a differential diagnosis, measured, and documented in two planes. The position of any lesion within the breast should be provided as precisely as possible, for example in the left upper outer quadrant. Additionally, lesions/abnormalities may be described as represented on a clock face, e.g. 1 o'clock, 9 o'clock etc., and the distance from the nipple given.
- Mammographic and clinical findings should be correlated when appropriate.

STORING AND VIEWING ULTRASOUND IMAGES

It is now common practice for images of the examination to be produced and stored in radiology PACSs for ease of access. Some systems still facilitate printing of paper copies as well. The equipment used for PACS should be compatible with the ultrasound system.

Quality assurance and quality control are of paramount importance for any imaging modality, and the printer should be included when checks are undertaken.

BREAST LESION LOCALISATION

Before the National Health Service breast screening programme was introduced in 1988[1] most breast cancers were only found when a palpable lump had formed, i.e. they were clinically detectable. The fact that the surgeons could feel these tumours meant that during breast-conserving surgery assistance was seldom necessary to locate the area to be excised; unfortunately, this also meant that tumours were more likely to be more advanced in their growth than those found via a screening mammogram.

Breast screening has increased the rate of diagnosis of breast cancers so small or so deep within the breast tissue that they are impalpable. In order for surgeons to remove these lesions accurately and achieve good cosmesis, the tumours need to be 'localised' under either X-ray or ultrasound guidance.

In most cases 'localisation' involves the insertion of a localisation needle into the breast under image guidance so that the tip is positioned just beyond and adjacent to the tumour. A flexible localisation wire is then passed through the needle and fixed in position with a hook or barb, depending on the type of localisation wire used (there are many different types). The wire remains in the breast with its tip acting as a landmark for the surgeon, who will surgically remove the lesion in question. In addition, the wire tip can often be seen ultrasonically; this can therefore be used to identify the lesion's area in relation to the skin surface to further improve surgical accuracy.

Ultrasound in localisation

If a lesion is visible ultrasonically localisation is relatively straightforward; it is very accurate, as the 'real-time' imaging means the needle and its relationship to the lesion can be monitored as the needle is positioned and the wire deployed. Ultrasound guidance should be the method of choice for localisation if possible; it is faster than X-ray guidance and adjustments for movement or incorrect needle placement can be made immediately. The patient is spared the discomfort of breast compression and is able to lie supine for the duration of the procedure. Moreover, further irradiation of the breast is avoided.

Stereotaxis in localisation

If a lesion cannot be seen clearly under ultrasound, X-ray guidance using a stereotactic device is necessary. There are currently two types of stereotactic device available: one involves the patient lying prone on a biopsy table and the other is an attachment to an upright mammography unit. Figures 26.9A,B and 26.10 demonstrate the position of the localisation needle in the attached stereotactic unit. For the purposes of this chapter, the upright method will be described, as this is the type most commonly encountered in the UK.

The number of staff involved in the procedure should be kept to a minimum, but there should be sufficient to ensure a high-quality procedure and no compromise to patient safety, i.e. consideration must be given to the fact that the patient must never be left alone. An ideal number of staff is three: the mammographer, the practitioner performing the localisation and a second mammographer or nurse.

Before bringing the patient into the room it is important to ensure that everything is ready for the procedure to begin, thereby minimising any anxiety and distress the patient may feel. Ideally, the procedure should also be explained to the patient before she enters the room. She is then seated in front of the mammography unit and made as comfortable as possible; once positioned in the stereotactic device she will be required to stay still in order to reduce the margin of error when inserting the needle.

The breast position for localisation will have been determined by assessing the location of the lesion from previous mammograms. The patient is then appropriately positioned in the machine and the compression paddle is applied. Once positioned, the patient's comfort is ensured and maintained and the outline of the compression window is marked on her breast. If there is any subsequent movement of the breast this will be easily seen and repositioning can be performed if

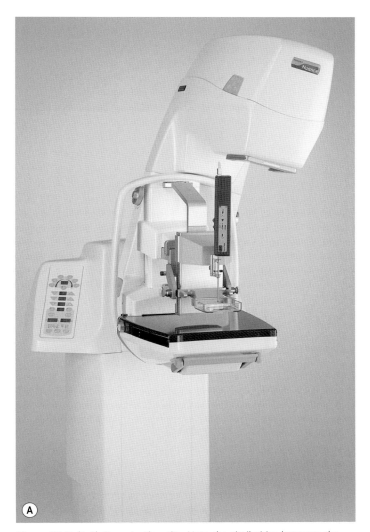

Figure 26.9 (A,B) Stereotactic units. Note the similarities between the two units.
Reproduced with permission from Xograph Imaging Systems.

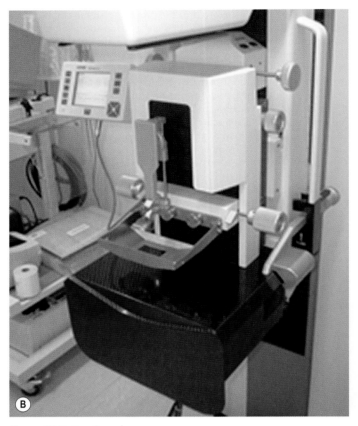

Figure 26.9, Continued

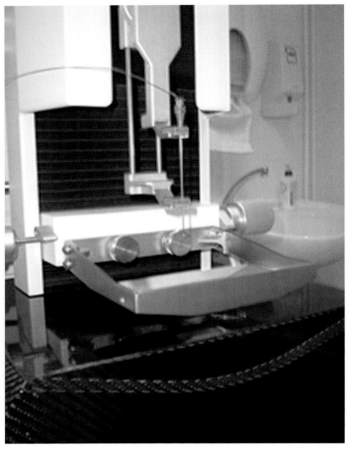

Figure 26.10 Localisation needle and guidewire positioned in stereotactic unit.

necessary. It is not easy for the patient to maintain her position as she may have to move her head to facilitate the swing of the X-ray tube. Two stereotactic images of the breast are required, with the tube being moved through an angle of 30° in between each exposure, and the patient position supported and maintained during the tube movement. The two images are displayed next to each other on the digital monitor. The images are checked to ensure that the abnormality is clearly demonstrated on both screens of the monitor. If necessary, the breast is repositioned and further images are taken. Once satisfactory stereotactic images have been obtained the abnormality is 'targeted' on each image and the coordinates of the target are then transmitted to the stereotactic device. The skin is cleansed and local anaesthetic administered before the needle is inserted into the breast through needle guides attached to the unit. The wire is then deployed so that the tip lies just beyond the lesion, and check images are taken in the craniocaudal and lateral positions to check its position. The wire tip must be positioned beyond the lesion so that the surgeon can follow the wire down to the area that needs to be removed. If the wire stops short of the abnormality, the surgeon may have difficulty in locating it.

Once the wire is deemed to be positioned satisfactorily the procedure is complete and sterile dry dressings are applied over the entry site and the wire itself. A detailed report is then written for the surgeon to inform them of the relation of the lesion to the wire tip and the length of wire within the breast. It can be helpful to include a diagram in the report demonstrating the position of the wire within the breast. The surgeon can also view the check images in the operating theatre. The patient is then escorted back to the ward to await surgery.

After surgery the excised tissue is returned for X-ray assessment. The tissue is imaged and, after comparison with the preoperative mammograms, the surgeon is informed by imaging department personnel about the presence of the abnormality within the excised tissue and the proximity of the abnormality to the borders of the tissue. A PACS will also enable the surgeon to view images from theatre. This stereotactic procedure is also used to obtain core biopsies of the breast for histological assessment. Lesions biopsied usually include microcalcification clusters and isoechoic masses that may not be visible ultrasonically.

REFERENCES

1. Department of Health. The NHS Plan: a plan for investment, a plan for reform. London: HMSO; 1 July 2000.

2. Department of Health. Radiography skills mix: A report on the four-tier service delivery model. London: HMSO; June 2003.

3. Banks E, et al. Influence of personal characteristics of individual women on sensitivity and specificity of mammography in the Million Women Study: cohort study. BMJ 2004;329(7464): 477.

4. National Institute for Health and Clinical Excellence. Understanding NICE guidance.

Women with breast cancer in the family. Clinical guideline 41. Issue date: October 2006.

5. Forrest AP. Breast cancer: the decision to screen. Journal of Public Health Medicine 1991;13:2–12.

6. International Agency for Research on Cancer. Mammography screening can reduce deaths from breast cancer. Geneva: World Health Organization; Press release 139: 19 March 2002.

7. Department of Health. Cancer Reform Strategy. London: HMSO; December 2007.

8. Lee L, et al. Fundamentals of mammography. 2nd ed. London: Churchill Livingstone; 2003: 143.

9. Bjurstram N, et al. The Gothenburg Breast Screening Trial. First results on mortality, incidence and mode of detection for women aged 39–49 years at randomisation. Cancer 1997;80:2091–9.

10. Nystrom L, et al. Breast cancer screening with mammography; overview of Swedish randomised trials. Lancet 1993;341:973–8.

11. Shapiro S, et al. Periodic screening for breast cancer: the health insurance plan project and its sequelae, 1963–1986. London: Johns Hopkins University Press; 1988.

12. Pritchard J. Quality assurance guidelines for mammography. Report of a Sub-committee of the Radiology Advisory Committee of the Chief Medical Officer. Oxford: NHSBSP Publications; 1990.

13. Breast Cancer Care. Breast cancer – the facts. Available from: http://www.breastcancercare.org.uk/breast-cancer-breast-health/breast-awareness/breast-m8s/breast-cancer-the-facts/; 2009.

14. Cancer Research UK. What do 'grade' and 's-phase' mean? Available from: http://www.cancerhelp.org.uk/about-cancer/cancer-questions/what-do-grade-and-sphase-mean; 2010.

15. National Health Service Breast Screening Programme. Review of Radiation Risk in Breast Screening. 2003; Publication No. 54.

16. Hendrick R, et al. Comparison of acquisition parameters and breast dose in digital mammography and screen-film mammography in the American College of Radiology Imaging Network Digital Mammographic Imaging Screening Trial. AJR 2010;194:362–9.

17. Department of Health. Cancer Reform Strategy. Available from http://www.dh.gov.uk/en/Publicationsandstatistics/Publications/PublicationsPolicyAndGuidance/dh_081006; 2007.

18. Mann R, et al. Breast MRI: guidelines from the European Society of Breast Imaging. European Radiology 2008;18:1307–18.

19. Pater J, Parulekar W. Sentinel lymph node biopsy in early breast cancer: has its time come? Journal of the National Cancer Institute 2006;98(9):568–9.

20. Poplack S, et al. Digital breast tomosynthesis: initial experience in 98 women with abnormal digital screening mammography. American Journal of Roentgenology 2007;189:616–23.

21. Gur D, et al. Digital breast tomosynthesis: observer performance study. American Journal of Roentgenology 2009;193:586–91.

22. NHS Breast Cancer Screening Programme. Tomosynthesis trial. Available from: http://www.cancerscreening.nhs.uk/breastscreen/research-tomosynthesis.html; 2010.

23. Lee L, et al. Fundamentals of mammography. 2nd ed. London: Churchill Livingstone; 2003.

24. NHS Cancer Screening Programmes. Commissioning and routine testing of full field digitial mammography systems. NHSBSP equipment report 0604. Version 3; Available from: http://www.cancerscreening.nhs.uk/breastscreen/publications/nhsbsp-equipment-report-0604.pdf; 2009.

25. Ciatto S, et al. The contribution of ultrasonography to the differential diagnosis of breast cancer. Neoplasma 1994;41(6):341–5.

26. NHSBSP Ultrasound Working Group. Review of the use of ultrasound scanners in the UK Breast Screening Programme. Publication 43 February 1999.

27. Teh W, Wilson ARM. The role of ultrasound in breast cancer screening. A consensus statement by the European Group for Breast Cancer Screening. European Journal of Cancer 1998;34(4):449–50.

FURTHER READING

Madjar H. The practice of breast ultrasound. Stuttgart, New York: Thieme; 2000.

Stavros AT. Breast ultrasound. Philadelphia, New York, London: Lippincott Williams & Wilkins; 2004.

Section | 6 |

Paediatric imaging

Chapter 27

Paediatric imaging in general radiography

Donna Jane Dimond, Tim Palarm

INTRODUCTION

Paediatric patients presenting for radiographic imaging range from the very small, such as neonates and premature babies, to teenagers and young adults. Regardless of age, each group has unique differences and presents separate challenges to the examining radiographer. Most children will first encounter the hospital environment through an attendance at the emergency department of a local general hospital, despite the presence of specialist paediatric units throughout the country. As a consequence, children are likely to meet radiographers who are more at home examining adults, using equipment and surroundings designed for that purpose.

It has been decided to include key examinations likely to be encountered in independent practice as opposed to those regularly carried out in paediatric radiology departments. Some of the radiographic techniques explored will need to be cross-referenced with the relevant chapter elsewhere in this book. Details of invasive procedures and specialised examinations are therefore not included, and readers are encouraged to refer to specialist paediatric texts for in-depth information. This chapter is not designed to be definitive or exhaustive, but provides a general overview of techniques which from the authors' experience have been shown to work well. It is recognised that alternative methods may be used which can also achieve desired results.

Radiographers are encouraged to formulate collaborative approaches through interprofessional working with other healthcare professionals and contact with colleagues at dedicated paediatric units throughout the country. The Association of Paediatric Radiographers (APR) is an excellent initial contact.[1] Not only will this be of direct benefit to patients but it will also contribute to the radiographer's continuing professional development. The specialty of paediatric imaging provides potential scope for the introduction of advanced and consultant radiographer practitioners for those aspiring to a career in this area.

SPECIAL CONSIDERATIONS WHEN IMAGING CHILDREN

The key factor in obtaining a high-quality diagnostic image is undoubtedly the gaining of the child's trust prior to the commencement of the examination.[2] With such trust follows the development of the patient–radiographer relationship that will result in compliance by the child and positive feelings about the imaging experience. Positive feelings are invaluable in the paediatric age group, as a large proportion of children are likely to return for X-rays in their formative years.

The Kennedy Report,[3] in the context of heart surgery, advises that all children should be treated in a paediatric environment by paediatric specialists and healthcare professionals. Clearly this is unachievable in many general hospitals. It is likely that most will agree that radiology departments should have at the very least a named lead radiographer and a core team of staff that are specially trained, competent and keen to examine children.[4] It is not unreasonable to strongly suggest that all undergraduate diagnostic radiography students should be provided with learning opportunities in dedicated paediatric departments. Most radiographers will examine children as early as their first appointment as a radiographer. Therefore, a sound knowledge and understanding of the paediatric specialty gained during placement will be of great benefit to all radiographers commencing their careers.

Anxiety is a common emotion in patients of any age, but is often heightened in children due to unfamiliar surroundings, adults, and sometimes the reactions of their parents/carers. The radiographer needs to appear friendly, positive and self-assured and able to instil a sense of confidence in both the child and the parent/carer (Fig. 27.1).

Ensuring that the physical environment is favourable to imaging children is an important factor, although this is often dependent upon additional funds and the backing of management. Child-friendly decor and furnishings with toys and books, ideally away from the adult waiting area, helps to achieve a welcoming, relaxed and warm atmosphere (Fig. 27.2).

Understanding the different stages of child development is vital in order to tailor the examination for the individual: make the examination fit the child rather than vice versa. Some helpful tips are as follows:

- Enabling the child to make choices, such as selection of a lead gown for their parent/carer, will give them a degree of feeling in control over their surroundings.
- Allowing the child to bring a favourite toy or comforter into the examination room helps dispel fears. On occasions taking an X-ray of the toy can prove a worthwhile venture to help the child understand what the examination involves.

requirement to obtain images of maximum diagnostic quality with no artefact, if avoidable, for example removal of nappies for abdominal and pelvic imaging.

Parents/carers play a pivotal role in the imaging of the young child, particularly the preschool age group. Babies and toddlers have very strong attachments to family members and resent any form of separation. When examining older children the radiographer may need to make a decision regarding the degree of involvement of the parent/carer and their location in the room. In addition to any anxieties, the older child is more aware of him/herself and understands how refusal to cooperate can control a situation to their liking. With regard to parental role, there is a risk that some parents will assert themselves and attempt to orchestrate the proceedings. It is therefore important that the radiographer carefully manages the imaging environment and the examination.

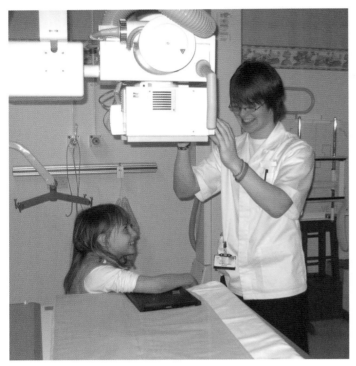

Figure 27.1 An explanation of the examination to take place.

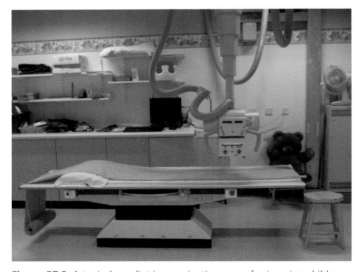

Figure 27.2 A typical paediatric examination room for imaging children.

- Likening the patient's position for the examination to a normal everyday occurrence can be extremely advantageous. For example, asking a child to breathe in as they would do to blow up a balloon or swim under water is likely to result in a better effort than the instruction to breathe in alone.
- Rewards, be it stickers or certificates, have proved to be excellent incentives, particularly for children likely to return for regular imaging. Many children look forward to receiving another sticker for their collection.
- Consideration should be given to ensure the child's privacy and dignity are maintained throughout the examination. This applies to all examinations, and needs to be balanced alongside the

RADIATION PROTECTION AND DOSE LIMITATION

Radiation exposure in the first 10 years of life may have an attributable lifetime risk three to four times greater than that after 30 years of age.[5] As such, there is a greater opportunity for potential harmful effects to manifest themselves. The rationale in this chapter is to offer suggestions for radiation dose reductions; however, optimisation of the exposure factors may be more realistic. The choice of radiographic exposures should be in accordance with the 1996 CEC guidelines,[5] taking weight, age and size into account. For examinations conducted using the X-ray table or bucky, automatic exposure devices may be used. The radiographer needs to consider the size of the selected chamber in comparison with the child's anatomical size. In these instances it is important that the correct ionisation chamber and X-ray tube potentials are selected. Information on exposure factors should be readily available throughout the department, including mobile apparatus. It is essential that there is close working alongside clinical scientists to ensure that the appropriate balance between dose and image quality are maintained. Although practitioners may become involved in the evaluation of computed/digital radiography systems, it is important that consideration is given to dose, particularly when used for imaging children.[6] Added consideration may need to be given to the optimisation of paediatric doses in non-specialist centres where digital imaging is already in place.

In keeping with the Ionising Radiation (Medical Exposure) Regulations[7] prior to carrying out a diagnostic radiographic examination, all requests must be clinically justified. It is not uncommon for junior clinicians to over-request X-rays on children through inexperience with image interpretation or difficulties encountered during the initial assessment. Radiographers need to fully understand the RCR guidelines[8] and enlist the assistance of a radiologist colleague if necessary.

Checking previous images is an essential part of any radiographer's role. In paediatrics, such an assessment can provide useful information regarding the technique employed, in addition to the exposure used and the exact image series obtained.

Radiographers will need to confirm the pregnancy status of any female of child-bearing age before undertaking a radiographic examination.[7] The lower age limit for pregnancy status is considered to be 12 years; however, some girls commence menstruation as young as 10. The issue of ascertaining pregnancy status is complex and delicate. A simple and uncomplicated approach is recommended as one that is likely to achieve an honest answer. First, the radiographer should ask whether the patient has started her monthly periods. If the answer is confirmatory, the radiographer needs to ask whether there is any possibility that the patient could be pregnant. Ideally this conversation should take place away from the parent/carer, and make clear to the patient that it is an important part of the radiographer's responsibility to ask such questions. Proof of pregnancy status should be retained permanently, either electronically or on paper.

A common error by radiographers who do not undertake X-ray examinations on children regularly is the failure to tightly collimate the primary beam. This may be through fear of missing the area of interest off the image. The use of effective immobilisation, be it with devices or a holder, coupled with ongoing learning and skill development, should enable the radiographer to feel confident about collimating more appropriately and thereby limiting radiation. A holder can be defined as anyone who supports and immobilises a patient during a radiographic exposure.[2] Different centres may use varying approaches in their recommended choice or preference of holder, be it the child's parent, carer or healthcare worker. Debate and appropriate recommendations on this subject should be encouraged, but the radiographer must be aware that immobilisation is a potentially contentious issue, in that there is a difference between immobilisation and restraint. It is therefore recommended that radiographers are fully conversant with the hospital's holding policy.

Care should be taken to ensure that any parent/carer remaining within the X-ray room and/or providing immobilisation is adequately protected (lead or equivalent apron). There must also be clear instruction by the radiographer how to put the apron on properly and the importance of good posture to avoid injury. Before enlisting the assistance of any female parent/carer, the radiographer should consider the possibility of pregnancy. Radiographers should provide the holder with clear instructions to avoid the need for repeat exposures.

The holder's fingers should always be excluded from the primary beam. Should the fingers be close to the primary beam, lead gloves/mittens should always be worn, although they will not provide complete protection at higher beam energies (Fig. 27.3). It is recommended that records are kept of any radiographers or healthcare personnel who hold children for X-ray examinations to avoid the same individual regularly undertaking this role.[1]

RADIOGRAPHIC EXAMINATIONS IN THIS CHAPTER

This chapter will examine standard imaging requested on paediatric patients. It will provide the undergraduate and less experienced radiographer with a fundamental understanding using a commonsense approach. Depending upon the area examined, it will be necessary to offer specific descriptions of techniques that differ in their approach from that of adult examinations of the same area. Other examinations may require only an observation on possible differences that may be relevant to immobilisation strategies and positioning that requires a supine approach for babies and very young children.

Subjects included in this chapter are as follows:

- Chest (including ingested/inhaled foreign bodies)
- Abdomen
- Appendicular skeleton
- Axial skeleton
- Skeletal surveys

FACILITATING THE RADIOGRAPHIC EXAMINATION

Before commencing any imaging examination the radiographer must undertake a holistic assessment, considering the child's physical state, and their emotional, cognitive and educational needs. Often talking to the child is sufficient in itself as a distraction technique.

As previously mentioned, immobilisation or clinical holding is sometimes unavoidable to obtain diagnostic images in a safe and controlled manner. Most hospitals will have a patient restraint policy document, often called a 'clinical holding policy'. It is important that a copy is kept in the radiology department. It is essential that all radiographers likely to be involved in immobilising children are adequately trained and aware of alternative approaches to gaining a child's cooperation. This may include distraction techniques (Fig. 27.4), play therapy, improved explanations or simple persuasion. Non-cooperation may be due to the child having a bad day or sensing their parent/carer's anxieties. On occasions having a break or time out can work wonders. Children who have undergone a seemingly endless series of examinations may benefit from returning on another day, provided this does not jeopardise their clinical management.

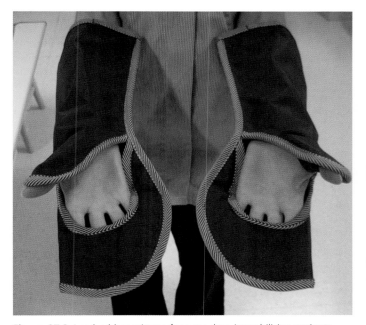

Figure 27.3 Lead rubber mittens for use when immobilising patients.

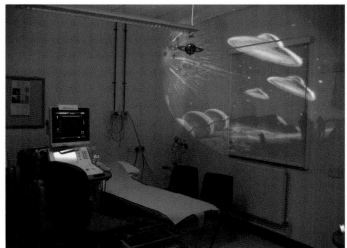

Figure 27.4 Image projector in an imaging room used as distraction.

Samples of tried and tested techniques are as follows:

- Prepare the examination room with several sizes of image receptor (IR), immobilisation pads and sandbags, protective lead aprons.
- Employ methods to reduce the potential for cross-infection.
- Select a preliminary imaging exposure prior to inviting the child into the room.
- Introduce yourself to the child and their family using your first name. Make eye contact and smile. Asking who the child has brought with them today will make them feel important and also act as a means of establishing the identity of the adult without mistake or embarrassment!
- Upon entering the examination room, ask them how they are today, whether they have had an X-ray before. Encourage them to talk about it if they are happy to do so.
- Look for conversation topics such as birthdays, holidays, sports (particularly if a sports shirt is being worn), or favourite television programmes (characters are often featured on clothing).
- Demonstrating the position required is often more effective than a description. Enlisting the help of the parent/carer can be particularly beneficial.
- Consider a practice run to limit the need for a repeat examination, for example for chest X-rays to avoid over inflation of the lungs.
- The child watching the light and announcing when it has gone out has proved to be a useful game. The child feels important in being given a job and is likely to be more compliant.
- Encourage the child to count while the X-ray is being taken. This may assist in maintaining the correct position.
- Children requiring comfort and reassurance from their parent/carer are best examined close to these adults. Clinicians carrying out patient assessment and examinations on children undertake as many required tests as possible while the child is seated on the lap of their parent/carer.[9] This approach works equally well with children in the X-ray room.
- If two projections are required and one is likely to be easier or less distressing than the other, it often pays to perform the easier one first.

COMMON MISTAKES AND ERRORS IN PAEDIATRIC RADIOGRAPHIC EXAMINATION

General errors that can occur during paediatric examinations, and the reasons for them, are detailed in Table 27.1. Common errors are also identified for some individual projections, when there may be additional considerations or common faults associated particularly with paediatric examinations; otherwise errors and their correction can be assumed to be the same as those for adults.

CHEST

The chest X-ray is one of the most commonly requested radiographic images in children but is often difficult to obtain and can be of poor quality, particularly in the younger age group.[10]

It is imperative that any clothing is removed so as to avoid the presence of artefact (embroidery, transfers on garments) on the resulting image. We strongly advise that long hair should be moved away from the area of interest, as should any monitors or leads, providing it is not detrimental to the patient to do so.

The posteroanterior (PA) erect projection is preferred by radiologists, although in practice the anteroposterior (AP) is more readily

Table 27.1 Common errors noted in paediatric radiography

Common errors	Possible causes
Too large an X-ray field size	Overestimation of a child's anatomical proportions/area of interest
Insufficient demonstration of anatomical area	Incorrect centring points – using those appropriate for adults that may not be suitable for child examinations (e.g. chest radiography in neonates)
Images of the parent's/holder's hands, or other parts in the region of interest	Extremities in the primary beam due to immobilisation attempt – often due to insufficient communication from the radiographer
Movement unsharpness or some/all area under examination moved outside collimated field	Inadequate immobilisation technique used
	Patient movement, crying, respiration, too long an exposure time
	Increased cardiac motion in babies for chest imaging
	Generator unable to support short exposure times. This may be more evident where mobile equipment is used
Gonad or lead protection obscuring the area of interest	Misplacement of item by the radiographer
	Movement of the child
	Movement of item by the parent has also been noted!
Under- or overexposure of the resultant image through the use of an automatic exposure device	Similarly to adults, incorrect selection of the ionisation chamber
	Movement of the child, removing required area away from ionisation chamber
Additional radiographic artefacts	Clothing image artefact
	Body piercing jewellery in situ
	Foam support pads/sandbags not radiolucent 'comforters' (e.g. dummy)

performed in infants and young children as they are more likely to cooperate with this style of examination. This patient preference can be attributed to the need of the child to see their surroundings and their parent/carer. Unfortunately, the choice of technique often relies heavily upon the confidence of the radiographer: the less capable individual may elect to use the AP projection when careful assessment and communication might have established that a PA could have been achievable. In other words, it may be more 'convenient' for the radiographer to undertake a supine AP projection in preference to an erect AP. It should be remembered that the majority of children reach their sitting milestone at approximately 6 months of age. The implication here is that at the very least erect projections should be performed from this age, or before.[2]

PA erect chest

The adult technique is appropriate for use in older children and reference should be made to Chapter 23.

AP erect chest

IR is vertical for this examination; size must be appropriate for the child

Positioning

- A stool is placed in front of the erect unit. A rubberoid material, e.g. Dycem, can be placed on the seat to prevent the child slipping
- The child is encouraged to sit on the stool with their back against the IR. The upper border of the receptor should be visible above the shoulders if a cassette-type IR is used
- A 15° radiolucent pad (if using digital radiography check the pad does not cause an artefact) may be placed behind the child's back, in front of the receptor, to limit the degree of lordosis and to act as a soft cushion to protect the back of the head
- A Velcro band may be useful to assist in maintaining the optimum position
- Both arms should be flexed at the elbow and raised to the side of the head. where they may be supported by the child's parent/carer or escort

Beam direction and focus receptor distance (FRD)

Horizontal, with a 5–10° caudal angle to reduce lordotic appearance on the image
2 m FRD

Centring

For babies: in the midline between the sternal angle and the xiphisternum
For older children: use the same centring point as for adults

Collimation

Apices, lateral margins of both lungs, cardiophrenic and costophrenic sulci

Respiration
Observe the child's breathing and make the exposure on inspiration if they are unable to comply with instructions.

Supine AP

An appropriately sized cassette-type receptor is placed on the table or in the cot/bed/incubator. Incubator sides should be opened for the absolute minimum of time to avoid temperature changes, which can adversely affect the patient. Evidence suggests that neonates are also susceptible to noise and vibration, which should be kept to a minimum. Be aware that incubators need to be separated by a distance of at least 60 cm in order to reduce the cumulative scatter dose to neighbouring isolettes.[11]

- The child is placed on the receptor with the shoulders and head resting upon a 15° pad, to reduce lordosis and aid patient comfort
- If not detrimental to the child's wellbeing, the arms should be extended, abducted anteriorly, raised and immobilised by the side of the head. Most efficient immobilisation is achieved by the arms held against the head by the elbows
- Some assistance may be required to avoid rotation of the child's lower body
- When examining a child in an incubator, strips of lead rubber can be arranged to form a 'window', providing radiation protection to the child and holder while improving image quality

Beam direction and FRD

Vertical, with a caudal angle of 5–10° at a distance of at least 100 cm. Longer FRDs should be utilized, but this is often unachievable owing to available tube height and/or incubator limitations

Centring

For babies: in the midline at the level of the sternal angle or nipples
For older children: use the same centring point as for adults

Collimation

Apices, lateral margins of both lungs, cardiophrenic and costophrenic sulci

A baby's diaphragm is anatomically higher than that of older children and adults as the bifurcation of the trachea occurs at the level of T3/4 as opposed to T5/6 in the older child.

Respiration
Observe the child's breathing and make the exposure on inspiration if they are unable to comply with instructions.

Criteria for assessing image quality

In essence the criteria for assessing a paediatric chest image are the same as those for an adult, with the additional considerations. It is essential, particularly in neonates, that reproducible exposure factors are consistently used.

- Image is as free as possible from artefact
- Sharp visualisation of the heart and lungs
- Mandible and chin must not obscure the lung apices
- Adequate penetration (appropriate kVp) to demonstrate the retrocardiac area
- No evidence of rotation – scrutiny of rib symmetry
- The chest does not appear lordotic

For general errors please refer to the introductory section of this chapter.

Common errors	Possible causes
Lordotic image – anterior ribs appear horizontal or lie above the posterior ribs	Hyperextension of the child's arms *or*
	child has arched their back during exposure
Left to right asymmetry of the anterior and posterior ribs	As for adults, rotation of the area – small children are far more 'cylindrical' in shape than older children and adults, making this fault more common
Soft tissue opacification over one or both of the apices	Neck is insufficiently extended, the soft tissues of the chin or mandible are overlying the area of interest. More frequently encountered in children than adults
Hyperinflated chest	Exposure has been made during a large intake of breath by the child during crying or over-enthusiasm
In cases of incubator baby images: circle overlying the image	'Porthole' of incubator lid overlies the area of interest
Excessive amount of abdomen included on the chest image	Centring too low – often encountered in neonates
Spine appears curved/scoliotic	Slouched position
Vertical streaking artefact	Hair artefact

If requested together, mobile chest and abdomen examinations should be performed separately. Tempting though it may be to take one projection to include both chest and abdomen, this must be avoided as this method produces an image of poor quality with a lordotic chest and uses an exposure only suitable for one area. The only exception is in the case of assessment for a 'central line' placement, and for this purpose collimation should be refined to a rectangular area that demonstrates the line only.

Lateral chest

For older children, please refer to the appropriate chapter on adult chest radiography, as adult technique is used for this group.

Positioning

- Where possible, children should be imaged erect, either standing or sitting, as for adults
- Very young children should be examined lying on their left side on the receptor with their head supported on a foam pad
- Infants being nursed in incubators may require a horizontal beam lateral while the receptor is safely supported vertically at one side
- Arms should be raised to either side of the head, away from the area of interest
- The neck needs to be adequately extended in order to prevent superimposition of the soft tissues of the chin or mandible upon the resultant image

Beam direction and FRD

Horizontal or vertical at 90° to the IR
FRD issues are as for the AP chest but it is likely that a 1.8–2 m FRD will be achievable for an older child examined erect

Centring point

Young children: midway between the anterior and posterior margins of the thorax at the level of the sternal angle
Older children: as for adults

Collimation

As for adults

Criteria for assessing image quality

As for adults

Ingested or inhaled foreign bodies

Young children will frequently attend emergency departments after swallowing or inhaling small objects. Usually clinicians will have taken a detailed history and excluded the presence of the item in clothing or other body cavities prior to referral for imaging. Ideally a duplicate of the item believed to have been inhaled/ingested will have been brought by the parent/carer to hospital, but unfortunately this does not always occur. This is helpful in order to assess the likelihood of the item being demonstrated radiographically.

A commonsense approach to the radiographic management of such patients has been chosen for this chapter. The emergency department staff will have already made a clinical decision regarding patient management, and some units use a metal detector to localise objects if they are ferrous in nature. This helps prioritise the order and number of images required. The first image should be studied before moving on to the next, as appearances will dictate whether another projection is required or not.

For suspected inhaled foreign bodies a chest X-ray is required. Even if the item is not purported to be radio-opaque the chest X-ray is still of value in identifying any possible associated collapse or air trapping and/or consolidation of the lung.

For ingested foreign bodies an abdominal X-ray should only be performed if the swallowed foreign body is suspected to be sizeable, sharp, toxic, or leakage is possible. An area of anatomical overlap must be ensured.

On the chest image it is useful to include the neck in the collimated field (patient's head turned to one side) to ensure the foreign body is not located in the nasopharanx or oropharynx.

ABDOMEN

The abdominal X-ray is routinely requested despite the advent of imaging modalities such as ultrasound and magnetic resonance imaging that use non-ionising radiation. Although undertaken frequently on neonatal units, this practice is not recommended on the ward for older children, owing to image quality and radiation protection issues. Because of the marked radiation dose imparted to the patient, all requests for abdominal imaging must be clinically justified and consideration given to the other imaging investigations that may be more appropriate as a primary examination. Radiographic techniques such as the lateral or dorsal decubitus, and erect abdomen, are seldom undertaken but may be justified in specific cases after discussion with consultant radiologists. It is not uncommon for imaging of both the chest and abdomen to be requested simultaneously.[6] This can be justified for the reasons outlined in the chest section above, although the effective dose has been reported to be 5% greater.[6]

Before carrying out abdominal radiography the child must always be undressed, including the nappy, and any potential artefacts removed from the area. Particular care should be taken with baby vests that have poppers: both the front and the back need to be removed from the area of interest.

AP abdomen

IR is horizontal
An appropriately sized IR is positioned with the long axis in line with the child's medial sagittal plane (MSP). For smaller children it is not necessary to use a scatter reduction device or grid.

Positioning

- The child is positioned supine on the examination table as for the adult abdomen examination
- When using a cassette-type receptor, babies and small children not requiring a secondary radiation reduction device (grid) are placed in direct contact with the IR
- For children unable to remain still, the femora and upper torso are supported (holding arms and legs) by an assistant to prevent rotation and lateral flexion of the trunk
- The arms are raised onto the pillow to enable the humeri to be shielded from the primary beam
- For portable examinations on the neonatal unit, the incubator lid can be used as placement for lead rubber strips (see procedure for paediatric chest examination)
- The exposure should be made on arrested respiration

Radiation protection

- Do not use secondary radiation grids for small children.
- Use X-ray tube potentials between 60–65 kVp with short exposure times.[5]

Beam direction and FRD

Vertical

100 cm FRD

Centring point

In the midline at the level of the iliac crests. The umbilicus is approximately at the same level and is a reliable centring point for babies

Collimation

* Use shadow shielding wherever possible
* Collimate to include the diaphragm, upper border of the symphysis pubis and lateral walls of the abdomen

Criteria for assessing image quality

* Diaphragm, upper border of the symphysis pubis and lateral walls of the abdomen
* Symmetry of the pelvic structures; the spinous processes should be demonstrated down the centre of the vertebral bodies
* There should be clear contrast between the skeleton and soft tissues, enabling clear demonstration of bowel gas

Appendicular skeleton

HAND AND FINGERS

The same principles for X-ray examination of the area are applied here as for adult radiography. The only differences relate to the variations in technique due to the child's age and level of cooperation. Hand and finger imaging is regularly undertaken to rule out bony injury or the presence of a foreign body in the soft tissues.

As previously mentioned, small children are more likely to be content sat on their parent/carer's lap, where they can feel secure as well as be able to see around them. However, circumstances may dictate that the child is happier being examined in a supine position.

The greatest challenge of examining this area is ensuring that the fingers remain extended and the correct position is maintained. Various methods have been described to obtain an optimum dorsipalmar (DP) image.[2] A useful strategy is to use a small radiolucent ruler to immobilise the fingers (Fig. 27.5); but, equally, having the parent/carer hold the child's hand in the desired position and removing the restraint at the moment of exposure can be successful and less traumatic for the child.

A lateral projection can prove equally as challenging. The use of a foam pad to gently separate the affected finger from its fellows can help maintain the position for the image to be obtained.

Suggested projections for conditions affecting the hands in children:

Polydactyly

* DP to assess the number of metacarpals present.

DP, obliques and lateral projections of the fingers/hand

Positioning should be as for adults whenever possible.

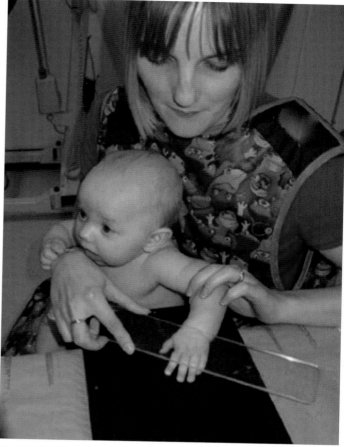

Figure 27.5 Positioning for a hand X-ray using a radiolucent plastic ruler as immobilisation aid.

Beam direction, FRD, centring point, collimation and criteria for assessing image quality

As for adults (see Chapter 5)

WRIST AND FOREARM

Alongside falls onto outstretched hands, a significant number of upper limb injuries in all ages are associated with particular recreational activities, for example the inappropriate use of trampolines[12] and monkey bars.[13]

It is regarded as poor practice to obtain one image of the entire upper limb, even in cases where clinical examination has been difficult.[14] The only exception to this rule is for surveys undertaken to assess and characterise skeletal dysplasias. Should any abnormalities be present, they will be visualised neither easily nor accurately owing to compromises in positioning and centring of the beam.

For forearm requests, both wrist and elbow joints should be visualised on one image. This is particularly relevant in cases where there is a seemingly isolated fracture of either the radius or the ulna. Scrutiny of the wrist and elbow is essential to rule out a Monteggia or Galeazzi injury. Overlooking these injuries can have considerable impact on the child's prognosis and result in a negligence claim against the hospital.

For suspected scaphoid injuries it is prudent to first perform and re-projection the DP and lateral projections of the wrist prior to undertaking additional scaphoid imaging. Scaphoid injuries are relatively rare in children compared to wrist injuries, and the radiation burden can be significantly reduced by taking this approach. Arguably it may be routine in some centres to undertake all four projections at one sitting.

PA and lateral wrist

Positioning should be as for adults whenever possible.

Beam direction, FRD, centring point, collimation and criteria for assessing image quality

As for adults (see Chapter 5)

Common error	Possible cause
Radius and ulna not superimposed on the lateral projection	Incorrect positioning for the lateral projection due to under- or over-rotation from the DP. This is often the result of the height of the X-ray table being inappropriate to facilitate patient positioning

Please also refer to the common mistakes and errors section of this chapter.

AP and lateral forearm

Positioning should be as for adults whenever possible.

Beam direction, FRD, centring point, collimation and criteria for assessing image quality

As for adults (see Chapter 6)

ELBOW

The elbow remains one of the most complex areas injured in children, a source of great concern to radiographers and clinicians alike. Complications can range from brachial artery damage manifesting as a compartment syndrome and Volkmann's ischaemic contracture to median nerve damage, malunion and myositis ossificans.

The technique used will depend on the age of the child and the nature of the injury if trauma is involved. The majority of elbow injuries occur in the 3–10-year age group[15] and involve the supracondylar area of the distal humerus, proximal to the trochlea and capitellum (Fig. 27.6). Fractures may be complete or incomplete, but involve a break in the anterior cortex with posterior displacement of the distal fragment. Other elbow injuries involve avulsion of the epicondyles and dislocations. In dislocations the distal humerus slides over the coronoid process, often with associated fractures.

The paediatric elbow is notoriously difficult to interpret owing to the six centres of secondary ossification. The order and approximate timing of ossification are given in Table 27.2. Careful assessment of the image and identification of the ossification centres present should identify most fractures, but the expert opinion of a consultant orthopaedic surgeon or consultant radiologist is often required. Requests for comparison projections of the unaffected elbow should never be accepted unless cleared by a consultant radiologist.

Where the child is in severe pain it is advisable to proceed only if they have had sufficient pain relief. The child may prefer to sit alone,

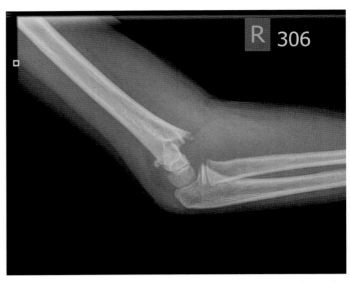

Figure 27.6 Incomplete supracondylar fracture with accompanying soft tissue effusion.

Table 27.2 Centres of ossification in the paediatric elbow (data from Children's Orthopaedics and Fractures[16])

	Approximate age (years)	Ossification centre
C	1	Capitellum
R	3	Radial head
I	5	Internal (medial) epicondyle
T	7	Trochlea
O	11	Olecranon
L	13	Lateral external epicondyle

on the lap of their parent/carer, or to lie down. It is good practice to obtain and re-projection a lateral of the elbow before attempting the AP projection. This is to enable the radiographer to be aware of the extent and severity of the injury prior to positioning for the often difficult and painful AP projection. The positioning of the lateral projection needs to be accurate to enable evaluation of the soft tissue fat pads (within the joint capsule) of the distal humerus (anterior and posterior) that often will indicate the presence of a fracture in the absence of bony signs. An AP projection may be achieved by externally rotating the arm from the shoulder joint, which will move the elbow into the desired position. An axial projection of the joint if held in a flexed position may be used as an alternative to the AP projection, as is described in the relevant adult section of this book.

A common misconception is that injuries to the proximal radius will involve the head of the bone. Although common in adults, paediatric injuries in this region are more likely to affect the radial neck owing to the presence of the epiphysis, and are reported to account for 10–15% of all presenting elbow injuries.[17]

AP and lateral elbow

Positioning

- If feasible, the child should be positioned as for adults, using supine or erect (sitting or standing) positioning and a horizontal beam direction when deemed appropriate. Assistance may be required to support the limb should foam pads and sandbags be insufficient

Beam direction, FRD, centring point, collimation and criteria for assessing image quality

As for adults (see Chapter 5)

Common errors	Possible causes
Good lateral projection not obtained	Incorrect positioning – usually due to the level of the forearm being at a different height to the humerus
Poor visualisation of one or both fat pads	Inappropriate exposure factors selected

Please also refer to the common mistakes and errors section of this chapter.

HUMERUS, SHOULDER AND CLAVICLE

Injuries of the shoulder and humerus are common in the older child, particularly those engaged in sporting activities. In the first instance, trauma cases should be examined in an AP and lateral position. As in adults, axial projections of the shoulder are only of benefit if the child is able to cooperate and may be better suited to non-trauma situations when the patient is sufficiently comfortable.

The clavicle remains one of the most frequently injured areas in children, particularly in contact sports.[18] It is often diagnosed clinically owing to the superficial position of the clavicle and the degree of local swelling that occurs immediately after injury. The majority of injuries are midshaft, either complete (overlapping of the two fragments) or incomplete (superior apical angulation). They are commonly caused by a direct fall onto the front of the shoulder. An audit of clavicle injuries at the authors' centre has demonstrated that a single 20° cranially angled projection of the clavicle will demonstrate the majority of injuries; AP projections of the shoulder are therefore only undertaken should this initial projection show no abnormality. The justification for this is that more clavicle injuries are easily identified than on the conventional AP projection. Further research needs to be undertaken with respect to the efficacy of this protocol. Requests for specialised projections of the acromioclavicular and sternoclavicular joints should be discussed with a consultant radiologist as they seldom yield additional diagnostic information.

AP shoulder and humerus

Positioning

- Wherever possible, position in a similar technique to adults (Chapter 6)
- The patient can be seated on a stool or stand depending on their level of cooperation; it will be useful to consider using a supine position when examining babies
- The amount of shoulder or proximal humerus to be included depends on the nature of injury and clinical examination
- The arm of the injured side can be supported by the patient's other arm or held by the parent/carer
- A small radiolucent pad may be placed between the trunk and the arm of the affected side to abduct it sufficiently and avoid superimposition of adjacent structures
- Ideally the exposure is made on arrested respiration

Beam direction, FRD and centring point

As for adults, but may be modified to accommodate the required clinical information

Collimation

Humerus: as for adults
Shoulder: include the entire shoulder girdle and proximal third of the humerus. On some occasions the entire length of the humerus will need to be visualised, including the glenohumeral and elbow joints (for injuries that extend to include the midshaft, e.g. in the case of spiral fractures)

Common errors	Possible causes
The shaft of the humerus superimposed over the thorax	The arm has not been sufficiently abducted, if collar and cuff support is in situ. Appropriate advice should be sought from medical personnel
The clavicle is overlapped by the lung apices and first ribs	Patient is leaning back – requires cranial angulation of the beam to correct this
The clavicle appears foreshortened	Patient is over-rotated towards the affected side

Please also refer to the common mistakes and errors section of this chapter.

FEET AND TOES

Dorsiplantar (DP) and dorsiplantar oblique (DPO) projections are routinely undertaken for trauma and orthopaedic referrals. Young children are examined either seated on the examination table or supine with a parent/carer supporting them to remain correctly positioned for the examination.

The toes need to remain extended so that the correct position is maintained. A small radiolucent ruler to immobilise the toes can be useful, but equally having the parent/carer hold the child's foot in the desired position and removing the restraint at the moment of exposure can be successful and less traumatic for the child. The lateral projection may be required for the assessment of the foot for specific conditions. On occasion standing projections will be requested to demonstrate the foot weightbearing (e.g. pes planus and coalitions).

Axial projections of the calcaneum may be indicated following trauma when the patient lands on their feet from a significant height. These are performed in the same way as for adults.

Suggested projections for conditions affecting feet in children:

Congenital talipes equinovarus (club foot)

- DP with the patient standing or simulated standing if non-ambulant. It is essential that the talus remains vertical for accurate assessment
- Two lateral projections, one taken in maximum dorsiflexion, one in extension to assess the mobility of the mid- and hindfoot. These can be achieved with the use of a radiolucent ruler to effect and maintain plantar flexion or dorsiflexion

Polydactyly

- DP to assess the number of metatarsals present

Hallux valgus

- DP with the patient standing to enable accurate evaluation of the deformity when weightbearing

Pes planus

- DP projection and a standing lateral to assess loss of the medial longitudinal arch and degree of rigidity
- Coalitions: DP, DP oblique and lateral (sometimes an axial) projections to demonstrate abnormal join between tarsal bones

DP, oblique and lateral foot and toes

- Position as for adults (Chapter 8)
- The parent/carer will need to support or immobilise younger children and babies

Beam direction, FRD, centring point, collimation, criteria for assessing image quality

As for adults (Chapter 8)

KNEE

Unlike in adults, there is little to be gained by performing radiographic examinations of the child's knee in a standing position, unless directed by an orthopaedic specialist. Standing projections are appropriate for demonstrating the extent of degenerative changes, of which there is a low incidence in paediatrics.

The patella does not commence ossification until the age of 3 years, and specific projections such as the axial or skyline are of limited value unless in cases of skeletal dysplasia that directly affect the development of the knee joint, such as nail–patella syndrome (Fong's disease).

A bipartite patella can sometimes mimic a fracture. They occur in the upper outer quadrant of the patella, are smooth edged, and will not be accompanied by the soft tissue signs of swelling, an effusion or lipohaemoarthrosis (fat–blood interface) that would be seen alongside the majority of fractured patellas.

AP and lateral projections of the knee

- Position as for adults
- The parent/carer will need to support or immobilise younger children and babies
- Consider using a horizontal beam to obtain the lateral projection to demonstrate a lipohaemoarthrosis

Beam direction, FRD, centring point, collimation, criteria for assessing image quality

As for adults (Chapter 9)

Additional projections

Additional projections are sometimes required, usually requested by orthopaedic specialists needing to visualise specific aspects of the knee and patellofemoral joint.

Osteochondritis of the tibial tuberosity (Osgood–Schlatter's disease)

- A traction apophysitis involving the tibial tuberosity and in essence should be a clinical diagnosis
- A lateral projection *only* should be undertaken unless otherwise directed by an orthopaedic specialist
- *Osteochondral defect or osteochondritis dissecans*
- The formation of a loose body within the joint space which initially appears as a flattened area of the distal femur, usually the lateral aspect of the medial condyle
- The intercondylar notch projection (see Chapter 9) is effective at demonstrating the stage of abnormality and amount of bone involved. The projection for the posterior notch should be used (full tunnel)

Common error	Possible cause
On the AP projection a lucent line is present, traversing the proximal tibia	This is the tibial tuberosity projected as such due to over- or under-rotation of the lower limb

Please also refer to the common mistakes and errors section of this chapter.

ANKLE, TIBIA AND FIBULA

It should be remembered that it is regarded as poor practice to obtain one image of the entire lower limb. Should abnormalities be present they will be visualised neither easily nor accurately. The 'toddler's fracture' affects the tibia in young children; this is a minimally displaced midshaft fracture and occurs after low-energy trauma.[19]

AP and lateral ankle

Positioning

- Position as for adults
- The parent/carer will need to support or immobilise younger children and babies
- Consider using a horizontal beam to obtain a lateral projection in cases of obvious deformity through trauma

Beam direction, FRD, centring point, collimation, criteria for assessing image quality

As for adults (Chapter 8)

AP and lateral projections of the tibia/fibula

Positioning

- Position as for adults
- The parent/carer will need to support or immobilise younger children and babies
- Consider using a horizontal beam to obtain a lateral projection in cases of obvious deformity through trauma
- Include both joints on the initial visit or in cases of trauma. This may be reduced to the joint nearest the site of injury on subsequent visits, provided the referrer is in agreement

Beam direction, FRD, centring point, collimation, criteria for assessing image quality

As for adults (Chapter 8)

Axial skeleton

The newborn spine is relatively straight, developing its curvatures as the child reaches the relevant milestones of holding up their head and starting to bear weight.

The vertebral column may require imaging after significant trauma or in the event of the development of deformity, known complications or pain of a chronic nature. Chronic pain is managed conservatively in adults, but in children any spinal tenderness or discomfort is treated as a genuine and serious ailment until proved otherwise.[20] Imaging is undertaken to rule out causes such as leukaemia, osteomyelitis, discitis or spondylolysis.

In cases of trauma, radiographers must ensure that precautionary measures (cervical collar and sandbags) are undertaken to the same extent as with adults until possible fractures have been excluded.

CERVICAL SPINE

AP and lateral cervical spine, AP C1/2

Positioning

- Positioning should be as for adults, whenever possible
- For the lateral projection it is advisable to sit the ambulant child on a stool, as opposed to implementing the standing position
- In small children a supine position with horizontal beam is a useful means of obtaining a lateral projection
- To ensure the rami of the mandible (lateral projection) do not overlie the anterior vertebral bodies, the chin should be gently lifted and supported in that position with the assistance of a parent/carer if necessary
- As for adults, an AP (C1/C2) open mouth projection should always be obtained in cases where acute injury is suspected. For younger children and babies, secondary radiation grids are not required for this projection

Beam direction, FRD, centring, collimation and criteria for assessing image quality for all projections

As for adults (Chapter 11)

Suggested projections for specific clinical histories

Torticollis

- AP (C3–7/T1) and lateral (C1–C7/T1)

Atlanto-occipital instability

Seen in some patients with trisomy 21 (Down's syndrome) and mucopolysaccharidosis type IV (Morquio's syndrome)

- Lateral projections should be obtained, in both flexion and extension
- Care should be taken to ensure that neither position is forced

Fixed rotary subluxation

- Three AP projections of C1 and C2, one taken with the neck in a neutral position and the remaining two with the head rotated 15° in each direction

THORACIC SPINE

AP and lateral thoracic spine

Positioning

- Positioning should be as for adults whenever possible
- For younger children and babies, secondary radiation grids are not necessary

Beam direction, FRD, centring, collimation and criteria for assessing image quality

As for adults (Chapter 12)

LUMBAR SPINE

AP and lateral lumbar spine

Positioning

- Positioning should be as for adults whenever possible
- For younger children and babies, secondary radiation grids are not necessary
- A lumbosacral junction (L5/S1) is not routinely undertaken unless specifically requested, as the area is adequately demonstrated on the lateral projection. An example of when this projection is useful is in cases of spondylolisthesis or spondylolysis; a tightly collimated projection of the lumbosacral junction (L5/S1) will demonstrate any abnormalities specific to this area

Beam direction, FRD, centring, collimation and criteria for assessing image quality

As for adults (Chapter 13)

Common errors	Possible causes
Bony anatomy on AP projection not sufficiently demonstrated	Overlying bowel gas can cause this problem and is particularly found in babies
Longitudinal artefact demonstrated over spine	Umbilical clip in situ
Artefact over anatomy in C1/2 open mouth projection	Artefact caused by orthodontic brace

Please also refer to the common mistakes and errors section of this chapter.

WHOLE SPINE FOR SCOLIOSIS

Scoliosis is a lateral curvature and rotation of the spinal column, often alongside a thoracic hypokyphosis (Fig. 27.7). Non-structural curves can be postural or caused through habit, others as a complication of a leg length discrepancy or pelvic obliquity.

The presence of vertebral malformation, such as a hemi- or butterfly vertebra, will produce a sharp scoliosis at the site of the deformity. A structural scoliosis can be metabolic, neuropathic, myopathic or idiopathic in origin. Most scoliosis cases are believed to be idiopathic with an incidence of 85%,[21] primarily affecting adolescent girls.

Scoliosis imaging must demonstrate the spine in its functional state and include from C3 to the sacroiliac joints. Demonstration of calcification of the iliac apophyses (Risser's sign[22]) is also essential in order to show the patient's remaining growth potential. Patients able to stand should be positioned for a PA projection in order to limit radiation exposure to the breast tissue, thyroid gland and gonads. For those unable to stand, every attempt must be made to obtain the image in an AP sitting position. Depending upon the degree of kyphosis and lordosis connected with the scoliosis, a lateral projection may also be required. The magnitude of the curve is assessed by the Cobb angle, a measurement of the angles between the planes of the spine.[23] By definition, a scoliosis is any curve with a measurement >10°.

It is essential that the images are reliable and reproducible. Treatment is driven by the curve magnitude and currently includes bracing to arrest the progression of developing curves and surgical rodding or fixation for curves of >40°.[24]

PELVIS AND HIPS

X-ray examinations of the pelvis and hips are frequently undertaken on children; therefore, it is crucial that such patients are properly protected from the hazards of radiation.[25] Although the amount of radiation absorbed by the body for a single X-ray is relatively small, paediatric patients with hip problems are likely to be monitored for some time, thereby becoming more susceptible to risk through the cumulative effect of regular X-rays.

Gonad shields of varying sizes made of solid lead encapsulated within plastic prove to be useful, especially as they are resilient and easily cleaned (Fig. 27.8A,B,C). Correct location of the device for girls is made simpler by the shape of the plastic flange which, when suitably aligned with the anterior superior iliac spines, will place the lead element of the shield accurately within the pelvis. For boys, the device can be inverted with the edge of the shield aligned with the inferior border of symphysis pubis. Shielding should be used in all cases, other than for the initial AP projection of the pelvis for emergency and medical cases. This is to ensure that no bony or soft tissue pathology is overlooked.

Fractures of the hip account for less than 1% of all paediatric fractures and are caused by severe trauma;[26] 80–90% of these patients will have multiple injuries to their head and/or abdominal viscera, where the likelihood of major blood loss is high.[27] On these occasions a pelvic X-ray is performed as part of the advanced trauma life support (ATLS) series carried out in the resuscitation room. Traumatic dislocations are also unusual and only occur when a considerable amount of force is involved, such as that encountered in some road traffic incidents. Depending on the history given it may be pertinent to perform a lateral hip projection, which may take the form of a turned lateral or a shoot-through horizontal beam.

X-ray imaging of the hips to assess development in neonates is of limited value as the ossification of the femoral capital epiphysis does not begin until the age of 4–6 months. Ultrasound is the preferred means of assessing the hip in this age group. Radiography should only take place if there is a suspicion of osteomyelitis or septic arthritis, and then only after referral from a consultant orthopaedic surgeon.

Developmental dysplasia of the hip

Developmental dysplasia of the hip covers a spectrum of hip problems ranging from the frankly dislocated hip at birth to a dislocatable hip, general hip laxity or abnormalities of the acetabulum that render it insufficient to contain the femoral head. Associated risk factors documented include a positive family history, breech presentation, first

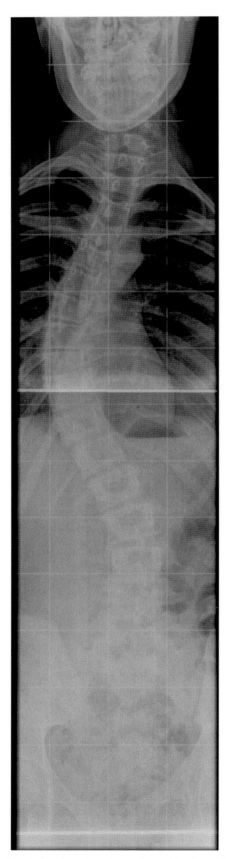

Figure 27.7 PA whole-spine view of a patient with idiopathic scoliosis.

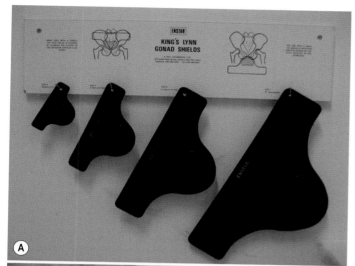

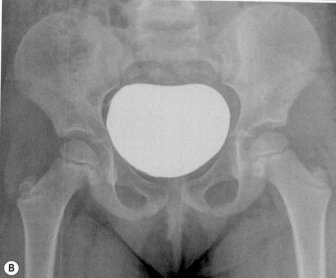

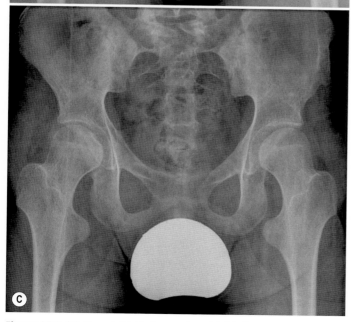

Figure 27.8 (A) Gonad shields for use in pelvis/hip imaging; (B) correct placement of gonad shield for a girl; (C) correct placement of gonad shield for a boy.

pregnancy, and the presence of other skeletal abnormalities such as neck torticollis and congenital talipes equinovarus (club foot).

Irritable hip

This is an acute onset of hip pain and stiffness in the 3–9-year age group. Hip X-rays are often unremarkable and effusions are best demonstrated by ultrasound. X-rays should only be performed should an ultrasound be normal and to exclude other causes of hip pain, such as Perthes' disease.

Legg–Calve–Perthes' disease, or Perthes' disease

Perthes' disease is a hip disorder involving ischaemia and necrosis of the femoral epiphysis with eventual remodelling. It is usually seen in the 4–8-year age group but can occur as early as the age of 2 or as late as 9 years. Bilateral Perthes' occurs in 10–12% of cases, though such patients demonstrate different stages of the disease on each side.[28] Boys are affected more than girls.

Slipped capital femoral epiphysis

A SCFE is movement of the epiphysis inferiorly and posteriorly from the proximal femur. SCFE can be either acute or chronic in nature and is seen predominantly in boys aged 9–15 years; 25% of cases will have a slippage of the other side within 6 months,[28] therefore it is essential that all examinations include an AP pelvis and frog lateral of both hips.

AP pelvis and hips

Positioning

- The child is initially positioned supine, as for adults
- The legs are extended and knees placed together with the patellae anterior (not with knees internally rotated)
- To aid immobilisation the parent/carer should be instructed to place a hand over the knees to prevent the child from bending their knees and twisting their trunk
- For younger children and babies, secondary radiation grids are not necessary

Beam direction and FRD

Vertical central ray
100 cm FRD

Centring

In the midline, at the level of the femoral heads. This lies midway between the upper border of the symphysis pubis and anterior superior iliac spines

Collimation

As for adults. It is especially important that the entire pelvis is demonstrated, to avoid missing avulsion fractures of the anterior superior iliac spine

Criteria for assessing image quality

As for adults (Chapter 10); these areas are of particular importance:

- Periarticular soft tissue planes must be demonstrated
- Symmetry of trochanters

Frog lateral for both hips

IR is horizontal

Positioning

- The child is placed in a supine position with the legs extended and the ankles touching
- The knees are flexed to draw the feet towards the trunk
- Keeping the feet together, the thighs are externally rotated to separate the knees until the lateral aspects of the femora are in contact with the table-top
- After such external rotation the plantar aspects of both feet should be in contact with each other
- Should the child experience discomfort and be unable to abduct the affected hip to the same extent as the unaffected hip, care must be taken to avoid compensatory pelvic tilt. In severe cases separate laterals of each hip are preferable
- For younger children and babies, secondary radiation grids are not necessary

Beam direction and FRD

Vertical central ray
100 cm FRD

Centring

As for the AP projection detailed above.

Collimation

The hip joints and proximal femora

Criteria for assessing image quality

As for adult AP pelvis (Chapter 10); the following areas are of particular importance:
- Symmetry of obturator foramina (if unachievable, single lateral projections should be performed)
- Symmetry of trochanters
- Periarticular soft tissue planes should be demonstrated

Common errors	Possible causes
Asymmetry of obturator foramina, greater trochanters and femoral necks on frog lateral projections	Unequal abduction of one of the limbs; usually the non-affected side is externally rotated further than the affected side
The femoral neck appears foreshortened	Often due to the patient raising the thigh from the table-top; this also can allow the knees to be 'drawn up' towards the trunk

Please also refer to the common mistakes and errors section of this chapter.

SKULL AND FACE

The incidence of skull imaging in paediatrics has largely diminished since the advent of NICE guidelines[29] and acknowledgement that the absence of a skull fracture on the X-ray image does not rule out an intracranial injury.[27]

Conventional skull radiography is requested as part of a skeletal survey for suspected non-accidental injury, skeletal dysplasia and oncology referral. It may also be requested for the assessment of craniosynostosis, in which a premature closing of the skull sutures leads to the development of an unusually shaped head. Patients with cochlear implants also require imaging to demonstrate the petrous portion of the temporal bone to ensure the structure is correctly positioned postoperatively. For older children all skull and face positioning is in keeping with that used for adults (Chapters 16–20).

Despite the increased radiation dose to the lenses of the eyes, for younger children it is normal practice to produce a fronto-occipital (FO) projection as opposed to the occipitofrontal (OF) projections selected for adults and older children. Usually young children are less anxious and disorientated by not having the IR close to their face. The positioning described below is aimed at these younger children and may involve the use of two assistants to aid immobilisation.

FO cranium

IR is horizontal

Positioning

- The child is placed supine. To prevent movement of the arms, legs and trunk, small children can be swaddled in a blanket and supported
- A secondary radiation grid is not required for small children and babies
- Care should be taken to ensure the mandible does not drop down towards the chest, as this will project the upper border of petrous temporal above the superior orbital margins, resembling an OF 30° (Towne's) projection
- To help maintain the position an assistant (usually a parent or carer) wearing lead rubber mittens/gloves may use two 45° pads placed on either side of the head

Beam direction and FRD

Vertical
100 cm FRD

Centring point and collimation

As for adults (Chapter 17); it is especially important in collimation to ensure that the hands of the person effecting immobilisation are outside the collimated field

Criteria for assessing image quality

As for adults (Chapter 17); the following is of particular importance:
- Exposure factors must ensure that the fontanelles are adequately demonstrated in babies

Lateral cranium

Positioning

- From a supine position the child's head is gently turned to the affected side (if an injury is involved). Some limited rotation of the trunk will assist in positioning the head so that it lies with the MSP parallel to the IR. It is suitable to use a blanket wrapped around the child for this projection to aid immobilisation, as outlined for the FO projection

- An assistant wearing protective mittens/gloves may use a 45° pad to maintain the position of the back of the head; at the same time the anterior aspect of the head is immobilised by gentle pressure to the child's jaw using a thumb
- An alternative option is to use a horizontal beam technique with the IR supported vertically next to the child's head and the head supported on a non-opaque pad. The MSP is maintained parallel to the IR using a 45° pad pushed against the vertex of the skull and by using a thumb to elevate and support the chin

Beam direction and FRD

Vertical if IR is horizontal; horizontal if IR is supported vertically at the side of the head
100 cm FRD

Centring point and collimation

As for adults (Chapter 17); it is especially important in collimation to ensure that the hands of the person effecting immobilisation are outside the collimated field

Criteria for assessing image quality

As for adults (Chapter 17); the following is of particular importance:
- Exposure factors must ensure that the fontanelles are adequately demonstrated in babies

Common error	Possible cause
Asymmetry of vault	Usually due to rotation (as for adults) *but* if the child's cranial vault is misshapen due to craniosynostosis, or effects of delivery on the neonate (e.g. ventouse extraction), this will be unavoidable

Please also refer to the common mistakes and errors section of this chapter.

PARANASAL SINUSES AND POSTNASAL SPACE

Sinus projections may be occasionally requested for children with a history of acute infection if they are not considered suitable for computed tomography (CT) or magnetic resonance imaging (MRI).

The formation and pneumatisation of the sinuses occurs gradually during early childhood and is not complete until puberty. Therefore, particular care must be taken to ensure that any requests for sinus projections are clinically justified.

A single occipitomental (OM) projection with 15° caudal angulation taken with the mouth open provides the best overall assessment of the four groups of sinuses. The OM projection is described in Chapter 19.

The lateral postnasal space is commonly examined in children with a history of snoring, adenoidal speech and/or difficult nasal breathing. The mouth should remain closed at the time of exposure. Exposure factors should be selected in order to demonstrate the soft tissues of the adenoidal pad; this will facilitate assessment of their size. Technique for this projection can be found in Chapter 19.

SKELETAL SURVEYS

Skeletal survey for non-accidental injury (NAI)

NAI in children and the associated skeletal survey are topics that remain at the forefront of paediatric radiography. National reports of several high-profile cases[30,31] and speculation that the incidence of child abuse may be increasing[32] have led to an increased awareness among clinical professionals.

Although skeletal fractures seldom pose an immediate threat to an ill-treated child, they remain the most robust radiological indicator of abuse in babies and toddlers.[33]

The aims of carrying out such a skeletal survey are threefold: diagnosis of known or suspected injuries, injury as yet unnoticed by the health professionals in charge of the child's care, and justification of actions (if necessary) to prevent a child being returned to a dangerous environment. In addition to providing the imaging of such patients, radiographers are required to call upon interpersonal skills to manage angry and/or distressed parents/carers while maintaining a child-friendly environment in this potentially volatile atmosphere.[34]

It is recommended that departments undertaking NAI examinations should have a written protocol outlining the entire procedure from the clinical referral to the radiological report.[35,36] An example of such a process is outlined below.

- *Referral.* Requests for skeletal surveys may only be accepted by consultant radiologists. The parents/carers should have had an explanation of the skeletal survey and the reasons for it explained to them by the clinical team *prior* to the examination.
- *Prioritisation.* Although NAI cases are not clinical emergencies, current recommendations from the Royal College of Radiologists[36] are that the skeletal survey should only be performed during the normal working day and within 24 hours of the time of the request, excluding weekends and bank holidays.
- *Medicolegal issues.* It should be remembered that all skeletal surveys in cases of suspected NAI could potentially be presented as evidence in a criminal law court. It is essential that all images are of optimal diagnostic standard, with correct centring, exposure, appropriate collimation, and accurately marked with the patient's demographic details and date with correct anatomical markers placed in the primary beam. Ideally two radiographers will undertake the examination; should this not be possible, an additional health professional (usually a qualified nurse) should be present to act as a witness to the proceedings and assist with any immobilisation when required.
- *Image quality and projections.* 'Babygrams' or whole-body images are not acceptable under any circumstances. The imaging of the right and left lower limbs together in one exposure should also be avoided. Table 27.3 outlines the suggested projections for a skeletal survey of suspected NAI as recommended by the British Society of Paediatric Radiology (BSPR).[1]

Upon completion of the examination the projections should be checked by a consultant radiologist before the child leaves the department. Any suspicious appearances, such as periosteal reaction, will require additional projections, usually lateral projections and coned APs of the area in question. It is not uncommon for children to return for follow-up limited surveys to enable a review of such areas at a later date.

The Association of Paediatric Radiographers[1] advocates the use of a checklist to be completed by the examining radiographer(s) to ensure that all the appropriate image checks are carried out. It may also act

Table 27.3 Suggested projections for NAI

Area	Projection
Chest	PA/AP, left and right posterior obliques
Abdomen	AP to include the entire pelvis and hips
Hands	DP of left and right
Forearm	AP of left and right
Humeri	AP of left and right
Whole spine	Lateral
Cranium	AP and lateral
Feet	DP of left and right
Tibia/fibula	AP of left and right
Femora	AP of left and right

Table 27.4 Suggested projections for skeletal dysplasias

Area	Projection
Chest	PA/AP
Pelvis	AP
Hand	DP to include wrist for bone age assessment
Upper limb	AP of humerus and forearm
Whole spine (cervical, thoracic and lumbar regions)	AP and lateral
Cranium	Lateral
Lower limb	AP of femur and tibia/fibula
Foot	DP

as a record of who was present, types of immobilisation used, exposures, radiation dose, final number of images, and name of the radiologist reporting on the images.

Skeletal survey for skeletal dysplasias

Skeletal dysplasias are a heterogeneous group of over 200 disorders characterised by abnormal cartilage and bone growth. Many forms are detectable antenatally during routine ultrasound screening or at birth. A significant number will not become apparent until the child is older. Patients will have an abnormally structured skeleton, sometimes in conjunction with disorders of other systems. Cases vary from the minimally affected, such as the epiphyseal dysplasias, to those with high mortality and morbidity such as osteogenesis imperfecta. Radiology plays an important role in the diagnosis and classification of skeletal dysplasias. Please note that this is the only scenario when it is acceptable to obtain a single projection of an entire limb. This can be justified by the need for identification of bone density and growth plate anomalies only, as opposed to the detail required in cases of trauma or suspected NAI.

Suggested projections for survey of skeletal dysplasias are given in Table 27.4.

For any projections of the long bones, both associated joints must be demonstrated to enable thorough scrutiny.

Occasionally a skeletal survey may be carried out for oncology and rheumatology referrals. Image series is suggested as in Table 27.4, with the addition of a fronto-occipital projection of the skull.

REFERENCES

1. Society and College of Radiographers. London: Association of Paediatric Radiographers [cited 2011 March 3]. Available from http://wwwsor.org/members/sigsandnets/index.htm.

2. Hardy M, Boynes S. Paediatric radiography. Oxford: Blackwell Science Limited 2003.

3. Department of Health. Learning from Bristol: The Department of Health's response to the report of the public inquiry into children's heart surgery and the Bristol Royal Infirmary 1984–1995. [cited 2011 March 3]. Available from http://www.dh.gov.uk/en/Publicationsandstatistics/Publications/PublicationsPolicyAndGuidance/DH_4002859.

4. Cook J. Radiation protection and quality assurance in paediatric radiology. Imaging 2001;13:229–38.

5. European guidelines on quality criteria for diagnostic radiographic images in paediatrics. The European Commission, EUR 16261 EN, CEC. Luxemborg; 1996.

6. Jones N, et al. Neonatal chest and abdominal radiation dosimetry: a comparison of two radiographic techniques. British Journal of Radiology 2001;74(886):920–5.

7. The Ionising Radiation (Medical Exposure) Regulations 2006. London: HMSO; 2006.

8. Royal College of Radiologists.ac.uk. London: Defining standards in imaging and cancer treatment [cited 2011 March 3]. Available from http://www.rcr.ac.uk/content.aspx?PageID=667.

9. Barrett T, Booth I. Sartorial eloquence: does it exist in the paediatrician-patient relationship? British Medical Journal 1994;309:1710–2.

10. Englemann D, et al. Quality of ambulatory thoracic radiography in the child – a pilot study. Radiologe 2001;41(5):442–6.

11. Trinh A, et al. Scatter radiation from chest radiographs: is there a risk to infants in a typical NICU? Pediatric Radiology 2010;40:704–7.

12. Wootton M, Harris D. Trampolining injuries presenting to a children's department. Emergency Medicine Journal 2009;26(10):728–31.

13. Kelley S. The response of children to trauma. Mini-symposium: basic science of trauma. Orthopaedics and Trauma 2010;24:29–41.

14. Gyll C, Hardwick J. Radiography of children: A guide to good practice. London: Elsevier Churchill Livingstone; 2005.

15. Greenspan A. Orthopaedic imaging: A practical approach. 5th ed. International: Lippincott Williams and Wilkins; 2010.

16. Benson M, et al. Children's orthopaedics and fractures. London: Springer-Verlag; 2010.

17. Eberl R, et al. Galeazzi Lesions in children and adolescents: treatment and outcome. Clinical Orthopaedics 2008;466(7):1705–9.

18. Pecci M, Kreher J. Clavicle fractures. American Family Physician 2008;77(1):65–70.

19. Dunbar J, et al. Obscure tibial fracture of infants – the toddler's fracture. Journal of the Canadian Association of Radiology 1964;15:136–44.

20. Kriss V. Handbook of paediatric radiology: Handbooks in radiology series. St Louis: Mosby; 1998.

21. Manaster B. Handbook of skeletal radiology: Handbooks in radiology series. 2nd ed. St Louis: Mosby; 1997.

22. Risser J. The iliac apophysis: an invaluable sign in the management of scoliosis. Clinical Orthopaedics 1958;11:111–9.

23. Cobb JR. Scoliosis: Quo Vadis? Journal of Bone and Joint Surgery. American volume 1958;40:507–10.

24. Drummond D. Back pain. In: Pediatric orthopaedic secrets. 2nd ed. Philadelphia: Staheli L Hanley & Belfus; 2002.

25. Sikand M, et al. Study on the use of gonadal protection shields during paediatric pelvic X-rays. Annals of the Royal College of Surgeons of England 2003;85:422–5.

26. Begg J. Accident and emergency X-rays made easy. London: Churchill Livingstone; 2004.

27. Quayle K, et al. Diagnostic testing for acute head injury in children: when are head computed tomography and skull radiographs indicated. Pediatrics 1997;99(5):E11.

28. Anderson L, et al. Sequelae of Perthes disease: treatment with surgical hip dislocation and relative femoral neck lengthening. Journal of Pediatric Orthopedics 2010;30(8):758–66.

29. National Institute of Health and Clinical Excellence. Head injury- triage, assessment, investigation and early management of head injury in infants, children and adults guidelines. June 2003 [cited 2011 March 3]. http://guidance.nice.org.uk/CG56/ReviewProposal.

30. Department of Health. London: The Victoria Climbie Inquiry report of an inquiry by Lord Laming. January 2003 [cited 2011 March 3]. Available from http://www.dh.gov.uk/en/Publicationsandstatistics/Publications/PublicationsPolicyAndGuidance/DH_4008654.

31. Care Quality Commission. London: Care Quality Commission publishes report on the NHS care of Baby Peter. May 2009 [cited 2011 March 3]. Available from http://www.cqc.org.uk/newsandevents/newsstories.cfm.

32. Horner G. Physical abuse: recognition and reporting. Journal of Pediatric Health Care 2005;19(1):4–11.

33. Mandelstam S, et al. Complementary use of radiological skeletal survey and bone scintigraphy in detection of bony injuries in suspected child abuse. Archives of Disease in Childhood 2003;88(5):387–90.

34. Hancock V, et al. Child protection and radiography: social and emotional context. Child Abuse Reprojection 1998;6(4):283–90.

35. The British Society of Paediatric Radiology. Standard for skeletal surveys in suspected non-accidental injury (NAI) in children [cited 2011 March 3]. Available from http://www.bspr.org.uk/nai.htm.

36. Royal College of Radiologists. London: Standards for radiological investigations of suspected non-accidental injury. Ref. No. 2008. BFCR(08)1 [cited 2011 March 3]. Available from http://www.rcr.ac.uk/publications.aspx?PageID=310&PublicationID=282.1

Section | 7 |

Contrast studies

Chapter 28

Contrast media

Susan Cutler

Contrast media are substances used to highlight areas of the body in radiographic contrast to their surrounding tissues. Contrast media enhance the optical density of the area under investigation so that the tissue/structure absorption differentials are sufficient to produce adequate contrast with adjacent structures, enabling imaging to take place. There are numerous types of radiographic contrast media used in medical imaging, which have different applications depending on their chemical and physical properties. When used for imaging purposes contrast media can be administered by injection, insertion or ingestion.

HISTORY OF RADIOGRAPHIC CONTRAST MEDIA

Radiographic contrast has been used for over a century to enhance the contrast of radiographic images. In 1896, in the year after X-rays were discovered, inspired air became the first recognised contrast agent in radiographic examinations of the chest. In 1898, the first contrast studies were carried out on the upper gastrointestinal tract of a cat using bismuth salts. These salts were very toxic, and by 1910 barium sulphate and bismuth solutions were being used in conjunction with the fluoroscope, barium sulphate having been used with differing additives ever since for imaging of the gastrointestinal tract.

Images of the urinary system were achieved in the early 1920s. In the early 1920s, syphilis was treated with high doses of sodium iodide. During this treatment the urine in the bladder was observed to be radio-opaque owing to its iodine content. In 1923 the first *angiogram* and opacification of the urinary tract was performed using sodium iodide. Sodium iodide was too toxic for satisfactory intravenous use, necessitating a need to find a less toxic iodinated compound.

The first iodine-based contrast used was a derivative of the chemical ring pyridine, to which a single iodine atom could be bound in order to render it radio-opaque. Iodine-based contrast media have been used ever since. These media, however, produced varying adverse reactions, and it was realised that a contrast agent was needed that was both safe to administer and enhanced the contrast of the radiographic image. Modern ionic contrast agents were introduced in 1950 and were derivatives of tri-iodo benzoic acid; this structure enabled three

atoms of iodine to be carried, rendering it more radio-opaque. However, the agents still caused adverse effects, as they were still of high osmolarity; the term is explained below.

Ionic media dissociate in water; their injection into the blood plasma results in a great increase in the number of particles present in the plasma. This has the effect of displacing water. Water moves from an area of greater concentration to an area of lesser concentration by the process of osmosis, the physical process that occurs whenever there is a concentration difference across a membrane and that membrane is permeable to the diffusing substance. Osmolality (which is generally considered interchangeable with the term 'osmolarity') is defined as the number of solute particles, i.e. the contrast medium molecules, dissolved in 1 L (1000 g) of water. These media exert tremendous osmotic activity on the body. The osmolality of normal human blood is given as around 290–300 mOsm/kg (milliosmoles per kilogram).

There remained a need to find a water-soluble iodine-based contrast agent with reduced toxicity but which still produced satisfactory radio-opacity on images. In the 1970s and 1980s non-ionic low-osmolality contrast media became widely available, with the first non-ionic contrast medium being introduced in 1974, representing a major advancement in diagnostic imaging. Most recently the non-ionic dimers have emerged. These media are highly hydrophilic, resulting in lower chemotoxicity, and they are iso-osmolar with the respective body fluids, meaning they can be used for examinations such as angiography and computed tomography (CT) arteriography, which require high doses of contrast media to be administered and where low toxicity is essential.

REQUIREMENTS OF 'THE IDEAL' CONTRAST MEDIUM AND TYPES OF CONTRAST AGENT

There is currently no contrast medium on the market that is considered to be ideal, but the ideal contrast medium should fulfil certain requirements for safe and effective application. It should be:

• easy to administer
• non-toxic
• a stable compound

- concentrated in the required area when injected
- rapidly eliminated when necessary
- non-carcinogenic
- of appropriate viscosity for administration
- tolerated by the patient
- cost-effective.

Contrast media are divided into two main categories. The first is *negative* contrast media, which are radiolucent and of low atomic number, causing the part in which they are placed to be more readily penetrated by X-rays than the surrounding tissue; as they attenuate the X-ray beam less effectively than body tissue, they appear darker on the X-ray image. Gases are commonly used to produce negative contrast on radiographic images. The second type is *positive* contrast media; these are radio-opaque and of a high atomic number, causing the part in which they are placed to be less readily penetrated by X-rays than the surrounding tissue. Consequently, this contrast agent-filled area appears denser than body tissue.

Barium- and iodine-based solutions are used in medical imaging to produce positive contrast. Both positive and negative contrast can be used together in double-contrast examinations to produce a radiographic image. Double contrast is used primarily in the alimentary tract, but is also used in arthrography of joints. The positive contrast medium is used to coat the walls of the cavity and the negative contrast, in the form of a gas, is used to distend the area being imaged. Double-contrast examinations permit optimum visualisation by producing a high inherent contrast while allowing adequate penetration of the area under examination. Use of a small amount of contrast agent in conjunction with the distended cavity allows coating of the structures in the cavity (or in the case of the alimentary tract, the mucosal lining), which provides better detail of the area when the thin coating is shown in contrast to the gas-filled area, rather than using large amounts which may be dense enough to mask important information.

NEGATIVE CONTRAST MEDIA

The following gases create negative contrast on radiographic images:

- *Air*: Introduced by the patient during a radiographic examination, e.g. inspiration during chest radiography, *or* can be introduced by the radiographer as part of the examination in a double-contrast barium enema
- *Oxygen*: Introduced into cavities of the body, for example in the knee during arthrography to demonstrate the knee joint
- *Carbon dioxide*: Introduced into the gastrointestinal tract in conjunction with a barium sulphate solution to demonstrate the mucosal pattern, e.g. double-contrast barium meal. For the barium meal it is formulated as effervescent powder (e.g. 'Carbex' granules) or ready-mixed carbonated barium sulphate (e.g. 'Baritop'). Carbon dioxide can also be introduced into the colon when performing a double-contrast barium enema. It has been recommended that carbon dioxide be used as the negative contrast agent in a double-contrast barium enema, rather than air, as it causes less immediate abdominal pain[1] as well as less post-procedural pain and discomfort.[2] However, some studies have shown that carbon dioxide produces inferior distension and additional insufflations are required to maintain adequate quality distension.[3] Carbon dioxide can also be used as an alternative contrast to iodinated contrast for diagnostic angiography and vascular interventions in both the arterial and the venous circulation. The gas produces negative contrast owing to its low atomic number and low density compared with adjacent tissues.

POSITIVE CONTRAST MEDIA

Barium and iodine solutions are used to create positive contrast on radiographic images.

Barium sulphate solutions (BaSO₄) used in gastrointestinal imaging

Barium solutions are the universal contrast media used for radiographic examinations of the gastrointestinal tract. The following characteristics make barium solutions suitable for imaging of the gastrointestinal tract:

- High atomic number (56) producing good radiographic contrast
- Insoluble
- Stable
- Relatively inexpensive
- Excellent coating properties of the gastrointestinal mucosa

Barium suspensions are composed from pure barium sulphate mixed with additives and dispersing agents, held in suspension in water. Compounds to stabilise the suspension are added; these act on the surface tension and increase the viscosity of the solution. A dispersing agent is added to prevent sedimentation, ensuring an even distribution of particles within the suspension. Also added to the suspension is a defoaming agent, used to prevent bubbles that may mimic pathology in the gastrointestinal tract. Flavourings are usually added to oral solutions, making them more palatable for patients.

The concentration of barium in the solution is normally stated as a percentage weight to volume ratio (w/v). A 100% w/v solution contains 1 g of barium sulphate per 100 mL of water; the density of the barium solution is therefore dependent upon the weight/volume. There are many varieties of barium suspension available and the type used depends on the area of the gastrointestinal tract being imaged. It also depends greatly upon the individual preferences of the practitioner.

Patients rarely have allergic reactions to barium sulphate but may react to the preservatives or additives in the solutions. Barium sulphate preparations are usually safe as long as the gastrointestinal tract is patent and intact. A severe inflammatory reaction may develop if it is extravasated outside the gastrointestinal tract; this is most likely to occur when there is perforation of the tract. If barium sulphate escapes into the peritoneal cavity, inflammation and peritonitis may occur. Escaped barium in the peritoneum causes pain and hypovolaemic shock and, despite treatment which includes fluid replacement therapy, steroids and antibiotics, there is still a 50% mortality rate; of those who survive, 30% will develop peritoneal adhesions and granulomas.[4] Aspiration of barium solutions during upper gastrointestinal tract imaging is considered to be relatively harmless, most frequently affecting the elderly patient. Physiotherapy is usually required to drain the aspirated barium and should be performed before the patient leaves the department.

Oral barium sulphate should not be administered in cases of obstruction as it may inspissate behind an obstruction, compounding the patient's condition. Sedated patients should not undergo radiological examinations of the upper gastrointestinal tract as their swallowing reflex may be diminished, increasing the risk of aspiration.

When preparing barium solutions for administration it is important to check expiry dates and ensure the packaging is intact. Solutions administered rectally should be administered at body temperature to improve patient tolerability and also reduce spasm of the colon. It is important that the administrator knows the patient's full medical history and checks for any contraindications prior to administration. Barium sulphate solutions are contraindicated for the following pathologies:

- Suspected perforation
- Suspected fistula
- Suspected partial or complete stenosis
- Paralytic ileus
- Haemorrhage in the gastrointestinal tract
- Toxic megacolon
- Prior to surgery or endoscopy
- If the patient has had a recent gastrointestinal wide bore biopsy (usually within 3–5 days) or a recent anastomosis

When barium sulphate solutions are contraindicated for gastrointestinal imaging, a water-soluble iodine-based contrast medium (e.g. Gastrografin or Gastromiro) should be used. These can be administered orally, rectally or mechanically, e.g. via stomas. The iodine concentration of Gastrografin is 370 mg/mL and of Gastromiro 300 mg/mL. When used for imaging the gastrointestinal tract, water-soluble contrast produces a lower-contrast image than barium owing to its lower atomic number.

The patient's consent must be given prior to the administration of barium contrast solutions. The patient should be given a full explanation, be reassured about the examination and given the opportunity to ask questions. It is important when using barium sulphate solutions that associated pharmacological agents such as buscopan and glucagon are fully understood and the indications and contraindications ensuring their safe application adhered to.

Iodine-based contrast media used in medical imaging and their development

The largest group of contrast media used in imaging departments are the water-soluble organic preparations in which molecules of iodine are the opaque agent. These compounds contain iodine atoms (iodine has an atomic number of 53) bound to a carrier molecule. This holds the iodine in a stable compound and carries it to the organ under examination. The carrier molecules are organic, containing carbon, and are of low toxicity and high stability. Iodine is used as it is relatively safe and the K edge = 32 keV (binding edge of iodine K-shell electron), thus being close to the mean energy of diagnostic X-rays. Selection of kVp for imaging examinations using iodine-based contrast plays a part in providing optimum attenuation. The absorption edge of iodine (35 keV) predicts that 63–77 kVp is the optimal range. The iodine-based compounds are divided into four groups (Fig. 28.1) depending on their molecular structure, as follows:

1. Ionic monomers
2. Ionic dimers
3. Non-ionic monomers
4. Non-ionic dimers

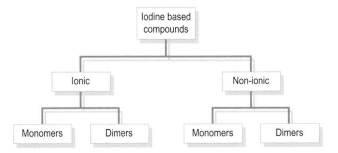

Figure 28.1 Classification of ionic contrast media.

Ionic monomers – high osmolar contrast media (HOCM) (Fig. 28.2)

The basic molecule of all water-soluble iodine-containing contrast media is the benzene ring. Benzene itself is not water soluble; to make it soluble, carboxyl acid (COOH) is added. Three of the hydrogens in this molecule are replaced by iodine, rendering it radio-opaque, but it still remains quite toxic. The remaining two hydrogens (R_1 and R_2 in Fig. 28.2) are replaced by a short chain of hydrocarbons, making the compound less toxic and more acceptable to the body. The exact nature of these compounds differs between different contrast media, but they are usually prepared as sodium or meglumine salts as these help to provide solubility.

Ionic compounds dissociate (dissolve) into charged particles when entering a solution. They dissociate into positively charged cations and negatively charged anions. For every three iodine molecules present in ionic media, one cation and one anion are produced when it enters a solution. Their 'effect' ratio is therefore 3 : 2. These solutions are highly hypertonic, with an osmolality approximately five times higher than human plasma (1500–2000 mOsm/kg H_2O compared with 300 mOsm/kg H_2O for plasma).

Ionic dimers – low osmolar contrast media (LOCM) (Fig. 28.3)

As contrast agents developed in the 20th century, it was acknowledged that a contrast medium with reduced osmotic effects was needed. As previously stated, the higher the 'effect' ratio the lower the osmolarity of the contrast media. An attempt was made to increase the 'effect' ratio and produce a contrast medium with lower osmolarity. This was achieved by linking together two conventional ionic contrast media

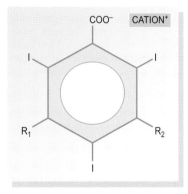

Figure 28.2 Molecular structure of an ionic monomer (HOCM).

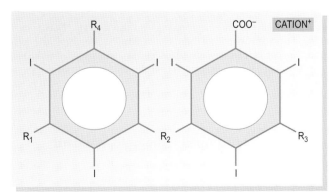

Figure 28.3 Molecular structure of ionic dimer (LOCM).

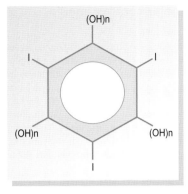

Figure 28.4 Molecular structure of non-ionic monomer.

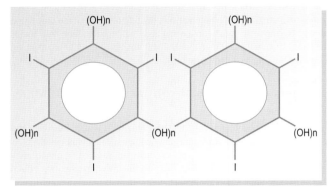

Figure 28.5 Molecular structure of non-ionic dimer.

molecules. The resulting dimeric ionic contrast medium was an improvement on the HOCM. Reduced osmolality (600 mOsm/kg H_2O) made the contrast more tolerable for patients. The ionic molecule still dissociates into two particles, a positive cation and a negative anion. However, there are now twice as many particles in solution with twice the osmolarity. Each molecule carried six iodines (as opposed to three in the HOCM), hence there is an iodine atom-to-particle ratio of 6:2; so only half the number of molecules are needed to achieve the same iodine concentration. This means a lower volume of contrast medium is therefore required for an examination.

Non-ionic monomers (LOCM) (Fig. 28.4)

These are low osmolar agents and do not dissociate into two particles in a solution, making them more tolerable and safer to use than ionic contrast. For every three iodine molecules in a non-ionic solution, one neutral molecule is produced. Non-ionic contrast media are therefore referred to as 3:1 compounds. They substitute the sodium and meglumine side chains with non-ionising radicals $(OH)_n$. Two major advantages arise through the change in chemical structure: the first is that the negative carboxyl group is eliminated, thereby reducing the neurotoxicity; and the second is that the elimination of the positive ion reduces osmolality to 600–700 mOsm/kg H_2O. Non-ionic LOCM is recommended for intrathecal and vascular radiological procedures.

Non-ionic dimers (isotonic) – the gold standard
(Fig. 28.5)

Clearly, the closer the osmolality of a contrast agent is to that of blood plasma, and the better an isotonic solution, i.e. that the contrast solution has similar osmolality to blood plasma (approximately

300 mOsm/kg H_2O), is a most ideal option. Non-ionic dimers are dimeric non-dissociating molecules; for every one molecule there are six iodine atoms. The ratio is therefore 6:1, double that of the non-ionic monomers. An important feature of these is that they are *isotonic*. Their iso-osmolality, combined with a slower diffusion of the larger molecules across vessel walls from the vascular space, plays a significant role in imaging venous phase images following arterial injections (and arterial phase images following venous injections). These compounds represent a gold standard water-soluble iodine contrast medium.

The percentage solution

The percentage solution indicates the amount of solute in the solvent. The percentage solution does not indicate the percentage iodine content, as demonstrated in the following table.

Percentage iodine content in contrast media		
Contrast media	Percentage solution	Iodine concentration of solution
Urografin 150	30	146 mg/mL
Urografin 370	76	370 mg/mL
Gastrografin	76	370 mg/mL
Niopam 370	75.5	370 mg/mL

The solvent affects the viscosity of the contrast agent. Viscosity is the resistance to flow of a contrast medium and relates to the concentration, molecular size and temperature of the contrast. The volume and density of contrast used is dependent upon the examination being undertaken, the pathology being investigated, the age of the patient and the patient's medical status.

Essential criteria for the 'ideal' intravenous contrast agent

- Water soluble
- Heat/chemical/storage stability
- Non-antigenic
- Available at the right viscosity and density
- Low viscosity, making them easy to administer
- Persistent enough in the area of interest to allow its visualisation
- Selective excretion by the patient when the examination is complete
- Same osmolarity as plasma or lower
- Non-toxic, both locally and systemically
- Low cost

POSSIBLE SIDE-EFFECTS OF IONIC-BASED CONTRAST MEDIA

Any water-soluble ionic contrast introduced into the vascular system can potentially cause physiological adverse effects. These effects are caused by the high osmolarity and chemotoxic effects of the medium. Although both ionic and non-ionic iodine media have physiological effects on the body, ionic media are of higher osmolarity and potentially cause more side effects in the patient. An ionic contrast has approximately five times the osmolarity of human plasma. Water-soluble organic iodine contrast media have two effects: the desirable primary effect of attenuating X-rays and providing the radiographic image with adequate contrast, and the unwanted secondary effect of inducing potential side effects in patients.

Primary effect – image contrast

Optimum attenuation is achieved by selecting the appropriate concentration of iodine in solution for the planned examination. Two solutions with the same iodine content should provide the same iodine concentration in blood after intravenous injection. This is not the case, however, and the concentration may be affected by small molecules diffusing out of the blood vessel lumen, or by solutions of high concentration within the blood vessel drawing water out of adjacent cells by osmosis (therefore diluting the solution), as mentioned in the introduction to this chapter. To illustrate this, remembering that osmolality is defined as the number of solute particles (e.g. the contrast media molecules) dissolved in 1 L (1000 g) of water, a comparison between normal blood plasma osmolality and different contrast agents is shown below:

- Normal blood plasma ~300 mOsm/kg water
- Ionic monomer ~1200–2400 mOsm/kg water, making it very hypertonic
- Ionic dimers, and non-ionic monomers and dimers (LOCM) are still hypertonic but to a much lesser degree, reducing the osmotic activity. They are, however, more expensive. Isotonic iodixanol (Visipaque) has approximately a third the osmolality of the non-ionic media and a sixth of that of the monomeric ionic media.

When comparing two contrast media with the same iodine concentration, a higher venous concentration of iodine is obtained when diffusion of contrast medium is slowed down by using large molecules (dimers) and osmotic effects are reduced by reducing the number of molecules/ions in solution (monomers).

Secondary effect – adverse events

Contrast media are specifically designed to minimise secondary effects or adverse reactions. The 'perfect' contrast agent would cause no adverse effects at all. Although reactions to contrast media are rare, it is essential that every effort is made to minimise the risk. Acute adverse reactions do occur and are defined as reactions that occur within 1 hour after administration of a contrast medium. Adverse reactions to contrast media or drugs are generally classified into two categories:

1. Idiosyncratic reactions are dose dependent and usually anaphylactoid in nature. These are unpredictable, having a prevalence of 1–2% (0.04–0.22% severe), and are fatal in 1 in 170 000.[5]
2. Non-idiosyncratic reactions are divided into chemotoxic and osmotoxic. Chemotoxic effects can be minimised through the use of LOCM. As LOCM are available at a reasonable cost the use of higher-toxicity substances could be challenged medicolegally.[6] These reactions are predictable and more likely to occur in debilitated patients or those in poor medical health. They are dose dependent and are caused primarily by osmotic effects causing shifts in fluids from the intracellular to extracellular structures, leading to cell dehydration and dysfunction.

The onset of reactions is variable: 70% of reactions occur within 5 minutes of injection, 16% occur more than 5 minutes after the injection, and the remaining 14% occur within 15 minutes of the injection. It is therefore advisable that a suitably qualified staff member remains with the patient for at least 15 minutes after injection.

Contrast media affect specific organs or systems of the body; the following is a summary of some of the major systemic effects of contrast media.

Cardiovascular toxicity

Pain can occur at the injection site during intravascular contrast administration. Thrombus formation and endothelial damage may occur, and contrast may impair platelet aggregation and blood clotting, possibly provoking a painful sickle cell crisis. Osmotic effects of the contrast media can also cause vasodilatation with associated hot flushing. Fluid shifts, as already discussed, can produce an intravascular hypervolaemic state, systemic hypertension and pulmonary oedema. Contrast media can lower the ventricular arrhythmia threshold and precipitate cardiac arrhythmias or cause an angina attack. In rare cases this may lead to cardiac arrest, necessitating urgent medical intervention.

Nephrological toxicity

Ionic contrast may affect renal output, causing renal impairment; this is usually temporary. Contrast medium nephrotoxicity is defined as an impairment in renal function (an increase in serum creatinine by more than 25% or 44 mmol/L) following the intravascular administration of contrast medium in the absence of an alternative aetiology. The following conditions may increase the incidence of nephrotoxicity in patients who receive an intravascular contrast medium:

- Pre-existing kidney disease
- Diabetes mellitus
- Multiple myeloma
- Dehydration
- Large volume of contrast injected
- Age of patient

Nephrotoxic effects can be minimised by ensuring that the patient is hydrated and by using low or iso-osmolar contrast media. In patients with known renal impairment alternative imaging strategies need to be considered that do not require the administration of iodinated contrast media.

Special consideration must be given to diabetic patients on oral metformin (Glucophage). These patients often have associated renal impairment and are more prone to developing lactic acidosis if iodine-based contrast media are administered. Advice from the Royal College of Radiologists (RCR) on the uses of iodinated contrast media in patients taking metformin is based on guidance from the European Society of Urogenital Radiology, stating that metformin is not recommended in diabetic patients with renal impairment.[7] Continued intake of metformin after the onset of renal failure results in a toxic accumulation and subsequent lactic acidosis. However, if serum creatinine levels are within the normal range a low volume of contrast medium (up to 100 mL) can be administered intravenously. There is no need to stop metformin after contrast administration in patients with serum creatinine within the normal range. However, if creatinine levels *are* raised metformin must be withheld 48 hours before and 48 hours after the administration of the iodinated contrast media. Renal function in patients taking metformin should be assessed after contrast administration, and if it is within normal limits after 48 hours, metformin intake can be resumed. Anecdotal evidence shows that in many imaging departments *all* patients taking metformin are advised to withhold this medication for 48 hours prior to and after administration of contrast agents, and it is suggested that this protocol be revisited in light of RCR advice.

Neurotoxicity

The incidence of serious neurotoxic effects is low following the administration of intravascular contrast media; neurotoxicity of contrast media is related to the osmolality of the solution. Entry of contrast media into the central nervous system is normally limited, but may be increased by the osmotic opening of the blood–brain barrier. The blood–brain barrier provides protection for the brain by acting as a selective barrier; it regulates the amount and composition of the brain's cerebrospinal fluid, in order that exchanges across the barrier between the blood and cerebrospinal fluid, which would harm the brain, are reduced, whereas exchanges of essential substances are facilitated. Ionic media are hyperosmolar with respect to human plasma and may dehydrate the cerebral endothelial cells, causing them to dysfunction and breach the barrier, resulting in depolarisation of cerebral neurons and leading to possible seizures. Seizures are more likely to occur in patients with brain tumours, abscesses and other processes that disrupt the blood–brain barrier. Convulsions may also occur as secondary to cerebral hypoxia (caused by hypotension), cardiac arrest or anaphylaxis, which may be induced after administration of a contrast medium. Neurotoxicity can be reduced by using a low osmolar contrast medium as these are less likely to breach the blood–brain barrier.

What happens during a reaction and how reactions may be prevented

Improvements in the chemical structure of modern contrast medium molecules have resulted in a significant reduction in the number of acute reactions. Severe reactions are a rare occurrence and previous allergic reactions to contrast material, asthma and known allergies are factors associated with an increased risk of developing a reaction. An injection of contrast medium causes the release of histamine from the basophils and mast cells in the blood. Some patients release more histamine than others, and the reason for this is still not fully understood. Another possible mechanism for reactions to contrast media is thought to be the inhibition of enzymes, e.g. cholinesterase, which deactivates and hydrolyses acetylcholine, causing symptoms of vagal overstimulation resulting in bronchospasm and cardiovascular collapse.

Patients must be assessed and past medical history ascertained before any contrast medium is administered. Any patient with a medical history that raises concern can be given prophylactic treatment to prevent potential reactions. Intravenous administration of a hydrocortisone may be given before the contrast agent to suppress inflammatory and allergic responses. This reduces the chance of allergic reactions, including anaphylaxis, renal failure or a possible life-threatening emergency. Prophylactic drugs should be administered in a separate syringe as they may cause crystallisation when they come into contact with contrast media. Serious reactions still occur, and awareness of and treatment for the different types of reaction is paramount for any staff member involved in intravenous administration of contrast media. Owing to the unpredictable nature of contrast reactions it is essential that appropriate resuscitation drugs are available in the examination room. In addition, professional guidelines and departmental protocols also recommend a clinician be available to deal with any potential severe reaction that may occur if the contrast medium is being administered by a radiographer.

Non-ionic versus ionic contrast media

As already discussed, ionic media dissociate in solution, altering the sodium balance in the body, whereas non-ionic media, which are made of compounds, do not dissociate in solution. Non-ionic contrast agents do not give the extra ion load that ionic contrast media do and are therefore more 'in tune' with body homeostasis and physiology. Non-ionic contrast media are usually safer to administer and better tolerated by patients. Ionic contrast is less expensive and is

usually used for examination such as cystograms, when contrast is introduced into a body cavity and not directly into the circulatory system. Non-ionic contrast is used primarily in examinations where the contrast is administered directly into the circulatory system. Advantages of non-ionic contrast media include:

- Reduction in the number of side-effects; reactions prove to be 3–10 times lower with non-ionic contrast, owing to the fact that it stimulates less histamine release
- Decreased vasodilatation, producing less alteration in the body haemodynamics and causing less damage to the vessel endothelium
- Reduced effect on the blood–brain barrier
- Improved tolerability for the patient

ADMINISTRATION OF INTRAVENOUS CONTRAST MEDIA

All personnel employed in the imaging department must be aware of the legal and professional regulations relating to the administration of contrast media as part of a radiological examination. All staff employed should have the appropriate training, and hospital trusts and departments should have protocols and procedures in place to ensure a safe and effective procedure for all parties concerned.

LOCM should be administered intravenously to all patients, but *especially* to:

- infants
- the elderly
- those with cardiac or renal impairment
- diabetics
- patients with a history of asthma or severe allergy
- patients with a history of a previous reaction to contrast media.

If a patient presents with a history of a previous reaction to a contrast agent, there is a serious danger of producing a severe and possibly fatal reaction if the examination is undertaken. Allergic patients who have previously tolerated an injection of contrast media may have become sensitised, and great care must be taken on any subsequent examination. The referrer should evaluate the risk involved against information to be gained from the examination being undertaken, and alternative imaging modalities used if deemed more appropriate.

Precautions taken before administration of contrast media

Reactions to the administration of a contrast medium are not predictable and all patients should be monitored closely during the procedure. The importance of assessing the patient before the procedure cannot be over-emphasised. This will give the radiographer a baseline value from which to measure the patient's condition throughout the procedure. The radiographer should be familiar with the symptoms of the various adverse events that may occur. The following is a summary of general advice and precautions to be taken before, during and after the administration of an intravenous contrast medium.

Before injection:

- Know the patient and their medical history
- Reassure the patient and obtain their consent
- If the patient is a high-risk patient administer a low osmolar contrast medium
- Consider the following high-risk factors which are associated with the administration of intravenous contrast medium:

- a previous severe adverse reaction to contrast medium
- asthma or a significant allergic history
- proven or suspected hypersensitivity to iodine
- severe renal or hepatic impairment
- severe cardiovascular disease
- epilepsy
- hyperthyroidism
- multiple myeloma
- pre-existing thyrotoxic symptoms
- severe respiratory disease
- diabetes
- sickle-cell anaemia

- check the batch number and expiry date of the contrast
- ensure the contrast medium is administered at body temperature
- check the correct contrast volume, dose and strength for the procedure being undertaken
- check the sterility of the packaging and that the contrast agent does not contain crystals or is cloudy
- know the procedure and be aware of the possible adverse effects that might occur
- check emergency equipment and be familiar with its application
- obtain a positive identification check on the patient

During the injection

- Know where the radiologist/administering doctor may be reached
- Evaluate the patient's vital signs and observe respiration, pulse, patient colour and level of consciousness, being aware of any changes

After the injection

- A suitably qualified person should remain with the patient for at least 15 minutes
- All relevant documentation regarding the contrast agent used should be correctly completed upon completion of any contrast administration. All relevant information regarding the contrast agent and its administration must be included in the patient's permanent medical record:
  - contrast medium used
  - volume administered
  - density
  - batch number
  - who performed the injection
  - any adverse effects and any treatment or drug therapy given
- In the event of any serious adverse reactions this should be reported to the manufacturing company to coordinate worldwide data collection on similar recent reactions. This ensures a global perspective
- On completion of the examination check that the patient is fit to travel home and do not allow them to leave if there is any doubt. If any concerns are identified the patient should be checked by a doctor before leaving the department

Radiographers performing intravenous administration

It is well documented that the clinical role of the radiographer has been evolving rapidly in recent years. Given the drive for role expansion in radiography, it is now common practice for radiographers to administer intravenous contrast media in their clinical roles. Although these extended roles bring increased job satisfaction and responsibility for radiographers, they equally bring associated legal and professional accountability. Radiographers are actively involved in clinical procedures where performing intravenous injections is entirely within the role development framework outlined by the RCR.[8] It is paramount that radiographers undertaking this role be adequately trained and aware of the professional issues. They must operate under an agreed protocol and a written scheme of work. The employing authority should be informed in writing and be assured of the competency of any radiographer undertaking this role; it is recommended that intravenous training should be via a local training course or a nationally recognised qualification that allows transferability between employers.

Before performing any intravenous administration it is important that the radiographer is aware of the:

- Related anatomy, physiology and pathology
- Correct choice and disposal of any equipment used
- Criteria for choosing the vein, aseptic techniques
- Indications and contraindications for any contrast media used
- Potential problems that may arise, including management of adverse reactions
- Health and safety issues relating to intravenous administration

Aseptic technique must be maintained throughout the procedure. The circulation is a closed sterile system and venepuncture can provide a method of entry for commensals into the system. Intravenous-related infection is a major cause of mortality and morbidity in hospitalised patients. A reduction in hospital-acquired infections is at the forefront of government policy, as the majority of these infections are both preventable and an expensive drain on finances. Patients with cannulae in situ are prone to developing nosocomial infections, and as the majority of acute patients in hospital are cannulated, the potential to develop an infection is high if careful technique and protocols are not observed. Any intravenous cannulation can potentially cause infection to the patient. Commensals can be transmitted from contaminated equipment such as the distal tip of the needle or Venflon, hubs or connectors or from the healthcare worker's hands. All departments have a hand-washing policy that must be adhered to in order to minimise risks, as bacteria can invade the site where the needle is inserted and local infection may develop in the skin around the needle. Bacteria can also enter the blood through the vein and cause a generalised systemic infection. These potential harmful infections can be reduced by:

- being aware of touch contamination of equipment
- ensuring all packaging is intact before opening
- checking expiry dates
- choosing insertion sites carefully
- minimal manipulation of connections
- following hand-washing procedures
- investigating mild pyrexias that may develop and treating them immediately
- observing and recording intravenous sites regularly

Health and safety

Owing to the increase in bloodborne viruses it is necessary for the professional administering the contrast medium to protect themselves from any potential blood spills. Good-quality gloves should be worn when performing venepuncture; these will protect from blood spillage but will not prevent a needlestick injury, long known to be hazardous for healthcare workers. Needlestick injuries account for a high number of accidents to staff in hospitals. Hepatitis B is more easily transmitted than human immunodeficiency virus (HIV), so any healthcare professional working with body fluids and performing intravenous injections should be vaccinated for hepatitis B and have their antibody levels checked as recommended. The impact for a staff member who suffers a needlestick injury can be devastating in terms of health effects, and the waiting period for results of blood tests following such injury can be psychologically traumatic.

Needlestick injuries most often occur when:

- the needle misses the cap (sheath) and accidentally enters the hand holding it
- the needle pierces the cap and enters the hand holding it
- the poorly fitting cap slips off of a recapped needle and the needle stabs the hand.

Recapping can account for 25–30% of all needlestick injuries among nursing and laboratory staff. There is no substitute for careful technique when performing any venepuncture procedure. Used needles should be discarded directly into a sharps container without being re-sheathed.

Treatment of needlestick injuries

Recent campaigns have targeted improved infection control, better management and staff training to reduce exposure to bloodborne pathogens. However, although these methods can remove human error, they cannot remove the primary risk – the needle or sharp itself.

If a needlestick injury occurs, departmental safety policy should be followed, and in any case the following steps should be followed immediately:

- Bleed the puncture site immediately
- Wash the needlestick injury site under running hot water
- Report the incident to your supervisor and occupational health department
- Seek medical treatment if necessary

Vein choice

The choice of vein is vital when performing an intravenous contrast injection. Painful, sore or bruised sites should be avoided as these may be irritated as a result of previous use, or they may be sclerosed. Always use veins with the largest diameter possible: these are easily palpable and have good capillary refill. If at all possible, use veins on the non-dominant side; veins that cross joints or bony prominences or have little skin cover (e.g. the wrist) should be avoided if at all possible. The area selected should have no broken skin, infection, lymphoedema, arteriovenous shunts or fistulae.

There are also some practical considerations to consider: for example the purpose of the cannulation and the length of time the needle is to remain in situ. Always choose the injection device after assessing the condition and accessibility of the individual patient's veins. The sites of choice on the upper limb are branches of the basilic, cephalic or median cubital vein. Preference should be given to veins that are patent and healthy and are easily detectable, visually or by palpitation, as already discussed.

Arterial administration of contrast media

In arteriography, a contrast medium is introduced via a catheter into an artery, rendering the lumen of the vessel opaque to X-rays. As the contrast is delivered as a bolus under high pressure, a pressure injector is usually used for administration. In angiography the femoral artery is the most frequent approach to the arterial system, using the Seldinger technique. Low osmolar contrast media should be used for all angiographic studies and isotonic contrast is recommended as it has improved tolerability for patients when high doses are administered. The quantity and strength of the contrast used is dependent upon the area of the vascular system being investigated.

Magnetic resonance angiography (MRA) is an emerging modality that examines blood vessels, using magnetic resonance imaging (MRI) technology to detect, diagnose and aid the treatment of heart disorders, stroke and vascular disease. MRA can provide detailed images of blood vessels without using any contrast medium, although contrast is usually administered to enhance image quality, and this will be discussed later in the chapter.

Preparation of injection site

Care should be taken in preparing the site for injection. Asepsis is vital, as the skin is being broken and a foreign device introduced into the sterile circulatory system. The two major sources of microbial contamination are:
- cross-infection from the practitioner to the patient
- skin flora of the patient

Good hand-washing and drying techniques are essential and gloves must be worn for each patient. The skin around the injection site should be cleansed with a preparation such as isopropyl alcohol or 1% iodine. In practice, alcohol swabs are usually used, and several types are available. To reduce the risk from the patient's own flora, the area should be cleansed for at least 30 seconds and it is important that swabbing is in one direction only. Once the site is swabbed it should not be touched again and should be allowed to dry for approximately 30 seconds before insertion of the needle to facilitate coagulation of organisms ensuring disinfection. Allowing the area to dry also prevents stinging. The injection site should not be touched after disinfection.

Needle insertion technique for administration of an intravenous contrast injection (for IVU)

- Ensure all the equipment required is ready and available prior to commencement of the procedure
- Approach the patient in a confident manner and explain the procedure; ensure that the patient is comfortable and is aware of the procedure – this reduces anxiety
- Allow the patient to ask questions
- Obtain consent
- Ascertain medical history and check allergies
- Support the chosen limb on a pad
- Apply a tourniquet to the upper arm on the chosen side to assess the injection site (tourniquets and pads are potentially a mechanism for cross-infection that staff need to be aware of). The patient may assist by clenching and unclenching their fist
- Select a vein using the criteria already discussed
- Wash and dry hands
- Put on gloves
- Clean the skin carefully for at least 30 seconds using the appropriate preparation. Do not palpate the vein or touch the skin after cleansing
- Anchor the vein by applying manual traction to the skin a few centimetres below the chosen injection site
- Insert the needle smoothly at an approximately 30° angle; look out for blood flashback and then advance the cannula slowly. Do not attempt repeated insertions with the same cannula. If the first insertion is not successful the procedure should be repeated with a new cannula
- Release the tourniquet
- To eliminate air from the system and ensure accurate positioning in the vein, it is common practice to draw blood into the syringe. However, use of a 'closed system' should be considered, where

the syringe is connected to the needle or Venflon and flushed with contrast medium. This is because it has long been suggested that thrombus may form if blood mixes with the contrast agent[9]
- Inject the contrast medium
- Place a sterile cottonwool ball over the site
- Remove the needle
- Apply pressure to the site after the needle has been removed and continue to apply pressure for approximately 1 minute until bleeding has stopped
- Ensure the patient has no allergies to plasters. Inspect the injection site before firmly applying a dressing
- Discard waste in the correct manner
- Remove gloves and wash hands

Treatment of adverse reactions to contrast medium

It has already been stated that all patients must be kept under constant observation during and after contrast medium administration and emergency drugs and oxygen should be available should they be required. All staff working in the area should be trained in cardiopulmonary resuscitation and know how to initiate an emergency call. Contrast media should be administered at body temperature and the manufacturer's optimum doses should not be exceeded. This minimises the risk of an adverse reaction. Before initiating any treatment the severity of the event should be carefully evaluated; this ensures the appropriate treatment can be given. Reactions to intravenous administration of contrast media can be classified into three categories:

- Mild
- Moderate
- Severe

Mild reaction

Mild reactions simply require careful observation of the patient. Most of the symptoms will pass within a few minutes. Some schools of thought have postulated that a great many mild adverse effects are the result of the patient's fear and apprehension.[5] Mild adverse reactions are encountered in as many as 15% of patients after administration of intravenous ionic HOCM and up to 3% of patients after non-ionic LOCM.[10]

Signs and symptoms of a mild reaction include:

- nausea
- a warm feeling that may be associated with hot flushing
- sneezing
- rhinorrhoea
- a metallic taste in the mouth
- headache
- pallor
- pruritus (itching)
- diaphoresis (sweating)

Treatment of mild reactions usually only involves observation of the patient and reassurance. Usually no medical treatment is required and the reaction does not interfere significantly with the examination procedure being undertaken.

Moderate reaction

This is a more severe reaction in which medical treatment is necessary and/or where the examination procedure is delayed or otherwise affected. Signs and symptoms of a moderate reaction include:

- erythema
- urticaria
- pruritus
- chest pain
- abdominal pain
- vasovagal syncope
- facial swelling due to oedema

Treatment of a moderate reaction may vary. Compression and tight clothing should be released and the patient reassured. The patient will need to be seen by a clinician, and the adverse reaction should be documented in the patient's permanent medical record. All documentation should be completed according to department protocols. Drug therapy may be required, such as antihistamine (e.g. Piriton 10 mg) intravenously, or adrenaline (epinephrine) 0.5 mL 1 : 1000 solution subcutaneously, to reduce the symptoms.

Severe reaction

Seek medical advice immediately; medical treatment with hospitalisation is necessary. The examination is terminated. The management of severe adverse reactions, including drug treatments, should be handled by the resuscitation team.[11] Signs, symptoms and effects of a severe reaction may include:

- paralysis
- seizures
- pulmonary oedema
- bronchospasm
- laryngeal oedema
- anaphylactic shock
- respiratory arrest
- cardiac arrest

It is important that the radiographer recognises the significance of certain signs:

- *Pulmonary oedema*: dyspnoea and cyanosis; the patient develops a cough with white frothy sputum, accompanied by dyspnoea.
- *Anaphylactic shock*: dramatic onset; pallor, sweating, nausea, syncope. A weak pulse due to hypotension, bradycardia or tachycardia may be observed. In severe cases cardiac arrest may occur.
- *Cardiac arrest*: dramatic onset; absence of palpable pulse, dilated pupils, pallor, cyanosis.
- *Respiratory arrest*: abrupt onset of cyanosis with cessation of breathing.
- *Cerebral oedema*: the accumulation of excessive fluid in the substance of the brain leading to convulsions and possible coma.

Administration of oxygen by mask (6–10 L/min) is vital and should be performed as soon as possible when a severe reaction occurs, as hypoxia may develop. Severe reactions require immediate recognition and evaluation of the patient's cardiopulmonary status. Cardiopulmonary resuscitation (CPR) equipment should be readily available in any area where contrast media are used. The radiographer should be trained in the techniques of CPR. Treatment of a severe reaction should follow the 'ABCD system':

- Airway open
- Breathing restored
- Circulation maintained
- Drug and definitive therapy

Contrast media should never be injected by anyone unfamiliar with resuscitation procedures. Radiology staff and management should continually review departmental protocols to ensure all staff are aware and are able to carry out their roles should an event occur.

Potential complications for the patient after intravenous cannulation

Any patient who undergoes intravenous cannulation has the potential to develop any of the following complications. Some are preventable, others are not:

- Infection
- Phlebitis and thrombophlebitis
- Emboli
- Vasovagal response
- Pain
- Haematoma/haemorrhage
- Extravasation
- Unintended arterial cannulation
- Allergy

Tissue damage from extravasation of contrast material is caused by the direct toxic effect of the agent. This is usually absorbed fairly quickly; cream such as Lasonil, which is anti-inflammatory, can be applied to the injection site to facilitate this. Compartment syndrome may occur if enough contrast material leaks into surrounding tissue. Compartment syndrome occurs when swelling takes place within a compartment of a limb and increases pressure on arteries, veins and nerves. In addition to causing extreme pain, this slows circulation to the muscles and nerves and may cause permanent damage to these tissues. This may lead to impaired blood flow and muscle and nerve damage. Compartment syndrome is a medical emergency requiring immediate treatment to prevent tissue death and permanent dysfunction.

CONTRAST MEDIA USED IN BILIARY AND HEPATIC IMAGING

Contrast examinations of the biliary system are very rarely undertaken have been superseded by cross-sectional imaging techniques such as CT and ultrasound. The molecule of biliary contrast media features two vacant binding sites that bind with serum albumin to form a molecule that is too large to be filtered by the kidneys. Biliary contrast media are tri-iodo benzoic acid derivatives. The oral contrast media have a single benzene ring (Biloptin); the intravenous medium (Biliscopin) is a dimer with a polymethylene chain connecting the two rings.

Oral cholecystography

This examination is very rarely undertaken in a modern imaging department. For its success it requires the contrast medium, usually sodium ipodate (Biloptin), to be absorbed from the gut. It is then bound to albumin and transported to the liver via the portal vein. The contrast is then excreted from the liver with the bile and concentrates in the gallbladder. The usual dose of contrast for this examination is six capsules of Biloptin, each containing 500 mg of sodium ipodate. Imaging of the gallbladder takes place 10–12 hours after the contrast has been administered.

Intravenous cholangiogram

This examination has been superseded by other imaging modalities such as ultrasound, CT and endoscopic retrograde cholangiopancreatography (ERCP).

The examination requires an infusion of meglumine iotroxate (Biliscopin) and conventional tomography for imaging.

Table 28.1 Contrast media used in the biliary system

Examination	Contrast media	Rationale for use
Preoperative cholangiography	HOCM or LOCM 150 5 mL and then 20 mL usually used	Low iodine content to avoid obscuring any stones
Postoperative cholangiography (T-tube)	HOCM or LOCM 150 approx. 20–30 mL	Low iodine content to avoid obscuring any stones
Percutaneous transhepatic cholangiography	LOCM 150 20–60 mL	Low iodine content to avoid obscuring any stones
Biliary drainage	LOCM 200 20–60 mL	Low iodine content to avoid obscuring any stones

ENDOSCOPIC RETROGRADE ERCP

This examination is a collaborative technique undertaken by an endoscopist but requires radiological screening and imaging. After the endoscope has been introduced, the ampulla of Vater is located and the contrast introduced. Low-density water-soluble contrast is used to prevent any calculi that may be present in the biliary system being obscured. Strictures can be accurately identified and, if required, interventional procedures such as stenting or stone removal can be performed. Other biliary examinations requiring contrast media are listed in Table 28.1.

IODISED OILS AS A CONTRAST MEDIUM

These are used very infrequently in the imaging department today. The examinations that use these contrast media have in the main been superseded by cross-sectional imaging modalities. They are used in examinations where water-soluble agents are contraindicated or where a viscous compound is required:

- Sialography 0.5–2 mL of Lipiodol per side
- Dacrocystography 0.5–2 mL of Lipiodol per side

These contrast agents are not easily absorbed and in some cases may carry a risk of oil embolus.

CONTRAST MEDIA USED IN OTHER RADIOGRAPHIC EXAMINATIONS

Table 28.2 highlights some of the other radiographic examinations undertaken in the imaging department that use contrast media.

CONTRAST MEDIA USED IN ULTRASOUND

Contrast agents can improve the image quality of sonography, either by reducing the reflectivity of undesired interfaces or by increasing the back scattered echoes from the desired regions. Use of contrast media

Table 28.2 Contrast media used in other examinations

Examination	Contrast media, dose, strength and volume	Comments
Hysterosalpingography	HOCM or LOCM 10–20 mL	LOCM has no advantage. Using non-ionic dimers is associated with decreased procedural and delayed pain[8]
Contrast venography	Approx. 30 mL LOCM	Use to image possible deep vein thromboses. It is invasive and is dependent upon cannulation of a vein often in a swollen foot
Arthrography	4–10 mL HOCM or LOCM. Air or oxygen can also be used to create a double contrast image	Volume of contrast used dependent upon joint under investigation
Cystography and micturating cystourethrography	HOCM or LOCM can be used	Volume used dependent upon the size of the structure and also patient tolerance
Renal imaging including retrogrades, nephrostomy, percutaneous nephrolithotomy	LOCM is frequently used	IVU: 50 mL 370 mg/mL standard for adult.[4] Other areas: volume dependent upon anatomical area. HOCM can be used dependent upon radiologist

in ultrasound has been well established for cardiac imaging since the 1980s, for example air being used to demonstrate atrial septal defects. Blood was taken from the patient, shaken to introduce air bubbles and then reinjected and imaged. The problem with this technique was the reproducibility and homogeneity of the contrast effect owing to variations in bubble size. This led to the development and manufacture of specialised products, e.g. Echovist, an echo-rich microbubble, microparticle suspension. The gas microbubbles reflect ultrasound almost totally, resulting in a strong echo enhancement.[12] The use of contrast media in abdominal ultrasound is still in its infancy; it is particularly useful in demonstrating portal vein thrombosis, alleviating the need for conventional, more invasive angiographic examinations. Also, intravenous vascular contrast agents can aid the imaging of malignant tumours in the liver, kidney, ovary, pancreas, prostate and breast. Tumour angiogenesis and Doppler signals from small tumour vessels may be detectable after an injection of contrast medium. As already discussed, however, these contrast media can cause adverse reactions.

can develop nephrogenic systemic fibrosis (NSF). NSF is a rare multi-systemic fibrosing disorder that mainly affects the skin, but may affect other organs in patients with renal insufficiency. Links have been made in the literature between the administration of gadolinium and NSF.[14] Gadolinium can be nephrotoxic in patients with existing renal impairment, and delayed excretion of gadolinium may cause acute renal failure. This current evidence does raise safety issues over the use of gadolinium as a contrast medium in MRI examinations.

Clinical indications for MRI contrast use:

- Central nervous system tumours
- Spinal imaging
- Brain abscess, in which MRI will demonstrate ring enhancement
- Assessment of the blood–brain barrier to see if it is intact
- Demyelinating diseases
- Staging disease progression in multiple sclerosis and malignant disease
- More accurate delineation of tumour margins from oedema
- Cardiac/aortic imaging

CONTRAST MEDIA USED IN MRI

Contrast enhancement plays a major role in MRI. MRI generates high natural contrast in images but contrast media are still used to improve tissue characterisation. Contrast media in MRI improve the potential for examining the function of systems and structures. MRI contrast is used to improve the image quality as well as the sensitivity and specificity of abnormalities and pathologies identified.[13] In some brain pathologies little difference exists in signal intensity between healthy and diseased tissue, hence the need for a contrast medium to enhance image quality. The contrast material used in MRA examinations must have magnetic properties and the most common agent used is gadolinium, a paramagnetic agent that allows positive contrast enhancement. Gadolinium is a rare earth metal, is paramagnetic and provides contrast between the lesion or pathology and the surrounding tissue by shortening the T1 relaxation time. Gadolinium has to be chelated with diethylenetriamine penta-acetic acid, as free gadolinium ions are toxic. It is hydrophilic, having very low lipid solubility, and so does not cross the blood–brain barrier. There are several categories of MRI contrast agent available, and the choice depends on the pathology being investigated.

Gadolinium has a relatively favourable safety profile, but recent research has identified patients who have gadolinium administered

CONTRAST MEDIA USED IN CT

Contrast media are used to enhance the quality of images produced during CT examinations. The contraindications, which have already been discussed, apply to the use of contrast in these examinations. Contrast media for CT examinations are administered in four different ways:

1. Intravenous injection
2. Oral administration
3. Rectal administration
4. Inhalation: This is a relatively uncommon procedure in which xenon gas is inhaled for a highly specialised form of lung or brain imaging. The technique, xenon CT, is only available at a small number of locations worldwide and is used only for rare cases

Almost all CT examinations of the abdomen and pelvis require the administration of oral contrast agents to opacify the gastrointestinal tract. Good bowel opacification helps differentiate between the lymph nodes, tumour masses and unopacified loops of bowel. Contrast enhancement in CT scanning of the abdomen and pelvis requires the patient to ingest oral contrast medium, which is usually a dilute barium sulphate solution. Patients usually need to drink at least

1000–1500 mL to fill the stomach and intestines sufficiently. An alternative to barium sulphate solution is an oral water-soluble iodine-based contrast medium, e.g. Gastrografin. Scanning is usually performed 1 hour after drinking the contrast to allow time for it to pass into the intestine. Although this may seem inconvenient, the oral contrast makes an essential improvement in the quality of the CT study and results in a more accurate diagnosis by providing delineation of low-contrast structures. Contrast can be administered rectally to help distinguish anatomical areas in the lower abdomen.

Water can be used as a negative agent, which is useful for assessment of carcinoma of the stomach. Another approach to negative contrast is, when scanning a female pelvis, to place a tampon in the vagina, which allows radiolucent air to distend the vagina, creating additional contrast between the reproductive organs. Air is used in CT colonoscopy for contrast purposes and to distend the bowel to unfold the mucosa. This procedure of the large bowel produces 3D images of the entire colonic mucosa similar to those obtained during colonoscopy. Patients undergo full bowel preparation, an intravenous smooth muscle relaxant is administered, and the colon is then insufflated with room air until it is fully distended. Once satisfactory distension has been achieved, CT is performed to image the entire colon. There has been mention of the use of CO_2 in this chapter relating to double-contrast barium enemas, which has the advantage of improved tolerance compared to air but also has the disadvantage of requiring reinsufflation during the procedure. Reinsufflation renders the use of CO_2 inappropriate for some CT scanners, but rapid multislice scanners are likely to be fast enough to allow the use of CO_2 for virtual colonoscopy. Additional information on CT colonoscopy is found in the chapter in gastrointestinal imaging.

Non-ionic water-soluble isotonic contrast agents are used in CT to highlight blood vessels and to enhance the tissue structure of various organs such as the brain, spine, liver and kidneys. CT angiography has developed rapidly and increased greatly since the early to mid-1990s, and most UK imaging departments undertake CT angiography as an adjunct to axial scanning. With CT contrast examinations the ability to time image acquisition to coincide with peak contrast enhancement was in the past a challenge for practitioners working in this imaging modality. The use of a pressure injector, coupled with current CT software, addresses this issue while ensuring that the radiographer is distanced from the CT scanner during exposure.

REFERENCES

1. Farrow R, Stevenson GW. In: Armstrong P, Waistie ML, editors. A concise textbook of radiology. London: Arnold; 2001.

2. Farrow R, et al. Air versus carbon dioxide insufflation in double contras barium enemas: the role of active gaseous drainage. British Journal of Radiology 1995;68:838–40.

3. Holemans JA. A comparison of air, carbon dioxide and air/carbon dioxide mixture as insufflations agents for double contrast barium enemas. European Radiology 1998;8;274–6.

4. Chapman S, Nakielny R. A guide to radiological procedures. 4th ed. London: WB Saunders; 2002.

5. Lalli AF. Urographic contrast media reactions and anxiety. Radiology 1974;112: 267–71.

6. Bush WH, Albright DE, Sather JS. Malpractice issues and contrast use. Journal of the American College of Radiology 2005;4:344–7; livepage.apple.com.

7. http://www.rcr.ac.uk/docs/radiology/pdf/bfcr(10)4_stand_contrast.pdf.

8. http://www.sor.org/public/document-library/sor_learning_development_framework_clinical.pdf.

9. Robertson HJ. Blood clot formation in angiographic syringes containing nonionic contrast media. Radiology. 1987;162(3): 621–2.

10. Thomsen HS, Morcos SK. Management of adverse reactions to contrast media. European Radiology 2004;14(3):476–81.

11. O'Neil JM, Bride KDM. Cardiopulmonary resuscitation and contrast media reactions in a radiology department. Clinical Radiology 2001;56(4):321–5.

12. Harvey CJ, et al. Developments in ultrasound contrast media. European Radiology 2001;11(4):675–89.

13. Leiner T, et al. Contemporary imaging techniques for the diagnosis of renal artery stenosis. European Radiology 2005;15: 2219–29.

14. Chewing RW, Murphy KJ. Gadolinium-based contrast media and the development of nephrogenic system fibrosis in patients with renal insufficiency. Journal of Vascular and Interventional Radiology 2007;18:331–3.

Chapter | 29 |

Gastrointestinal tract

Joanne Rudd, Michael Smith, Darren Wood

The gastrointestinal (GI) tract has traditionally been examined using radiography, barium sulphate suspension (commonly referred to as 'barium' and used interchangeably) and gas as a double-contrast agent. Accessory organs of the tract (Chapter 30) have traditionally been examined using iodine-based contrast agents. However, the rapidly changing field of medical imaging, with the development of faster image acquisition, higher resolution, better computing power and improvements in post-processing software, now sees the tract examined by a variety of methods, some of which supersede conventional contrast radiography.[1,2] Recent advances in the technology of multidetector computed tomography (CT) systems have increased the use of CT in the diagnosis of the small bowel.[3] CT enterography and magnetic resonance (MR) enterography are now proving accurate in defining the extent and severity of small bowel inflammation and neoplasms, and detecting extraluminal pathology. Capsule endoscopy is another developing imaging modality used to examine the GI tract. It is highly sensitive but has a lower specificity, and there is also the risk of capsule retention.[4-6] Virtual colonoscopy, primarily using CT (although MR may be used), is another advancing technology.[7] Endoscopic ultrasound and positron emission tomography are also emerging supplementary technologies that may find a role in imaging of the GI tract.[8,9] Some of these newer imaging techniques are complementary as opposed to alternatives to traditional barium studies.[10] The use of videofluoroscopy or the 'modified barium swallow' is, however, a barium examination that has increased in popularity.

Besides examination of the tract itself, other contrast-enhanced X-ray imaging procedures provide studies of the abdominal region, namely angiography and arteriography. Angiography is an injectable contrast agent-based technique used to provide a 'road map' that shows the arterial or venous supply to the entire abdominal cavity. Arteriography is mainly used to assess tumour resectability or demonstrate suspected GI haemorrhage. The superior mesenteric artery, inferior mesenteric artery and coeliac axis are filled with a contrast agent in order to show the entire region. Venography is used in assessment of the portal venous system and is generally used for preoperative demonstration of varices. The use of CT and MR angiography and Doppler ultrasound is reducing the need for these procedures.

NOTES ON POSITION TERMINOLOGY FOR FLUOROSCOPIC EXAMINATION

In the UK, positioning terminology tends to describe positions in relation to the image receptor (IR). This concept is generally easily understood when the traditional position of the IR is described (e.g. under the examination table) but can become confusing when over-couch IRs are used; fluoroscopic units often fall into this category. Further confusion occurs when it is realised that fluoroscopy units may have over- or under-couch IRs; this then makes it even more difficult for an author to ensure that their readers fully understand position descriptions.

For example, if a patient is initially supine on a *conventional radiography examination table* (over-couch *tube*, under-couch *IR*) and their right side is then raised, the position is described as a left posterior oblique (LPO), as the patient is oblique with the posterior aspect of their trunk still in contact with the table-top (Fig. 29.1); on a *fluoroscopy table* with under-couch *tube* and over-couch *receptor*, this same body position is usually described as a right anterior oblique (RAO) as the right anterior aspect of the body is nearest the IR. Simpler projections such as anteroposterior (AP) change to posteroanterior (PA) with over-couch receptor and under-couch tube. Students in particular become very confused by this, and many radiographers resort to describing the positions as 'right side raised' or 'left side raised' to avoid confusion.

For the purpose of this chapter and to avoid this confusion, the authors have decided to use the *traditional under-couch receptor and over-couch tube descriptor*, identical to that used for general under-couch IR over-couch tube radiography. Figure 29.1 identifies the positions in full. We hope that this proves less confusing than using the traditional fluoroscopy description technique.

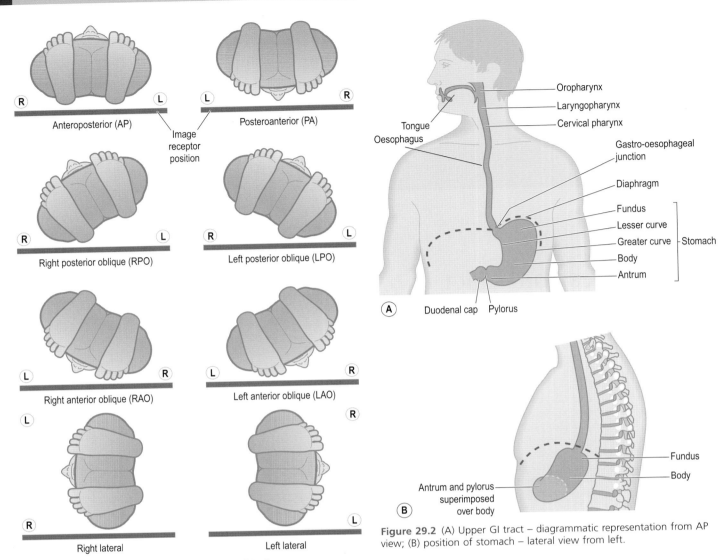

Figure 29.1 Positioning descriptions for use in this chapter.

Anteroposterior (AP)

Image receptor position

Posteroanterior (PA)

Right posterior oblique (RPO)

Left posterior oblique (LPO)

Right anterior oblique (RAO)

Left anterior oblique (LAO)

Right lateral

Left lateral

Oropharynx
Laryngopharynx
Cervical pharynx
Tongue
Oesophagus
Gastro-oesophageal junction
Diaphragm
Fundus
Lesser curve
Greater curve — Stomach
Body
Antrum

(A) Duodenal cap Pylorus

Fundus
Body
Antrum and pylorus superimposed over body
(B)

Figure 29.2 (A) Upper GI tract – diagrammatic representation from AP view; (B) position of stomach – lateral view from left.

UPPER GI TRACT

The upper GI tract consists of the oropharynx, hypopharynx, oesophagus, stomach and first part of the duodenum (for a general appraisal of the layout of this part of the GI tract see Figure 29.2). The aim of a contrast examination is to outline these structures in single and/or double contrast to obtain optimum visualisation. The most common contrast agent used is a barium sulphate suspension, although ionic and non-ionic contrast agents can be used.

Most patients who have upper GI symptoms are referred primarily for oesophagogastric duodenoscopy (OGD), but this may be used in conjunction with other tests so that a 'gold standard' approach is applied.[11] For some symptoms there is, as yet, no acknowledged standalone gold standard.[12] There are, however, sometimes reasons why contrast-enhanced X-ray studies are required: for example when patients cannot tolerate an OGD due to medical constraints; when patients simply refuse an OGD procedure; or when their symptoms persist after OGD results are found to be negative. Contrast examinations are the examination of choice in suspected cases of high dysphagia (above the sternal notch) and when motility issues such as achalasia are suspected.[13]

REFERRAL CRITERIA FOR EXAMINATION OF THE UPPER GI TRACT

Barium swallow

- Sensation of 'lump in throat' (globus)
- Regurgitation of unaltered food
- Dysphagia
- Gastro-oesophageal reflux (GOR)
- Assessment of oesophageal perforation (water-soluble contrast must be used)
- Known hiatus hernia – anatomical roadmap required prior to surgery
- Patient refuses OGD

Barium meal

- Anaemia
- Suspected carcinoma
- Upper abdominal mass

- Normal OGD but persistent symptoms of dyspepsia, weight loss, recurrent vomiting or epigastric pain
- Patient refuses OGD
- Assess transit to small bowel postoperatively
- Anastomosis check postoperatively

PATIENT PREPARATION – ALL EXAMINATIONS OF THE UPPER TRACT

The patient should be starved for at least 6 hours before the examination,[14] but 5 hours has been considered adequate.[15] It is suggested that this should be the case even if only a barium swallow is indicated, in case views of the stomach are found to be required; this avoids the patient having to return for a second examination. However, medications must be taken as normal. This is because some diseases affect the swallowing process and effective medication often improves the mechanism of swallowing. One example of this is in the case of Parkinson's disease. If drug therapy is suspended, swallowing may be compromised, resulting in inadequate imaging of the swallowing process.

- The patient should cease smoking for 6 hours. Smoking can increase the amount of stomach secretions, which can prevent the barium sulphate from coating the stomach mucosa adequately
- All jewellery or artefacts (e.g. hearing aids) should be removed
- Patient clothing should be removed and a radiolucent gown should be worn
- The patient should then be informed of the procedure (they should have received information with their appointment prior to attending) so they can give their consent
- Compliance with instructions on the starvation period should be checked

BARIUM SWALLOW AND MEAL

Historically, this examination has been carried out on patients as a complete examination. With the development of radiographer-led procedures there is a move towards giving a direct answer to a set of clinical indications and questions and so tailoring the examination to fit this need. The barium swallow and meal can therefore reasonably be split into a number of 'sub-examinations' when the clinical picture has a definite direction.

Upper ('high') barium swallow

This examination is used for patients who have high dysphagia or definite oesophageal symptoms, or quite often have had a normal OGD but are still symptomatic; often a motility disorder may be the cause.

Contraindications

- Known aspiration during ingestion (although this can be overcome by using non-ionic water-soluble contrast)
- Suspected perforation

Contrast agent

- Barium sulphate suspension 250% w/v[14,15] or water-soluble contrast medium

Additional equipment

- Disposable cup
- Tissues

Technique

If there is any query that the patient may aspirate the contrast agent, the initial swallow is best carried out using a water-soluble contrast, although aspiration of barium sulphate has been considered by some to be relatively harmless.[14] Aspiration may not be suspected but unsuspected 'silent aspiration' may be found. Otherwise use the following technique (ensure that you have understood the notes on fluoroscopic examination positioning descriptors earlier in this chapter before considering technique descriptors):

- The patient is initially asked to stand erect in the AP position on the fluoroscopic table and hold the cup of barium sulphate in their hand, usually the left, as further turning of the patient is usually to the left. The arm will then lie clear of the trunk, without the patient having to negotiate its movement around the intensifying screen carriage.
- The patient is turned into the left lateral position in order to commence with routine assessment of possible aspiration. They are asked to take a 'normal' (for them) mouthful of the liquid and hold it in their mouth until asked to swallow. This is to give the operator a chance to centre on the area of interest, the pharynx, and optimise the collimation. This view allows the posterior wall of the hypopharynx to be optimally viewed (Fig. 29.3). It also clearly shows the larynx and trachea, thereby allowing demonstration of laryngeal penetration and/or aspiration should it occur.
- If the radiographic equipment allows, a frame rate of 3 per second is suggested as an initial choice; modern digital equipment can allow recording of the screened image. This offers a reduction in radiation dose by allowing retrospective and repeated study of the patient's swallowing action without returning to rescreen missed actions, and also allows a more real-time assessment to take place.

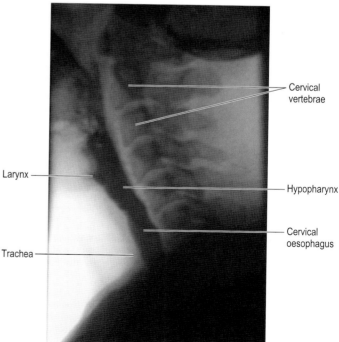

Figure 29.3 Lateral view of hypopharynx and cervical oesophagus.

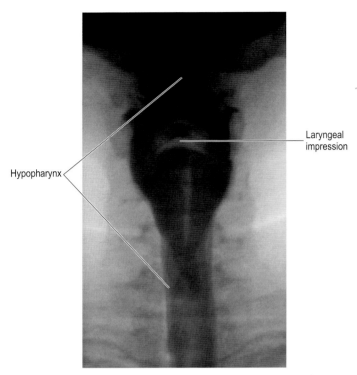

Hypopharynx

Laryngeal impression

Figure 29.4 AP barium swallow showing normal hypopharyngeal anatomy.

- The patient is then asked to swallow and the exposure is initiated. Real-time recording (exposure) is terminated when the barium bolus passes beyond the screened image or point of interest. This lateral pharynx view is then repeated, as some pathologies such as cricopharyngeal spasm may be transient and may not occur on every swallow.
- The patient is then turned back to AP, ideally standing with their chin raised so that their symphysis menti is superimposed over the occiput. The AP view is the optimum for hypopharyngeal anatomy;[16] it will be seen in both single- and double-contrast images (Fig. 29.4). This view may be repeated at least once more to ensure there is consistency in the images, making it easier to definitively identify pathology.
- Depending on the patient's history and the individual imaging department protocols, the examination may be terminated at this point, or the lower oesophagus may be imaged with a check for reflux. Some lower oesphageal pathologies such as hiatus hernia and GOR may mimic 'high' pathology such as globus (see barium swallow and reflux assessment below).

The most common abnormalities in the pharynx are persistent cricopharyngeal impressions or diverticula, the most common diverticulum type being Zenker's; this occurs in the mid-hypopharynx and is more common in the older population. They are quite often termed hypopharyngeal pouches.[16] The pouches can become quite large, often causing patients to be referred because of regurgitation of undigested food some time after they have eaten. They are also often difficult to endoscope, as the scope enters the pouch and cannot be passed further; the barium swallow can thus quite often be the most appropriate test for confirming the presence and extent of this pathology.

Oesophageal webs are also best seen on the lateral projection, shown on the anterior wall, although they are best viewed with rapid imaging sequences; they have been noted in 1–5% of asymptomatic patients and 12–15% of dysphagia patients.[16]

Barium swallow and reflux assessment

Patients for this type of study often present with clinical symptoms of GOR. They often have a feeling of retrosternal discomfort and no other symptoms. Although pH monitoring is an effective way of evaluating GOR, there is not as yet a gold standard test.[12] The barium study can still be useful as an adjunct to other tests, as some GOR patients may have small hiatus hernias that are not seen on endoscopy. These patients may have mucosal changes in the distal third of the oesophagus, such as oesophagitis or Barrett's oesophagus. Barrett's oesophagus is a premalignant condition known to be caused by GOR,[17] so the swallow is used to view the region closely and observe the fundus to check for herniation.

Patient preparation

Patient preparation and contraindications are as for the upper swallow.

Contrast agent and pharmaceutical aids

- 250% w/v barium sulphate suspension
- An effervescent agent will be required, e.g. a combination of sodium bicarbonate and citric acid, to produce carbon dioxide to distend the stomach. This will also act as double contrast against the barium, to enhance visualisation of the mucosa[15]

Additional equipment

- Disposable cup
- Small cup for effervescent agent
- Tissues
- A straw may be required for ingestion of barium sulphate when the table is horizontal (if needed)

Technique

(Ensure that you have understood the notes on fluoroscopic examination positioning descriptors earlier in this chapter before considering technique descriptors.)

- AP and lateral projections can be taken of the hypopharynx and upper oesophagus as previously described for the barium swallow
- A more useful view of the mid and distal thirds of the oesophagus is provided by the erect left posterior oblique, taken after the patient is asked to swallow. In this position the oesophagus does not lie over the thoracic spine and the gastro-oesophageal junction (GOJ) is opened out, thereby ensuring clearer visualisation. The barium bolus is imaged as a column and spot films are taken to show the distal third of the oesophagus. This allows mucosal rings and peptic strictures to be shown well.[16] As the column passes and the mucosa relaxes, spot films can be taken; this may show oesophagitis
- The patient is then asked to take the effervescent granules (either dry or mixed with a small amount of water if dry is too difficult) or other effervescent aid, followed by the citric acid. It is important to impress on the patient that these will produce gas in the stomach and may give them the feeling that they need to belch; it is imperative they do not succumb to temptation, and the best way to avoid this is to tell them to keep swallowing. Advance explanation of this, giving reasons for its importance, will maximise compliance
- The patient is then asked to swallow another mouthful of barium while in the LPO position (Fig. 29.5) and images can be taken of the lower oesophagus (either spot image recording or 1 frame per second is likely to be adequate). This will give a double-contrast examination of the oesophagus, allowing a good view of mucosal detail

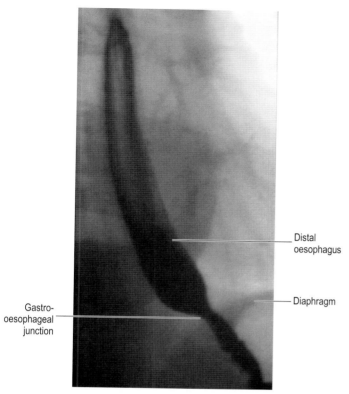

Figure 29.5 Distal oesophagus and gastro-oesophageal junction (GOJ) (LPO).

Labels on figure: Distal oesophagus; Diaphragm; Gastro-oesophageal junction

- To detect signs of a hiatus hernia (if one has not been noted so far) or GOR, the fluoroscopic couch is then placed horizontally and the patient turned to their right to assess reflux. Spot images of the area are taken
- A prone swallow may also be undertaken at this point. The patient lies either completely prone with their head turned to one side or in the RAO position, which throws their oesophagus away from their spine. The patient then drinks some barium through a straw and the barium bolus is screened as it travels along the oesophagus. Spot films are also taken. This view maximises oesophageal distension and can also produce well-coated double-contrast views of the oesophagus and gastro-oesophageal junction. It is a particularly good view to demonstrate oesophageal varices. A prone swallow must *never* be attempted if aspiration or laryngeal penetration is evident when erect
- The patient is then asked to rotate through 360° at their own pace; this will ensure that all aspects of the gastric mucosa are coated ready for assessment of the stomach. Ideally the patient turns to the left: this helps to prevent the barium from spilling into the duodenum before the stomach is coated and obscured by barium-filled small bowel. While they are performing this movement it is best to screen periodically in case any additional lower oesophageal pathology is noted so that a spot image of the lower oesophagus and GOJ can be taken. On completing this manoeuvre, further images of the stomach are taken at key stages:
  1. the patient is asked to turn to their left (LPO) where a spot image is taken of the antrum
  2. turned back to supine (AP) (stomach body and greater curve)
  3. turned to their right (RPO) (body and lesser curve)
  4. turned completely to the right (right lateral) to image the fundus
  5. the patient is returned to the erect position, turned slightly to their left and an erect (LPO) film is taken to show the distal oesophagus and the fundus of the stomach
- To show reflux actually occurring, the patient can be tilted head downwards (Trendelenburg position) as this mimics stress reflux, but as this is an artificial position it may have limited bearing on the accuracy estimation of the true extent of reflux. The patient can also be asked to cough while turning on to their right side, again to mimic reflux
- If reflux is demonstrated the freedom with which it occurs and the level it attains should be noted (e.g. free reflux to the cervical region), as this will be an aid to the clinician in the assessment of the patient. It is noted, however, that reflux may only occur in about a third of symptomatic patients[5]

Barium meal

This examination is performed to show the stomach and duodenum. It is becoming less frequently requested owing to the increase in the use of endoscopy as the front-line examination, and is recommended for use in a very limited number of circumstances. These include: if endoscopy proves negative and symptoms persist; after (healed) surgery to assess afferent loop, narrowed anastamoses, and closed loops or internal hernias,[18] or to assess complications after bariatric surgery.[19] It therefore can be seen that the barium meal can still be useful for those patients who are not considered fit for, or refuse, OGD.

Patient preparation

Patient preparation is as for all upper tract examinations.

Contraindications

- Complete large bowel obstruction[14]

Contrast agents and pharmaceutical aids for the examination

- Barium sulphate suspension 250% w/v
- Effervescent granules and citric acid, or other gas-producing agent
- An antispasmodic agent such as hyoscine-*N*-butyl bromide (Buscopan) may be used intravenously. These help to reduce peristalsis in the stomach and prevent rapid progress of the barium into the small bowel[14]

Additional equipment

- Disposable cup
- Small cup for effervescent agent
- Tissues
- A straw may be required for ingestion of barium sulphate when the table is horizontal (if needed)

Technique

(Ensure that you have understood the notes on fluoroscopic examination positioning descriptors earlier in this chapter before considering technique descriptors.)

If required, the patient may given the antispasmodic agent immediately prior to commencing the examination, although some practitioners prefer to give the antispasmodic during the examination when the barium is just beginning to leave the pylorus. Administration of an antispasmodic should not give false results during the reflux check.

- The patient is asked to stand on the step of the fluoroscopic couch and then the procedure for ingesting the gas-producing agent is explained. The importance of keeping the gas in the stomach is emphasised, and an explanation of a strategy to prevent belching (dry swallowing) is given
- The patient is given the effervescent agent (dry, or mixed with a small amount of water if this is more tolerable for the patient); they are then asked to drink the citric acid, to produce carbon dioxide and distend the stomach
- The patient is turned slightly to their left and asked to swallow a mouthful of the barium; the barium column is screened and spot images are taken of the distal oesophagus with single and double contrast
- After three or four reasonable mouthfuls of barium have been ingested, the table is tilted horizontally and the patient asked to rotate (at least once) through 360° to enable the barium to coat the stomach mucosa. A prone swallow may also be undertaken at this point. Periodic screening during this movement allows for images to be taken if the radiographer feels it is necessary, especially if a small hiatus hernia or GOR are noted. This also enables the operator to note which positions show the anatomy most effectively, in preparation for other spot images. Quite often the most difficult region to image well can be the duodenal cap, owing to the peristaltic action of the small bowel (which can occur even after administration of intravenous muscle relaxant); therefore, if the duodenal cap is well visualised during the patient's initial movements, there may be an opportunity to obtain the spot images required
- Once the patient has completed their rotation and good mucosal coating and distension of the stomach have been noted, it is possible to obtain the spot images. If coating is poor, give the patient more barium or ask them to perform another 360° rotation; if distension is inadequate then repeat the dose of effervescent agent. Because this is a dynamic investigation it is best to take the spot images as quickly as possible, and if the chance arises and an area is well shown while moving the patient, take the opportunity
- The following positions are a general guideline to how best to show the anatomy of the stomach and duodenum in double contrast:
  1. the patient with their right side raised (LPO) demonstrates the antrum and the greater curve (Fig. 29.6)
  2. if the patient is supine this demonstrates the antrum and the body of the stomach and also the lesser curve (Fig. 29.7A,B)
  3. turning the patient into the RPO position demonstrates the lesser curve en face (Fig. 29.8)
  4. moving the patient into the right lateral position with head tilted up shows the fundus (Fig. 29.9A,B)
- A combination of the following positions will help to best demonstrate the duodenal loop and duodenal cap. It may be necessary to use magnification at this point to optimise the view:
  1. LPO (Fig. 29.10)
  2. supine
  3. RPO, centred on and collimated to the duodenal loop
  4. prone
- The patient can then be tilted erect and turned slightly to the left to show the fundus (Fig. 29.11). If visualisation of the duodenal cap has been poor during the earlier (table horizontal) stages of the examination, turning the patient in both directions (while they are standing) may provide better views of the duodenal cap

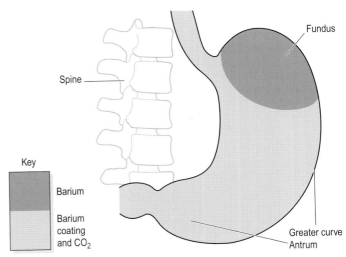

Figure 29.6 LPO position for antrum and greater curve. The stomach is turned to the left: the barium drops into the fundus and obscures it; CO_2 rises into the body and antrum to act as double contrast for good visualisation of these areas. The greater curve is also visualised.

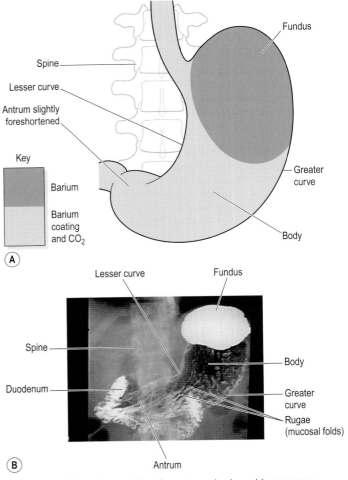

Figure 29.7 (A) Supine position for antrum, body and lesser curve – barium pools in the lowest point, which in the supine position is the fundus, allowing CO_2 to rise into the body and antrum which are coated with barium; (B) supine stomach.

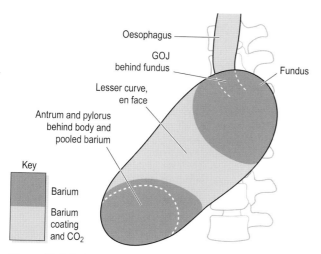

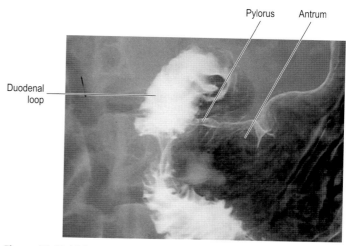

Figure 29.8 RPO position to show lesser curve en face. Obliquity moves the lesser curve to turn it from profile to an en face position; it is seen through the CO_2-filled body. Barium will pool in the fundus and antrum as these are the lowest points of the stomach in this position.

Figure 29.10 LPO – antrum and duodenal loop.

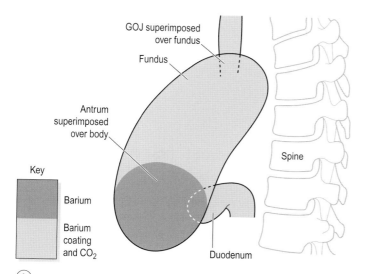

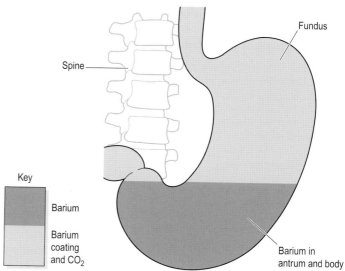

Figure 29.11 Erect (slight LPO) position to show fundus. Barium sits in the antrum and body; CO_2 rises into the fundus.

Aftercare

- A damp tissue should be provided for the patient to clean their mouth
- The patient should be informed that their stools will be paler or white for a few days, and to keep their fluid intake up to reduce any chance of constipation. Encourage a high-fibre diet for several days
- Ensure that the patient knows how to obtain their results
- If a muscle relaxant is used, the patient must remain in the department until any blurring of their vision has passed

Possible complications

- Leakage of barium from an unsuspected perforation
- Constipation
- Partial bowel obstruction becoming complete obstruction due to barium impaction[14]

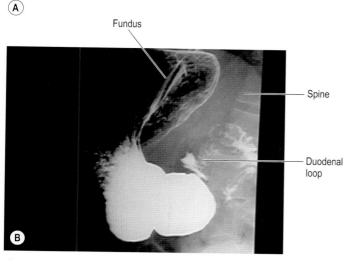

Figure 29.9 (A) Right lateral position, head tilted up, to show fundus – barium pools in the antrum as it is now the lowest positioned part of the stomach and CO_2 rises to the fundus; (B) right lateral, head tilted up.

- Aspiration of barium: as previously mentioned, each patient must be carefully questioned before the procedure to ensure the examination is tailored for that individual. If a patient coughs during or shortly after meals, or has a recent history of chest infections, then aspiration must be considered a risk. Some patients are at a higher risk of aspiration than others. These include patients who have had a previous cerebral vascular accident, Parkinson's disease, multiple sclerosis, motor neurone disease, dementia, Huntington's chorea, previous head injury, other progressive or acquired neurological disorders, acute exacerbation of chronic obstructive pulmonary disease (COPD), history of recurrent chest infections, history of head or neck carcinoma with associated surgery or radiotherapy, or recently extubated patients

If mild aspiration occurs during an examination, encourage the patient to cough and expectorate the barium. No more barium should be given, but the examination may be continued if appropriate and safe to do so. If severe aspiration occurs then the examination must be terminated and the patient referred for physiotherapy. The patient should not leave the radiology department until a physiotherapist has assessed their condition. A referral to the speech and language therapy department for a future appointment may also be appropriate.

Supplementary techniques

For patients with dysphagia it may be necessary to undertake the swallowing section of the examination using an imitation 'food bolus', as liquid may show no abnormality. Common examples of imitation food bolus are marshmallow coated in barium or pieces of fresh bread coated in barium. If a patient is unable to ingest the barium rapidly the relaxing effect of adding ice to the barium could be used.[16]

Videofluoroscopy

This is usually undertaken in conjunction with speech therapists. Its aim is to assess patients who have swallowing dysfunction due to mechanical or neuromuscular problems, with the result that they are at increased risk of aspiration and inevitable associated chest problems.

Images may be recorded on video, but digital exposure recording at several frames per second (e.g. 4–6) is now very valuable. Recording of the fluoroscopy image acquired with at least 3 pulses a second is also a way of reducing patient radiation dose while collecting image data. Fluoroscopic recording of the swallow at up to 30 frames per second can be valuable, but this may use up the entire memory of the screening unit for just one patient, whilst increasing the radiation dose to the patient. This therefore may not be a workable option.[20]

Criteria for referral for videofluoroscopy include:

- When silent aspiration is suspected but not clearly confirmed on bedside assessment
- When the degree of aspiration as a result of ingestion of different food consistencies needs clarification
- When the degree of dysphagia appears mild but the patient suffers from recurrent chest infections
- When long-term non-oral feeding, e.g. percutaneous endoscopic gastrostomy, is being considered
- When postural or procedural swallowing techniques will benefit the patient

Most referrals are for patients who have suffered:

- cerebrovascular accident
- motor neuron disease
- multiple sclerosis
- Parkinson's disease
- previous head or neck surgery, e.g. partial laryngectomy

The technique requires the patient to swallow small amounts of liquid, semi-solids and solids in order to ascertain their safety in eating and drinking after discharge from hospital. The patient is screened in the lateral pharynx position as they swallow the various consistencies, and the process is recorded on video, PACS (picture archiving and communication system) or CD to allow close examination of the process. Occasionally an AP pharynx view is taken, for example, to define asymmetries of pharyngeal residue and which side is affected.[21] As well as demonstrating aspiration at different consistencies, videofluoroscopy also allows coping strategies to be tried; for example, using a chin tuck on swallowing, or turning the head to one side, may prevent aspiration. The aim of the process is to decide on the best strategy compatible with nutrition, to help the patient cope with their problem.

SMALL BOWEL

The small bowel (from the duodenojejunal flexure to the ileocaecal valve) can be examined by one of two methods: the barium follow-through (BaFT) or the small bowel enema. The aim is to produce a continuous column of barium suspension outlining the small bowel.[3]

Referral criteria

- Anaemia
- Diarrhoea
- Persistent pain
- Crohn's disease
- Meckel's diverticulum

Barium follow-through (BaFT)

During this examination the patient has to drink a volume of barium sulphate suspension, and images (fluoroscopy and/or permanent image recording) are taken as the small bowel fills. The examination frequently takes 2 hours, and in some instances can take most of the day.[22]

Contraindications

- Suspected perforation
- Complete obstruction

Patient preparation

Patient preparation is usually the same for both follow-through and small bowel enema, and imaging department protocols do vary. Generally the patient is not allowed to eat or drink for 5–6 hours prior to the examination. Some centres may give the patient a mild laxative and/or a clear fluid diet the day before the examination.

Contrast agent

- At least 300 mL 100% w/v barium sulphate suspension is required for an adult BaFT.[14] The constituents of the drink are:
  1. Barium sulphate suspension
  2. Effervescent agent (may be carbonated barium sulphate suspension)
  3. Water
  4. Accelerator, e.g. Gastrografin or metoclopramide hydrochloride (Maxalon)

Additional equipment

- Disposable cup
- Small cup for effervescent agent
- Tissues

Technique

- The patient is asked to drink the barium sulphate suspension steadily. Drinking too quickly can cause nausea; drinking too slowly causes the barium sulphate suspension to flocculate and the small bowel does not distend adequately to obtain diagnostic images
- The imaging technique used depends on the equipment available, the preference of the practitioner or local imaging department protocol. The actual timing of imaging depends on each individual patient and the motility speed of the bowel. Transit of barium through the proximal bowel (jejunum) is usually rapid, whereas transit through the distal bowel (ileum) is often less rapid[22]
- A series of over-couch abdominal radiographs (see Chapter 31 (Fig. 31.9A) for prone positioning) may be taken at predetermined time intervals, e.g. every 30 minutes, or alternatively each image is individually assessed in order to determine the timing of the subsequent image. The radiographs are often taken prone, as the pressure on the abdomen helps to separate the bowel loops.[14] The first image is usually taken 15–20 minutes after drinking commenced. When the barium has been seen to reach the terminal ileum, fluoroscopy is used to image the ileocaecal area, although over-couch images can be taken if necessary (Fig. 29.12)

  The terminal ileum will be shown on a prone image of the abdomen. The patient lies prone and a radiolucent pad is placed in their right iliac fossa; for the pad to be inserted correctly the patient must lie on their left side and the pad placed and held firmly in the right iliac fossa. The patient then rolls prone to prevent small bowel falling back against the caecum and obscuring the terminal ileum. Prone positioning then follows as for the prone abdomen/KUB (kidneys, ureters, bladder) as described in Chapter 31, with collimation to include the whole of the small bowel.

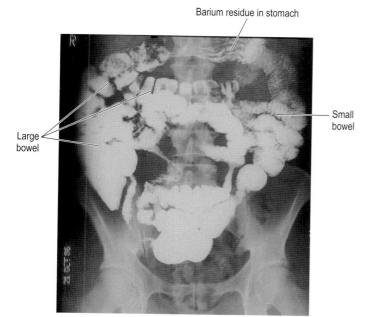

Barium residue in stomach

Large bowel

Small bowel

Figure 29.12 Prone abdomen – BaFT.

Alternatively, fluoroscopy may be used to image the small bowel at the necessary intervals. With fluoroscopy the proximal jejunum is often imaged supine or in the RPO position. All the other loops are usually imaged supine until the terminal ileum is reached.

- Regardless of imaging modality, all bowel loops should be palpated (using lead rubber gloves with hands outside the primary beam) or the abdominal wall compressed with a radiolucent pad during imaging. Barium does not move into areas of adhesions, which are difficult to spot anyway, as they are often subtle and can be obscured by overlapped loops of barium-filled bowel
- Fluoroscopy of the terminal ileum frequently requires an LPO position, but sometimes RPO or prone positions are more satisfactory
- An erect abdominal view may be required to show fluid levels, usually required when jejunal diverticulosis is present.[3] This is usually imaged with fluoroscopy, but an over-couch image may be taken

Complications

- Constipation
- Abdominal pain
- Transient diarrhoea (due to a large volume of fluid)

Patient aftercare

- Ask the patient to increase their fluid intake over the next 48 hours to prevent constipation
- Warn the patient about white stools

There are certain criteria and common errors that relate to all small bowel barium studies – see below.

Criteria for assessing image quality

- All barium-filled loops of bowel (area of interest) are included on the film
- Sharp image clearly demonstrating valvulae conniventes
- Adequate penetration to demonstrate detail in the contrast-filled bowel

Common errors – BaFT	Possible reasons and strategies to overcome these
Image is pale and valvulae conniventes are not demonstrated	Image is under-penetrated. Increase the kVp. A high kVp technique increases the range of densities visualised (as well as reducing exposure time and radiation dose)[15]
Slow barium transit of the proximal bowel	Ask the patient to lie in the right lateral decubitus position to promote gastric emptying[22]
Slow barium transit of the distal bowel	Give the patient a hot drink. If the patient has been in the department for a long time, a small snack can be given to try to encourage small bowel movement[14]
Overlying loops of bowel	If the overlying loops of bowel are deep within the pelvis ask the patient to avoid micturition, as a full bladder may push up and separate the loops of bowel. If the bladder is already full and the bowel loops are overlapping, ask the patient to empty their bladder. Alternatively, the patient can lie prone over a radiolucent pad to displace the loops[14]

Small bowel enema (Fig. 29.13A,B)

During a small bowel enema the duodenum is intubated and a contrast agent introduced. This is arguably the ideal method for imaging the small bowel as it results in improved visualisation of the bowel loops.[14,15] This is because the infusion of contrast agent avoids segmentation of the barium column and the small bowel is unobstructed by the overlying barium-filled stomach and duodenum. This method also avoids pyloric control over the rate of transit.[22] However, it is invasive for the patient and time-consuming, and can be technically difficult for the operator.

The small bowel enema may also be used after a BaFT to localise a lesion or examine a particular section of small bowel.[14]

Contraindications

- Facial surgery or trauma
- The patient is prone to nose bleeds
- Active Crohn's disease (especially of the duodenum)
- Severe gastro-oesophageal reflux/hiatus hernia
- Suspected perforation
- Complete obstruction

Patient preparation

- As for BaFT
- The procedure must be carefully explained, as it is often difficult for the patient to tolerate[14]

Contrast agent

For single contrast, typically 1000 mL of fluid is used.[15] The mixture comprises barium sulphate suspension and water; the ratio of barium sulphate to water tends to vary according to the preferences of the examining radiographer or radiologist. For double-contrast examination 150–200 mL barium sulphate suspension is followed by up to 2 L methylcellulose 0.5%.[15]

Additional equipment

- Nasogastric or duodenal catheter
- Lubricating jelly for the tube
- Anaesthetic spray
- Tissues
- Sterile gloves
- Swabs to wipe the tube after removal

Technique

- The patient lies supine and, under fluoroscopic control, the duodenal or nasogastric catheter is inserted until the tip of the catheter is shown in the duodenojejunal flexure. The anaesthetic spray may be used to numb the throat, but this prevents the examination continuing by follow-through if the intubation is unsuccessful
- The guidewire within the catheter acts as a stiffener to prevent coiling and enables manipulation into the correct position
- The barium solution is infused by gravity or by an enteroclysis pump
- Imaging is usually by fluoroscopy, but spot films can be taken as well. The terminal ileum may need prone imaging as for BaFT
- For a double contrast study methylcellulose solution is infused after the barium sulphate suspension until the terminal ileum is demonstrated in double contrast
- During a single-contrast examination air may be introduced at the end of the examination to demonstrate the terminal ileum in double contrast. Air may be introduced via the duodenal catheter or by a rectal catheter
- All the loops of bowel are usually imaged supine until the terminal ileum is reached and oblique views may be needed

Potential complications and post-procedure care

- As for BaFT

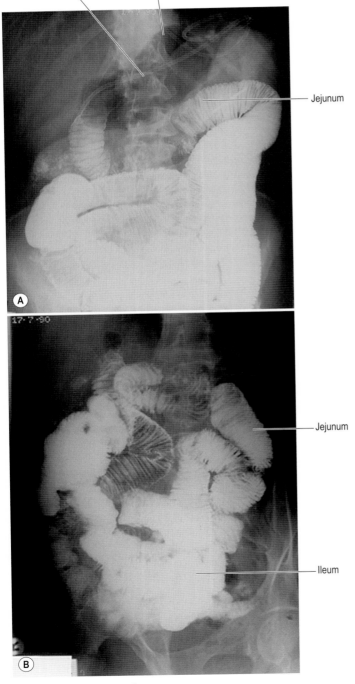

Figure 29.13 Small bowel enema.

Lower GI tract

LARGE BOWEL

The large bowel comprises the colon, rectum and caecum and is usually examined by the double-contrast barium enema. At the point of publication (2012) CT colonoscopy is rapidly overtaking the barium enema as a mainstream examination.

Referral criteria

- Change in bowel habit
- Iron deficiency anaemia
- Rectal bleeding
- Tenesmus
- Left iliac fossa pain
- Palpable mass
- Documented cancer on endoscopy: to exclude synchronous lesions

Double-contrast barium enema (DCBE)

The aim of this examination is to image the entire large bowel in double contrast, using gas (CO_2 or air) to distend the bowel, to facilitate a fine coating of barium on the bowel mucosa and to act in extreme contrast with the dense barium.

Contraindications

- Biopsy via rigid sigmoidoscope within 7 days[14]
- Incomplete optical colonoscopy[23]
- Toxic megacolon
- Incomplete bowel preparation
- Suspected perforation
- Obstruction

Patient preparation

- There are various preparations available but the most commonly used method is to instruct the patient to follow a low-residue diet and take laxatives 48 and/or 24 hours before the examination. However, cleansing enemas can be given and some centres also restrict fluids for 4–6 hours prior to the examination. Fluid restriction exacerbates the dehydrating effects of the laxative, which is potentially dangerous for all patients. In certain cases laxative use is contraindicated (ileostomy, currently clinically active inflammatory bowel disease) or should be used with caution, as in patients with a colostomy
- Elbow pads may be provided immediately prior to the examination to reduce the risk of skin damage in the frail or elderly

Contrast agents

- Barium sulphate suspension. Warm water is added to the barium sulphate powder/liquid to ensure a high-density low-viscosity suspension. The powder is usually supplied in an enema bag
- Air or carbon dioxide

Additional equipment/pharmaceuticals

- Funnel to fill enema bag with water or barium sulphate suspension
- Additional clamp (although rare, clamps supplied on enema bags may fail)
- Rectal catheter with additional gas insufflation line
- Drip stand for barium bag
- Air or CO_2 insufflation device
- Lubricating jelly
- Gauze swabs for application of lubricant to catheter
- Wide adhesive tape to help maintain position of catheter
- Latex or vinyl gloves
- Muscle relaxant, needle and syringe

Technique

(Ensure that you have understood the notes on fluoroscopic examination positioning descriptors earlier in this chapter before considering technique descriptors.)

As the aim of the examination is to provide clear images of the whole bowel, the natural variations in bowel orientation will necessitate the selection of a method of barium coating and patient positioning which varies. Selection of the most suitable technique may rest solely upon the individual but may also be based on variations around an agreed protocol. The routine presented here is one option only:

- The patient lies on their left side with their knees and hips flexed and a lubricated catheter is inserted into the rectum. The catheter is then taped in place. A hypotonic agent (also known as a smooth muscle relaxant), e.g. Buscopan or glucagon, is frequently given at this point to reduce bowel spasm. Contraindications for buscopan include cardiovascular disease and glaucoma, so glucagon may be given instead[24]
- The bag or bottle of barium sulphate suspension is suspended on the drip stand about 1 m higher than the patient. The patient remains on their left side and the table is tilted slightly (with the patient's head down); the clamp on the barium sulphate suspension is released and the fluid is slowly run into the colon
- The first phase of the study is to introduce enough barium and air to coat the bowel mucosa. Introduction of too much barium increases the likelihood of barium reaching the caecum and refluxing into the terminal ileum, where it will obscure sigmoid loops before spot images of the sigmoid can be recorded. Not enough barium will mean that the entire length of the colon will not be coated. Under fluoroscopic assessment the flow of the barium is monitored
- When the barium sulphate suspension reaches the splenic flexure the patient turns prone until the barium sulphate suspension has filled half of the transverse colon. At this point the patient turns back onto their left side and the bag/bottle of barium sulphate suspension is placed on the floor to enable excess fluid to drain back out of the patient
- Air or carbon dioxide is then gently insufflated into the rectum and the imaging sequence begins. The gas is insufflated throughout the examination as required to ensure double contrast throughout; as CO_2 is absorbed by the colon, it is more likely to require additional insufflation than air
- It can be difficult to move barium and air around the bowel, and some strategies are available to achieve this:
  1. Tipping the patient head down (supine position) clears barium from the caecum

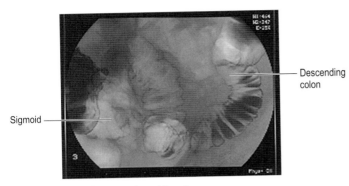

Sigmoid

Descending colon

Figure 29.14 LPO – rectosigmoid region.

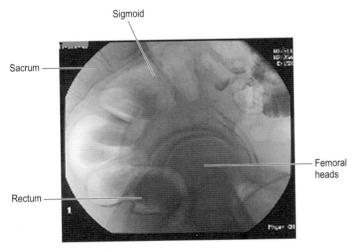

Sigmoid

Sacrum

Femoral heads

Rectum

Figure 29.15 Lateral rectum.

2. Lying the patient on their left side, turning them to prone then back to the left side also clears the caecum. However, if the ascending colon is long and the caecum lies in the midline or left of the midline it may be necessary to turn the patient from supine to lie on their right side and then back to supine

3. Turning the patient 360° to coat the mucosa effectively. This will only work if enough barium is in the region of interest, and may require additional barium to be run into the region, or rotation of the patient to bring barium to the area

• Once the bowel is coated and adequately gas-filled, projections are taken and may include:

1. LPO of the rectum and sigmoid (Fig. 29.14)
2. RAO of the rectum and sigmoid (any areas obscured by barium sulphate suspension in the LPO view should now be outlined with air)
3. Prone rectum
4. Lateral rectum (Fig. 29.15)
5. RPO descending colon
6. Supine and erect (Fig. 29.16A,B) transverse colon
7. Erect RPO splenic flexure (Fig. 29.17)
8. Erect LPO hepatic flexure (Fig. 29.18)
9. LPO ascending colon and caecum
10. Slight RPO and supine caecum with palpation. The table may be tilted slightly head-down for these views
11. Left lateral decubitus (positioned with left side down and right side raised). This view demonstrates the medial wall of the rectum, sigmoid, descending colon; the superior and inferior wall of the transverse colon; the lateral wall of the caecum, ascending colon and hepatic flexure

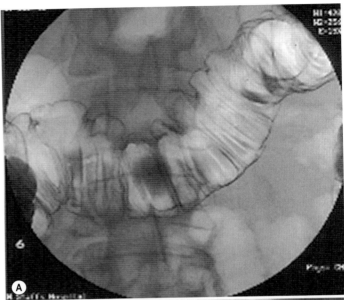

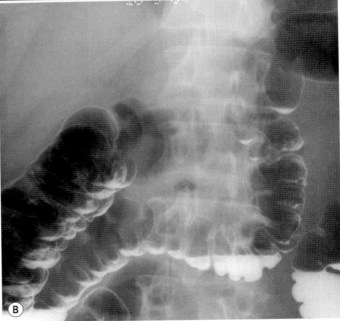

Figure 29.16 (A) Supine transverse colon; (B) erect transverse colon.

12. Right lateral decubitus (right side down). This view demonstrates the lateral wall of the rectum, sigmoid and descending colon; the superior and inferior walls of the transverse colon; the medial wall of the caecum and ascending colon
13. When the rectum is included on lateral decubitus views it is not always possible to include the splenic flexure. It is preferred that the rectum be included in preference to the splenic flexure, which should have been included on spot images
14. For additional information on the distal descending colon and sigmoid, use the prone 30–35° projection (described later in this section and shown in Figures 29.21 and 29.22)
15. The examination is not complete until the appendix and ileocaecal junction are adequately demonstrated.

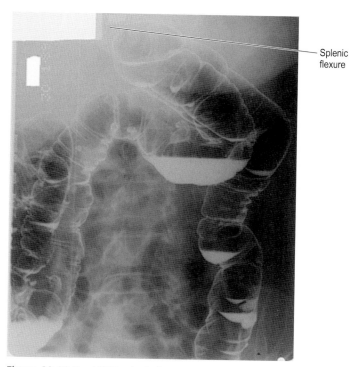

Figure 29.17 Erect RPO splenic flexure.

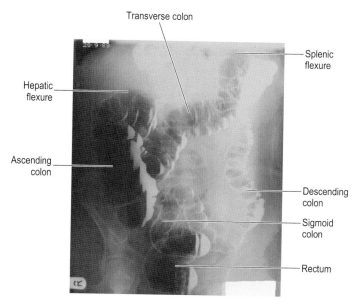

Figure 29.19 Left lateral decubitus.

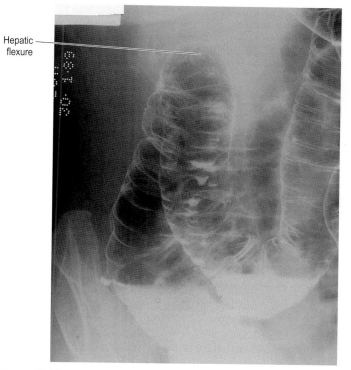

Figure 29.18 Erect LPO hepatic flexure.

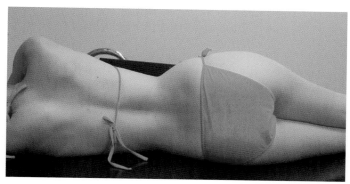

Figure 29.20 Left lateral decubitus (positioning).

Lateral decubitus abdomen (Fig. 29.19, 29.20)

The lateral decubitus projection is most frequently used as part of the barium enema examination but is also useful to demonstrate free extraperitoneal air in acute cases when the patient cannot sit erect. The patient is examined on both sides as for barium enema, the projection affording demonstration of lateral aspects of the large bowel mucosa. The raised side ensures that air rises above the barium, showing mucosal detail.

Unfortunately, some confusion can arise when describing the decubitus projections: the right side raised will demonstrate the right side of the bowel, and because of this it is often incorrectly referred to as a 'right lateral decubitus'. As the patient is lying on their left side for this the correct term is actually 'left lateral decubitus', and vice versa for the left side raised position, which is the 'right lateral decubitus'.

An IR with grid is placed vertically at the side of the patient, its longitudinal axis parallel to the coronal plane of the patient.

Positioning

- The patient lies on the table-top on a thick radiolucent pad and turns to a lateral position with their back to the radiographer, with the right or left side raised. The arms are raised onto a pillow and the knees flexed to aid stability
- The tube side of the IR will now be in contact with the patient's abdomen and its long axis coincident with the median sagittal plane (MSP). The MSP is perpendicular to the IR
- A PA anatomical marker is applied within the primary beam

The radiolucent pad will bring the spine into a position where it is more likely to be coincident with the midline of the IR. Difficulties do arise when trying to insert the pad under the patient, in addition to asking the patient to lie on their side. The concept is somewhat alien to patients and the complications of catheter retention and barium/air retention only compromise cooperation. Instructions should be given clearly, and also step by step, only moving to the next instruction once an action has been successfully completed. It is vital that the catheter remains in place during positioning, as last-minute reinsufflation may be required to ensure optimum image quality.

Beam direction and focus receptor distance (FRD)

Horizontal, 90° to the IR
100–120 cm FRD

Centring

Over the fourth lumbar vertebra, in the midline at the level of the iliac crests

Collimation

Symphysis pubis, as much upper abdomen as possible, lateral soft tissue or bowel outlines

Note that no AP positioning has been described above. Although it is common practice to undertake the lateral decubitus images for barium enema by turning the patient first AP and then PA (or vice versa), it is actually advantageous to position both in the PA position, by moving the patient's head to the opposite end of the table. The advantages of this are:

1. The large bowel is positioned relatively anteriorly in the peritoneal cavity and magnification of this is reduced on both projections to ensure maximum coverage of bowel area with the minimum number of exposures made to demonstrate the whole of the large bowel
2. As radiosensitive organs are generally positioned more anteriorly, the PA projection affords some dose reduction to these organs as the posterior tissue attenuates a proportion of beam energy
3. The abdominal tissue can be compressed gently against the IR, allowing a reduction in exposure factors in the PA position and reduction of scatter

Unfortunately, the suggested procedure is somewhat difficult for the patient with rectal catheterisation, especially as the typical barium enema patient is over 45 years old, but careful consideration for assistance and instruction may result in success.

> Expose on arrested respiration, but careful consideration for assistance and instruction may result in success

Variation in abdominal tissue thickness over the area of interest ('belly sag')

Adipose tissue in the abdomen has a tendency to sag towards the table-top, creating a variation in tissue thickness which is thicker on the side nearer to the table-top and thinner on the raised side. Undertaking both projections in the PA position is likely to partially address this by compressing the tissue against the IR.

Other methods to compensation for this variation in density include the use of a high kVp to reduce the range of densities on the image, or the application of a wedge filter over the light beam diaphragm (LBD).[15] However, as the recommended kVp for fluoroscopic examination using barium is a minimum of 100, it is likely that kVp in use will already be relatively high. The wedge filter is positioned coincident with the raised side of the patient, the tapering edge pointing towards the table-top. It is tempting to position the top of the wedge level with the superior edge of the LBD, but this will often place the useful wedge thickness above the bowel. For this reason the radiographer should ensure the thickest part of the wedge lies level with the thinnest part of the patient; in practice this often means that the wedge appears to be in a relatively low position on the LBD housing.

AP lateral decubitus

If AP positioning is required the MSP is still positioned as perpendicular to the IR and centring is as for the AP abdomen, using a horizontal beam and AP marker. The centring point is in the midline, level with the iliac crests. The beam is horizontal and at 100–120 cm FRD.

Criteria for assessing image quality: all lateral decubitus positions

- Rectum, descending colon, splenic and hepatic flexures, ascending colon and caecum are included on the image
- Spinous processes of vertebrae are seen coincident with the midline of the image and centralised and aligned down the middle of the vertebral bodies
- Sharp image demonstrating air in the bowel and in contrast with barium-coated mucosa

Common errors (lateral decubitus)	Possible reasons
Region/s of bowel omitted from field	Large patient, patient possibly not positioned in contact with IR, or AP rather than PA position has been used; may need additional examination of missed area, or undertake in PA position. If a radiolucent pad is not used under the patient, the lateral portion of the bowel on the lowered side is also likely to be omitted from the field
Over-penetrated/ overexposed, air-filled area on raised side, possibly under-penetrated/ underexposed on area nearest table-top	Wedge filter not used, or not used correctly (see paragraphs relating to varied tissue thickness, above)
Grid 'cut-off'	Grid cut-off is caused if the IR is allowed to tilt from its vertical position

Prone 30–35° to demonstrate the sigmoid colon: Hampton's projection (Figs 29.21, 29.22)

In the case of the barium enema examination, if additional information on the *sigmoid colon* is required, the Hampton's projection may be used.

An IR with grid is used horizontally for this projection.

Positioning

- The patient is prone, head turned to the side and arms raised onto the pillow for stability and comfort
- The MSP is coincident with the long axis of the table
- For males, lead rubber or lead gonad protection is applied below the buttocks to protect the gonads
- ASIS (anterior superior iliac spines) are equidistant from the table-top

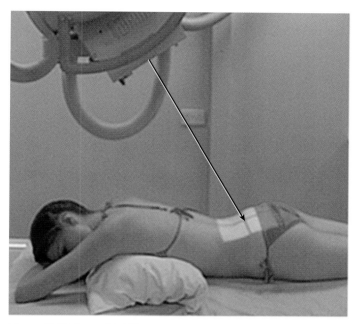

Figure 29.21 Prone 30–35°.

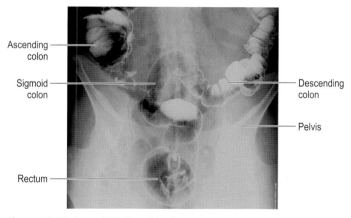

Ascending colon

Sigmoid colon

Rectum

Descending colon

Pelvis

Figure 29.22 Prone 35° sigmoid colon.

Beam direction and FRD

A vertical central ray is angled 30–35° caudally
100 cm FRD
The IR is displaced until its centre is coincident with the central ray.

Centring

Over a point in the midline, at the level of the first sacral segment

Collimation

Rectum, sigmoid colon. It has been noticed that this projection has sometimes been undertaken using the full field available on a large IR and irradiating the whole abdomen and even the upper femora. As the projection is specifically intended to demonstrate the sigmoid colon, rectum, rectosigmoid junction and distal descending colon, *only* these areas should be included in the field of radiation.

Expose on arrested respiration?

At the level of the sigmoid, the abdominal organs are less likely to be affected by diaphragmatic movement and exposure need not be made after expiration. In fact, it is likely that the image may not show movement unsharpness even if exposure was to be made during gentle respiration.

Criteria for assessing image quality

- Rectum and sigmoid colon are included on the image
- Spinous process of upper sacral segments seen coincident with the midline of the image and centralised and aligned down the middle of the sacrum
- Sigmoid colon is no longer superimposed upon itself in a craniocaudal direction, but 'opened out' along its length by the effect of caudal angulation
- Sharp image demonstrating air in the bowel and in contrast with barium-coated mucosa

The examination is not complete until the ileocaecal junction is adequately demonstrated.

Common error	Possible reason
Sigmoid not demonstrated centrally on the image	Inaccurate centring of beam or centring of IR to central ray

Patient aftercare

- Remove the catheter and escort the patient to the toilet
- Warn the patient about constipation; encourage a high-fibre diet and plenty of fluids over the next 48 hours
- Warn the patient about white stools
- Ensure the patient knows how to obtain results
- If a muscle relaxant has been used, warn of the possibility of blurred vision and ensure that the patient does not leave the department until any blurring of vision has resolved

Complications

- Constipation
- Impaction
- Obstruction
- Barium appendicitis

Modifications to the barium enema

- A water-soluble contrast agent may be used to demonstrate a recent bowel anastomosis or in cases of suspected bowel perforation
- Patients with an ileostomy or colostomy may require a barium examination to examine their proximal bowel. A soft Foley catheter is gently inserted into the stoma and the barium sulphate solution is slowly infused into the colon

CT colonography (CTC)

The DCBE was a long-standing first-choice radiographic investigation of the large bowel, but it has largely been superseded by CTC, which is minimally invasive and better tolerated by the majority of patients. Evidence has also established that CTC sensitivity to polyps >10 mm is between 91% and 100%[25] compared to DCBE, which has a variable detection rate of between 48%[26] and 81%.[27] It also has the advantage of being able to detect extracolonic lesions, particularly beneficial when the patient presents with vague symptoms relating to the large bowel.

Colorectal cancer is the third most common cancer in the UK, with 100 new cases being reported as diagnosed daily.[28] Early detection is essential to survival, and the 5-year survival rate has increased from 23% to 50% in the last 30 years. Although the extent to which CTC is used still varies across the National Health Service in the UK, it has become more widely available with improvements in both training and technology. CTC is better tolerated than DCBE and has therefore been used for elderly and immobile patients, but because pathology detection rates are superior for CTC, its use is rapidly increasing. Radiation dose for CTC is comparable to that for DCBE,[29,30] and if sinister colonic pathology is detected the patient does not need to undergo dual examination (DCBE and staging CT scan), thus a dose reduction is offered in such cases. It is also advantageous because patients with positive findings will not have to wait for a CT staging scan, thereby accelerating treatment times.

Indications

CTC is indicated for the same reasons as DCBE and, in addition:
- Incomplete optical colonoscopy[24]
- To evaluate the colon proximal to an obstruction
- If optical colonoscopy is contraindicated

Contraindications

- Risk of perforation
- Following colonic biopsy
- Inflammatory bowel disease

Note that contraindication to contrast media is *not* a contraindication to CTC, as CTC may be performed without contrast. If findings prove positive for the colon, ultrasound may be used to exclude liver metastases. Some centres perform non-contrast CTC and only administer contrast if CTC indicates sinister colonic pathology.

Patient preparation

Laxative use for bowel preparation prior to CTC has commonly been replaced by a technique know as 'faecal tagging'. This requires the patient to follow a low-residue diet 2 days prior to the examination and ingest oral contrast the day before (100 mL of Gastrografin in two separate doses of 50 mL, at 0800 and 1600 hours). The faeces and contrast agent combine and help differentiate faeces from lesions in the colon when imaging takes place. The technique is also useful if the patient has had an incomplete colonoscopy, particularly due to suboptimal bowel preparation, as the patient can return for CTC the following day without having to undergo rigorous bowel preparation again. It has become more widely used in any case, particularly as both radiologists and radiographers gain more experience in assessing the scan. Because the instruction to 'follow a low-residue diet' may not be meaningful to those without a good understanding of food-stuffs and fibre, it is sensible to offer patients examples of foods they may eat, and those to be avoided. 'Allowed' foods and drinks given as examples can include milk (up to half a pint per day), eggs, plain yoghurt, cheese, butter, margarine, tofu, white pasta and rice, grilled white fish, grilled chicken breast, breads made with white flour, mashed or boiled potato, clear soup (e.g. with no meat, vegetables, noodles or barley), Bovril, Oxo, clear fruit juice such as apple or grape, fruit squash, fizzy pop or water, tea, coffee, jelly without fruit, ice cream, sugar, honey, artificial sweetener, salt and pepper. Banned food examples can be given as fruit jams, chutneys, pickled onions, breads made with brown flour, brown rice and pasta, fruit, vegetables other than potatoes as given in the 'permitted' list, cereals, bran, beans, nuts,

lentils, beef, pork, lamb, salmon. It is important to emphasise that drinking plenty of fluids is advisable, as with any bowel preparation method.

Contrast agents

Gastrografin (see section on patient preparation, above); non-ionic water soluble contrast agent, e.g. Niopam 300 (Iopamidol 61.2% w/v). Some centres do not use intravenous contrast agent unless sinister pathology is noted during CTC.

Additional equipment

- Automatic CO_2 insufflator (preferable) *or* air or CO_2 hand insufflation device
- Rectal catheter to attach to CO_2 insufflator
- Lubricating jelly
- Gauze swabs for application of lubricant to tip of catheter
- Vinyl or nitrile gloves
- Antispasmodic agent (hyoscine butylbromide 20 mg/mL IV, e.g. Buscopan)
- 2 mL syringe and filter needle
- Intravenous cannula (Venflon) for administration of contrast medium and muscle relaxant
- 10 mL saline and 10 mL syringe (optional)

Preparation immediately prior to the examination

- All radio-opaque objects should be removed from the patient's chest, abdominal and pelvic region
- Check all equipment is readily available. Plug in the CO_2 insufflator and switch on. Open the valve to the insufflator using the spanner provided, ensuring that there is sufficient CO_2 in the cylinder (gauge on the insufflator) to commence the examination
- The rectal catheter is attached to the CO_2 insufflator in accordance with the manufacturer's instructions
- Informed consent should be obtained from the patient prior to the examination, therefore it is necessary to give a full and detailed account of the procedure so that the patient can make an informed decision to proceed. Their agreement to proceed should be documented

Technique

- The patient lies in the supine position on the CT scanner table
- An intravenous cannula (or 'Venflon') is inserted into a suitable vein; its position and stability can be checked using normal saline flush. An antispasmodic agent can then be administered if not contraindicated (see barium enema technique for contraindications to Buscopan), but glucagon is not recommended as an alternative[31]
- The patient then lies on their left side with their knees and hips flexed, and the lubricated catheter is introduced. CO_2 is then insufflated automatically at a pressure of 25 mmHg until 1.2 L have been administered. With the patient on their left side, gas is allowed to rise into the right colon. The patient is then turned into the supine position with their arms raised above their head (to reduce the possibility of artefact)
- The scanner table is then moved into position, ensuring that the start position is above the level of the patient's diaphragm. At this point it should be ensured that the height of the scanner table has been adjusted so that the longitudinal positioning beam is level with the midpoint of the abdominal tissue

- The tube from the contrast injector is now connected to the Venflon and secured. The injector syringe is positioned to allow for maximum movement of the scanner table. A 'scout' view (terminology will vary according to the scanner manufacturer) is then performed with the patient supine, from a level just above the patient's diaphragm to a level just below the symphysis pubis. The scout view should also be assessed at this point to assess adequate colonic distension. This is extremely important, as distension is essential to ensure adequate visualisation on the scan (for additional information see under problem solving – inadequate distension); but how is adequate distension defined? One piece of published research suggests that it should be assessed for all bowel segments, using a scale of 'no distension' (therefore totally inadequate) to the 'optimum' of 2 cm distension or more.[32] Using the scout view as a baseline, the scan is then planned from above the diaphragm to just below the symphysis pubis and the patient scanned craniocaudally, still lying supine. A scan start delay of 50 seconds is required from initiation of the contrast injection to ensure that the liver is imaged in the portovenous phase. This is necessary, particularly if sinister colonic pathology is encountered, for the exclusion of liver metastases and to exclude extracolonic pathology[33]
- Once the supine scan has been completed, the contrast injector can be disconnected and the patient turned into the prone position. The Venflon can be left in situ, but care must be taken that it is not compromised during repositioning. Patients can experience delayed reaction to contrast injections and it is important to maintain venous access for this reason, so that emergency or counteractive drugs can be administered without delay
- The patient is aligned again with a start position just above the level of the diaphragm, and terminating at a level just below the symphysis pubis. The scout view is performed and colonic distension assessed again. If the CO_2 insufflator should terminate (usually at 4.0 L CO_2) this should be restarted. A prone scan is then planned from above the diaphragm to just below the symphysis pubis and the patient is again scanned craniocaudally. The scan parameters should be adjusted to a lower dose (e.g. effective mAs of 50). Although this results in a slight reduction in image quality it is sufficient to confirm or exclude any pathology that may have been observed on the supine component of the examination
- The total dose length product for the examination should then be recorded
- Once both scans have been completed the CO_2 insufflation should be terminated immediately and the rectal catheter removed

Acquisition parameters

Supine: 120 kV
160 mAs (effective)
16 collimation × 0.75 mm
Prone: 120 kV
50 mAs (effective)
16 collimation × 0.75 mm

Image assessment: area of interest

Both supine and prone scans are checked to ensure the whole of the colon, rectum and beyond the anal verge have been imaged, and that the whole of the liver is included. It is particularly important to include all solid abdominal organs so that other abdominal pathology, including metastases, can be excluded.

Problem solving

- *Inadequate distension.* This must be assessed on the scout view, and if the colon and rectum are not adequately distended further insufflation must take place. The initiation of the scan should be delayed until distension is sufficient. If necessary, repeat the scout view. Although this involves a small radiation dose it is extremely important that the bowel is distended fully before starting the scan. Inadequate distension will affect the ability of the observer to detect colonic lesions, particularly small polyps, and will be insufficient if a 3D 'fly-through' is required.
- *Patient movement artefact.* Motion artefact is generally encountered during the examination if the patient is unable to hold their breath for the duration of the scan (although patient movement may be encountered, especially if the patient is agitated or restless). Scan times vary, but can be between 25 and 30 seconds (although at the time of writing technological advances are reducing times considerably), which can be a particular problem for the elderly and those with existing chest conditions, e.g. COPD, asthma or pneumoconiosis. Ideally, if the patient can hold their breath for the first 15 seconds of the scan time this will enable the majority of the solid abdominal organs to be adequately visualised. It is preferable to scan the patient craniocaudally so that the abdominal section is scanned first; it is this region that is most affected by motion artefact due to respiration, and therefore it is important that it is captured sooner rather than later. In the pelvis, motion artefact due to inadequate arrested respiration is less of an issue as pelvic organs are less likely to move during respiration. It is therefore important to stress the need for the patient to remain relatively still and to hold their breath when instructed to do so, for the duration of the scan if possible.
- *Other artefacts.* Metal objects can cause streaking artefact and this can result in degradation of the resulting images.[34] It is important to ensure that patients are prepared for the examination by removing any metal objects from the area to be scanned. If the patient is unable to raise their arms above their head (see section on positioning) then all metal objects should be removed from this region. It may be that some metal objects cannot be removed, e.g. hip replacements. Streak artefact from this source is difficult to avoid, and although techniques such as gantry angulation and thinner acquisition sections can be used in some types of CT examination, this is not a recommendation for CTC.

Patient aftercare

The patient should remain in the department for at least 15 minutes after contrast agent injection to ensure that no delayed adverse events occur, and during this time the Venflon should be left in situ. The images should be reviewed by a suitably qualified radiographer or a radiologist prior to the patient leaving the department.

Complications

With CTC there is a small risk of colonic perforation, and this should be excluded before the patient leaves the department: the CT scan is reviewed to ensure that there is no free air in the abdomen and, as the patient should remain in the department for 15–20 minutes after a contrast agent injection, they can be assessed periodically for signs and symptoms of perforation; these signs and symptoms include severe abdominal pain, nausea and, in extreme cases, fever and vomiting.

The patient may also experience mild symptoms of abdominal cramping after colonic insufflation; if this occurs they should remain in the X-ray department until the symptoms subside. Wherever possible CO_2 should have been used in the examination, as opposed to room air, to reduce or even eliminate these symptoms. CO_2 is readily absorbed, and therefore the colon is distended for a shorter period.

If Buscopan is used patients should be advised to seek medical attention if they develop painful blurred vision after leaving the imaging department.

Additional information

It is essential that a multidetector CT scanner is used so that detailed image reconstruction can take place. Ideally there should be access to 3D software to allow the images to be reviewed and to assist with problem solving. It is also essential that dual-position scanning is used. This is vital to help distinguish between actual pathology and faecal residue. If the patient is unable to lie in the prone position, lateral decubitus imaging should be used. CTC is limited in its detection of colitis, and optical colonoscopy remains the 'gold standard' for diagnosis of ulcerative colitis.

REFERENCES

1. Frøkjær JB, et al. Imaging of the gastrointestinal tract-novel technologies. World Journal of Gastroenterology 2009;15(2):160–8.

2. Maglinte D, et al. Advances in alimentary tract imaging. World Journal of Gastroenterology 2006;12(20): 3139–45.

3. Engin G. Computed tomography enteroclysis in the diagnosis of intestinal diseases. Journal of Computer Assisted Tomography 2008;32(1):9–16.

4. Moscandrew ME, Loftus Jr EV. Diagnostic advances in inflammatory bowel disease (imaging and laboratory). Current Gastroenterology Reports 2009;11(6): 488–95.

5. Masselli G, et al. Small bowel neoplasms: prospective evaluation on MR enteroclysis. Radiology 2009;1(3):743–50.

6. Swain P. The future of wireless capsule endoscopy. World Journal of Gastroenterology 2008;14(26):4142–5.

7. Buchner AM, Wallace MB. Future expectations in digestive endoscopy: competition with other novel imaging techniques. Best Practice and Research Clinical Gastroenterology 2008;22(5): 971–87.

8. Ponsaing LG, et al. Diagnostic procedures for submucosal tumors in the gastrointestinal tract. World Journal of Gastroenterology 2007;13(24):3301–10.

9. Leighton JA, Loftus Jr EV. Evolving diagnostic modalities in inflammatory bowel disease. Current Gastroenterology Reports 2005;7(6):467–74.

10. Saibeni S, et al. Imaging of the small bowel in Crohn's disease: a review of old and new techniques. World Journal of Gastroenterology 2007;13(24):3279–87.

11. Chua TS, et al. Validation of ^{13}C-urea breath test for the diagnosis of *Helicobacter pylori* infection in the Singapore population. Singapore Medical Journal 2002;43(8):55–7.

12. Moayyedi P, et al. New approaches to enhance the accuracy of the diagnosis of reflux disease. Gut 2004;53:55–7.

13. Eckardt AJ, Eckardt VF. Current clinical approach to achalasia. World Journal of Gastroenterology 2009;15(32):3969–75.

14. Chapman S, Nakielny R. A guide to radiological procedures. 4th ed. Edinburgh: Saunders; 2001.

15. Whitley AS, et al. Clark's special procedures in diagnostic imaging. Oxford: Butterworth Heinemann; 1999.

16. Ott DJ. In: Sutton D, Young WR, editors. A short textbook of clinical imaging. St Louis: Mosby; 1995.

17. Smith CM, et al. MicroRNAs, development of Barrett's esophagus, and progression to esophageal adenocarcinoma. World Journal of Gastroenterology 2010;16(5): 531–7.

18. RCR Working Party. Making the best use of clinical radiology services: referral guidelines. 6th ed. London: The Royal College of Radiologists; 2007.

19. Varghese JC, Roy-Choudhury SH. Radiological imaging of the GI tract after bariatric surgery. Gastrointestinal endoscopy 2009;70(6):1176–81.

20. Logemann J. Evaluation and treatment of swallowing disorders. 2rd ed. Austin, Texas: Pro-Ed; 1998.

21. Logemann J. Videofluoroscopy conference, Royal Preston Hospital, April 2008.

22. Carver E, Carver B, editors. Medical imaging: techniques, reflection and evaluation. Edinburgh: Churchill Livingstone; 2006.

23. Yucel C, et al. CT Colonography for incomplete or contraindicated optical colonoscopy in older patients. American Journal of Roentgenology 2008;190: 145–50.

24. Bryan G. Diagnostic radiography: a concise practical manual. 4th ed. Edinburgh: Churchill Livingstone; 1987.

25. Bogoni L, et al. Computer-aided detection (CAD) for CT colonography: a tool to address growing need. British Journal of Radiology 2005;78:S57-62.

26. Winawer SJ, et al. A comparison of colonscopy and double-contrast barium enema for surveillance after polypectomy. New England Journal of Medicine 2000;342:1766–72.

27. Steine S, et al. Double-contrast barium enema versus colonoscopy in the diagnosis of neoplastic disorders: Aspects of decision-making in general practice. Family Practice 1993;10:288–91.

28. http://cancerresearch.org/cancerstats/types/%20bowel.

29. Hodler J, et al. Diseases of the abdomen and pelvis: Diagnostic imaging and interventional techniques. New York: Springer; 2006.

30. Neri E, et al. CT colonography versus double-contrast barium enema for screening of colorectal cancer: comparison of radiation burden. Abdominal Imaging 2010;35(5):596–601.

31. Burling D. CT colonography standards. Clinical Radiology 2010;65(6):474–80.

32. Keshav K, et al. Quality assessment for CT colonography: validation of automated measurement of colonic distention and residual fluid. American Journal of Roentgenology 2007;189:1457–63.

33. Tolan DJM, et al. Replacing barium enema with CT colonography in patients older than 70 years: the importance of detecting extra colonic abnormalities. American Journal of Roentgenology 2007;189: 1104–11.

34. Barrett JF, et al. Artifacts in CT: recognition and avoidance. RadioGraphics 2004;24: 1679–91.

Chapter 30

Accessory organs of the gastrointestinal tract

Darren Wood, Elizabeth Carver

SALIVARY GLANDS

Plain radiography imaging alone cannot be considered an accurate imaging method as only 50% of parotid gland and 20% of sub-mandibular gland sialoliths are radio-opaque.[1] Therefore, contrast enhancement of the ducts is required or other imaging modalities must be considered: computed tomography (CT), ultrasound (US), magnetic resonance imaging (MRI) and radionuclide imaging (RNI) all have increasing roles to play in demonstrating this area and will be discussed briefly later in this chapter. In addition to diagnosis, imaging is also a precursor to interventional techniques, such as basket removal of sialoliths.

Contrast-enhanced X-ray imaging of the salivary glands has traditionally remained relatively constant in its technique; usually only parotid and submandibular glands are imaged using contrast agents, as it is considered more difficult to cannulate the sublingual gland. Submental occlusal radiography can be used to assess the sublingual region but will only show radio-opaque calculi (see Chapter 21).

Referral criteria

- Pain
- Swelling

Both symptoms are often noted on or after eating.

Sialography

Contraindications

Acute infection or inflammation[2,3]

Contrast agent

- High or low osmolar water-soluble contrast agent with an iodine content of 240–300 mg/mL *or* 480 mg/mL in an oily contrast agent. Neither contrast agent appears to be more advantageous than the other

Additional equipment

- Small syringe (2 mL)
- Filling cannula
- Lacrimal dilator (sterile)
- 18 G blunt needle with catheter (sterile)
- Sterile gloves
- Gauze swabs
- Sialogogue (used to stimulate salivation and help dilate the salivary duct for cannulation). This may be in the form of lemon juice, a citrus-flavoured sweet or sherbet
- Wooden spatula
- Mouthwash and disposable cup

Patient preparation

- Removal of artefacts, including false teeth
- After plain radiography has been undertaken, the sialogogue is administered to promote salivation and maximise visualisation of the salivary duct
- Explain to the patient that it will be necessary for them to indicate when the salivary duct feels full of contrast agent. Arrange for a distinctive sign to be given by the patient (e.g. raising a hand) when the relevant area feels tight or full. It is important that the patient understands the process *before* the procedure starts, as explanation while undergoing cannulation often proves ineffective
- Explain to the patient that it will be necessary for them to keep their lips closed gently over the cannula, to ensure it stays in place in the duct

For all areas, control images are taken prior to administration of the contrast agent; basic information on head positioning can be found in corresponding position descriptors in relevant chapters on radiography of the head or teeth (Chapters 16–22), although centring and collimation differ for sialography. Some slight modifications from basic head positions will be outlined, if relevant.

Parotid glands

Control images for sialography can be taken prior to application of the sialogue, for preassessment of any radio-opaque calculi.

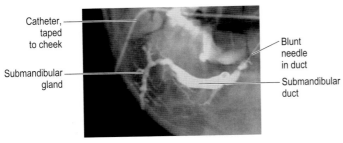

Figure 30.1 AP – submandibular gland.

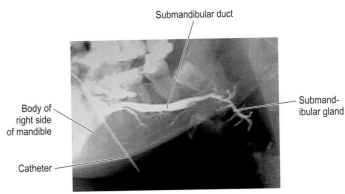

Figure 30.3 Lateral oblique – submandibular gland.

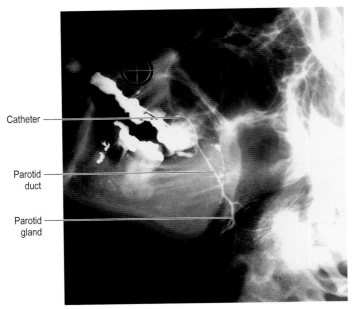

Figure 30.2 Lateral – parotid gland.
From Ryan S, et al. Anatomy for diagnostic imaging. 2nd ed. Edinburgh: Saunders; 2004.

Image receptor (IR) position is dictated by patient position during the procedure, as patient or investigator preferences influence whether a supine or erect sitting position is used.

Control images required:

1. *Anteroposterior (AP) (fronto-occipital (FO) position)* projection with the head rotated 5° away from the side under investigation. Centre midway between the symphysis menti and the angle of the mandible on the side under examination. Collimate to include soft tissues of the neck and face, symphysis menti and zygoma on the side under examination. Figure 30.1 shows an AP projection (of the right submandibular gland) after contrast injection
2. *Lateral,* centred to the angle of mandible. Collimate to include soft tissues of the neck and under the chin, external auditory meatus, zygoma, and to level with the ala of the nose anteriorly. Figure 30.2 shows a lateral projection (of the right parotid gland) after contrast injection
3. *Lateral oblique* with the patient's head tilted 15° towards the side under investigation. Tube angle of 10–15° cranially, centre midway between the angles of mandible. Figure 30.3 shows a lateral oblique projection (of the right submandibular gland) after contrast injection

Technique

- If the gland is not visible, the sialogogue may be used to promote salivation
- Saliva is blotted away from the duct area using a gauze swab and the duct is dilated with a lacrimal dilator
- The duct is cannulated, using the blunt-ended sialographic needle/catheter apparatus
- Following cannulation, up to 2 mL of contrast are injected until the patient indicates that the gland feels 'full' (see the preparation section with regard to a signal for this)
- The catheter tubing is taped to the skin surface, away from the duct and gland area
- The precontrast images are repeated
- After the images have been taken the patient is given a mouthwash to promote saliva secretion and a lateral view can then be taken to demonstrate drainage of the duct and any sialectasis if present

Submandibular gland

Control images required:

1. A *lower occlusal* image, with the IR possibly displaced over to the side in question
2. *Lateral,* as for the parotid gland, centred to the angle of mandible with the floor of the mouth depressed by a wooden spatula
3. *Lateral oblique,* as for the parotid gland

Technique

- The procedure then follows that described for the parotid gland, but the occlusal film is not required after contrast introduction and it is not necessary to use a spatula in the lateral projection. A post-sialogogue lateral film is required

Aftercare: parotid and submandibular glands

- Provide further mouthwash, if the patient requires it
- Advise the patient that they may experience an unusual taste (which may occur intermittently) until the contrast has fully drained

Possible complications: parotid and submandibular glands

- Infection
- Duct orifice damage
- Duct rupture

OTHER IMAGING TECHNIQUES FOR THE SALIVARY GLANDS

Digital subtraction sialography

On the whole this technique is as described for traditional sialography with contrast agent but using digital subtraction. It is similar in its imaging process to arterial radiography by the fact that an increased frame rate (usually approx. 2 frames per second) is used and the resultant image is subtracted; therefore, only the contrast-enhanced area is visualised. This method has been shown to be of high quality compared to CT, MRI and US, particularly in demonstrating pathology in the parenchymal part of the gland.[4] There is, however, an increase in patient radiation dose compared to conventional technique, therefore the benefit of image quality versus radiation dose should be considered when using this technique.

Magnetic resonance sialography

This is a non-invasive technique and, with advances in equipment and availability, is becoming more popular. Indeed, it has been stated that it is now 'routinely' used to image the salivary parenchyma but that contrast X-ray is still mainly used to show the ducts.[5] It has long been compared favourably to conventional techniques.[6] Its obvious advantage is that it uses hydrographic technique (relying on the presence of the patient's own saliva), so no cannulation is required, and of course there is no ionising radiation. However, to combat the spatial resolution difference a number of methods have been used: these include the use of a sialogogue for dynamic studies and also the use of small surface coils.[7,8] A recent study showed that using a sialogogue and a passive occlusion device (a pad used to compress and occlude the opening of the duct) is comparable with interventional methods, particularly when assessing the parotid gland;[5] however it must be noted that the investigators had undertaken research on volunteers, recognising that further study on patients was required in order to assess diagnostic performance and the practicality of this technique.

CT

With duct cannulation and contrast enhancement, CT is also being used more frequently. It is considered to be most useful in imaging (without contrast) for tumour enhancement or in patients who have a mass lesion. Radiation dose plays an important factor, especially compared to all other techniques, but image quality is high.

Ultrasound

This has an increasing role in assessing the salivary glands, particularly when using Doppler. All major pathologies exhibit classic signs of hypoechoic, anechoic or inhomogeneous areas that can be recognised and aid in differential diagnosis.[9] Owing to its non-invasive nature and capability in detecting numerous pathologies, ultrasound can be extremely useful as a front-line investigation but it is known to be difficult to detect sialoliths with ultrasound, or in chronic cases where the gland does not function.[9]

It is particularly useful for assessing solid mass salivary gland pathology, and also effective in conjunction with fine needle aspiration because of the high resolution that can be attained. It has also been advocated as a quick and simple process to use in assisting fine needle aspiration of tumours.[6]

RNI

Particularly useful as a safe and reliable method to assess gland function. It is also proving to be reliable in the differential diagnosis of patients with suspected Sjögren's syndrome.[10]

GALLBLADDER AND BILIARY TREE

Oral cholecystography

Oral cholecystography remains an excellent method of gallstone detection but its role has diminished, mainly due to the advantages of alternative imaging methods (especially ultrasound[11]). It is rarely carried out in the UK but is still considered to be an option in some imaging departments.

The examination has three phases:

1. Control plain radiography
2. Contrast images
3. Gallbladder showing drainage of contrast after fatty meal (AFM)

Referral criteria

- Suspected gallbladder pathology

Contraindications

- Hepatorenal disease
- Serum bilirubin levels in excess of 34 μmol/L
- Acute cholecystitis
- Dehydration
- Previous cholecystectomy

Contrast agent

- There are a number of agents on the market, all producing the required result. The most common are sodium iopodate (Biloptin) and iopanoic acid (Telepaque)

First stage of the examination and patient preparation

- Prior to the examination a *control image* is taken. Its use was advocated by Twomey et al.,[12] who estimated that it could aid in the diagnosis of up to 5% of calculi. The projection used for this is the 20° left anterior oblique (LAO) described in the second-stage examination procedure and positioning technique
- An information sheet and contrast agent are given to the patient to take home; this provides instructions on appointment time for the second stage of the examination, contrast agent and dietary preparation
- The patient is instructed to follow a light, fat-free diet on the day before the examination and to fast from 6 pm the night before their cholecystogram appointment.[2] They are encouraged to drink water to ensure hydration
- They are then instructed to take the contrast agent 12 hours prior to their appointment and are asked not to smoke

Second stage: examination procedure and positioning technique

For prone and supine projections the IR is horizontal, employed with an antiscatter grid

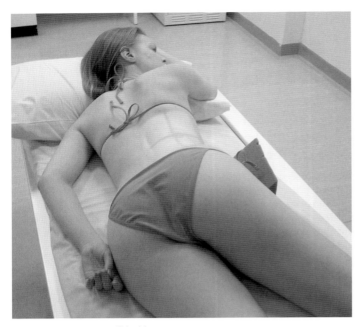

Figure 30.4 LAO – gallbladder.

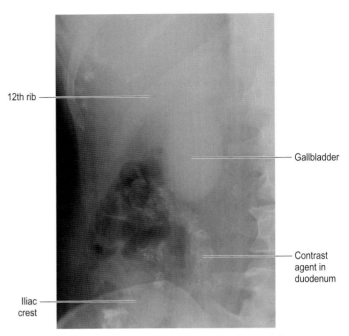

Figure 30.5 LAO – gallbladder. The position and shape of the gallbladder will vary according to patient build. This example is of an 'average build' patient. In hypersthenic patients the gallbladder will be rounder and sit higher in the abdomen; it will also tend to lie more obliquely towards the lateral abdominal wall, or even horizontally. In asthenic patients the gallbladder will be longer and lie lower in the abdomen; it is also likely to lie closer to the spine. As a result, centring should be modified according to patient build.[8]

Prone 20° LAO to show the fundus (Figs 30.4, 30.5)

- From the prone position, the right side is raised 20° and radiolucent pads are used to support the abdomen
- The right arm is placed on the pillow and the left knee flexed, to aid immobilisation

Central ray and focus receptor distance (FRD)

Vertical central ray
100 cm FRD

Centring

Level with the spinous process of L1, midway between the spine and the right flank

It is acknowledged that patient build will affect centring quite significantly. Slim patients will require centring to fall lower, closer to the spine, and well-built patients will require centring to lie higher and further from the midline (closer to the flank).[13]

Collimation

Collimate to include the soft tissue on the right of the abdomen, spine, 11th rib, iliac crest

For second 20° LAO after ingestion of contrast agent

- Mark the posterior abdominal wall over the point used for centring, to aid positioning later in the examination. It will be necessary to explain the reason for this to the patient and gain consent. Document that consent has been given

---

Expose on arrested expiration

Exposing after full expiration will ensure that the gallbladder always lies in the same position in the abdomen for every exposure.

Supine 20° right posterior oblique (RPO) to show the gallbladder neck (Fig. 30.6)

- From the supine abdomen position, the patient is rotated 20° to their right
- The left side is supported on radiolucent pads

This projection may also clear appearances of faeces or bowel gas, which can obscure detail over the gallbladder.

Central ray and FRD

Vertical central ray
100 cm FRD

Centring

In the right midclavicular line, approximately 5 cm above the lower costal margin (but possibly varying with patient build)

Collimation

Collimate to include the soft tissue on the right of the abdomen, spine, 11th rib, iliac crest

---

For all projections expose on arrested expiration; expiration ensures that the gallbladder lies in a more constant position for comparison of images.

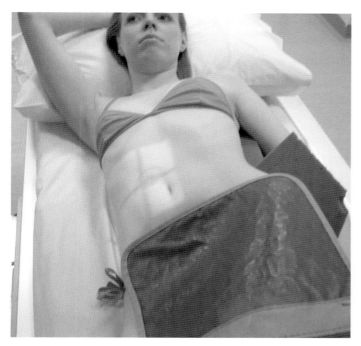

Figure 30.6 Supine RPO – gallbladder.

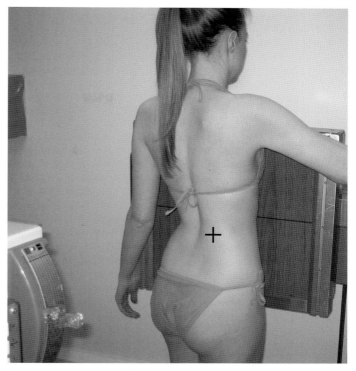

Figure 30.7 LAO erect gallbladder.

Erect 20° LAO (Figs 30.7, 30.8) **for possible floating gallstones**

For erect projections the IR is vertical, used with an antiscatter grid
• From the erect posteroanterior (PA) position, the right side is turned 20° away from the IR
• The right arm is placed on top of the IR unit

Central ray and FRD

Horizontal central ray
100 cm FRD

Centring

Using the centring mark made after the prone 20° projection, centre 2–3 cm below and 2–3 cm medially to the mark. This allows for the change in gallbladder position that the erect position causes. Note that there may be no shift in gallbladder position for the hypersthenic patient

Collimation

Collimate to include the soft tissue on the right of the abdomen, spine, 12th rib, iliac crest
   If there are any overlying bowel shadows, fluoroscopic assessment may be made while the patient's trunk is rotated to clear the image of the gas from the gallbladder. If this method fails, conventional tomography may be required.

Third stage: AFM

The images for this stage should show that the gallbladder is emptying satisfactorily and is not obstructed by calculi. After satisfactory contrast images have shown the gallbladder, the patient is given a fatty meal (e.g. chocolate bar or a fat emulsion drink).

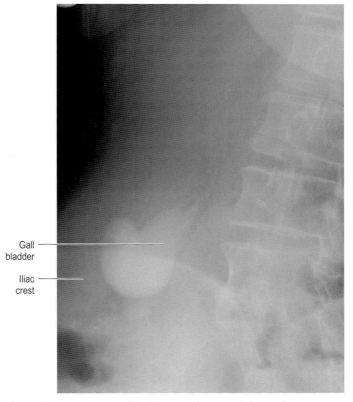

Gall bladder

Iliac crest

Figure 30.8 LAO erect gallbladder. Note how much lower the gallbladder is in this position compared to the prone LAO image in Figure 30.5.

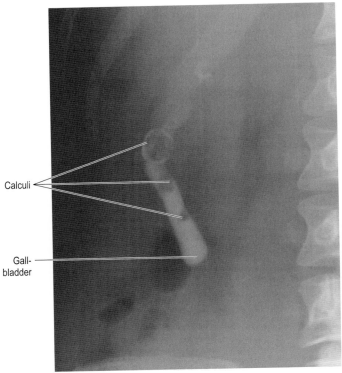

Calculi

Gall-
bladder

Figure 30.9 Calculi in the contracting gallbladder (prone 20° LAO) AFM.

- Patients fast for only 6 hours
- No contraindications
- Pain on scanning can be related to acute cholecystitis (Murphy's sign)
- No complications
- No use of ionising radiation
- Less time-consuming for the operator and patient
- Other structures can be imaged at the same time (e.g. bile duct, liver, pancreas)

RNI

Cholescintigraphy (or HIDA (hepatobiliary iminodiacetic acid) scan) is a useful adjunct to assess function (often after normal ultrasound has been performed for right upper quadrant pain) because a normal ^{99m}Tc-IDA scan excludes the diagnosis as it provides a direct assessment of cystic duct patency. This technique has high sensitivity and specificity, particularly for the diagnosis of acute cholecystitis (97% and 94%, respectively).[14]

CT

CT can be used to visualise the gallbladder but is not always as accurate as ultrasound in the diagnosis of gallstones, and has additional risks associated with the use of ionising radiation. CT can be useful in the very obese patient, as these patients prove difficult to image with ultrasound.

Patients can be scanned without contrast to show a dilated bile duct system. Infusion of contrast agent before the scan will produce a CT cholangiogram. Recent studies indicate that CT cholangiography may have an increased role to play in the imaging of the biliary tree.[15]

MRI

This technique is constantly finding new applications as technology and expertise continue to grow in the field. The most common examination is the magnetic resonance cholangiopancreatogram (MRCP), which will be mentioned in more detail later in comparison with endoscopic retrograde cholangiopancreatography.

Intravenous cholangiography (IVC)

This examination is almost never undertaken in the 21st century thanks to safer imaging via ultrasound, endoscopic retrograde cholangiopancreatography (ERCP) and MRCP.[2]

Operative cholangiography

The radiographer undertakes this examination under sterile conditions in the operating theatre.

Referral criteria

- During cholecystectomy and/or bile duct surgery, if there is concern that calculi remain in the biliary tract

Contraindications

- There are no contraindications

Contrast agent

- Low iodine content, e.g. Niopam 150

At this stage the images may be more strictly collimated, as the second-stage images can be studied to ascertain the exact gallbladder position; the radiographer uses the marks made over the second-phase centring points, adjusting the third-phase centring if the gallbladder has not been shown in the centre of the radiation field at the second phase. The gallbladder will also have contracted.

30 minutes after ingestion of the fatty food, a well-collimated prone 20° LAO image is taken (Fig. 30.9). It may be necessary to repeat the 20° erect LAO and/or the supine RPO.

Complications[2]

- Nausea*
- Diarrhoea in up to 50% of patients
- Headache*
- Urticaria*

*These complications are rare.

OTHER DIAGNOSTIC TECHNIQUES FOR THE GALLBLADDER

Ultrasound

Ultrasound has a high degree of accuracy for the diagnosis of gallstones, similar to that of oral cholecystography, but with a number of significant advantages. It is also an excellent method of evaluating the common bile duct and common hepatic ducts without the use of contrast. Advantages of ultrasound are:

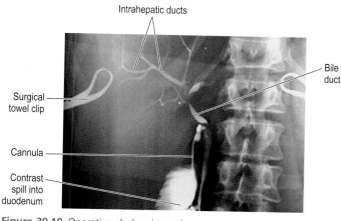

Intrahepatic ducts

Bile duct

Surgical towel clip

Cannula

Contrast spill into duodenum

Figure 30.10 Operative cholangiography.

Technique

• This is a sterile procedure performed in the operating theatre. The surgeon will cannulate the cystic duct and introduce approximately 20 mL of the contrast agent. The aim is to show contrast flow into the duodenum and outline the length of the common bile duct (CBD) with minimal filling of the intrahepatic ducts (Fig. 30.10). Images of the area are taken using a mobile X-ray machine or, more frequently, using a mobile image intensifier (this can negate the need for further injections and reduces the risk of missing the information required by taking subsequent plain films). Sterile towels cover the abdomen and the surgeon generally indicates the region of interest by pointing or putting a spot of sterile water on the towel to aid correct centring. No radiographic positioning is necessary. The area is viewed and/or images are taken after 10 mL of contrast agent have been injected, and then exposure is repeated after a further 10 mL have been injected

Complications

• If the biliary tract is obstructed there is a risk that injection of contrast under pressure could cause septicaemia

Postoperative (T-tube) cholangiography
Referral criteria

• To demonstrate or exclude calculi in the biliary tract if it is suspected that calculi remain in the tract after gallbladder surgery

Contraindications

• There are no contraindications

Contrast agent

• As for operative cholangiography

Additional equipment

• Syringe and needle
• Filling cannula
• Antiseptic
• Gauze swabs
• Sterile gloves
• Clamp

Technique

• The examination is carried out using fluoroscopy, 7–10 days postoperatively
• The patient lies supine on the fluoroscopic couch and a fluoroscopic spot control film may be taken to show the position of the internal drain
• The external drainage tube is cleaned with antiseptic and clamped. A needle is inserted into the tube, between the clamp and the skin surface. Contrast agent is then injected until the ducts are demonstrated fluoroscopically
• Images are then taken, as required, after turning the patient until optimum visualisation of the area is achieved. Alternatively, if a C-arm intensifier is used, the tube may be rotated to achieve the same effect. It may be necessary to elevate the patient's head, shoulders and trunk (using table tilt) to assess duct drainage

Complications

• As for operative cholangiography

Percutaneous transhepatic cholangiography (PTC)

This involves the introduction of contrast agent into the hepatobiliary system via a needle technique, through the lateral abdominal wall and into the liver. Needle insertion takes place using spot fluoroscopy for guidance.

Referral criteria

• Jaundice: to check for hepatic bile duct obstruction
• Prior to interventional procedures, e.g. biliary drainage or stenting

Contraindications

• Tendency towards bleeding, platelets <100 000 or prothrombin time more than twice the control figure
• Infection of the biliary tract
• Hydatid disease

Contrast agent

• High or low osmolar contrast media with an iodine concentration of 150–300 mg/mL

Additional equipment

• 22 G flexible, long needle
• Small syringe and needle for administration of local anaesthetic
• Local anaesthetic
• Sterile gloves
• Antiseptic skin wash
• Gauze swabs
• Filling cannula
• Suturing equipment or skin sealant spray and skin dressing for after the procedure

Patient preparation

- Results of blood tests must be available and checked to ensure they are within acceptable limits, because of the risks associated with bleeding
- The patient should also be given prophylactic antibiotics prior to the procedure (and also afterwards) to reduce the risk of infection
- Dietary preparation should include 'nil by mouth' to reduce the chance of nausea and/or vomiting
- It is recommended that the patient be given sedative premedication as the procedure can be uncomfortable
- As this is an invasive procedure and there are risks associated with it, written informed consent should be obtained

Technique

- The patient is positioned supine on the fluoroscopic couch. If a C-arm intensifier is being used, their right arm can be placed on an arm board and extended out to allow for the lateral C-arm movement and so that the lateral projection can be taken more easily. Using a C-arm intensifier means that the patient will not be required to turn during the procedure
- Initial screening of the region with the patient in full inspiration and expiration will allow the clinician to make a decision as to the best point to enter the liver
- Using aseptic technique, the area is cleansed and local anaesthesia given
- The flexible needle is inserted through the skin and into the liver with the patient in arrested respiration. The patient is then asked to breathe in a more shallow fashion to reduce needle movement and hence discomfort. The needle is advanced into the centre of the liver
- Contrast agent can then be injected into the liver as the needle is slowly withdrawn; this process can be repeated while moving the needle tip in any direction until the ducts begin to fill with contrast. The more dilated the ducts are, the easier cannulation will be. When the hepatic duct system is filled the needle can be withdrawn, unless access is still required for a therapeutic procedure
- Images taken may vary but often include:
  - supine
  - 45° lateromedial angle (from left and right); this will require 45° rotation of the patient in each direction if the C-arm is not available
  - right lateral
- Because contrast is heavier than bile it may be necessary to tilt the patient head down (Trendelenburg position) to ensure filling of the system. The patient can then be tilted more erect to check for obstruction or to see if contrast flows into the duodenum

Aftercare

- After withdrawal of the needle, the area is sealed (or sutured) and a clean dressing is applied
- After the procedure, pulse and blood pressure should be taken every 15 minutes for the first hour and then half-hourly for 5 hours
- The wound site is monitored
- Abdomen size is monitored

Complications

- (Morbidity is approximately 4%)
- Pyrexia
- Pancreatitis
- Perforation of the T-tube[2]

ERCP (Figs 30.11, 30.12)

Referral criteria

- Extrahepatic biliary obstruction
- Jaundice
- Post-cholecystectomy patients who remain symptomatic
- Pancreatic disease
- Other diffuse biliary tract diseases

Contraindications

- HIV/AIDS
- Australia antigen positive
- Previous gastric surgery (affects the normal anatomy)
- Acute pancreatitis
- Severe cardiorespiratory disease

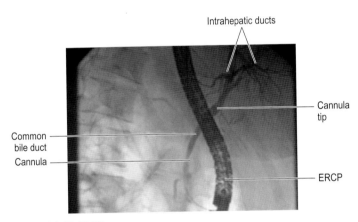

Figure 30.11 ERCP.

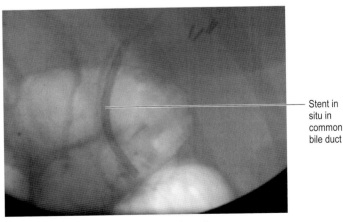

Figure 30.12 ERCP – following stent insertion.

Contrast agent

- Low osmolar contrast with an iodine concentration of 240–300 mg/mL is considered optimal. This is generally diluted to half strength with saline when cannulation has been confirmed to reduce the risk of obscuring any calculi and decrease the possibility of pancreatitis

Patient preparation

- Nil by mouth for 4–6 hours prior to the procedure
- Antibiotic cover to reduce any infection risk
- As this is an invasive procedure which may need further therapeutic intervention, written informed consent must be obtained. Advance explanation is important as the patient will be sedated immediately before the examination

Technique

- In the past, this procedure has generally been carried out by surgeons or gastroenterologists under fluoroscopic control, within a medical imaging department. Although this remains the more usual scenario, radiographers and nurses are increasingly carrying out this procedure.
- The patient's pharynx is anaesthetised using anaesthetic spray (to aid the passage of the endoscope); an intravenous sedative (e.g. diazepam or Hypnovel) is administered
- The patient is then asked to lie prone with their right side raised 30–45° and radiolucent pads are used to support the right side; the endoscope is then introduced
- During the procedure the patient is monitored for pulse and oxygen saturation to ensure their safety
- The endoscopist passes the scope into the duodenum and locates the ampulla of Vater (the bile duct orifice). Once located, a small catheter is positioned in the entrance and contrast agent introduced and viewed under fluoroscopic control. It is possible at this point for the endoscopist to cannulate the pancreas and obtain images, although repeated cannulation and introduction of contrast is to be avoided due to an increase in the risk of pancreatitis
- As contrast agent begins to fill the common bile duct, images can be taken which will demonstrate any calculi that might be present
- As for the PTC, the patient may be tilted (a) into the Trendelenburg position to fill the intrahepatic ducts and (b) semi-erect to fill the distal end of the CBD and gallbladder
- If there is no need to progress to a therapeutic procedure, or a sphincterotomy has been performed (thereby aiding in the ease of recannulation of the duct), the scope may be removed; this will allow a better view of the duct, over which the scope may have been lying

Aftercare

- The patient should continue to starve until sensation in their throat has returned
- The patient should have their pulse, temperature and blood pressure monitored half-hourly for 4–6 hours
- If pancreatitis is suspected, serum amylase tests should be undertaken

Complications

- Damage caused by the endoscope (e.g. to the ampulla, distal ducts and the oesophagus)
- Acute pancreatitis 0.7–7.4%[2]

Comparison of ERCP with PTC

ERCP has three main advantages over PTC:[9]
1. ERCP enables visualisation of the ampulla, which can be the site of a tumour, and allows for biopsy during the procedure
2. ERCP can demonstrate both the biliary tree and the pancreatic duct
3. There are better therapeutic possibilities via ERCP, e.g. sphincterotomy, removal of stones via basket or balloon, drain or stent insertion

However, these do not negate PTC, which:

- Has a growing role as a precursor for interventional procedures that cannot be achieved via ERCP
- Generally shows the intrahepatic ducts better than ERCP, although the use of balloon catheters during ERCP means the endoscopist can improve their view of the area

SUPPLEMENTARY TECHNIQUES FOR THE BILIARY TREE

Ultrasound

Whereas PTC may have been a primary investigation for obstructive jaundice in the past, ultrasound has now established itself in that role; it is non-invasive, involves no ionising radiation and has no complications. Ultrasound has become very accurate in assessing the level and cause of biliary obstruction; even early studies showed that the level of biliary obstruction was correctly noted in 95% of cases and the cause correctly noted in 88%,[16] and ultrasound equipment and techniques have improved significantly since that time.

CT

This has also proved itself an appropriate modality for the diagnosis of obstructive jaundice. Studies have shown multislice CT to have long had a role in the assessment of cholangiocarcinoma, although MRI is also considered useful.[17]

MRI

MRI has become increasingly useful for assessment of the biliary tree with MRCP (Fig. 30.13). Compared to endoscopy this is a

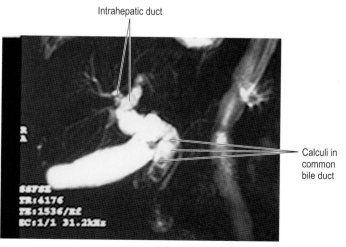

Intrahepatic duct

Calculi in common bile duct

Figure 30.13 MRCP.

non-invasive technique that negates the need for contrast injection. A study as long ago as 2002 showed that MRCP had a high accuracy rate in evaluating common bile duct stones (choledocholithiasis).[18] It did, however, advocate that patients with a high probability of disease should undergo ERCP, as some form of therapeutic procedure might be required. Since this investigation, other literature has concluded that MRCP has an extremely high sensitivity and specificity and is therefore an important imaging modality in this patient group.[19]

PANCREAS

In X-radiography the pancreas is only visualised via ERCP with direct injection of contrast, but if a patient is suffering acute pancreatitis this is contraindicated. Ultrasound, CT and MRI are the best methods for imaging the pancreas as they are non-invasive and also have the bonus of being able to show the involvement of surrounding structures.

REFERENCES

1. Greenberg MS, et al. Burket's oral medicine. 11th ed. Ontario: BC Decker Inc; 2008.

2. Chapman S, Nakielny R. A guide to radiological procedures. 5th ed. Edinburgh: Saunders; 2009.

3. Whitley AS, et al. Clark's special procedures in diagnostic imaging. Oxford: Butterworth Heinemann; 1999.

4. Kalinowski M, et al. Comparative study of MR sialography and digital subtraction sialography for benign salivary gland disorders. American Journal of Neuroradiology 2002;23(9):1485–92.

5. Hugill J, et al. MR sialography: the effect of a sialogogue and ductal occlusion in volunteers. British Journal of Radiology 2008;81(967):583–6.

6. Daneva S, et al. Ultrasound and fine needle aspiration of the salivary glands. ECR presentations; 1999: lecture ref. 8–008.

7. Takagi Y, et al. Fast and high resolution MR sialography using a small surface coil.

Journal of Magnetic Resonance Imaging 2005;22:29–37.

8. Wada H, et al. High resolution MR sialography of the parotid gland: comparison of microscopy coil and conventional small surface coil. Proceedings of the International Society for Magnetic Resonance in Medicine 2005;13:1078.

9. Bialek J, et al. US of the major salivary glands: anatomy and spatial relationships, pathologic conditions and pitfalls. Radiography 2006;26:745–63.

10. Keyes J, et al. Best scintigraphic measures of parotid gland dysfunction in Sjogrens syndrome. Arthritis and Rheumatology 2010;62(Suppl. 10):1887.

11. Gregory A, et al. Gallbladder stones: imaging and intervention. Radiographics 2000;20:751–66.

12. Twomey B, et al. The plain radiograph in oral cholecystography: should it be abandoned? British Journal of Radiology 1983;56(662):99–100.

13. Unett EM, Royle AJ. Radiographic techniques and image evaluation. London: Chapman & Hall; 1997.

14. Zeisseman HA. Nuclear medicine hepatobiliary imaging. Clinical Gastroenterology and Hepatology 2010;8(2):111–6.

15. Morosi C, et al. CT cholangiography: assessment of feasibility and diagnostic reliability. EJR 2009;72(1):114–7.

16. Gibson RN, et al. Bile duct obstruction radiologic evaluation of level cause and tumour respectability. Radiology 1986;160:43–7.

17. Schima W. Biliary malignancies: multi-slice CT or MRI? Cancer Imaging 2003;3(2):75–8.

18. Calvo MM, et al. Role of MRCP in patients with suspected choledocholiathiasis. Clinical Proceedings 2002;77:422–8.

19. Hekimoglu K, et al. MRCP vs ERCP in the evaluation of biliary pathologies: review of current literature. Journal of Digestive Diseases 2008;9(3):162–9.

Chapter | **31** |

Investigations of the genitourinary tract

Elizabeth Carver, Darren Wood

As outlined in Chapter 28, contrast-enhanced imaging of the urinary tract was originally developed in the early 1920s, when suitable contrast agents were first used. For the most part of the 20th century contrast conventional radiography was the only option for imaging of the tract, but all complementary imaging methods, and especially ultrasound, now offer a significant contribution to imaging the area.

Ultrasound is an excellent imaging method that will show or estimate renal volume, parenchymal thickness, kidney shape and size, congenital development abnormalities, cysts, benign prostatic hypertrophy or carcinoma, hydronephrosis and tumours of the renal system. Use of colour Doppler will demonstrate the renal vascular system. The list is by no means exhaustive but does serve to show why ultrasound came to the forefront of imaging in this area.

The advent of low radiation dose computed tomography (CT) of kidneys, ureters, bladder (KUB) has now moved towards extra-low dose CT KUB (equivalent dose to a plain radiography KUB exposure), making CT a suitable option in this area.[1] Comparison has been made between ultra-low dose (contrast-enhanced) CT and KUB (particularly relating to renal colic assessment), finding CT to be comparable in diagnostic yield to KUB.[2] MRI also has a place in imaging the urinaryly system, thanks to its superior ability to demonstrate differences in soft tissue appearances. There is additional information on imaging methods for the urinary system at the end of the section on the urinary tract below.

As a result of these developments in imaging, the use of intravenous urography (IVU) has slowly receded since the 1980s, mainly because of the increased availability and use of ultrasound. However, it may still be used in some centres, in emergency cases, or where there may still be difficulties using or accessing other imaging modalities (more specifically CT). According to the Royal College of Radiologists (RCR), the unavailability of CT is the only reason for performing an IVU.[3]

COMMON PATHOLOGIES AND CLINICAL INDICATIONS FOR IMAGING OF THE URINARY SYSTEM

This is not an exhaustive list and any suggested imaging methods are based on current UK guidelines.[3]

Calculus/calculi

Renal calculi are formed in the urine and create problems for patients when they lodge in the urinary tract, causing severe pain (renal colic) and, potentially, ureteric obstruction, hydronephrosis and haematuria. Stones as small as 0.4 cm can cause renal colic. The constituents of calculi vary, but the most common are calcium oxalate and calcium phosphate; they are often radio-opaque (but can also be radiolucent and not visible via X-ray imaging) and can therefore be visualised on the plain radiographic image. However, owing to their (usually) small size they may not always be well visualised; this is also complicated by the surrounding (possible superimposition of) soft tissue structures of the abdominal viscera, and also mesenteric nodes and phleboliths. This obviously means that plain radiographic imaging of the abdomen, albeit a reasonable tool for imaging renal stones, is not as useful to determine ureteric stones and their position. Current UK guidelines suggest unenhanced low-dose CT as the investigation of choice, with IVU indicated only when CT is unavailable.[3]

Large radio-opaque calculi may occupy the space within the pelvicalyceal system, filling it in almost exactly the same shape as the system; these are known as staghorn calculi (Fig. 31.1) and can mimic the appearance of a contrast-filled pelvicalyceal system. They can be an incidental finding seen on abdomen images.

Benign and malignant prostatic disease

Although the prostate gland is not located within the urinary tract itself, prostatic disease affects urinary tract imaging by its extrinsic effects on the system. A large proportion of men from late middle age onwards will have an enlarged prostate due to benign prostatic hypertrophy/hyperplasia (BPH).[4] Symptoms of this include frequency of micturition, poor urine stream and dysuria. Extreme forms can cause bladder outlet obstruction. Although a benign condition, BPH will often require treatment in order to alleviate its symptoms, as they often significantly affect the patient's quality of life. It is important to differentiate between BPH and carcinoma of the prostate, which can cause similar symptoms.

If the urinary tract contains contrast agent, if prostatic enlargement of any type is present the bladder appears to have a depression at its base, in the shape of a mushroom. Bladder ultrasound with

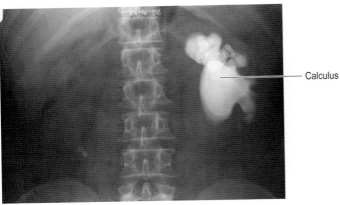

Figure 31.1 Staghorn calculus on control image. The radio-opaque calculus has filled the pelvicalyceal system, almost mimicking a hydronephrotic kidney filled with contrast agent.

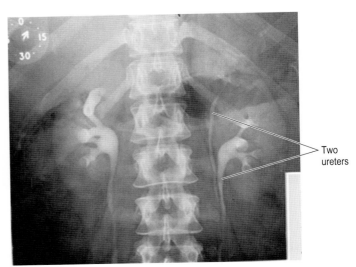

Figure 31.2 Duplex system. In this case the pelvicalyceal systems are duplicated, but most duplex systems are not so extensive.

measurement of postvoid residual volume is the examination of choice when investigating BPH and the extent of its effect, and contrast radiography is not indicated for this condition.[3] Ultrasound will help differentiate between BPH and prostatic carcinoma and is usually used in conjunction with assessment of blood levels of prostate-specific antigen (PSA); an elevated PSA level may indicate malignancy.

Commonly encountered malignant tumours

The most common type affecting the intrinsic system is transitional cell carcinoma, and the most common location is the bladder. A common method of imaging assessment for bladder malignancy is ultrasound; however, cystoscopy is considered to be the optimum method. Epithelial cell tumours also affect the renal tract and are best demonstrated by contrast-enhanced CT. At one time the IVU was considered to be superior to CT for demonstration of these tumours but advances in multislice CT technology led to a change in opinion.[5]

Nephroblastoma (Wilms' tumour) is a malignant tumour affecting children: ultrasound is the first-line imaging test to identify the condition, with CT used to assess extent of the mass; MRI may also be useful.

For the diagnosis of suspected renal cell adenocarcinoma or transitional cell carcinoma, the optimal methods of imaging have long been considered to be ultrasound or CT; however, MRI is now known to be sensitive and is being used increasingly, especially if contrast administration is contraindicated.[3]

Duplex system

This is a duplication of part or parts of the urinary system involving the kidney and ureter. The most extensive form presents as a single kidney which has two sets of calyces, two renal pelves and two ureters (Fig. 31.2); this may be unilateral or bilateral. Less extensive forms of the variant may show as two renal pelves entering a single ureter, or two pelves entering two ureters, which later fuse before entering the bladder. The variant is usually an incidental finding but is monitored in children because of its relationship to recurrent urinary tract infection (UTI).

Ectopic kidney

The kidney is found in an area away from the usual site, sometimes on the opposite side to where it should lie (crossed ectopia).

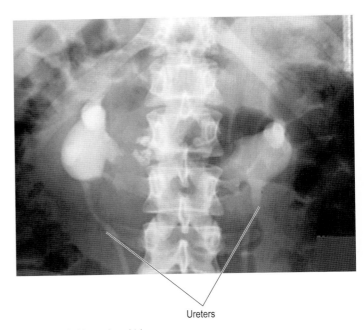

Figure 31.3 Horseshoe kidney.

Floating kidney

The kidney may appear to be in a normal position or poses as a fixed ectopic kidney, which then moves as an examination progresses.

Horseshoe kidney

A relatively rare variant. The two kidneys are joined at their upper or lower poles, the latter being by far the most common. Each kidney has its own ureter, and if the kidneys are joined at their lower pole X-ray contrast images show the calyces appearing similar to those in a 'normal' kidney which has been placed in an oblique position (Fig. 31.3). In these cases the ureters cannot leave the kidney pelvis and hilum medially as in the normal kidney, and travel forward and over the adjoined lower poles. Ultrasound, CT and MRI will also identify this variant.

'Reflux' and pyelonephritis

More specifically known as ureteric or vesicoureteric reflux and reflux nephropathy; it commonly affects children. Urine flows backwards from the bladder owing to failure of the vesicoureteric valve. Reflux, in these cases, refers to backtracking of urine from the bladder into the ureter and upwards towards the kidney. This can lead to pyelonephritis, renal dysfunction and scarring, and in chronic cases renal failure. Vesicoureteric reflux can be assessed using micturating cystography and radionuclide imaging (RNI), which provides a non-invasive approach to diagnosis.[6,7]

Urinary tract obstruction

This can be due to a number of causes, either intrinsic or extrinsic. Obstruction affects the tract's ability to drain, potentially causing hydronephrosis, kidney enlargement and loss of renal cortex. If obstruction is caused by a calculus, unenhanced low-dose CT is the imaging modality of choice. Contrast-enhanced CT (CT urogram), ultrasound, Doppler ultrasound, RNI and MRI all have a place if considering intrarenal blood flow, renal function, or assessment of patients who are not suitable for administration of intravenous contrast agent. IVU is not recommended unless CT is unavailable.[3]

Renal transplant

Transplant patients will have one functioning kidney: the transplanted one, attached to a short ureter and placed in the right iliac fossa. The current recommendations for assessment of transplanted kidneys are for Doppler ultrasound with the use of RNI (can distinguish acute rejection) or MR/MRA (if ultrasound is equivocal).[3]

RADIOGRAPHIC EXAMINATION OF THE URINARY SYSTEM

INTRAVENOUS UROGRAPHY (IVU)

Although the current UK guidelines no longer consider the IVU a front-line examination, a description of the technique follows as some centres still use it on occasion in an emergency situation if CT is unavailable. It must be envisaged that in the near future this examination may no longer be carried out.

The aim is to demonstrate the renal cortex, calyces, renal pelvis, pelviureteric junction, ureteric drainage and the bladder (although demonstration of the bladder may not be required). Contrast agent is administered intravenously and images of the system are obtained through various stages, from glomerular filtration to urine and contrast collection in calyces, and then on to ureteric drainage and bladder filling.

A range of projections are used for the IVU, in various combinations to demonstrate the system, and appropriate selection of this combination will be discussed later in this section. Projections used are taken from the following list:

- Full-length KUB
- Prone KUB
- Cross-renal, collimated to the kidneys and upper ureters
- Oblique single kidney
- Bladder anteroposterior (AP) with caudal angle of approximately 15° to clear the bladder from the upper border of symphysis pubis
- Oblique bladder

Contrast agent can be seen almost immediately after injection, shown as a 'blush' in the renal cortex and known as a nephrogram

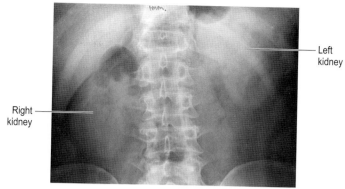

Figure 31.4 Nephrogram.

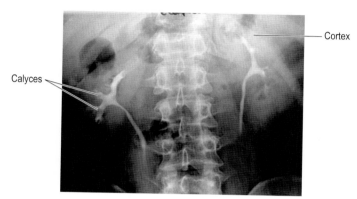

Figure 31.5 Contrast agent in renal cortex and pelvicalyceal system.

(Fig. 31.4). This shows glomerular filtration of the contrast agent before it reaches the calyceal systems. It is important to see the renal outlines, as changes in the smooth outline may indicate the presence of tumours, cysts or cortical scarring. It also provides early information on renal size. It is possible to see appearances of renal blush for some time after injection and it is not always considered necessary to show the first blush immediately after injection of contrast agent, as renal outlines can be assessed along with the calyceal systems at later stages in the examination.

Around 5 minutes after injection the calyces should be seen to fill with contrast agent (Fig. 31.5), which then passes down the ureters to fill the bladder. In some cases the calyces empty quickly, preventing adequate demonstration of the calyces and renal pelvis. To counteract this, compression over the abdominal area level with the iliac crests is required, which restricts the flow of excreted contrast down the ureters. This therefore retains contrast agent in the kidney for a longer period to ensure adequate imaging of the collecting systems. Compression is usually left in place for around 5 minutes before an image of the kidneys is taken, but it must be noted that excessive and prolonged compression may cause the calyces to appear slightly blunted and distended (imitating early hydronephrosis). It is recognised that compression is often applied routinely, often 5 minutes after injection, to ensure optimal contrast build-up in the calyces, but there are contraindications to the use of compression that must be considered. These include:

- renal colic
- known renal calculi
- abdominal tenderness
- recent abdominal surgery
- recent pregnancy
- renal transplant

In addition to fast drainage there may be other reasons for failure to demonstrate the cortex or calyces, and these are related to pathology or overlying bowel gas and faeces. Additional or supplementary projections/techniques may be necessary to improve visualisation in these situations. These include:

- images in the opposite phase of suspended respiration to potentially change the position of overlying appearances such as bowel gas, faeces or radio-opacities
- zonography to clear images of bowel gas and faeces
- tomography to provide more detailed information after calyceal and renal pelvis images suggest or cannot exclude filling defects.

Tomography (and zonography) should not be used routinely and most manufacturers now offer limited equipment with this capability.

Once the calyceal system has been demonstrated it is necessary to provide information on the ureters and bladder; evidence of ureteric drainage is especially important. A KUB projection (around 15–20 minutes after injection) will show most of the tract, including some early bladder information (Fig. 31.6). If the use of compression has been necessary it must be released before this KUB can be taken, in order to allow kidney drainage. Compression release usually allows for good visualisation of ureteric drainage, as the contrast-enhanced urine flows down the ureter. Some sections of the ureters may not be visible on the KUB, owing to the fact that urine is transported down these structures by peristalsis and portions of the ureters will be constricted; these portions will not be visible on the image. This in itself does not really pose a problem: if the ureter is obstructed then there should be other evidence to suggest this, including distended or blunted calyces, hydronephrosis (seen initially as delayed concentration of contrast agent and later as distended and club-shaped calyces), distended ureters (or even megaureter) and failure of contrast to pass the obstructed area on prone KUB or oblique bladder images. The prone KUB is particularly useful to show the ureteric obstruction site: the kidneys lie posteriorly in the retroperitoneal abdomen and the ureters extend from the kidneys anteriorly until they are approximately level with L4/L5 and then towards the bladder, which is situated anteriorly in the pelvis. Therefore, in the supine patient urine is moving in an upward direction for the first section of the ureter; turning the patient prone after sitting them upright for 5 minutes reverses this and allows the urine to drain towards the site of obstruction.

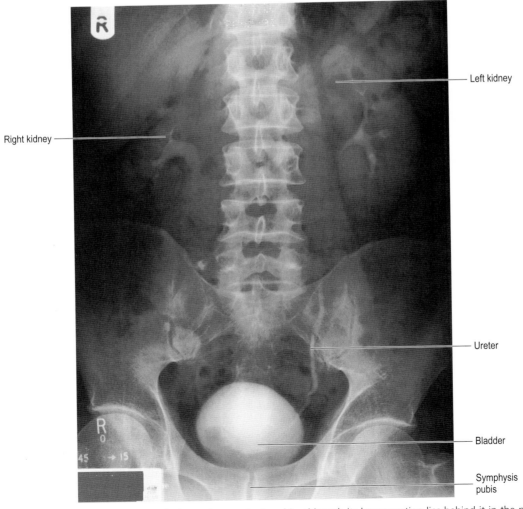

Figure 31.6 KUB projection. The bladder appears to sit above the symphysis pubis, although its lower portion lies behind it in the pelvic cavity. The appearance is a result of oblique rays at the lower periphery of the beam, which project the symphysis clear of the bladder.

SERIES OF PROJECTIONS FOR THE IVU

Texts describing excretion urography do vary on the suggested standard or routine 'protocol' for the examination,[7–10] but it must be accepted that owing to the decline in its use as a front-line examination a 'conventional' IVU series is no longer a valid concept. Providing a useful IVU series must be governed by the need to keep radiation dose to the patient as low as is reasonably practical, as stated in current regulations and guidelines,[3,11–13] and the need to use a series that will provide the best possible diagnostic images for each patient and their clinical history (or the appearances found as the examination progresses).

So, considering the range of projections available, strategies to improve visualisation of key areas and effects of pathology on the appearances of the system, it is difficult to present a set of instructions that are guaranteed to work every time for every patient. The most important point is that, even if a set 'protocol' has been agreed, it is essential that radiographers carrying out IVU examinations must have a thorough understanding of the aims of the examination to ensure that those aims are met. An example of a 'full' IVU procedure is outlined as follows:

1. Control KUB on inspiration for assessment of gross anatomy and presence of obvious pathology such as radio-opaque calculi
2. Position the patient for a cross-renal image
3. Injection of the contrast agent
4. Cross-renal 5 minutes after injection, to assess renal outlines and calyces and taken on arrested expiration. If calyces are not well demonstrated, apply compression if this is not contraindicated, and repeat the cross-renal 5 minutes later. If there is suspected pathology, or gas or faeces impair detail, undertake zonography or tomography of the renal area. Fulcrum heights selected for this will vary according to patient build, but three 'cuts' are usually taken from a range between 7 and 11 cm
5. If compression has not been applied, 15–20 minute KUB with contrast, taken on inspiration. If compression has been applied, release compression and undertake KUB after calyces have been adequately demonstrated
6. Collimated AP 15° caudal angle bladder image, taken after micturition

It is clear that this represents a significant number of exposures and it is increasingly rare to find that a full IVU series is undertaken in imaging departments. As the IVU is still undertaken in some centres, albeit with less frequency, it is necessary to outline how certain conditions may affect the IVU process.

Hydronephrosis (Fig. 31.7)

This may be known to pre-exist or may manifest itself during the examination as:

- Failure to demonstrate the calyces (especially easy to note when one kidney appears normal in comparison to a non-apparent kidney on the other side in the early stages of the examination). This is due to excessive urine, which dilutes the contrast agent, remaining in the kidney. Often there is concentration of the contrast agent later in the examination, but sometimes not for several hours. The cause of the hydronephrosis is impairment or obstruction of drainage at some point, from the pelviureteric junction down to the bladder, usually due to calculus or tumour. It can also be caused by bladder outlet obstruction

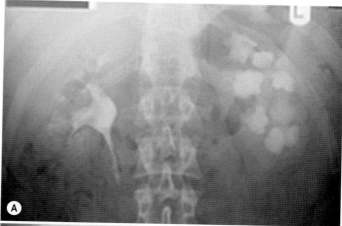
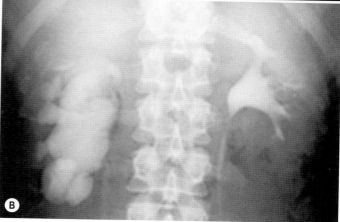

Figure 31.7 Hydronephrosis. Two cases of hydronephrosis: (A) shows the left side with late concentration of contrast agent in the blunt calyces; (B) shows the affected right side, but in this case the distended renal pelvis is also seen. Compare the hydronephrotic kidney in both cases with the normal kidney on the opposite side. KUB with contrast.

- Blunted and distended calyces
- Chronic hydronephrosis is likely to be accompanied by loss of renal cortex

Simple modification involves ensuring that there are delayed images of the affected kidney, initiated at around 20 minutes after injection, to allow for more contrast agent to mix with the urine and improve image contrast over the calyces and pelvis. If available, tomography may be useful, especially if gas and faeces make visualisation even more difficult. If the other kidney appears to be functioning the rest of the 'routine' aspect of the examination may continue, with further delayed images of the affected kidney being supplied at intervals (depending on how quickly concentration of contrast agent appears to be progressing). Micturition is delayed until adequate demonstration of both kidneys has been achieved, unless several hours pass and this is not possible.

Ureteric obstruction

Hydronephrosis will manifest itself as a result of obstruction, and the radiographer will therefore initiate modification for hydronephrosis, followed by methods to show the site of obstruction. These include:

- Sitting the patient for 5 minutes (or 10–15 minutes if the hydronephrosis is severe) and then undertaking a prone KUB image
- Tilting the patient (if a tilt facility is available) with their head up for 5–15 minutes and undertaking a cross-renal image in this position
- When the suspected site of obstruction is at or near the vesicoureteric junction (where the lower ureter lies behind the contrast filled bladder): oblique bladder, with affected side raised
- At post-micturition stage, undertaking a KUB image to show contrast and urine remaining in the ureter above the site of obstruction

Renal colic as an emergency

Exclusion of calculus is essential and a limited IVU series will offer this if the first choice of CT is unavailable. The acutely ill patient will present in the emergency situation. It is possible to keep radiation exposures to a minimum and a limited series is possible, suggested as:

1. Control KUB
2. Administration of contrast agent
3. KUB 15 minutes after injection

Radiation protection and the IVU

Protection is afforded as for the AP abdomen for the AP supine KUB projection; the supine or oblique projections of renal outlines require placement of lead rubber over the lower abdomen. As the edge of collimation for cross-renal, oblique and KUB projections falls next to breast tissue in adult women, it is recommended that lead rubber is also placed over the breasts for these images. The upper abdomen can be protected during the oblique bladder projection.

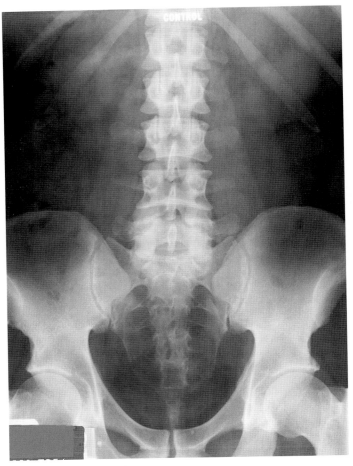

Figure 31.8 KUB control.

RADIOGRAPHIC PROJECTIONS FOR THE IVU

For all IVU projections the image receptor (IR) is horizontal, using antiscatter grid

Kidneys, ureters and bladder (KUB) (Fig. 31.8)

This projection may be undertaken as a 'control' image for the IVU examination (Fig. 31.8) or as a standalone projection to assess the position of existing radio-opaque calculi. Discussion on the AP abdomen in Chapter 24 carries many points which are also relevant to the KUB projection.

Positioning

- The patient is initially positioned as for the supine abdomen (see Chapter 24, Fig. 24.1)

Beam direction and focus receptor distance (FRD)

Vertical
100–115 cm or higher in tall patients

Centring

In the midline at the level of the iliac crests

Collimation

Symphysis pubis, upper poles of kidneys

The lateral borders of collimation can be brought in to coincide with the ASISs (anterior superior iliac spines), as information on the whole of the abdomen will not be needed for IVU unless additional general information on the abdomen is requested. This will avoid unnecessary irradiation of lateral portions of the abdomen.

Expose on arrested respiration

In the discussion on arrested respiration for the AP abdomen (Ch. 24) comments are made on the phase of arrested respiration during exposure. These are also relevant to the KUB projection, and exposure on suspended inspiration is recommended to ensure the whole of the system is included on this image.

Criteria for assessing image quality

- Symphysis pubis and renal outlines are included on the image
- Spinous processes of the vertebrae are seen coincident with the midline of the image, and centralised and aligned down the middle of the vertebral bodies
- Symmetry of the iliac crests
- Sharp image demonstrating soft tissue of the kidneys in contrast with bowel gas and bony structures

Common errors	Possible reasons
Symphysis pubis not included on the image	Inaccurate centring/positioning or tall patient? It may be necessary to undertake two projections to cover the area. It is suggested that these are (a) an image with symphysis pubis and as much upper tissue as possible is included, and (b) a cross-renal image. Excessive overlap of irradiated areas should be avoided
Upper abdomen not included; symphysis pubis is well above the lower edge of the film	May have been centred using the lateral borders of iliac crest rather than the highest point of crests at the back
Vertebral column is not coincident with the midline of the film	Xiphisternum to symphysis line is inaccurately positioned, or scoliotic patient
Spinous processes are not demonstrated in the midline of vertebral bodies	MSP not perpendicular to table-top; palpate ASIS to ensure it is equidistant from the table or patient is scoliosed

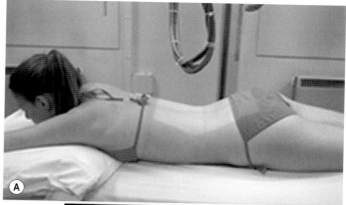

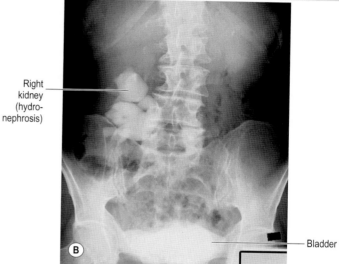

Right kidney (hydro-nephrosis)

Bladder

Figure 31.9 Prone KUB. (B) is a prone image which shows hydronephrosis on the right side. Note how the position affects the appearances of the pelvis and bladder compared to the supine KUB in Figure 31.7. The iliac crests appear flattened and much of the bladder now appears to lie behind the symphysis pubis (rather than above it as in the supine KUB). These differences are the result of the effects of oblique rays and change in position of the structures.

Prone KUB (Fig. 31.9A,B)

This projection is used to demonstrate the site of ureteric obstruction, draining the affected kidney so that contrast and urine lie at the lowest possible point (the site of obstruction). The patient should be asked to sit up for around 5 minutes to encourage kidney drainage, before turning prone for positioning. If the patient is unable to sit, their trunk can be propped up into a semi-recumbent position using pillows and sponges.

Positioning

- The patient is prone, head turned to the side and arms raised onto the pillow for stability and comfort. Care must be taken to ensure that any needle in situ is not moved
- The median sagittal plane (MSP) is coincident with the long axis of the table
- For males, lead rubber or lead gonad protection is applied, below the buttocks, to protect the gonads
- ASISs are equidistant from the table-top

Beam direction and FRD

Vertical
100–115 cm FRD or higher in tall patients

Centring

Over the spine, level with the iliac crests

Collimation

Symphysis pubis, renal outlines

Expose on arrested inspiration

Criteria for assessing image quality

- Symphysis pubis and renal outlines are included on the image. However, as this projection is intended to identify the location of ureteric obstruction, it may not be necessary to insist that all of the bladder and upper renal outlines are included

- Spinous processes of vertebrae seen coincident with the midline of the image, and centralised and aligned down the middle of the vertebral bodies
- Symmetry of iliac crests, which appear flattened out compared to their appearances on the supine AP image
- The symphysis pubis should appear to be deeper and the obturator foramina more open than in the AP projection
- Sharp image demonstrating contrast filled structures in contrast with bowel gas and bony structures

Common error	Possible reason
Rotation, demonstrated by asymmetry of the iliac crests and spinous processes not seen in the midline of the vertebral column	Trunk has been turned to one side as the patient turns their head for comfort. Often this is addressed by simply turning the patient's head the opposite way

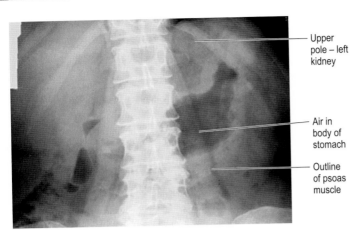

— Upper pole – left kidney

— Air in body of stomach

— Outline of psoas muscle

Figure 31.10 Cross-renal control.

Common errors	Possible reasons
Vertebral column not coincident with the midline of the film	Xiphisternum to symphysis line is inaccurately positioned, or scoliotic patient. Severe scoliosis may significantly alter the kidneys' positions and necessitate less stringent lateral collimation
Spinous processes not demonstrated in the midline of vertebral bodies	MSP is not perpendicular to the table-top; palpate ASIS to ensure it is equidistant from the table, or patient is scoliosed
Vertebral column not coincident with the midline of the film	Xiphisternum to symphysis line inaccurately positioned or scoliotic patient

Supine AP kidneys ('cross renal', 'cross kidney') (Figs 31.4, 31.10)

Positioning

- The patient is positioned as for the supine AP abdomen

Beam direction and FRD

Vertical
100 cm FRD

Centring

In the midline, at a point between the xiphisternum and the level of the lower costal margins

Collimation

Renal outlines
The lateral borders of collimation can be left as those used for the KUB projection, or modified after the KUB has been viewed.

Expose on arrested respiration

Exposure should be made on arrested expiration so that the renal shadows lie in a consistent position when exposures of the area are made at later stages in the examination.

Criteria for assessing image quality

- Renal outlines are shown on the image
- Spinous processes of vertebrae are seen coincident with the midline of the image, and centralised and aligned down the middle of the vertebral bodies
- Sharp image demonstrating renal outlines tissue in contrast with bowel gas and bony structures for this projection when undertaken without contrast enhancement. After injection of contrast agent, image contrast will be enhanced further and the renal outlines should still show in good contrast to other soft tissue; calyces and renal pelvis should also be seen in contrast with the renal cortex

Oblique kidney (Fig. 31.11A,B)

This projection is used at the control stage to ascertain the position of radio-opacities that appear to lie over the renal outline, or after injection of contrast to clear appearances of bowel gas or faecal matter from the renal image.

Positioning

- From the supine AP position the patient's trunk is rotated 30° *towards* the side under examination. Radiolucent pads are placed under the trunk to aid immobilisation and the arm on the lowered side is raised onto the pillow for comfort

Beam direction and FRD

Vertical
100 cm FRD

Centring

In the midline, midway between the xiphisternum and level of the lower costal margins

As the renal outlines generally lie with the left kidney slightly higher than the right, previous cross-renal images can be assessed to ascertain the exact kidney position before centring the beam for the oblique kidney projection. Note that centring is recommended as over the midline and not in the midclavicular line (sometimes erroneously quoted by students); this is due to the posterior position of the kidneys in the abdominal cavity – as the trunk rotates, the image of the kidney moves closer to the spine.

Collimation

Kidney under examination

Criteria for assessing image quality

- Kidney under examination is seen on image
- If contrast agent has been injected the calyces and renal pelvis should appear shortened in a lateromedial direction

Common error	Possible reason
Medial aspect of the kidney is omitted from the image	Centring over the midclavicular line rather than over the midline of the patient

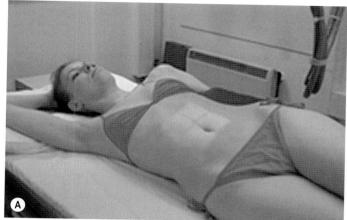

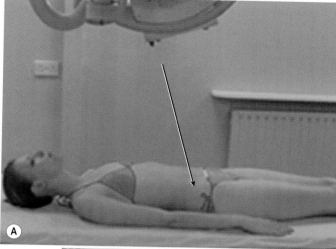

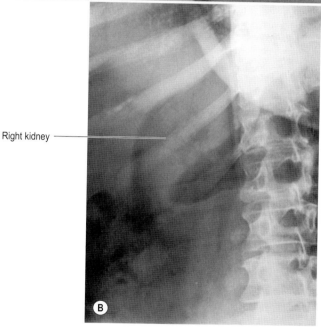

Right kidney

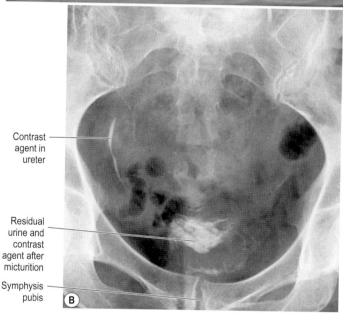

Contrast agent in ureter

Residual urine and contrast agent after micturition

Symphysis pubis

Figure 31.11 Oblique kidney. (A) Note that the central ray is in the midline, not the midclavicular line (which is sometimes wrongly believed to be the centring plane for this projection); (B) the oblique kidney projection is often used before injection of contrast agent (as in this case) to provide further information on the position of opacities which overlie the kidney on supine images. It can also be used after injection of contrast agent, at any stage thereafter.

Figure 31.12 15° bladder.

Centring

In the midline, midway between the upper border of the symphysis pubis and the level of the ASIS

IR displacement may be necessary to ensure that the image lies within its boundaries.

Collimation

Symphysis pubis, bladder, lower ureters

Criteria for assessing image quality

- Symphysis pubis, bladder and lower ureters are shown on the image
- Symphysis pubis is seen below and clear of the bladder
- Sharp image demonstrating the bladder in contrast with the surrounding soft tissue, if contrast has been used. This projection is less likely to be produced without contrast agent but is sometimes used as an additional control film if the lower abdomen has not been demonstrated on the KUB

Bladder: supine AP 15° caudal angle (Fig. 31.12A,B)

Positioning

- The patient is positioned as for the supine abdomen (KUB)

Beam direction and FRD

Initially vertical, angled 15° caudally
100 cm FRD

Common errors	Possible reasons
Top of bladder is close to the top of the image, or outside collimation/boundaries of the film	Centring too low, often found to be over the symphysis pubis or IR was not displaced correctly (too low)
Base of bladder is omitted from the boundaries of the film	Centring too high or IR was not displaced correctly (too high)

Posterior oblique bladder (Fig. 31.13A,B)

This projection is usually used to demonstrate the lower end of the ureter as it enters the bladder posteriorly and inferiorly. To achieve this, the area is brought into profile by raising the side of interest; note that this is opposite obliquity to that required for the oblique kidney. Caudal angulation is not vital as the area of interest is the vesicoureteric junction, which is not superimposed over the pubis in an AP direction. However, angulation may reveal more information if it is required.

Positioning

- The patient is initially positioned as for the supine AP KUB
- The affected side is raised 30° and the trunk is supported and immobilised with radiolucent pads
- The arm on the lowered side is placed on the pillow for support

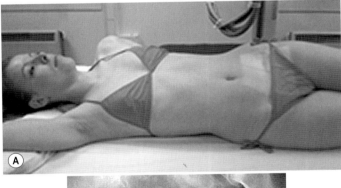

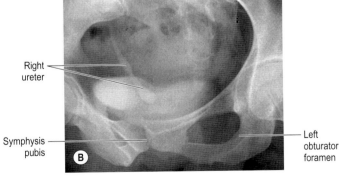

Right ureter

Symphysis pubis

Left obturator foramen

Figure 31.13 Oblique bladder. The oblique projection aims to raise the lower end of the ureter in question to bring it from behind the bladder. In this case the intention was to show the lower end of the left ureter, which has failed to be demonstrated as there does not appear to be contrast agent in this lower portion (possibly because there is actually no obstruction at this point). The right ureter is seen, however, projected behind the contrast-filled bladder. There does appear to be some distension in this ureter, and an oblique with the right side raised will help confirm or exclude obstruction.

Beam direction and FRD

Vertical or caudally angled 15°
100 cm FRD

Centring

Midway between the middle of the upper border of the symphysis pubis and the ASIS on the raised side. IR displacement is required if an angle is used

Collimation

Symphysis pubis, bladder

Criteria for assessing image quality

- Symphysis pubis and bladder are seen on the image
- Contrast-filled ureter on the raised side is seen at its site of entry into the bladder

Common error	Possible reason
Ischium of raised side is superimposed over lower ureter and bladder	Too much obliquity

BLADDER AND URETHRA: CYSTOGRAPHY AND URETHROGRAPHY

It must be mentioned that US offers high-quality information on the bladder and prostate, especially due to its ability to differentiate between benign and malignant prostatic disease. It is also more efficient in its representation of disease affecting anterior and posterior bladder walls. It has largely replaced cystography in the adult, but cystography may still have a place in the assessment of vesicoureteric reflux, which is especially relevant in patients with recurrent UTI. This condition is most frequently assessed in children.[6]

Cystography involves the administration of contrast agent via the urethra and into the bladder. Fluoroscopic investigation after surgery (e.g. radical cystoprostatectomy) is a quick and efficient method of identifying any possible leaks and is possibly the most common use for this particular examination. The examination is undertaken using fluoroscopic control, and bladder emptying and the urethra are also monitored while the patient micturates. This is termed *micturating cystourethrography* (MCU). Its potential for embarrassment is clear, and the radiographer has the usual responsibility to respect the patient's privacy and dignity during the procedure. In addition, the radiographer must clearly convey that they know this is important for the patient. The opportunity for this lies in clear explanation of the procedure before the examination.

MCU (Fig. 31.14A,B)

Referral criteria

- Stress incontinence
- Suspected vesicoureteric reflux
- Assessment of the urethra in micturition

Contraindications

- Cystitis or other UTI infection
- Urethral stricture

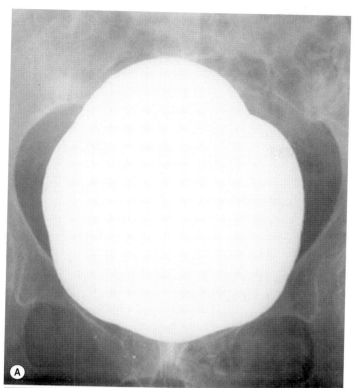

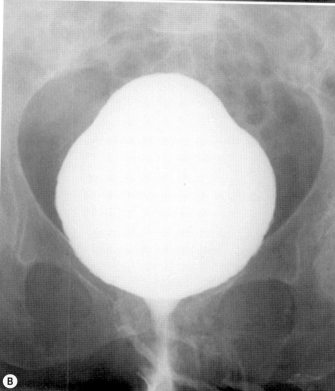

Figure 31.14 (A) MCU – full bladder; (B) MCU – during micturition.

Contrast agent

- High or low osmolar contrast agent – up to 300 mL of 150 mg iodine (mgI) per mL

Additional equipment

- Sterile towels
- Drip stand
- Saline
- Clamp
- Sterile gloves
- Gauze swabs
- Antiseptic skin wash and sterile receptacle
- Foley catheter
- Sterile anaesthetic jelly
- Incontinence pads
- Receptacle for receiving urine

Patient preparation

- Explanation of the procedure, paying particular attention to the fact that patient privacy is taken most seriously. Requirement for micturition during the examination should also be explained and that it will be necessary for the patient to let staff know when their bladder feels full. The patient will also need to mimic the action of 'straining' without passing urine, and this must also be explained in advance
- Micturition immediately prior to the examination

Technique

- The area around the urethral opening is cleansed and the urethra is catheterised
- The bladder is drained of any remaining urine via the catheter
- After connecting the contrast agent to the catheter, the contrast agent vessel is hooked onto a drip stand and agent is allowed to run into the bladder; the flow should be controlled initially to allow early filling to be assessed fluoroscopically (to ensure that the catheter is positioned in the bladder and not in the vagina or ureter)
- Contrast agent is followed by saline, until the patient indicates that their bladder feels very full; it may be necessary to tilt the patient's head down slightly to ensure that the bladder fills completely
- Spot images are recorded in a variation of positions which include:
  - any position where vesicoureteric reflux is seen
  - AP
  - right posterior oblique (RPO) and left posterior oblique (LPO) (as shown in normal positioning descriptor outlined in Chapter 29 and Fig. 29.1) which will show distal ureters
  - lateral to demonstrate a fistula
- Additional images are taken with the patient 'straining'. The lateral is considered to be useful as well as an AP; male patients may be able to use a urine receptacle in the lateral decubitus position. For females, sitting erect will allow them to sit on a bedpan. This may require special equipment such as a high platform, which is placed against the erect fluoroscopy unit that has had the step removed
- The catheter is removed and further images are taken during micturition

Patient aftercare

- The urethral area is wiped with a gauze swab
- The patient may wish to micturate further after the examination is complete
- The patient may wish to wash the genital area, and facilities should be available for this
- Antibiotic cover should be given to patients who have demonstrated vesicoureteric reflux

Possible complications

- UTI
- (Rarely) reaction to contrast agent
- Perforation of the tract by the catheter

Urethrography

Only the male urethra is examined by this method.

Referral criteria

- Urethral fistula
- Congenital abnormality
- Urethral stricture

Contraindications

- UTI
- Recent cystoscopy or catheterisation
- Contrast agent
- 5–20 mL high osmolar contrast media (HOCM) or low osmolar contrast media (LOCM), 200–280 mgI/mL

Additional equipment

- Sterile towels
- 20 mL syringe
- Filling tube for contrast agent
- Knuttson's (penile) clamp or urethral catheter with balloon
- Sterile water if a balloon catheter used
- 2 mL syringe for pushing water into the balloon
- Sterile gloves
- Gauze swabs
- Antiseptic skin wash and sterile receptacle
- Sterile anaesthetic jelly
- Incontinence pads
- Receptacle for receiving urine

Patient preparation

- Explanation of the procedure
- Empty bladder

Technique

- The area is cleansed with antiseptic and anaesthetic jelly inserted into the urethra
- The penile clamp is applied to the tip of the urethra *or* the catheter inserted into the fossa navicularis. If the catheter is used it is also necessary to expand its balloon using 1 or 2 mL of water
- Approximately 5–10 mL of contrast agent is injected into the urethra and checked by fluoroscopic control. Further administration of contrast agent may be required to fill the long urethra or filling defects

- Spot images in RPO, LPO and AP positions are taken (following normal positioning descriptor as outlined in Ch. 29 and in Fig. 29.1), plus additional images if they provide useful information
- Further contrast filling may be necessary in order to allow the patient to micturate enough contrast agent to show the urethra during bladder voiding. Spot images may also be recorded during this action

Patient aftercare

- Cleanse the area and allow the patient to micturate further if they wish

Possible complications

- UTI
- Urethral tear

OTHER METHODS FOR IMAGING THE URINARY SYSTEM

Ultrasound

In many cases this has replaced contrast radiography as a first-line examination for the urinary system, but features such as the site of ureteric obstruction or calculus size may still require alternative imaging. Along with CT it is the front-line investigation for the assessment of a renal mass,[3] and is also an extremely useful tool for the assessment of renal transplant patients, particularly when using Doppler.[14]

CT

As a standalone investigation CT has certainly improved with the combination of low-dose unenhanced and ultra-low dose techniques coming to the fore, especially in the acute situation.[1,2,15] Since the first edition of this book the need to discuss CT as a potential competitor in imaging the renal tract has diminished owing to its proven emergence as a main contributor to renal imaging, becoming the front-line recommendation for the detection of a renal mass.[16]

An obvious advantage of CT is its ability to produce diagnostic images without contrast agent (unenhanced CT) and its associated risks. Another big attraction of CT urography has to be the 3D image reconstructions now widely available. Advances in medical software mean that information obtained through coronal sectional imaging can be digitally reconfigured to produce accurate anatomy/pathology that can be viewed from any angle on a computer screen.

MRI

The role of MRI should not be forgotten, particularly with regard to the question of risk of radiation dose to the patient. MRI is a relative newcomer in urinary imaging and has been used to demonstrate ureteric dilatation and obstruction.[17] It is not as accurate as other modalities in the diagnosis of small calculi, owing to the bright signal received from urine, which can obscure tiny stones. The place of MRI in this type of investigation is governed mainly by the patient and their suitability, or unsuitability, for other techniques. If the use of contrast agent or ionising radiation is contraindicated (e.g. in children or pregnant women), then MRI has proved its worth, especially as it compares favourably with contrast-enhanced CT when assessing renal masses.[3]

RNI

Renal function is effectively assessed by radionuclide imaging, which is probably the most appropriate technique for this. It can differentiate between obstructive uropathy and non-obstructive dilation of the renal pelvis, delineate areas of renal scarring due to infection, and localise ectopic kidneys after ultrasound fails to find their location. Its ability to assess function is also useful in the assessment of transplanted kidneys.[3] It can also assess vesicoureteric reflux, providing a less invasive and less traumatic diagnostic tool than cystography, as it does not involve urethral catheterization.[7]

RADIOGRAPHIC EXAMINATION OF THE FEMALE REPRODUCTIVE SYSTEM

Hysterosalpingography (HSG)

This is assessment of the anatomy of the uterus and uterine (fallopian) tubes, undertaken under fluoroscopic control. Spot images are recorded.

Referral criteria

- Infertility – to check for patency of uterine (fallopian) tubes
- Recurrent spontaneous abortion (miscarriage)
- To assess patency of uterine tubes after reversal of female sterilisation
- It is possible that the procedure may have a therapeutic effect and clear obstructed uterine tubes

Contraindications

- Known or possible pregnancy
- Recent surgery
- Recent miscarriage
- Recent infection such as pelvic inflammatory disease or salpingitis

Contrast agent

- Approximately 20 mL HOCM or LOCM 280–300 mgI/mL

Additional equipment

- Sterile towels
- 20 mL syringe
- Filling tube for contrast agent
- Sterile gloves
- Gauze swabs
- Antiseptic skin wash and sterile receptacle
- Vaginal speculum
- Vulsellum forceps
- Uterine cannula or Foley catheter
- Incontinence pads
- A portable Anglepoise light will help with visualisation of the cervix
- Sanitary pad

Patient preparation

- Prior to attending for the examination the patient is advised to use contraception from their last period and up to the examination, or abstain from sexual intercourse. Alternatively,

the '10-day rule' is applied and the patient is only examined in this 10-day safe period after menstruation. However, some practitioners are reluctant to undertake the examination close to menstruation (i.e. within 4 days) to avoid the risk of extravasation or intravasation of contrast agent via the uterine endometrium.[9] If the 10-day rule is to be used in conjunction with this second rule, the patient can only be examined during days 5–10 of their menstrual cycle, providing a very narrow window of time for this examination. On arrival, the radiographer should ascertain that information on pregnancy status is correct
- The patient may feel more comfortable if she micturates before the examination
- The procedure is explained, stressing that staff will observe the privacy rights of the patient. It will also be helpful to indicate that the procedure may be uncomfortable, rather than painful

Technique

- The area is cleansed and the speculum inserted to allow for location of the cervix
- The vagina and cervix are cleansed
- It may be necessary to stabilise the position of the cervix with the Vulsellum forceps before using the cannula. The cannula or catheter is inserted into the external os of the cervix and the contrast agent injected into the uterus. The speculum is removed, though sometimes it may be left in place if secure cannulisation of the cervix is at risk
- Filling of the uterine cavity is observed under pulsed or intermittent fluoroscopy
- Spot images are recorded in the AP position when the contrast agent is seen to reach the uterine cornua, when it starts to fill the fallopian (uterine) tubes, and then when the contrast agent has filled the tubes, spilling into the peritoneal cavity (Fig. 31.15)
- The cannula or catheter is removed and the area is wiped with gauze swabs

Patient aftercare

- Give advice on using analgesia if the patient has low abdominal discomfort or slight cramps; advise that slight aching is not a matter for concern
- Provide the patient with a sanitary pad
- Explain that slight bleeding is possible and may last for a few days
- Advise that heavy bleeding or clotting is not normal and medical help should be sought if these occur

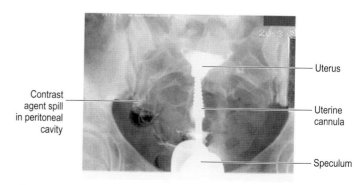

Contrast agent spill in peritoneal cavity — Uterus — Uterine cannula — Speculum

Figure 31.15 Hysterosalpingogram.

Possible complications

- Trauma to the vagina or cervix
- Severe abdominal cramps
- Extravasation/intravasation of contrast agent via the endometrium to the uterine veins; this creates the risk of embolus
- Infection

Other methods for assessment of fallopian tubes and uterine abnormalities

MR HSG

A recent study has shown that this examination can become a viable alternative to the traditional HSG.[18] However, as it does not use the traditional metal cannula but a plastic cannula with a balloon, it may be that this equipment aids in the result, although the improved spatial resolution of MR may still be consequential.

Ultrasound

Similar in principle to the HSG but the hysterosonogram uses saline instead of radio-opaque contrast. It is highly sensitive for identifying abnormalities in the uterus but cannot compete with the conventional method for assessing the fallopian tubes.

REFERENCES

1. Kluner C, et al. Does ultra-low-dose CT with a radiation dose equivalent to that of KUB suffice to detect renal and ureteral calculi? Journal of Computer Assisted Tomography 2006;30(1):44–50.

2. Fowler J, et al. Clinical evaluation of ultra-low dose contrast-enhanced CT in patients presenting with acute ureteric colic. British Journal of Medical & Surgical Urology 2011;4(2):56–63.

3. RCR Working Party. Making the best use of a department of radiology: guidelines for doctors. 6th ed. London: The Royal College of Radiologists; 2007.

4. Prezioso D, et al. Lifestyle in patients with LUTS suggestive of BPH. European Urology 2001;40(Suppl. 1):9–12.

5. Noroozian M, et al. Multislice CT urography: state of the art. British Journal of Radiology 2004;77:74–86.

6. Fefferman NR, et al. The efficacy of digital fluoroscopic image capture in the evaluation of vesicoureteral reflux in children. Pediatric Radiology 2009;39:1179–87.

7. Ziessman HA, Majd M. Importance of methodology on (99m)technetium dimercapto-succinic acid scintigraphic image quality: imaging pilot study for RIVUR (Randomized Intervention for Children With Vesicoureteral Reflux) multicenter investigation. Journal of Urology 2009;182(1):272–9.

8. Unett EM, Royle AJ. Radiographic techniques and image evaluation. London: Chapman & Hall; 1997.

9. Carver E, Carver B, editors. Medical imaging: techniques, reflection and evaluation. Edinburgh: Churchill Livingstone; 2006.

10. Chapman S, Nakielny R. A guide to radiological procedures. 5th ed. Edinburgh: Saunders; 2009.

11. The Ionising Radiation (Medical Exposure) Regulations 2006. London: HMSO.

12. Statutory Instrument 1999 No. 3232. The Ionising Radiations Regulations 1999. HMSO: United Kingdom.

13. European Commission Directorate-General for the Environment 2000.

Referral guidelines for imaging. Radiation protection 118.

14. Jimenez C, et al. Ultrasonography in kidney transplantation: Values and new developments. Transplantation Reviews (Orlando) 2009;23:209–13.

15. Rimondini M, et al. Effective dose in X ray examinations: comparison between unenhanced helical CT (UHCT) and intravenous urography (IVU) in the evaluation of renal colic. European College of Radiology; proceedings of ECR 2002: presentation C 0732.

16. Lee EY, et al. Renal cell carcinoma visible only during the corticomedullary phase of enhancement. AJR 2005;184:104–6.

17. Sudah M, et al. Patients with acute flank pain: comparison of MR urography with unenhanced helical CT. Radiology 2002;223:98–105.

18. Sadewski EA, et al. MR Hysterosalpingography with an angiographic time resolved 3D pulse sequence; assessment of tubal patency. AJR 2008;191(5):1381–5.

Chapter 32

Cardiovascular system

Mark Cowling, Colin Monaghan

INTRODUCTION

This chapter will consider diagnostic angiography and venography. There are now several non-invasive methods available for evaluation of the cardiovascular system, such as Doppler ultrasound, computed tomography angiography (CTA) and magnetic resonance angiography (MRA). However, intra-arterial catheter angiography and venography remain important diagnostic tools and are likely to remain in clinical use for some years. Indeed, although it is invasive, intra-arterial catheter angiography has the benefit of being able to proceed directly to intervention should that be appropriate.

EQUIPMENT

Digital subtraction angiography (DSA) has been available for over 20 years. It is noteworthy that in the 2000 NCEPOD (National Confidential Enquiry into Perioperative Deaths)[1] report on interventional vascular radiology it was stated that 8% of hospitals in the UK were still undertaking vascular work on barium screening systems. No recent, more up-to-date data are available, but it seems likely that this situation is now much improved, and certainly it should be considered unacceptable to be performing complex vascular imaging and intervention without access to DSA.

All dedicated DSA units have the X-ray tube and image intensifier mounted on a 'C-arm', allowing oblique views to be obtained easily without moving the patient. When angiographic images are acquired (often referred to as an angiographic run), a number of images are obtained before the intra-arterial injection of contrast; these are used as mask images. Contrast is then injected and the arteries are opacified. The mask image is then subtracted from the contrast images. All detail on the mask, such as bone, is thus removed from subsequent images, leaving only the contrast opacifying the vessels on the image. Although the spatial resolution of this technique is a little less than that for film-based angiography, this is more than compensated for by the much greater contrast resolution. In other words, the finer detail is not obscured by overlying structures such as bone. Digital acquisition of the image data means that the subtraction process is performed by computer, and the subtracted images are available in real time.

In general DSA is an excellent technique, but there can be problems with image quality, particularly due to patient movement. One method of dealing with this is to use a facility termed pixel shifting. This involves using the computer to move the mask and contrast images relative to one another such that they are properly aligned, thereby removing misregistration artefact (Fig. 32.1A,B). This method of image processing is most suited to movement in relatively simple anatomical structures such as a limb, and also in situations where movement has only been slight. More extreme movements can be very difficult, if not impossible, to correct by pixel shifting. This is because pixel shifting involves a simple translation of image data in two dimensions, whereas patient movement actually occurs in three dimensions, often involving a degree of rotation, rather than pure translation. Modern automated methods of pixel shifting can be of benefit where more extreme patient movement has occurred; however, there are still limitations to the technique, and attention to good patient positioning and explanation remains critical to obtaining good results.

Further degradation of image quality can be encountered owing to patient breathing and bowel peristalsis during an acquisition. The former can be problematic in both the chest and the abdomen, and pixel shifting is of little value. It may prove necessary to perform the angiographic run again, but if a patient is very ill (the most common reason for being unable to suspend respiration adequately) it is often more helpful to acquire a larger number of masks than normal while the patient is breathing gently and 'remask' each image to improve the diagnostic quality. This involves changing to a different mask while looking at a single contrast image. The mask giving the least degree of misregistration artefact is chosen.

Misregistration due to bowel movement can cause marked degradation of images of the abdominal aorta and its branches, as well as the iliac arteries. In addition, it is nearly impossible to obtain images of diagnostic quality when undertaking mesenteric arteriography for gastrointestinal bleeding. Misregistration caused by gut peristalsis can be largely prevented by administering Buscopan (hyoscine-*N*-butylbromide) 20 mg either intravenously or through the arteriography catheter. This abolishes peristalsis for about 15 minutes, thereby improving the quality of arteriographic images in the abdomen and

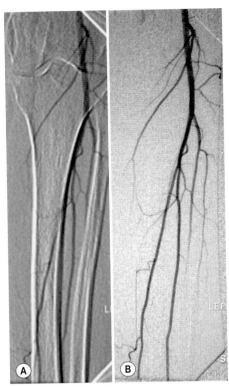

Figure 32.1 (A) Digital subtraction arteriogram of distal calf showing misregistration artefact due to patient movement; (B) after pixel shifting the image quality is much improved.

pelvis. With regard to images obtained during mesenteric angiography for acute gastrointestinal bleeding, misregistration of bowel loops can give the impression of contrast extravasation into the lumen where there is none. Buscopan can be very helpful and should be administered, but it is also important to review the images without subtraction in order to avoid misdiagnosis.

Other techniques have been used to try to avoid problems with gut misregistration. For example, bowel loops can be displaced laterally by using a balloon between the patient and the image intensifier to compress the abdomen. However, such methods can often no longer be used because of the presence of proximity sensors in the equipment that prevent it from moving if it is in contact with the patient or any other object.

TECHNIQUE

Points of access for arteriography

Arteriography is most commonly performed by introducing a catheter through the common femoral artery in the groin. If this is not possible, the preferred route is to use the brachial artery at the level of the elbow joint. Alternatives include the radial artery, high brachial and axillary routes. Translumbar aortography, involving direct puncture of the abdominal aorta, is no longer practised in the UK.

The transfemoral approach

This involves the administration of local anaesthetic into the skin and deeper tissues, followed by the insertion of an arterial puncture needle. A suitable guide wire is introduced through the needle into the vessel. It is usual to observe the passage of the wire proximally through the iliac arteries into the abdominal aorta using fluoroscopy. This is helpful because it is possible for the wire to enter the inferior epigastric artery rather than the external iliac artery. This problem is immediately obvious if observed on fluoroscopy, and can be corrected. It should be noted, however, that as operators become more experienced and used to the 'feel' of the guide wire in the vessel, they may undertake little or no screening during this part of the procedure unless they encounter resistance to the passage of the wire.

The guide wire may fail to advance satisfactorily for a variety of reasons. Sometimes this can be resolved simply by repositioning the needle tip so that backflow of blood is improved, indicating that the needle tip has been positioned more ideally within the vessel lumen. However, on other occasions it may be necessary to screen over the needle tip while the operator is manipulating the puncture needle, and possibly even injecting contrast. At such times the primary beam is very near the operator's hands. It is important that the screening radiographer remains vigilant and collimates as closely as possible to the needle tip to reduce the chances of the operator's hands entering the primary beam.

Once the guide wire has been correctly introduced into the aorta the needle is removed, leaving the wire in place, and a suitable catheter or sheath is introduced over the wire. The next stage in the procedure will depend very much on the examination to be performed, and will be dealt with below.

Complications of the transfemoral route are minimal during diagnostic arteriography; however, the recommended upper limit of complications for audit purposes is as high as 3%.[2]

The transbrachial route

This route is very useful if the femoral pulses are impalpable, but if a purely diagnostic study is required, CTA should be considered. The complication rate associated with this route of access is in fact quite low, and in the past it would have been quite reasonable to use it routinely, and it may even have had advantages for outpatient or day-case angiography. However, it is used much less frequently than the transfemoral route, probably because it is technically more demanding and therefore a little more time-consuming, and also because of concerns about placing a catheter across the origin of the left vertebral artery. The technique is very similar to that described above for the transfemoral route. However, a vascular sheath is used to facilitate the administration of antispasmodic and anticoagulant drugs during the procedure, as these are considered to reduce the incidence of brachial artery occlusion.

Most arterial territories can be examined using the transbrachial route, although the manipulations required are often more difficult because the catheters tend to be longer. In general the left brachial approach will be used wherever possible, as this avoids placing the catheter across the origins of the great vessels, with the associated potential for formation of pericatheter thrombus and consequent embolic stroke. Most frequently the femoral arteries will be examined, which involves placing the catheter inferiorly into the descending thoracic aorta and distally into the abdominal aorta. Although the initial brachial puncture and vascular sheath insertion can usually be achieved without fluoroscopy, when passing a pigtail catheter proximally into the brachial and subsequently axillary artery it is not at all uncommon for the catheter and guide wire to enter branches such as the circumflex humeral arteries. It is therefore necessary to use fluoroscopy to follow the passage of the catheter and guide wire.

It can be difficult to screen sufficiently laterally, and careful positioning of the patient before the start of the procedure is important. More modern angiographic tables are able to pivot laterally; moving the table in this way can be very helpful. Once the catheter and guide wire have reached the origin of the subclavian artery, the operator will manipulate the catheter into the descending aorta. Depending on the tortuosity of the vessels this may be relatively difficult. One of the issues is the proximity of aerated lung to the aortic arch, which can make the catheter very difficult to see. Use of filters, collimators and sometimes magnification can be very helpful in improving visibility. In addition, on modern angiographic units with pulsed fluoroscopy it can occasionally be helpful to raise the pulse rate, which will improve image quality.

Complications of brachial puncture for diagnostic arteriography are also said to be low, with a rate of up to 0.3% requiring surgery being reported.[3] Minor complications not requiring surgery and resolving spontaneously have been reported as 8–15%.[3,4]

Other routes of access

Other routes of access are now much less commonly used. The axillary and high brachial routes were associated with a relatively high incidence of haematoma formation and occasional consequent nerve damage (up to 2.4%),[5,6] owing to difficulty in achieving adequate compression. The translumbar route is no longer used in the UK because of the high incidence of retroperitoneal bleeding, the need for a general anaesthetic and lack of flexibility for performing selective arteriography. Of the other routes mentioned at the beginning of this section, the transradial approach has found favour with many cardiologists. However, although radiologists have used this approach for arteriography, it has not entered widespread use.[7]

Intravenous DSA

This technique is now rarely, if ever, performed, but is mentioned here for completeness. It involves the injection of a large bolus of contrast, typically 50 mL, into a catheter placed directly into the right atrium. Performing multiple runs, for example during a femoral arteriogram, can therefore involve giving very large volumes of contrast. In addition, in the presence of poor cardiac function the images are frequently suboptimal. In general the images are of less good quality than those obtained using a direct arterial injection, but when DSA first entered clinical use this method represented a less invasive alternative to using arterial access.

Non-invasive vascular imaging is now so improved that intravenous DSA is usually unhelpful in providing any additional information that may be required.

ARTERIAL TERRITORIES EXAMINED

A variety of arterial territories can be examined, and the indications for each vary slightly. This section will discuss the approach to the examination of the various different territories, and, where relevant, will describe differences in technique according to the indication for the examination. Where projections are referred to, they are described in relationship to the image receptor (IR). For example, PA is a supine position, and anterior obliques are supine obliques with the named side of the oblique being that nearest the over-couch IR.

Femoral arteriography

This describes examination of the abdominal aorta, iliac arteries and arteries of the lower limbs. Indications for femoral arteriography are:

- Intermittent claudication
- Critical limb ischaemia
- Acute limb ischaemia
- Trauma
- Preoperative, e.g. prior to free flap skin grafting

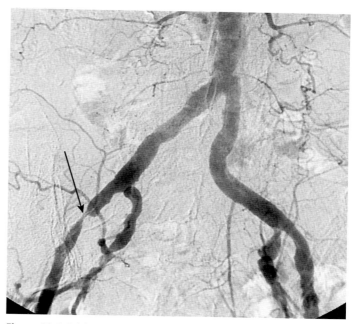

Figure 32.2 Pelvic view from a digital subtraction arteriogram showing a severe focal stenosis of the right external iliac artery (arrow).

The procedure is undertaken almost exclusively to demonstrate arterial stenoses and/or occlusions, and is the most commonly performed peripheral arteriogram at the time of writing (Fig. 32.2).

The patient lies supine on the angiographic table, legs placed as close together as possible. Some angiographic systems require the placement of lead rubber filters between and lateral to the legs. This reduces the variability in exposure across the field and will help to diminish flare. The filters also help to support the lower limbs and keep them still during acquisitions. Other devices for providing limb support, such as bean bags, are also available.

Having gained arterial access, the catheter, typically a pigtail, is positioned within the abdominal aorta. Contrast is then introduced using a pressure injector. Exact protocols for injection vary. A typical protocol is to administer 25 mL of a non-ionic iodine-based contrast medium, 300 mgI/mL, at 10 mL per second. The pressure is set at 750 psi with a rise time of 0.5 seconds.

With many angiographic systems it is necessary to image the lower limb vessels in sections. Thus an abdominal aortogram will be performed, followed by a pelvic view to image the iliac vessels, and so on until the entire lower limb down to the foot has been imaged.

This is a disadvantage compared to the traditional film changer systems, where a bolus of contrast was administered, a series of views taken in one position, the table then automatically moved to the next position, another set of films exposed, and so on until the whole lower limb was imaged. This allowed only about 70 mL of contrast to be used, rather than up to 150 mL, for an equivalent DSA examination acquiring images at individual levels.

Of course, the traditional non-subtracted film-based systems did not allow imaging in real time, meaning that if there were a significant difference in flow rates down the two lower limbs, only the vessels in one of them might successfully be imaged. In addition, it is possible to dilute the contrast used in a DSA examination, making the contrast doses similar.

Newer systems have attempted to address this issue with 'bolus chasing'. Precise protocols vary between manufacturers, but the principle involves obtaining mask images along the entire length of both legs and then injecting a single bolus of contrast and following this as it flows distally along the lower limb vessels. The flow of contrast can be monitored in real time, meaning that the table movement can be slowed or hastened appropriately. Some systems also allow the speed of table movement to be set up automatically, depending on the time taken for a test bolus of contrast to reach the popliteal artery. Regardless of the method used, however, the system will provide subtracted images along the entire length of the lower limbs.

Although this facility is useful, the image quality is less good than that provided by static images, examining a single area at a time, because the signal-to-noise ratio is reduced. However, by using bolus chasing to perform an overall 'survey' of the lower limb vasculature, followed by static images over areas of concern, it is possible to reduce the overall contrast dose.

The C-arm allows appropriate oblique views to be performed. This can be most useful in the iliac arteries, where either the posteroanterior (PA) view has shown no abnormality when a lesion is suspected clinically, or where there is a suspicion of a stenosis on the PA view and confirmation of its location and severity is required. If the right iliac arteries are to be imaged then a left anterior oblique (LAO) projection is used, and if the left iliac arteries are to be examined a right anterior oblique (RAO) projection is used. An angulation of approximately 30° produces the best results.

Another area that is often shown poorly on the standard PA images is the origin of the profunda femoris artery. In this instance, LAO is used for the left side and RAO for the right side, with an angulation of 25–30%.

Renal arteriography

The native renal arteries arise from the abdominal aorta. Their positions and number are variable, though they most frequently arise at the level of the L1/L2 vertebral bodies, and there is usually a single artery to each kidney. However, it is not at all unusual for a kidney to be supplied by two arteries, and they may be even more numerous than this. Furthermore, when the aorta is considered in cross-section, each artery may arise from either the anterior or the posterior quadrant. The most common arrangement is for the left renal artery to arise from the left posterior quadrant, and the right renal artery to originate from the right anterior quadrant. However, this is also very variable. Such anatomical variability requires scrupulous angiographic technique to ensure that every part of every renal artery is imaged.

Indications for renal arteriography include:

- Uncontrolled hypertension thought to be due to renal artery stenosis
- Rising serum creatinine thought to be due to renal artery stenosis or occlusion
- Bleeding after trauma, e.g. blunt trauma or renal biopsy

The commonest indication for renal arteriography is to search for possible renal artery stenosis. In the majority of patients the cause for this is atheroma, and such lesions are most frequently located at the origin of the renal artery. Therefore, flush aortography is used at least initially, and there may be no need to go on to selective arteriography for diagnosis.

The pigtail catheter is positioned in the abdominal aorta at about the level of the L1 vertebral body. The image is centred such that the entire abdominal aorta is imaged. Around 30 mL of a non-ionic iodine-based contrast medium, 300 mgI/mL, is administered at 15 mL/second, and images are acquired at two or three frames per second (Fig. 32.3). The first acquisition allows the number of renal arteries to be assessed, and may provide some information regarding the presence of stenoses. However, stenosis cannot be excluded until the renal artery origins have been satisfactorily visualised, and this almost always requires oblique views; magnification is also often

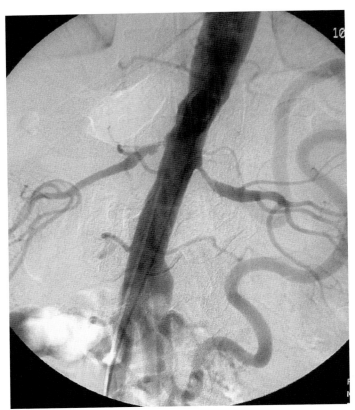

Figure 32.3 Frontal view from a digital subtraction abdominal aortogram showing severe bilateral renal artery stenosis.

helpful. Both LAO and RAO images centred on the renal arteries are obtained. Typically an angulation of 15° may be used, but sometimes different angulations are required.

If selective arteriography is required, for example if there is doubt about the presence of stenosis, especially if fibromuscular dysplasia is suspected, or because of bleeding from the kidney, a selective catheter will be introduced into the vessel origin, and having centred on the individual artery, contrast is injected by hand while images are acquired.

Occasionally arteriography is required for a renal transplant, for similar indications to those in native kidneys. The anatomy of transplant kidneys can produce some challenges for imaging. First, it is important to know whether the transplant is cadaveric or from a live donor. With the former, when the kidney is harvested it is possible to take a cuff of aorta so that the transplant kidney can be attached to the external iliac artery in one of the iliac fossae. It may require a number of obliques to profile the renal artery properly, as it may be quite tortuous. A kidney from a live donor will have a shorter artery, so will normally have been anastomosed to the internal iliac artery, but it will still lie in an iliac fossa.

Mesenteric arteriography

This examination is most commonly performed to identify a bleeding source, but may also be undertaken to identify stenoses or occlusions in the mesenteric vessels of patients suspected of suffering from bowel ischaemia (Fig. 32.4). In the latter case an abdominal aortogram is performed in the same way as for the renal arteries, but a lateral view is performed to profile the mesenteric vessel origins.

In the case of mesenteric arteriography performed for gastrointestinal bleeding, selective arteriograms are performed on each individual times and the volume of contrast administered. However, monoplanar rotational or 'spin' angiographic techniques can also be effective.[10] High acquisition frame rates are essential, with all major equipment manufacturers offering cardiac units with exposure rates of between 10 and 50 frames per second. Arterial access is traditionally via the femoral approach, although the radial artery approach is gaining in popularity.

Ventriculography

A pigtail catheter is guided across the aortic valve and positioned midchamber in the left ventricle. Correct positioning is essential to avoid complications (tachycardia or myocardial staining) or misleading results (forced mitral valve regurgitation).

Ventriculography is usually limited to two projections. RAO 30° and LAO 60° will demonstrate ventricular wall motion. A lateral projection is more useful in assessing mitral valve regurgitation.

A pressure injector should be used to deliver a bolus of contrast agent. 30 mL at 10 mL per second is usually sufficient to assess ventricular function.

Aortography

The same pigtail catheter can be withdrawn and positioned just above the aortic valve in order to perform an aortogram. Aortography is also usually limited to two projections.

LAO 60° or lateral projections are useful for demonstrating ascending aortic dissections. Both projections offer an open view of the aortic arch and the position of the neck vessels. RAO 30° is also helpful in delineating aortic dissections and can also demonstrate more of the descending thoracic aorta.

Two projections will also allow assessment of any aneurysmal dilatations and the competency of the aortic valve.

A pressure injection of contrast agent should be used. Parameters of 40 mL of contrast at 20 mL per second are not uncommon.

Coronary arteriography

The coronary arteries are cannulated using separate selective catheters. The positioning of the catheters is crucial to avoid occluding the artery or mimicking and/or camouflaging osteal diseases.[9]

The non-linear and oblique courses of the coronary arteries necessitate a number of different angiographic projections. The number of projections will vary from patient to patient. A combination of the following static projections is commonly used and will usually adequately demonstrate the coronary anatomy:

- Left coronary system: PA, lateral, RAO 30°, LAO 60°, RAO 30° with caudal 30°, LAO 60° with cranial 30°
- Right coronary artery: RAO 30°, LAO 60°, PA, lateral, LAO 60° with cranial 30°

Rotational angiographic projections often involve a dual axis rotation of the imaging system. The following swings should provide a comprehensive demonstration of the coronary tree:[11]

- Left coronary system: LAO 30° with cranial 30° via RAO 40° to LAO 40° with caudal 20°
- Right coronary artery: LAO 30° with cranial 30° via LAO 35° to RAO 30° with caudal 25°

Power injections of contrast can be used and are as safe as hand injections. However, hand injections offer advantages and flexibility for rapid repeat injections. 5–10 mL at 3–4 mL per second is commonly used for static acquisitions, and 3 mL per second can be used for rotational acquisitions.

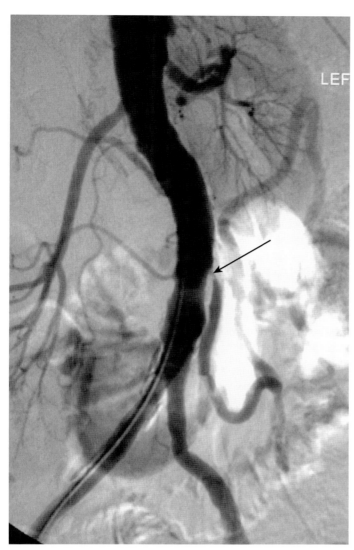

Figure 32.4 RAO view (70°) of the abdominal aorta showing a severe stenosis of the inferior mesenteric artery. The coeliac axis and superior mesenteric artery were occluded, and the patient was suffering from symptoms of mesenteric ischaemia.

vessel. Injection into the coeliac axis and the superior mesenteric artery is best performed with a pump, delivering around 20 mL of contrast medium at 6 mL per second. The inferior mesenteric artery is generally a smaller vessel, and is imaged using a hand injection. The operator may well advance the catheter more distally into the vessel to perform superselective injections. These will also be performed by hand, and will require magnified views.

Cardiac arteriography

This is the radiological demonstration of not only the heart's structure but also its function. Routinely only the left ventricle, ascending aorta and both coronary arteries are studied. In order to reduce complications and risks, cardiac studies require constant monitoring of arterial pressures and electrocardiogram (ECG) waveforms.[8,9] This often requires the presence of ECG technicians, and it is quite common for these examinations to be performed by cardiologists.

High-quality fluoroscopic imaging equipment is essential, preferably using a biplanar system. Biplanar systems can reduce procedural

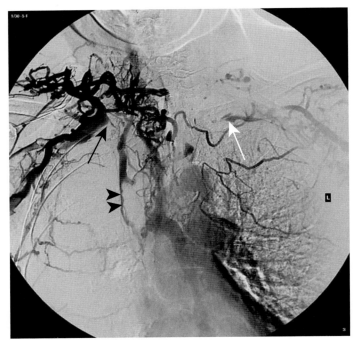

Figure 32.5 Digital subtraction superior vena cavagram showing occlusion of the right (black arrow) and left (white arrow) brachiocephalic veins. The superior vena cava is narrow and contains thrombus (double arrowheads). The underlying diagnosis was bronchogenic carcinoma.

Upper limb arteriography

This is required infrequently, as arterial pathology in the upper limb is much less common than in the lower limb. However, conditions such as subclavian steal (due to subclavian arterial occlusion), damage to the vessel because of trauma from cervical ribs or peripheral embolus may require arteriography. The examination will start with an arch aortogram, followed by selective catheterisation of the relevant subclavian artery, with views obtained along the length of the arm.

Venography

Until the 1990s venography was most commonly performed in the lower limb for diagnosis of deep vein thrombosis (DVT). DVT can now almost always be diagnosed or excluded on the basis of Doppler ultrasound, and venography is only rarely required. Once a vein on the dorsum of the foot has been cannulated, and tourniquets applied just above the ankle and just above the knee, contrast is injected and images of the calf are obtained in PA, RAO and LAO views. The knee tourniquet is then removed and views of the popliteal, femoral and iliac veins are obtained. It is also possible to perform arm venography and superior venacavography using similar techniques (Fig. 32.5).

FUTURE DEVELOPMENTS

As mentioned in the introduction to this chapter, there have been major developments in non-invasive vascular imaging in recent years. Doppler ultrasound provides a non-invasive and relatively cheap method of assessing the vasculature, but it does not produce an anatomical map for the surgeon or interventionist who will subsequently undertake treatment. CTA and MRA have improved considerably in

recent years, and may supplant purely diagnostic angiography in the near future.

With the advent of multislice technology, CTA can be undertaken over large anatomical areas, such as the entire thorax abdomen and pelvis, in a single breath-hold. It therefore has considerable advantages over DSA, such as being non-invasive, using a lower overall contrast dose when assessing large areas, and also demonstrating information about structures beyond the lumen of the vessel. Thus, in the assessment of aneurysmal disease the wall of the vessel and the true size of the aneurysm can be assessed. DSA can be misleading in this situation, as the presence of intramural thrombus can give a misleading impression of the size of the aneurysm. In addition, although CTA has the disadvantage over MRA of using ionising radiation, it has the advantage of being usable where MRI is contraindicated, e.g. if a patient has a pacemaker, and is less likely to cause claustrophobia. Multislice CTA also tends to be faster than MRA.

ALTERNATIVE TECHNIQUES

Intra-arterial catheter angiography is a well-established and relatively safe technique for imaging the arterial tree. Where there has been evidence of substantial risk either locally, such as in the case of axillary artery puncture, or in the territory to be examined, such as the carotid arteries, other techniques or approaches have been used.

The current mainstay of carotid artery imaging is Doppler ultrasound. However, this technique requires regular audit to ensure that there is minimal inter- and intraobserver variation. Such audit becomes difficult to undertake if, as in many centres, carotid arteriography is no longer performed and surgeons are prepared to operate on duplex findings alone. This approach has the benefit of removing the potential stroke risk associated with carotid angiography for an individual patient, but the hidden consequence is that if Doppler ultrasound results are inaccurate, some individuals may be treated inappropriately and some requiring treatment may not receive it.

Despite progress in non-invasive vascular imaging techniques such as MRA, a large number of invasive arteriograms are still carried out in the UK. This is at least on the surface undesirable, as the costs in terms of bed days of this strategy are relatively high. However, a significant number of patients will be unsuitable for MRI, for example due to having cardiac pacemakers, claustrophobia or other contraindications. Furthermore, MRA lends itself very much to planned outpatient-type work, such as may be undertaken in patients with intermittent claudication.

However, many such patients do not require imaging at all, as there is little evidence to support treatment in this group unless their exercise tolerance is less than 100 m. Patients with acute or chronic critical limb ischaemia require either urgent or, at the very least, prompt imaging and management to prevent limb loss. Owing to the pressure on MRI services and the consequent lack of availability of MRA in many places in the UK, most centres would find it difficult to provide such a non-invasive service on this basis. In addition, owing to its tendency to overestimate the severity of vascular lesions, there may be confusion between severe stenosis and occlusion in a vessel. Such a distinction can be critical in deciding whether to use open surgical or endovascular therapy.

Using intra-arterial angiography in this clinical situation has the advantages of better distinction of stenosis versus occlusion, although it can still prove difficult to identify distal vessels, and of being able to proceed directly to endovascular therapy if that is appropriate.

One area in which MRA has proved invaluable is in the evaluation of patients suspected of having atheromatous renal artery stenosis. MRA avoids catheter manipulations in the aorta and the potentially nephrotoxic contrast administration of intra-arterial angiography. Non-invasive imaging is very attractive in evaluation of the renal arteries, as there are no reliable clinical or biochemical tests for exclusion of atheromatous renal artery stenosis. Practice in this area is, however, changing: recent trials have indicated that outcomes from stenting for renal artery stenosis are not as good as many had previously thought, and in addition the use of gadolinium contrast agents in patients with significant renal impairment is contraindicated. Some institutions have seen a significant reduction in demand for renal MRA as a result.

REFERENCES

1. Callum K, et al. Interventional vascular radiology and interventional neurovascular radiology. A Report of the National Confidential Enquiry into Perioperative Deaths November 2000. London: NCEPOD; 2000.

2. Royal College of Radiologists. Standards in Vascular Radiology 1999. Ref. BFCR(99)9.

3. Gritter K, et al. Complications of outpatient transbrachial intra-arterial digital subtraction angiography. Work in progress. Radiology 1987;162:125–7.

4. Heenan S, et al. Transbrachial arteriography: indications and complications. Clinical Radiology 1996;51:205–9.

5. Chitwood R, et al. Surgical complications of transaxillary arteriography: a case control study. Journal of Vascular Surgery 1996;23:844–9.

6. McIvor J, Rhymer J. 245 transaxillary arteriograms in arteriopathic patients: success rate and complications. Clinical Radiology 1992;45:390–4.

7. Cowling M, et al. The role of transradial diagnostic angiography. Cardiovascular and Interventional Radiology 1997;20:103–6.

8. Noto T, et al. Cardiac catheterisation 1990: a report of the Registry of the Society for Cardiac Angiography and Interventions. Catheterization and Cardiovascular Diagnosis 1991;24:75–83.

9. Kern M. 2003. Cardiac catheterization handbook. 4th ed. Saunders.

10. Klein AJ, et al. Rotational coronary angiography. Cardiology Clinics 2009;27(3):395–405.

11. Horisaki T, et al. Feasibility evaluation of dual axis rotational angiography in the diagnosis of coronary artery disease. Medica Mundi 2008;52/2:11–13.

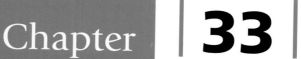

Chapter | **33** |

Vascular imaging of the head and neck

Patricia Fowler, Andrew Layt

The vasculature of the head and neck is now most commonly imaged using techniques other than conventional catheter angiography. The use of computed tomography (CT), magnetic resonance imaging (MRI) and ultrasound techniques allows these vessels to be visualised in a less invasive manner. Catheter studies are still performed in specialist centres, especially as part of endovascular treatment. In this chapter consideration will be given to the use of all these, with some examples of the common indications for imaging.

COMMON INDICATIONS FOR VASCULAR EXAMINATION

Cerebral aneurysm

This is the most common indication for cerebral angiography. Aneurysmal rupture occurs in 6–12 per 100 000 population and the presence of asymptomatic aneurysms is thought to be in the region of 2% of the population.[1] A ruptured aneurysm presents the commonest cause of subarachnoid haemorrhage (SAH) in adults. The most common type is the saccular or berry aneurysm. Typically, defects develop due to the pressure of systolic waves causing herniation of the vessel wall.[2]

The average age of presentation is 40 years. Below this age presentation is more common in men than in women, but this reverses from 40 years upwards.[1] Over 90% of saccular aneurysms occur in the anterior circulation at branch points in the carotid supply,[3,4] the remaining 10% being in the posterior circulation.[1] In the anterior circulation approximately 25% are located in the middle cerebral artery distribution, 35% around the anterior cerebral artery and 30% associated with the internal carotid artery.[1,4,5] Cerebral aneurysms can range from 1–2 mm to 1–2 cm,[5] with the risk of bleeding generally increasing with size.[1,4,6]

The clinical presentation of rupture leading to SAH includes:

- sudden severe headache[1,7,8]
- rapid loss of consciousness[7,8]
- vomiting[1,7]
- photophobia[6]
- nuchal rigidity[8]

Photophobia and nuchal rigidity result from meningeal irritation as a result of blood in the subarachnoid space.

Complications include:

- rebleeding[4]
- vasospasm with cerebral ischaemia[1]
- hydrocephalus resulting from clot or obstruction of arachnoid villi by blood products[1,9]

Arteriovenous malformation (AVM)

AVMs are the second most common cause of SAH in adults. They result from developmental abnormalities of arterial and venous vessels leading to the formation of fragile vascular walls[2] as well as the lack of development of a capillary bed.[1] Typically they are made up of three parts: a core of dysplastic vessels known as a nidus, arterial feeding vessels and draining veins.[10] The associated vessels are hypertrophic and hyperplastic. AVMs are typically 3–4 cm in diameter[2] and are usually symptomatic by the age of 40 years.[1]

Clinical presentation:[1,9]

- intracranial haemorrhage
- seizure
- headache
- progressive neurological deficits

Points of note

- A SAH occurs when blood escapes into the subarachnoid space, which is the space between the arachnoid and the pia mater. In this space it mixes with the cerebrospinal fluid
- A subdural haemorrhage is the presence of blood between the dura and the arachnoid mater
- An extradural haemorrhage is a bleed outside the dura mater, between the dura mater and the bony skull
- SAH may arise from a ruptured intracranial aneurysm, a bleeding AVM, or infrequently as a result of trauma. In contrast, subdural and extradural haemorrhages usually occur as a result of trauma

Stroke

The World Health Organization has estimated that, worldwide, there were 5.7 million deaths from stroke in 2005, equivalent to 9.9% of all deaths.[11] A first or recurrent stroke is experienced by 110 000 people in England each year,[12] and stroke accounts for 11% of all deaths in England and Wales.[13] In England there are more than 900 000 people living with the effects of stroke.[13]

Stroke may be divided into two main categories:

- Ischaemic 85%
- Haemorrhagic 15%[2,14]

Ischaemic stroke

This type may lead to regional infarction or to small isolated areas known as lacunar infarcts. It occurs as a result of a regional lack of blood supply to the brain and can be due to occlusion of an artery by any mechanism, such as thrombosis, emboli or dissection. Thrombus may form intracranially or more commonly at the region of the carotid bifurcation, a common site for atheromatous disease and from where distal emboli frequently occur.

Haemodynamic ischaemic stroke occurs following:

- a reduction in perfusion for any reason
- dissection of the vessels in the neck particularly following trauma.

Vasospasm, a common complication of SAH, may also lead to ischaemic stroke. This process can also be a complication of the use of some recreational drugs.

Lacunar infarcts occur as a result of occlusion of small penetrating arteries, usually around 1–15 mm in size, in subcortical areas or in the brainstem.[15]

Haemorrhagic stroke

This may result from bleeding into the brain tissue and may be the outcome of aneurysm rupture, AVM or head injury. It can also be spontaneous, e.g. as a result of a hypertensive bleed. Cocaine and heroin abuse also increases the risk of cerebral haemorrhage and may lead to stroke.

Clinical presentation[9]

- Vomiting
- Sometimes headache
- Deficits in the body area related to associated cerebral involvement. Associated pressure on the brain may lead the condition to deteriorate rapidly and patients can present in coma

Tumour

Preoperative examination of the layout of the vascular supply to tumours is now more usually undertaken by magnetic resonance angiography (MRA). Preoperative devascularisation (embolisation) is used in some centres.

IMAGING METHODS

Digital subtraction angiography (DSA)

DSA remains the gold standard in the examination of the cerebral vasculature for many abnormalities. However, the less invasive alternatives are now adequate for many situations, and so its use is now confined to specialist applications such as prior to endovascular or neurosurgical treatment. It is advantageous to use a biplanar C-arm mounted fluoroscopic system rather than a single-plane system, to enable a reduction in examination time and the amount of radiological contrast medium administered. Biplanar is preferred for diagnostic use, and is considered essential for interventional use. 3D rotational angiography is useful to depict intracranial aneurysms, providing the facility to rotate the resultant angiographic image to display the vessels under examination to their best advantage.

Procedure

Fully informed consent must be obtained. Patients who are acutely ill may be unable to give consent, and may be treated as an emergency. Those undergoing diagnostic investigation may later undergo interventional treatment and will need to give their consent for this separately. Preparation is as for standard peripheral angiography, with the addition of a baseline neurological observation. Studies are routinely carried out with the patient awake, or with mild sedation. General anaesthesia may be used in the case of a patient who is unwell, or unable to cooperate, or where interventional treatment is undertaken.

Arterial access is normally gained via the femoral artery. The catheter and guide wire are advanced via the aorta and each cerebral vessel is selectively catheterised. Catheters for cerebral angiography have pre-shaped tips to facilitate vessel access. More than one catheter type may be used if vessels are tortuous or stenosed and a different shape is required. The catheter is often connected via a three-way tap to a pressurised saline flush, which is maintained throughout the procedure to minimise the risk of thrombus formation in the catheter.

Physiological monitoring is maintained throughout the procedure, with neurological observations at 15-minute intervals. Bed rest is necessary for 4 hours after the procedure, and during this time neurological and catheter site observations are made every 30 minutes.

Complications

- Stroke: risk of between about 0.1% and 1%. This may result from vessel dissection, arterial spasm or embolus
- Haematoma around the catheterisation site
- Allergy to local anaesthetic or contrast media

Technique

Cerebral angiography

The routine examination is the 'four-vessel angiogram' (right and left internal carotid arteries, right and left vertebral arteries). Both internal carotid arteries are selectively catheterised, with the tip of the catheter placed above the carotid bifurcation in the internal carotid artery. Often only one vertebral artery is selectively catheterised, as the termination of the contralateral vertebral artery may be filled by reflux, thereby demonstrating both posterior inferior cerebellar arteries with a single injection. Some centres include selective injections into both external carotids, particularly if a dural fistula is suspected.

It is prudent to examine first the vessel most suspected of having an abnormality, in case the procedure needs to be terminated before completion. Non-selective runs, for example with the catheter in the common carotid artery, may be performed if vascular access is difficult, but the quality of the study will be degraded by the superimposition of vessels.

Limited studies, e.g. of a single vessel, may be performed at follow-up.

A standard set of projections will be taken for each patient. This will vary slightly, depending on the radiologist's preference and the angiographic equipment used.

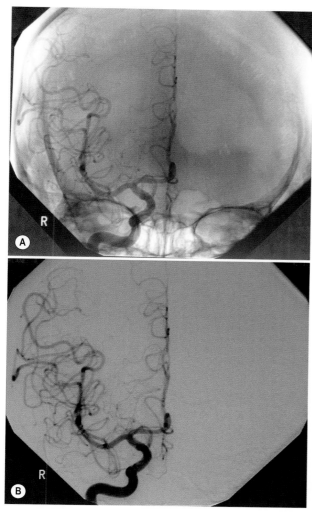

Figure 33.1 OF projection following injection into the right internal carotid artery: (A) unsubtracted; (B) subtracted.

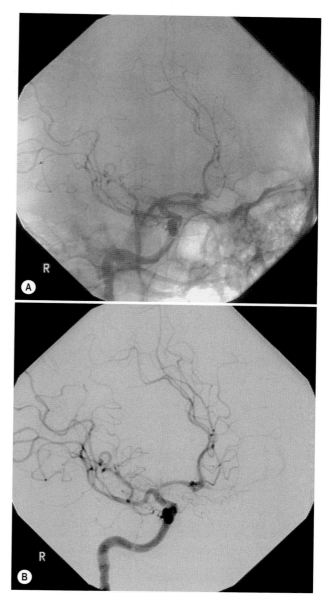

Figure 33.2 AO projection following injection into the left internal carotid artery: (A) unsubtracted; (B) subtracted image.

Internal carotid artery (Figs 33.1A,B, 33.2A,B, 33.3A,B)

Typical standard projections are shown in the following table.

Projection	Positioning guidelines	Field of view
Occipitofrontal (OF)	Petrous ridge viewed at the top of the orbit. Vertex at the top of the field of view	17 cm
Anterior oblique (AO)	From the OF position, oblique image intensifier to the side under examination 20–25°	17 cm
Lateral	Anterior of the skull at the top of the field, include from the skull base to the vertex, with as much of the rest of the cranium as possible	22 cm

Vertebral artery (Figs 33.4A,B, 33.5A,B, 33.6A,B)

Typical standard projections are shown in the following table.

Projection	Positioning guidelines	Field of view
FO 30° (Townes)	Posterior clinoids viewed through foramen magnum. Foramen magnum positioned at the lower third of the field	17 cm
OF 20°	Petrous ridge at bottom of orbits. Include occiput in field of view	17 cm
Lateral	Include all of the occiput. Position with C2 at the bottom of the field of view	22 cm

Final positioning adjustment is made under fluoroscopic control.

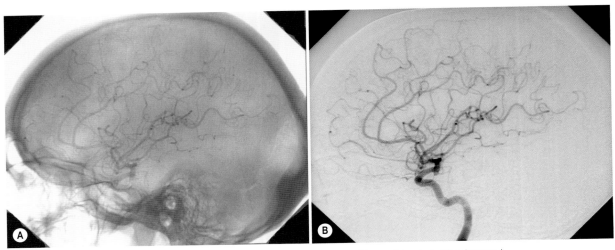

Figure 33.3 Lateral projection following injection into the left internal carotid artery: (A) unsubtracted; (B) subtracted.

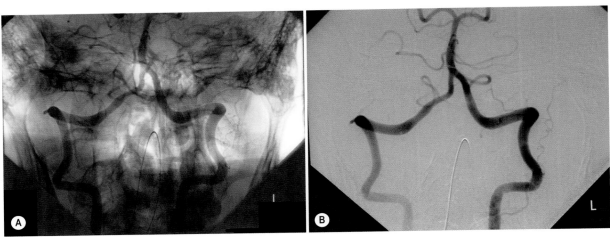

Figure 33.4 F0 30° projection following injection into the left vertebral artery: (A) unsubtracted; (B) subtracted.

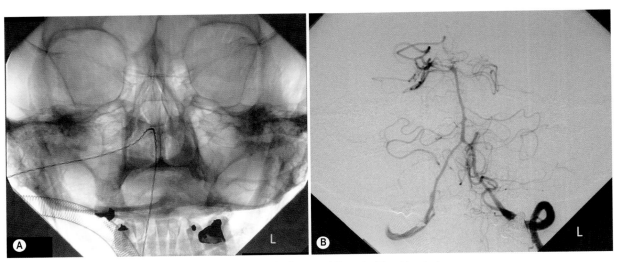

Figure 33.5 OF 20° projection following injection into the left vertebral artery: (A) mask; (B) subtracted.

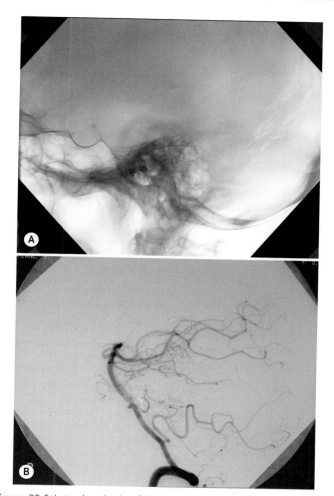

Figure 33.6 Lateral projection following injection into the left vertebral artery: (A) unsubtracted; (B) subtracted.

Supplementary projections may be taken to exclude or demonstrate pathology. These will depend on the patient's anatomy.

Supplementary projection	Positioning guidelines	Field of view
Orbital oblique	From the standard anterior oblique projection, angle caudally to project the petrous ridge at the bottom of the orbit	17 cm
Reverse oblique	Anterior oblique 20–25° to the side opposite to the vessel under examination	17 cm
Submentovertical	Raise the patient's chin as much as possible (the head support may be removed) and angle cranially as much as the equipment will allow	17 cm

It is often difficult, with limited projections, to distinguish normal vessels from those with pathology, because the arteries are complex 3D structures. For example, a normal vascular loop may be superimposed over another vessel and mimic an aneurysm. Supplementary projections will allow a full understanding of the anatomy, including which vessels supply or drain any abnormality. It is important to demonstrate fully the morphology of aneurysms to determine the

optimum treatment. Of particular interest is the ratio of diameter of the aneurysm body to the neck and the relationship of normal vessels to the aneurysm. The choice of projections, and the use of supplementary projections, is modified if 3D rotational angiography can be performed.

Neck vessels

Examination of the extracranial portion of the arteries may be performed. The catheter is placed in the proximal vessel and injections are made as described above. A common indication is atheromatous stenosis of the carotid bifurcation. Standard projections for the common carotid artery are lateral and 20° anterior oblique.

Hard copy imaging

If hard copy is to be produced, a representative selection of images from each run should be included. This should include the arterial images that best demonstrate the vessel, as well as venous images. Each sheet of film should have an image without subtraction included to permit orientation with bony landmarks.

3D rotational angiography

Rotational angiography is performed, using suitable equipment, by rotating the C-arm around the vessel of interest during contrast injection administered by injector pump. The catheter is positioned in the vessel as for a conventional angiogram. The vessel of interest is positioned at the isocentre under fluoroscopic control. The C-arm rotates to acquire a series of projections, typically over 5–10 seconds. Subtracted or non-subtracted images can be acquired. The resultant data set consists of a series of images taken at intervals around the vessel, which can be viewed and manipulated on a workstation. The images can be viewed as a multiplanar reformation, maximum intensity projection or volume rendered.

Manipulating the 3D reformat of the images on a workstation allows the vessel to be viewed from any angle, without the need for further acquisitions. An appreciation of the morphology of the vessel, and any abnormality, can be gained, which can add significantly to the information obtained from conventional projections. It allows the operator to determine the optimum working projection (the C-arm position) at which to perform embolisation.

The ability to perform rotational angiography with 3D reformatting often removes the need for conventional supplementary oblique projections. The standard projections may be limited, depending on radiological preference, to frontal, lateral and rotational acquisitions for each vessel. Alternatively, the rotational acquisition may be used only where an abnormality is demonstrated conventionally.

CT angiography (CTA) (Figs 33.7, 33.8)

CTA is acquired by obtaining CT images of a volume of tissue while a radiological contrast medium is flowing through it. The slice thickness used is dependent on the particular vessels of interest. A contrast medium is introduced intravenously via an automatic injector, the amount being dependent on the speed of flow and diameter of the vessels of interest, typically between 50 and 100 mL. The data obtained are reviewed as a maximum intensity projection or a 3D surface rendered image. Post-processing facilities enable extraction of surrounding data, and this, together with the ability to rotate the 3D image, enables optimum visualisation of the vessels under examination.

Although of lower resolution than conventional angiography, for most diagnostic purposes it is sufficient, and, although standard precautions for iodine-based contrast media must be observed, the

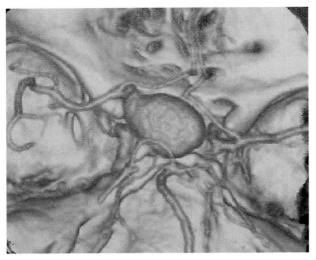

Figure 33.7 Volume rendered CTA demonstrating aneurysm.

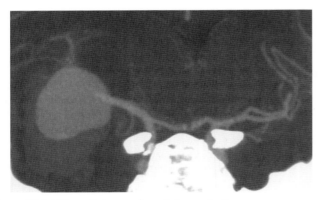

Figure 33.8 CTA multiplanar reformat demonstrating aneurysm.

advantage of being a less invasive technique means it is commonly used to image the cerebral and neck vessels.

As well as the arterial phase, delayed images can be used to image the cerebral venous system. Recent scanner developments mean that arterial and venous information can be easily obtained from a single acquisition, in conjunction with perfusion mapping.

The speed and simplicity of CTA means it is the method of choice to image vessels following trauma or other emergency presentations, with DSA being performed only if the CTA is inconclusive.

Magnetic resonance angiography (MRA)

(Fig. 33.9)

Several imaging options are available using MRA. As described in Chapter 36, the most commonly used are time-of-flight (TOF) angiography, phase contrast angiography (PCA) and contrast-enhanced MRA (CE-MRA). Each takes a different approach and has advantages and disadvantages in the investigation of the cerebral vessels. MRA techniques are still developing. MRA has the advantages of being minimally invasive with no radiation dose, and, with the exception of CE-MRA, can be performed without exogenous contrast media. This makes its use suitable for screening studies, such as ruling out aneurysms in subjects with family history as a risk factor, or where regular follow-up studies are required, such as monitoring an unruptured aneurysm. MRA is useful in the evaluation of the neck vessels to look for stenosis or dissection.

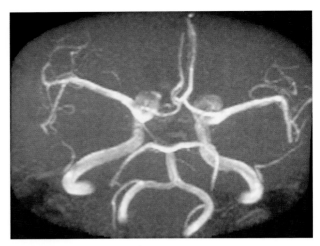

Figure 33.9 MR TOF angiography.

The use of MRI is difficult in emergency situations where it may not be easy to establish whether the patient has factors that contraindicate MR, and also difficult for patients who are critically ill, because of limited access to the patient.

Carotid artery Doppler ultrasound

Doppler ultrasound is a well-established method of imaging the extracranial carotid arteries, particularly following transient ischaemic attacks (TIAs) or for those at risk of stroke. The aim of the investigation is to determine the presence or absence of atherosclerosis and the related degree of stenosis, prior to making decisions on appropriate treatment.[16]

A common place for the build-up of atherosclerosis is the carotid bifurcation, and this is a region of particular interest in Doppler ultrasound because it is an area of turbulence as the flow divides between the external and internal carotid arteries. The peak velocity and the relative changes in systole and diastole in different sections of the common, internal and external carotid arteries are indicators of the degree of stenosis. The vertebral arteries are also assessed to complete the examination. The degree of vessel stenosis will influence the selection of treatment method, which may include carotid endarterectomy or carotid stenting.[17] The urgency of imaging depends on the individual's risk of stroke.[12]

Doppler ultrasound also has a role in the follow-up of patients after carotid endarterectomy, and in the imaging of pulsatile masses and carotid dissection.[16] Doppler ultrasound examination of the extracranial vessels is dependent on a combination of grey-scale imaging, Doppler and colour flow analysis.[18] MRA and CTA may also be used in the imaging of these vessels.

Transcranial Doppler ultrasound

Vessels in the cranium may be assessed by Doppler ultrasound using three possible approaches: transcranial, suboccipital or transorbital.[16] Transcranial Doppler ultrasound is widely used in perioperative carotid endarterectomy to determine the presence of emboli in the brain circulation, shown as high-intensity ultrasound signals.[19] It is also well established as a screening tool to determine the risk of stroke or TIA in those with sickle cell disease.[20–22] Other applications include the detection and assessment of vasospasm in patients with SAH[23,24] and the detection of circulating emboli in establishing the risk of stroke or TIA.[19] It has also been shown that clot lysis may be increased by combining transcranial Doppler ultrasound with thrombolytic drug therapy, particularly when combined with the use of microbubbles.[25–27] A newer development in clot lysis is the use of high-frequency ultrasound on a catheter tip to break up the clot.

IMAGING METHODS

Aim of imaging methods

- *Aneurysms*: to demonstrate the aneurysm neck and adjacent vessels to inform the choice of appropriate treatment methods: surgery or endovascular therapy.
- *Arteriovenous malformations*: to obtain information on the layout of the vascular anatomy to inform treatment decisions.
- *Stroke*: to establish the type of stroke and define the area of the vasculature involved, and to more accurately assess the endovascular anatomy of vessels, particularly in the context of vasculopathies.

Imaging methods used

Aneurysms

Cerebral angiography supplemented with 3D rotational angiography enables a more exacting presentation of anatomical details than other approaches. DSA with 3D capabilities remains the gold standard, although CTA provides a non-invasive and cheaper alternative and is now the standard method of initial assessment. DSA is performed only if the CTA is inconclusive.

Vasospasm may occur as a complication of SAH and will affect treatment decisions. It typically occurs 3–10 days after aneurysmal rupture.[6] In the imaging of vasospasm, CTA is more suited to the critically ill patient. CTA demonstrates anatomical configuration independent of the possible flow artefacts associated with MRA. Elevated velocities in transcranial Doppler ultrasound also have a role in confirming a clinical diagnosis.[15]

Arteriovenous malformations

In the management of AVMs the layout of the vascular anatomy will influence treatment decisions. Information is required on the size and location of the nidus as well as the feeding and draining vessels. MRI and CT both have a role in providing information on the location of an AVM, with CTA providing additional information on the vascular anatomy. In preoperative assessment of AVMs there is a role for the range of imaging methods, but DSA remains the definitive procedure and provides optimum resolution for differentiation between vessels (Fig. 33.10).

Stroke (Fig. 33.11A,B,C,D)

Brain imaging must be performed immediately after admission for an acute stroke. Imaging is important to determine the best treatment, especially the use of anticoagulant or thrombolytic therapies. Urgent treatment has been shown to improve outcome in stroke.[12]

The aim of imaging is to establish the diagnosis and to determine whether the event is purely ischaemic or has any haemorrhagic component. Haemorrhage will contraindicate anticoagulant or thrombolytic treatment. Treatment of an ischaemic stroke is based on how much brain tissue has suffered irreversible damage and how much of the surrounding ischaemic tissue can be saved.

MR with diffusion and perfusion weighted imaging, or CT with perfusion imaging, can be used. MR has some advantages over CT in terms of radiation dose, sensitivity and specificity. The volume covered

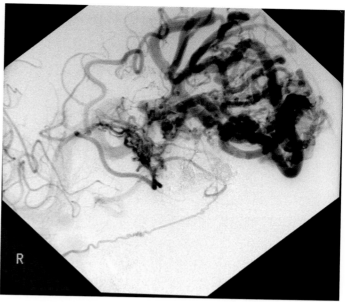

Figure 33.10 Lateral projection following injection into the right common carotid artery. Subtracted image demonstrating an arteriovenous malformation.

may be greater than is possible with CT perfusion techniques on some CT scanners, thereby allowing visualisation of, for example, small cortical lesions. However, MR may not be available in the emergency setting, is a difficult environment for patients requiring monitoring or ventilation, and is not suitable for patients with certain contraindications. The speed and wide accessibility of CT and an accuracy approaching that of MR makes it the most commonly used modality.

An unenhanced CT scan is first performed to rule out haemorrhage or other pathology. Perfusion CT can then be performed to evaluate an ischaemic stroke. A single bolus of contrast is injected while a volume of the brain is repeatedly scanned. The protocol will depend on the scanner configuration, with newer scanners offering wider coverage.

The change in attenuation caused as the contrast flows through the tissue is measured within each voxel and these data are used to produce different perfusion maps. Typically the mean transit time, the time the contrast takes to pass from the arterial to the venous phase (Fig. 33.11A), the time to peak, the time taken for the contrast to reach the maximum density, and the cerebral blood volume (CBV), volume of contrast within the blood vessels (Fig. 33.11B), are shown. From these measurements cerebral blood flow (CBF) can be calculated (Fig. 33.11C). Comparison can be made between the affected and normal hemispheres, and the different maps viewed in combination to establish the degree of reversible damage. An area with reduction in CBF and increased or maintained CBV suggests tissue with reversible ischaemia, as the blood vessels dilate in an attempt to maintain cerebral perfusion. An area with matched reduction in CBF and CBV suggests infarcted tissue.

CTA can be used to demonstrate the site of the occlusion. The current generation of scanners allow CTA to be obtained from the perfusion data set without the additional injection of contrast.

Perfusion weighted MR can be used in a similar manner to CT perfusion. Diffusion weighted MR is very sensitive to early stroke changes, but the problems of imaging the acutely ill patient may limit its use compared to CT. The use of arterial spin labelling techniques

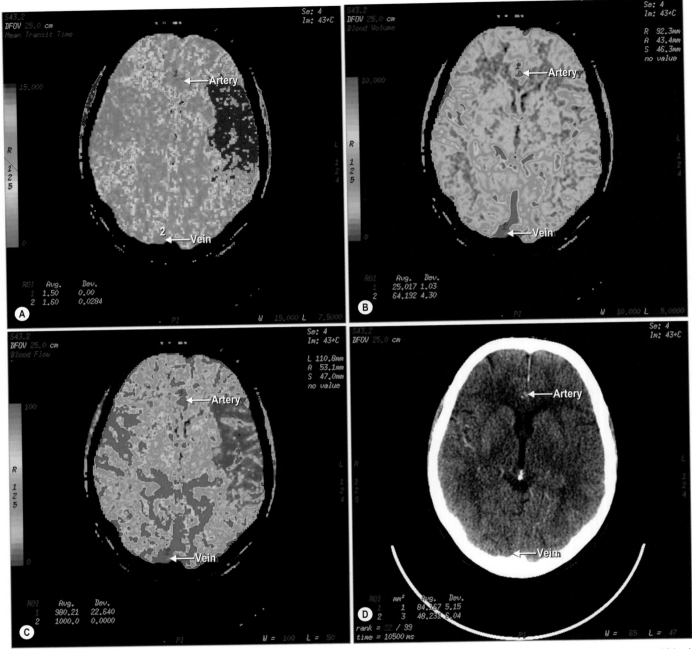

Figure 33.11 A patient with an acute onset of right sided weakness and dysphasia. The plain CT scan (D) shows small areas of hypodensity within the left cerebral hemisphere. The CT perfusion study demonstrates an extensive region of perfusion mismatch within the left middle cerebral artery.

allows perfusion imaging by magnetically 'labelling' blood during the scan. It therefore requires no injection of any contrast, so is completely non-invasive.

Transient ischaemic attack (TIA)

A transient ischaemic attack, sometimes described as a 'mini stroke', occurs when a cerebral artery is temporarily occluded, with the symptoms and signs resolving within 24 hours. Patients who have had a TIA are at high risk of stroke and should receive urgent assessment, including imaging. Diffusion weighted MRI is the best method of imaging the brain because of its sensitivity to subtle vascular changes, and is helpful in assessing which blood vessels may be involved. Imaging will help rule out other pathologies such as migraine or haemorrhage.[12] Carotid artery disease is a common cause of TIA, and imaging is important to determine whether carotid endarterectomy is required. Doppler ultrasound is the modality of choice, supplemented by MRA or CTA if inconclusive.

CONCLUSION

The gold standard for the demonstration of vascular abnormalities remains conventional catheter angiography. However, many conditions can now be adequately demonstrated using alternative techniques that are less invasive and quicker.

Continuing refinements in MRA mean that the use of this investigation will increase. With a range of different angiographic sequences available, this non-invasive non-ionising technique is ideal for imaging many vascular abnormalities, with the exception of acute haemorrhage. Acutely ill patients may be unable to cooperate with MRI scanning, and the restrictions of the MRI environment produce difficulties in imaging high-dependency patients.

Doppler ultrasound provides another non-invasive means of imaging the head and neck vessels, and is especially important in the management of patients presenting with TIAs or stroke.

The widespread availability of multislice CT scanners, with technology that continues to improve, means that CT has become the primary investigation for patients presenting with conditions such as SAH or stroke. Advances in hardware and processing software mean that diagnostic confidence in CTA compared to conventional DSA is high. Even relatively small vascular abnormalities, such as small aneurysms, can be demonstrated. This investigation can be performed on patients presenting from the A&E department, leading to rapid diagnosis, with demonstration of the morphology of vascular abnormalities, and subsequent expedition of effective treatment.

CTA is not suitable for all conditions: degradation due to metallic artefacts can make it unsuitable for patients with vascular clips or coils, and its demonstration of abnormalities such as small vessels in slow-flowing AVMs is inferior to that of conventional angiography. DSA will remain the investigation of choice for such conditions. DSA will continue to be performed where the results of other techniques are equivocal, but its use as a diagnostic tool has declined. The efficacy of interventional radiological treatment over conventional neurosurgery is accepted for many intracranial vascular abnormalities.[28] The use of intra-arterial thrombolytic drugs, administered under DSA control, to treat acute stroke is another example of how the DSA room is now more dedicated to treatment than diagnosis.

REFERENCES

1. Lindsay K, Bone I. Neurology and neurosurgery illustrated. 4th ed. Edinburgh: Churchill Livingstone; 2004.

2. Stevens A, Lowe J. Pathology. 2nd ed. Edinburgh: Mosby; 2000.

3. Rubin R, Strayer DS. Rubin's pathology: Clinicopathologic foundations of medicine. 5th ed. Philadelphia: Lippincott Williams and Wilkins; 2008.

4. Kumar V, et al. Robbins basic pathology. 8th ed. Phildelphia: Saunders Elsevier; 2008.

5. Reid R, Roberts F. Pathology illustrated. 6th ed. Edinburgh: Elsevier Churchill Livingstone; 2005.

6. Wiebers D, et al. Unruptured intracranial aneurysms: natural history, clinical outcome, and risks of surgical and endovascular treatment. Lancet 2003;362:9378:103–10.

7. Kumar P, Clark M. Clinical medicine. 5th ed. Edinburgh: Saunders; 2002.

8. Fitzgerald M, Folan-Curran J. Clinical neuroanatomy and related neuroscience. 4th ed. Edinburgh: Saunders; 2002.

9. Porth C. Pathophysiology. 6th ed. New York: Lippincott-Raven; 2002.

10. Lawton M, Spetzler R. Surgical management of acutely ruptured arteriovenous malformations. In: Welch K, et al., eds. Primer on cerebrovascular diseases. San Diego: Academic Press; 1997. p. 511–9.

11. World Health Organization. WHO STEPS Stroke Manual: The WHO STEPwise approach to stroke surveillance. Geneva: World Health Organization; 2006.

12. National Institute for Health and Clinical Excellence. Stroke: diagnosis and initial management of acute stroke and transient ischaemic attack (TIA). NICE clinical guideline 68:2008.

13. National Audit Office. Reducing brain damage: faster access to better stroke care. (HC 452 Session 2005–6). London: The Stationery Office; 2005.

14. Rothwell PM, et al. Change in stroke incidence, mortality, case-fatality, severity, and risk factors in Oxfordshire, UK from 1981 to 2004 (Oxford Vascular Study). Lancet 2004;363(1004);1925–33.

15. Losseff N, et al. Stroke and cerebrovascular diseases: In: Clarke C, et al. editors. Neurology: A Queen Square Textbook. Chichester: Wiley-Blackwell; 2009. p. 109–54.

16. Allan PL, Gallagher K. The carotid and vertebral arteries; Transcranial colour Doppler. In: Allan PL, et al. editors. Clinical Doppler ultrasound. 2nd ed. Philadelphia, Churchill Livingstone; 2006. p. 41–72.

17. Zwolak RM, Siegel JI. Follow-up after carotid endarterectomy and stenting. In: Zierler RE, editor. Strandness's duplex scanning in vascular disorders. Philadelphia: Lippincott Williams and Wilkins; 2010.

18. Henningsen C. Clinical guide to ultrasonography. St Louis: Mosby; 2004.

19. King A, Markus HS. Doppler embolic signals in cerebrovascular disease and prediction of stroke risk: A systematic review and meta-analysis. Stroke 2009;40:3711–7.

20. Verduzco LA, Nathan DG. Sickle cell disease and stroke. Blood 2009;114(25):5117–25.

21. Pavlakis SG, et al. Transcranial Doppler ultrasonogaphy (TCD) in infants with sickle cell anemia: Baseline data from the BABY HUG trial. Pediatric Blood Cancer 2010;54:256–9.

22. Roberts L, et al. Stroke prevention in the young child with sickle cell anaemia. Annals of Hematology 2009;88:10:943–6.

23. American College of Radiology. ACR Practice Guideline for the Performance of Transcranial Doppler Ultrasound for Adults and Children. American College of Radiology Practice Guideline: 2007.

24. Kinaid MS. Transcranial Doppler ultrasonography: a diagnostic tool of increasing utility. Current Opinion in Anaesthesiology 2008;21:5:552–9.

25. Csiba L. Ultrasound in acute ischaemic stroke. In: Brainin M, et al. editors. Textbook of stroke medicine. Cambridge: Cambridge Medicine; 2010. p. 58–76.

26. Rubiera M, Alexandrov AV. Sonothrombolysis in the management of cause ischaemic stroke. American Journal of Cardiovascular Drugs 2010;10:1:5–10.

27. Tsivgoulis G, et al. Safety and efficacy of ultrasound-enhanced thrombolysis: A comprehensive review and meta-analysis of randomized and nonrandomized studies. Stroke 2010;41:280–7.

28. Molyneux A, et al. International subarachnoid aneurysm trial (ISAT) of neurosurgical clipping versus endovascular coiling in 2143 patients with ruptured intracranial aneurysms: a randomised trial. Lancet 2002;360(9342):1267–74.

Chapter 34

Interventional and therapeutic procedures

Mark Cowling

INTRODUCTION

Interventional and therapeutic procedures undertaken in the medical imaging department locate body structures accurately before intervention and assess the progress of the procedure to follow. Interventional procedures often use a contrast radiology approach, but now almost equally often use computed tomography (CT) or ultrasound (US). Use of magnetic resonance imaging (MRI) is also being initiated or considered as a medium for vascular intervention. Interventional and therapeutic procedures include angioplasty, embolisation, dilation, stent or filter insertion, stone removal and biopsy.

Peripheral angioplasty was first carried out in the femoral artery by Charles Dotter in the USA in 1964. He used coaxial catheters of progressively increasing sizes to widen the lumen of the vessel. Initial results were not as good as would be expected today; however, the equipment available has progressively developed such that results of angioplasty are now vastly improved and a number of other techniques are available for treatment of vascular lesions. These include embolisation in various arterial or venous territories and stent grafting for aneurysms.

VASCULAR INTERVENTIONAL PROCEDURES

Indications

The most common indication for interventional vascular procedures is limb ischaemia, usually of the lower limb. This can present in a variety of ways, such as intermittent claudication (pain in the limb on exercise and relieved by rest), chronic critical limb ischaemia (e.g. causing rest pain, ulcers or gangrene) or acute limb ischaemia (causing pallor, coldness and numbness of the limb).

The common feature is the presence of stenoses or occlusions in the arteries supplying blood to the limb. In general, the greater the severity of the vascular disease, the greater the severity of the symptoms. Limb ischaemia considered suitable for management by interventional radiological techniques can be treated in a variety of ways, such as angioplasty, stent insertion or thrombolysis. It is important to

remember, however, that treatment is chosen on the basis of the symptoms, not simply the angiographic appearance.

Embolisation, on the other hand, may be undertaken for a variety of reasons. First, there may be uncontrolled bleeding: for example from the gastrointestinal tract, tumours in various sites and from the kidney, liver or other solid organs after trauma or biopsy. Embolisation is also useful in the treatment of some aneurysms. This is particularly true of aneurysms in the cerebral circulation, where coil embolisation may be used as an alternative to surgical aneurysm clipping to prevent recurrence of subarachnoid haemorrhage. Other indications include treatment of arteriovenous malformations and embolisation of the testicular vein for varicocoele. Uterine artery embolisation can be used for the treatment of uterine fibroids.

Stent grafting is used in the treatment of aneurysms. A true aneurysm describes a situation where the vessel is abnormally dilated because of expansion of all three layers of the vessel wall, making it prone to rupture. When such an aneurysm is present in the abdominal aorta, rupture causes bleeding and without emergency surgery is fatal. Therefore, if an abdominal aortic aneurysm measuring 5.5 cm or more in diameter is identified, it is usual for surgical aneurysm repair to be undertaken to remove the risk of rupture if the patient is sufficiently fit to undergo such major surgery. Since the 1990s, stent grafts have been, and continue to be, developed; this can provide an alternative to open surgical repair, particularly in patients who are at high risk from open surgery. True aneurysms may also arise at other sites, such as the thoracic aorta and iliac arteries, and may also be amenable to treatment by stent grafting.

A false aneurysm is not surrounded by normal vessel wall. Instead, it represents the persistent leakage of blood into a cavity surrounded by haematoma. These are most commonly seen as a result of trauma to the vessel, often iatrogenic, but may also arise due to erosion by tumours or the presence of infection in the vessel wall. Stent grafting may also be useful in the treatment of false aneurysms. However, if infection is thought likely to be present then a stent graft should be avoided if possible, as being of a foreign material its presence would make the infection impossible to eradicate. In deciding whether or not to use a stent graft the site of the false aneurysm should also be considered. For example, a false aneurysm arising from the common femoral artery (CFA) after arterial puncture is positioned directly over the hip joint: a stent graft implanted at this site would be subject to repeated stress and would eventually fail. False aneurysms at this site are therefore better treated with US-guided injection of thrombin, which thromboses the false aneurysm.

ANGIOPLASTY

The basic principles of angioplasty are the same in whichever vascular territory they are to be applied. These will be described first, followed by important caveats with respect to different arterial territories.

Once an arterial stenosis requiring treatment has been identified, it is traversed with a suitable guide wire and catheter combination. In very narrow stenoses, which can be very difficult to cross, it can be extremely helpful to use the 'roadmap' facility available on modern digital subtraction angiography (DSA) equipment. This allows contrast to be injected while screening, and the image of the vessels to be retained on the monitor. When the screening pedal is next depressed the image of the vessel remains superimposed over the real-time image of the catheter and guide wire as they are being manipulated.

Once the lesion has been crossed it is important that either a guide wire or a catheter should remain across it at all times until the procedure has been completed. When an angioplasty is undertaken, complications such as vessel dissection, occlusion due to acute thrombosis or distal embolisation, or even vessel rupture may occur. If a guide wire has been left across the lesion it is a comparatively simple matter to go on to manage the complication appropriately. If the guide wire has been removed it may be possible to cross the lesion again, but this is often highly complex, is not always successful, and may result in vessel dissection and irretrievable occlusion. At the very least time will be taken up in crossing the lesion again, which in an acute situation is highly counterproductive.

Angioplasty itself is undertaken using a balloon catheter designed for the purpose. Balloons are available in a wide variety of diameters and lengths to suit the vessel and lesion being treated. The majority of balloons have radio-opaque markers at each end to facilitate the correct positioning of the device in relation to the stenosis (some have a marker in the middle). The balloon catheter is inserted through the vascular sheath over the guide wire and advanced into the correct position. This can be done using the roadmap, or bony landmarks may be chosen to facilitate positioning. The balloon is then inflated to the correct pressure for 30 seconds in the first instance. It is then removed, leaving the guide wire in place, and an angiogram is performed to demonstrate the response. If the result of the angioplasty has been satisfactory, the guide wire can be safely removed. If the result is unsatisfactory, further balloon inflations may be undertaken, perhaps to a greater diameter or for a longer period of time, or, depending on the site, a vascular stent may be inserted.

Iliac angioplasty

The results of iliac angioplasty are generally very good, with a low complication rate.[1,2] The procedure is safe and successful, and in many centres it is offered to patients who have intermittent claudication after 100 m walking or less. It may also be of great value as an adjunct to surgery.[3] For example, if a lower limb bypass graft is to be undertaken, iliac angioplasty to a stenosis above the proposed site of the proximal anastomosis will improve the inflow of blood, making a successful bypass more likely and reducing the extent of the surgery required.

When undertaking an iliac angioplasty it is often possible to choose whether to approach the lesion ipsilaterally and retrogradely, or contralaterally and antegradely. An ipsilateral approach, puncturing the artery on the side to be treated followed by crossing the stenosis in a retrograde fashion, offers an advantage: should a vessel dissection occur it is unlikely to lead to vessel occlusion, as the blood flow distally along the vessel will tend to close the intimal flap. The alternative, which involves puncturing the contralateral femoral artery, crossing the aortic bifurcation and then traversing the lesion, is technically more demanding and if a dissection occurs the blood flow will tend to cause the intimal flap to extend distally, potentially causing vessel occlusion.

Superficial femoral artery (SFA) angioplasty
(Fig. 34.1A–D)

This procedure is most commonly undertaken for the management of critical lower limb ischaemia or short-distance intermittent claudication. Such ischaemia is most likely to be caused by SFA occlusion, rather than a simple stenosis; thus to perform an angioplasty one must first cross the occlusion with a guide wire. This can be difficult, but the use of a hydrophilic guide wire will facilitate successful crossing in the vast majority of cases, with many operators electing to pass the guide wire subintimally. SFA angioplasty is less commonly performed for treatment of intermittent claudication, as generally the results are inferior to those of iliac angioplasty,[4,5] and two randomised studies have shown that the results are no better over the long term than those observed after a supervised exercise programme.[6,7]

As with iliac angioplasty, SFA lesions can be approached either contralaterally or ipsilaterally. The contralateral approach is the same in technical terms as that used for the iliac vessels. However, the ipsilateral approach to the SFA is technically more difficult, as an antegrade puncture of the CFA is required. To perform an antegrade puncture, the femoral head is first identified under fluoroscopy and its position marked on the skin surface with a metal marker. Local anaesthetic is infiltrated into the skin over the femoral pulse as it is palpated at this level. A puncture needle is introduced first and a guide wire is then introduced along the SFA. It is possible that the guide wire may pass into the profunda femoris, and for this reason it is important to observe its progress under fluoroscopic control. If it proves difficult to enter the SFA, it may be necessary to screen over the needle tip while manipulating it into different positions to facilitate guide wire advancement. When doing this it is very easy for the operator to put their hands into the X-ray beam without realising. The radiographer can prevent or minimise this by centring only on the very tip of the needle, rather than its whole length, and using the collimators appropriately. Antegrade puncture is often used because the distance from the puncture site to the angioplasty site is short, avoiding the need to use very long guide wires. It also avoids any problems associated with catheter manipulation when dealing with tortuous iliac arteries or an acutely angled aortic bifurcation; in the event of a complication occurring, the subsequent management, e.g. aspiration embolectomy, is much more straightforward (Fig. 34.1C,D).

Popliteal artery and the tibial vessels

Lesions in these vessels will only be treated with angioplasty in the presence of critical lower limb ischaemia or short-distance claudication (Fig. 34.2A,B). The potential benefit of angioplasty at these sites in patients with uncomplicated intermittent claudication would be completely outweighed by the potential risk and the likely recurrence rate in the future.[8] Technically there is very little difference between angioplasty performed here and elsewhere in the lower limb. Smaller diameter balloons are used, and many operators prefer to use finer guide wires.

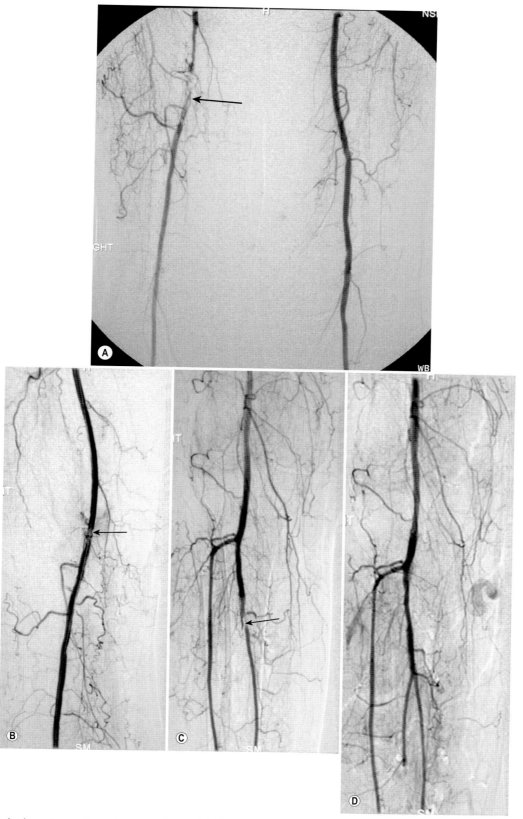

Figure 34.1 (A) Digital subtraction angiography (DSA) of superficial femoral and popliteal arteries – this image shows occlusion at the right adductor canal level (arrow) in a patient with critical ischaemia of the right foot. (B) Angioplasty – the occlusion seen in (A) was crossed easily and there was a good result from angioplasty (arrow). (C) Embolus in the peroneal artery – best practice involves obtaining views of the distal vessels to look for any possible complication. This image shows an embolus occluding the peroneal artery and projecting across the origin of the posterior tibial artery (arrow). (D) Peroneal artery post embolectomy – after aspiration embolectomy much of the embolus seen in (C) was removed. The posterior tibial artery is now patent, though it was not possible to clear the peroneal artery completely.

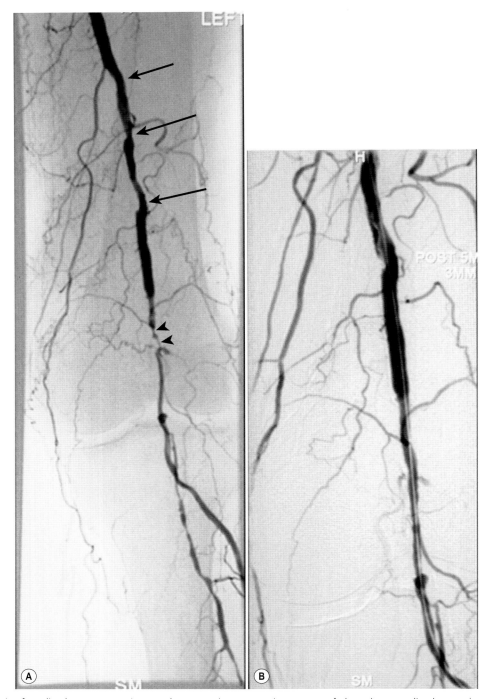

Figure 34.2 (A) Stenosis of popliteal artery – arteriogram demonstrating a stenotic segment of above knee popliteal artery (arrows) and a tight stenosis at the origin of the anterior tibial artery (arrowheads), which has an abnormally high take-off. (B) Arteriogram post angioplasty – a good technical result after angioplasty in the case shown in (A).

VASCULAR STENT INSERTION

The term 'stent' describes a device designed to keep a passage or conduit open. Vascular stents have become accepted as extremely helpful both in maintaining patency where the result of angioplasty alone has been suboptimal, and in certain locations where they provide such markedly superior benefits compared to angioplasty alone that they are considered to be the first line of treatment.

Vascular stents are metallic, commonly made either of stainless steel or nitinol. Nitinol is a nickel–titanium alloy which has great elasticity and 'shape memory', which allows it to return to its original state even after significant manipulation and bending. Stents may be self-expanding or balloon expandable. Prior to deployment, stents

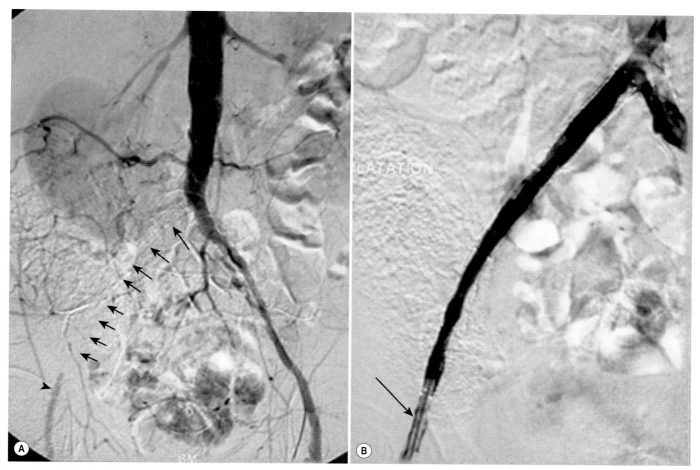

Figure 34.3 (A) Occluded common iliac artery – patient with rest pain in the right foot. A previous right common iliac stent is now occluded, along with the external iliac artery (arrows). There is reconstitution of the common femoral artery distally (arrowhead). (B) Stenting the occlusion – the patient in (A) was considered a very poor risk for surgery, therefore the occlusion was successfully stented despite the fact that there was concern that the distal end of the stent would be very near the hip joint and might be damaged during hip flexion. There is a filling defect distally caused by the vascular sheath (arrow).

are compressed onto a delivery catheter; each end of the stent either has radio-opaque markers on the device itself or on the catheter, to facilitate correct positioning. The technique used for deployment of a stent is much the same as that described for angioplasty, with the obvious difference that instead of performing simple balloon dilation, a stent is deployed instead. It will often prove necessary to perform angioplasty prior to stent deployment, and further angioplasty after deployment may be required to ensure that the stent is fully expanded.

Stents are used commonly in the iliac, renal and subclavian arteries. They are being used increasingly in the carotid arteries, although this remains experimental. In the UK, stents have only been used in the SFA as a 'bail-out' if angioplasty has resulted in vessel occlusion. However, stents have been used much more freely in the SFA elsewhere, and evidence is starting to show, at least with more modern stent designs, that concerns about low long-term patency rates of stents in the SFA (compared to those of angioplasty alone) may be unfounded. Stents are not used routinely in the popliteal or tibial vessels, though devices are available to be used in the event of a suboptimal result.

Stenting the iliac artery (Fig. 34.3A,B)

It has been shown that if iliac angioplasty is technically successful there is no advantage in terms of clinical outcome in adding a stent.[9–11] However, in about 50% of cases the outcome from angioplasty is suboptimal, perhaps due, for example, to elastic recoil of the vessel wall or dissection causing flow limitation. Many professionals would add to this and include failure to reduce the intra-arterial pressure gradient across the lesion to less than 10 mmHg as an indication.

The exception to this is the treatment of iliac artery occlusions where, if angioplasty alone is used, there is an incidence of peripheral embolisation of up to 50%.[9] For this reason, primary stenting is undertaken when treating iliac occlusions endovascularly. Thus, a self-expanding stent is first deployed across the occlusion and subsequently dilated using an angioplasty balloon.

Stenting the renal artery (Fig. 34.4A,B)

Renal artery stenosis is generally caused by one of two pathologies, either fibromuscular hyperplasia or atheroma. Fibromuscular

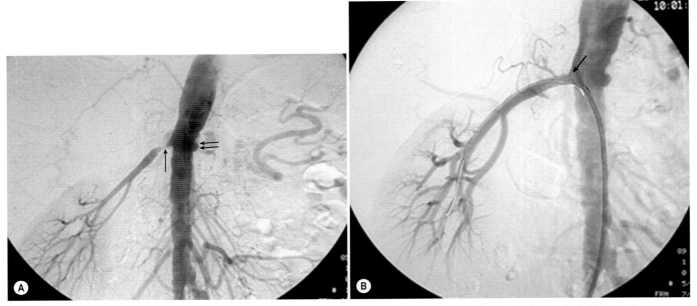

Figure 34.4 (A) Renal artery stenosis – abdominal aortogram showing severe right renal artery stenosis (arrow) and an occluded left renal artery (double arrow). (B) Renal artery stent – the patient was experiencing episodes of flash pulmonary oedema and had deteriorating renal function; a right renal artery stent was inserted (arrow) with good technical and clinical results, with improvement in cardiac failure and greatly improved renal function.

hyperplasia is an uncommon cause of uncontrollable hypertension and responds well to angioplasty alone. Atheromatous renal artery stenosis (ARAS), when it requires treatment, responds very poorly to angioplasty alone, and it has clearly been demonstrated that primary stenting is superior in both the short and the longer term.[12] This happens because the vast majority of ARAS occurs at the origin of the vessel and is caused by aortic atheroma rather than true atheroma of the renal artery. Therefore, an expansile force applied to the stenosis causes shear stresses within the aortic plaque, rather than an expansile force within the renal artery lumen. Once the angioplasty balloon is removed the stenosis will frequently recur as the aortic plaque moves back into position.

Balloon-expandable stents are favoured for the treatment of ARAS. In order to avoid the stent being compressed by the aortic plaques, it is necessary to position the stent so that it projects 2–3 mm into the aortic lumen. Such precision is much easier to achieve with balloon-expandable stents, as they do not shorten when they are deployed. Although much improved over older designs, even modern self-expanding stents show some shortening.

Subclavian stenting

Although stenoses or occlusions can occur in the subclavian arteries at any point, by far the commonest site of disease is the origin of the left subclavian artery. The majority of these lesions are asymptomatic. However, where there are symptoms of arm claudication or subclavian steal syndrome, intervention may be indicated. Stents are frequently used at this site, especially in the presence of arterial occlusion. However, there is little reliable published data in this area to allow firm conclusions to be drawn.

If there is occlusion at the origin of the left subclavian artery it is usually very difficult indeed to cross the lesion using a catheter inserted via the groin. It is therefore often helpful to use a transbrachial approach. Previously this often required a surgical cut-down onto the brachial artery for access, as 7 Fr or 8 Fr sheaths were required. Now sheaths of only 6 Fr in diameter can be used, which allows for true percutaneous puncture.

VASCULAR STENT GRAFTS

As previously mentioned, stent grafts are used in the treatment of true or false aneurysms. The technology continues to evolve, and it is not possible to say at this point whether stent grafting will replace open surgery in the treatment of aneurysmal disease. However, there is growing evidence to support the use of stent grafts in the treatment of thoracic aortic aneurysms, where the risks of surgery are considerably greater than those of open surgery for abdominal aneurysms.[13] Furthermore, there is some evidence to suggest that stent grafting may be of value in patients who would be at greater than average risk for abdominal surgery, for example if they have renal failure.[14-16] More recently, randomised data have shown a reduction in 30-day mortality when stent grafts are used for abdominal aortic aneurysm repair, compared to open surgery.[17,18]

When used for aortic aneurysms, stent graft delivery systems are large and require surgical exposure of one or both common femoral arteries. Smaller aneurysms, such as in the iliac arteries, can be treated without surgical exposure of vessels (Fig. 34.5A,B). Therefore, aortic stent graft procedures are frequently performed in the operating theatre with a mobile image intensifier. A better alternative, which is becoming increasingly available, is to use an angiographic suite that has been constructed to operating theatre standards. This provides a sufficiently sterile environment with a high standard of imaging.

Prior to the stent graft procedure the aneurysm is assessed for the diameter of the proximal and distal landing zones, as well as the overall length of the device. A number of 'off the shelf' devices are available, and several manufacturers are able to supply custom-made stent grafts for more complex cases.

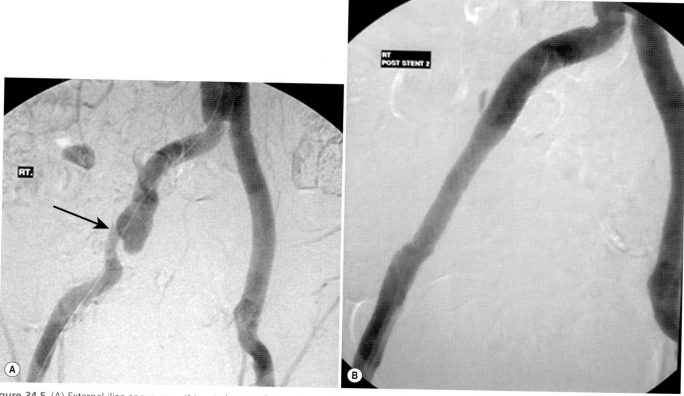

Figure 34.5 (A) External iliac aneurysm – this arteriogram shows a 3 cm diameter external iliac aneurysm arising at the distal end of an aorto-bi-iliac graft. (B) Treating the aneurysm with stent grafts – the aneurysm seen in (A) was successfully treated with two balloon expandable stent grafts.

Angiographic 'runs' are performed to ensure precise positioning of the device. For example, in stent grafting of abdominal aortic aneurysms it is clearly vital to avoid covering (and thereby occluding) the renal arteries with graft material. However, there are devices that have a bare stent at the proximal end which is designed to lie over the renal arteries. Once an image has been selected as the reference image for the deployment of the device it is vital that the C-arm is not moved. Even slight movement can cause errors due to parallax, which could cause misplacement of the stent graft.

EMBOLISATION

Commonly used embolisation agents include gelatin sponge (Fig. 34.6A–C) (for temporary embolisation), polyvinyl alcohol particles and coils (for permanent vessel occlusion). The full range of embolic materials available for clinical use is vast, complex, and includes materials that would require a whole chapter to describe and explain in detail. Embolisation procedures are often complex and time-consuming, and may require the use of superselective coaxial catheter systems; multiple magnified views of the area are needed.

The basic principle of embolisation is to identify the target vessel and place the catheter tip in the correct location prior to introducing the embolic material. Generally one wishes to place the catheter as far distally as possible to avoid embolisation of normal tissue. In addition, when delivering particulate materials it is important to avoid reflux of emboli. It is important, therefore, to use continuous fluoroscopy when injecting such materials.

Some embolisation procedures are relatively simple, such as treatment of varicocoeles. Varicocoeles normally affect the left testis, and occur because the valve at the confluence of the left testicular and the renal vein is incompetent, allowing reflux of blood at systemic venous pressure into the venous drainage of the testis. Treatment involves embolisation of the left testicular vein. The procedure involves placing a catheter in the left renal vein and injecting contrast while screening, and also saving the fluoroscopic image. Once valve incompetence has been confirmed and the anatomy demonstrated, the testicular vein is entered and embolisation coils are placed along its length. Generally patients requiring embolisation of the testicular vein are young, and it is clearly important to minimise radiation dose during this procedure.

Other procedures are more complex, such as embolisation for gastrointestinal bleeding (Fig. 34.7A–C), and require a more flexible approach to determine the precise anatomy and demonstrate the bleeding point accurately, followed by therapy. Highly complex situations, such as therapy for arteriovenous malformations, may be better referred to centres with a specialist interest in this area.

VENOUS INTERVENTIONS

Commonly undertaken venous interventions include placement of tunnelled venous lines and insertion of inferior vena cava (IVC) filters. Stents are also used in the venous system; however, the techniques used are very similar to those used in arteries, so it is not necessary to describe them in any greater detail.

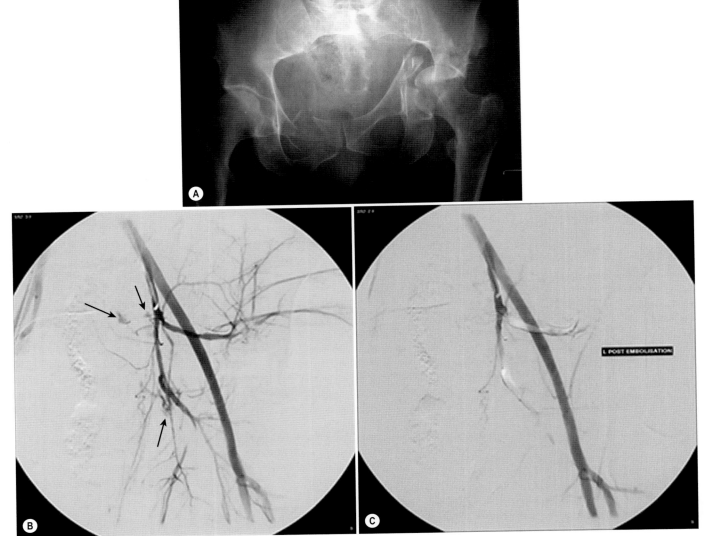

Figure 34.6 (A) Plain film showing very obvious pelvic fracture involving the left acetabulum and the pubic rami on the right. Pelvic fractures can be associated with severe bleeding, as was the case here, and angiography with a view to embolisation was performed. (B) Iliac arteriogram after pelvic fracture – selective left internal iliac arteriogram showing at least three bleeding points (arrows) on the case seen in (A). Appearances were similar on the right side as well. (C) Embolisation after trauma to internal iliac artery – the case seen in (A) and (B) after embolisation with gelatin sponge; no further bleeding is seen.

Tunnelled central venous lines

Tunnelled central venous lines are used for a variety of purposes, including administration of chemotherapy, total parenteral nutrition and temporary (and occasionally permanent) haemodialysis access. The line is tunnelled subcutaneously; near the point where the tunnel exits the skin it has a Dacron cuff attached to it which becomes incorporated into the tissues, making accidental dislodgement much less likely than with non-tunnelled lines. There are also port systems available in which the entire device can be placed subcutaneously and be accessed percutaneously with a needle for drug administration.

The most commonly accessed vessels are probably the internal jugular veins, followed by the subclavian veins. On occasion, these

vessels are occluded; this is particularly the case for patients who have had multiple central lines placed in the past, e.g. for haemodialysis. In these instances it may prove necessary to use alternative vessels, such as the external jugular vein, or even direct puncture of the IVC to provide venous access.

The best method of guiding the vessel puncture is US, which has the clear benefit of avoiding the use of ionising radiation and is recommended by NICE for jugular vein puncture.[19] When performing subclavian vein puncture it is possible to opacify the target vein with contrast, and guide the puncture in this way. Fluoroscopy is used to identify the catheter tip when positioning it in the superior vena cava (SVC). The first choice of vein for puncture is the right internal jugular. This vein follows an almost straight course into the right

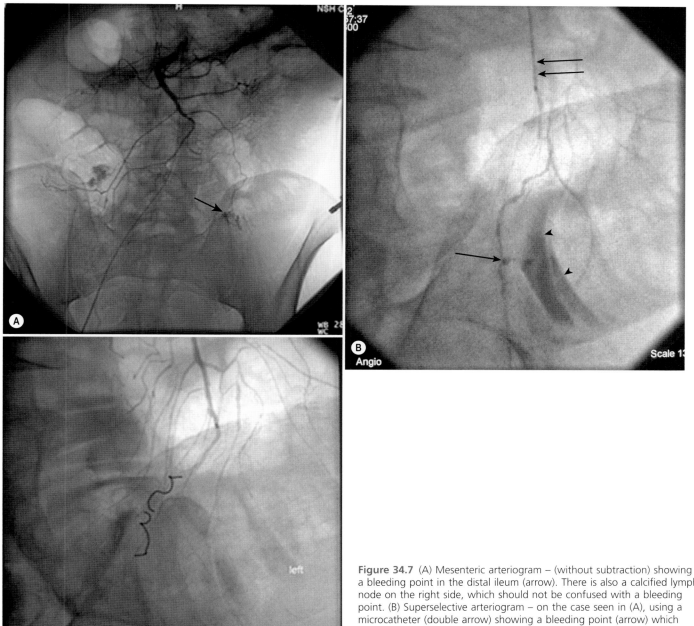

Figure 34.7 (A) Mesenteric arteriogram – (without subtraction) showing a bleeding point in the distal ileum (arrow). There is also a calcified lymph node on the right side, which should not be confused with a bleeding point. (B) Superselective arteriogram – on the case seen in (A), using a microcatheter (double arrow) showing a bleeding point (arrow) which is allowing extravasation of contrast material into the bowel lumen (arrowheads). (C) Embolisation – the bleeding vessel seen in (A) and (B) was successfully embolised using two microcoils.

brachiocephalic vein and subsequently the SVC, meaning that there is little potential for kinking of the introducer sheath during insertion. Use of the left internal jugular and subclavian veins is usually straightforward, whereas the use of the right subclavian vein can be difficult, as kinking of the introducer sheath can be a significant problem here.

The procedure is performed using local anaesthetic, often with light sedation. The target vein is punctured, under imaging guidance, and the guide wire introduced; passage of the guide wire through the heart into the IVC confirms that a venous puncture has been achieved. A short incision is made at the puncture point, and a tunnel measuring approximately 6 cm long is formed on the anterior chest wall. A specific tunnelling device is used for the purpose, and the catheter is then drawn through the tunnel and inserted through a peel-away sheath into the vein (depending on the manufacturer there is some variation in the precise technique used, which is beyond the scope of this chapter). The catheter tip is visualised on fluoroscopy and positioned in the lower part of the SVC. By using image guidance for the insertion of tunnelled central venous catheters, complications should be minimised. For example, pneumothorax rates with image-guided vein puncture have been reported as being as low as 0%, compared to 5% for blind puncture.[20]

IVC filters

IVC filters can be permanent or removable and are designed to prevent the passage of thrombus from the lower limbs into the pulmonary circulation, as prophylaxis against pulmonary embolism, which can be fatal. The standard treatment for deep vein thrombosis (DVT) is anticoagulation with heparin and subsequently warfarin. IVC filters are therefore only used in certain situations, such as when anticoagulation is contraindicated, when pulmonary embolism has occurred despite adequate anticoagulation, and on occasion as prophylaxis against pulmonary embolism during surgery for pelvic trauma. Although these are accepted by many as standard indications, the evidence surrounding the use of IVC filters is very weak,[21] and practice varies widely around the world.

Many types of IVC filter are available, and insertion via the internal jugular or femoral routes is possible. A number of retrievable filters are available on the market. The principles of filter insertion are relatively simple. Access to the venous system is achieved and an inferior venacavagram is obtained to document the size of the IVC and the location of the renal veins. Assuming that the IVC is not of an abnormally large diameter, the filter is deployed below the level of the renal veins. Although it is occasionally necessary to deploy above the renal veins, this is to be avoided wherever possible so that in the event of IVC thrombosis the renal veins do not also become occluded.

IVC filters have been shown to be effective at preventing pulmonary emboli[22] and have replaced the previous treatment of surgical ligation of the IVC. However, in the longer term IVC filters do not prevent recurrence of DVT. The complication rate of IVC filter insertion is low, but includes potential migration of the device, IVC thrombosis and IVC perforation.

FUTURE DEVELOPMENTS AND CURRENT IMPACT OF INTERVENTIONAL VASCULAR PROCEDURES

These minimally invasive procedures have had a massive impact in the management of patients with vascular disease. For example, iliac angioplasty or stent insertion has now replaced surgery for many patients who require treatment for iliac artery disease. In addition, where open surgery is required, adjunctive angioplasty or stent insertion can be of great value in reducing the complexity of surgery undertaken. This chapter has necessarily concentrated on the better-established techniques or devices. However, there is constant development in the devices industry, and there is little doubt that solutions will be found for some of the problems encountered with current technology. Perhaps one of the best publicised examples is the development of drug eluting stents. The stent surface is coated with a drug that inhibits endothelial cell growth, preventing in stent stenosis or occlusion by neointimal hyperplasia.[23,24]

Work is also progressing on the use of MRI for guidance when performing these procedures. Interventional MRI is becoming fairly well established in some areas, such as biopsy or image-guided surgery. However, the situation with vascular procedures is more complex, in that device movement needs to be monitored in real time. Work is being undertaken to allow catheter tracking to this end.[25]

REFLECTION ON ENDOVASCULAR THERAPY

The evidence concerning the use of endovascular therapy in the management of intermittent claudication is fairly clear. However, in the management of critical limb ischaemia the issues are more complex. The argument that is frequently advanced is that attempting an endovascular procedure does not preclude the subsequent use of surgery, which is usually true. However, consumables for these procedures are relatively expensive and if, to take an extreme, they were rarely successful, endovascular therapy in this arena would be highly wasteful of resources. The evidence for their use is often conflicting. The patients being treated in the various studies are, of course, a heterogeneous group, and the endpoints used are often different, making direct comparisons between studies very difficult.

In the 'real world' endovascular therapy is used by many as the first line, with surgery being held in reserve. Surgery for critical limb ischaemia, which will usually involve some form of distal bypass, is complex and may not be possible if there is no good vein available for use as a graft. Furthermore, wounds from open surgery may become infected, which in an already compromised limb can be disastrous, especially if infection is due to a multiresistant organism. Surgery may also be relatively contraindicated if there is pre-existing infection in the limb secondary to ischaemia. If revascularisation fails, amputation will inevitably follow. Not only is this expensive in terms of resources for rehabilitation, but many patients never actually manage to use their prosthetic limb, and the mortality from amputation is also very high. Therefore, there is a need for pragmatism in this area. Even if patency rates from endovascular therapy for critical limb ischaemia are far from perfect, avoiding amputation can only be regarded as a good thing.

With regard to stent grafts, the picture is becoming clearer. There is no doubt that anatomically suitable thoracic aortic aneurysms should be treated by stent grafting, as the mortality and morbidity from open surgery is so high. With regard to the abdominal aorta, two randomised trials have shown reduced 30-day mortality compared to open surgery.[17,18] There remains controversy about the longer-term outcomes, and further follow-up of these patient cohorts is ongoing. There is little doubt that, as technology improves to allow treatment of larger numbers of patients with challenging anatomy and to improve the durability of devices, the use of abdominal aortic stent grafting is likely to increase.

What of the future for conventional open vascular surgery? There has been much talk in the UK of the development of a single specialist with skills in both open and endovascular surgery. However, it has become apparent that the shortage of people wanting to enter both vascular surgery and interventional radiology requires that both groups of specialists remain at the present time. In addition, it is unlikely that there is sufficient time available in the training years to become competent in both. Elsewhere in Europe and the USA many vascular surgeons have adopted endovascular techniques. However, it is almost certainly true that individuals tend to concentrate on one or the other, as it is very difficult to remain highly skilled at both. For the foreseeable future there will be a continued need to use open surgical techniques, but as technology improves, endovascular therapy is likely to be used in ever-increasing numbers of patients.

NON-VASCULAR INTERVENTIONAL PROCEDURES OR THERAPIES

This sphere of interventional radiology is often referred to as non-vascular interventional radiology and encompasses techniques in the gastrointestinal tract, liver and biliary system, the urogenital system, the musculoskeletal system and the airways. Before considering the interventional techniques used in specific systems, it is worth examining the subjects of biopsy and drainage, which are very commonly used techniques that do not fit within a systems categorisation as they are used in many organs and cavities.

Image-guided biopsy

This term refers to any procedure conducted under image guidance that yields tissue for histological or cytological examination. Although not strictly therapeutic, it is a common invasive procedure that is frequently a prerequisite to some form of therapy. The principles of fine needle aspiration (FNA), where cells are sampled with a narrow-gauge needle for cytological examination, and core biopsy, where a larger core of tissue is obtained for histological examination, are the same. However, if FNA is to be undertaken the diagnostic yield is greatly enhanced by a technician or cytologist being present at the time of biopsy to ensure that the sample is diagnostic. If that is not possible, experience shows that it is better, wherever feasible, to obtain a core of tissue for formal histological examination. This applies even in the lung, where one might imagine that a thinner needle would produce lower complication rates.

Biopsies are perhaps most commonly performed under either US or CT guidance. It is also possible, using non-ferromagnetic needles, to perform biopsies using interventional MRI scanners. The principles governing image-guided biopsies are very similar, with CT requiring additional considerations regarding the use of ionising radiation.

Having chosen the most suitable modality for performing a biopsy, and ensured that there are no contraindications such as abnormal blood clotting, the first decision concerns the position the patient should be placed in. This will be based on where the skin entry point needs to be, not only to allow the needle to follow the shortest path to the lesion, but also to avoid important structures such as vessels. Patient comfort and stability are important in ensuring safe execution of the procedure. Supine or prone positions are commonly used, having the advantage of being fairly stable, meaning that patient movement during the procedure is rarely a problem. Some older patients do have problems with lying prone for prolonged periods, especially if they have arthritis of their cervical spine, which may give neck pain during the procedure. Lying patients on their side may sometimes be necessary, and if so it is important that suitable support is provided to eliminate movement during the biopsy.

One must be cautious when performing a biopsy in a different position from that of the diagnostic imaging, as the relationships of various structures can be altered. A good example is when performing CT-guided adrenal gland biopsy. When a patient has a CT scan in the supine position the upper abdominal organs and diaphragm tend to fall backwards, obliterating much of the posterior costophrenic recess, giving an apparently straightforward path to the adrenal glands. However, the adrenal glands are in the retroperitoneum and it is necessary to perform a biopsy with the patient in the prone position. This causes the organs of the upper abdomen and the diaphragm to displace anteriorly, widening the posterior costophrenic recess and extending it caudally. In the majority of patients this means that aerated lung will now lie between the target adrenal gland and the nearest skin entry point. It is therefore necessary to insert the biopsy needle with a cranial angulation in order to travel upwards towards the adrenal gland while avoiding the lung. The advent of CT fluoroscopy makes such manoeuvres more easily achievable as the needle can be viewed in real time.

In some situations there may be no immediately obvious path available. A good example is that of lesions in the chest positioned behind the heart. Clearly there is no path from the anterior chest wall, and trying to reach the lesion from a lateral approach would involve crossing a great deal of lung parenchyma, with the consequent risk of pneumothorax or even bleeding. It is possible to use a posterior approach by injecting normal saline paraspinally to produce a window through which the biopsy needle can pass. This avoids crossing lung parenchyma and any potential pneumothorax.

Percutaneous drainage procedures

A large number of drainage procedures are undertaken to treat abdominal or pelvic abscesses, as even in the antibiotic era, if pus is not drained from an abdominal or pelvic abscess cavity, the mortality rate remains high. Abdominal and pelvic abscesses may arise from a variety of causes, including as a complication of surgery, diverticular disease, Crohn's disease and pancreatitis. Pancreatitis may also cause pseudocysts in the pancreas itself, and abscesses may develop in the liver and occasionally the spleen. Drainage procedures are also increasingly being undertaken in the thorax, both for simple pleural effusions and for empyemas.

A variety of drains are available, varying from 6 Fr (2 mm) to 16 Fr (5.3 mm) in diameter. In general, the more viscous the material to be drained the wider the catheter required. If initial drainage with a catheter fails, it may be worth exchanging it for a larger one.

Drains can be inserted using US, CT, fluoroscopy or MRI for guidance. Clearly there are issues for MRI-guided procedures, related to the requirement to use non-ferrous materials.

The fluid collection or abscess is first identified via the chosen diagnostic imaging procedure and then the optimal position for intervention is decided upon in much the same way as for percutaneous biopsy. If a collection is relatively large and superficial it may be straightforward to insert a drain directly into it on a trocar, without the use of a guide wire. If this is to be done, it may be helpful to insert a narrow gauge Chiba needle first and check its position, to give an idea of the direction in which the larger drain needs to be inserted.

If the procedure is particularly complex it is often effective to insert an 18 G Chiba needle under CT guidance and, having checked that the needle tip lies within the collection, insert a guide wire over which the drain can be inserted. There is less chance of kinking the guide wire if the procedure is visualised in real time, so CT fluoroscopy is again useful. If CT fluoroscopy is not available it may be advantageous, once the Chiba needle has been inserted, to move the patient into a fluoroscopy suite for guide wire insertion and drain introduction, but as long as the procedure is undertaken with extreme care, insertion of the guide wire and drain without fluoroscopy ought not to cause problems.

When draining pancreatic abscesses or pseudocysts, one must take particular care to prevent the formation of a fistula between the pancreas and the skin. This is best achieved by using a transgastric approach; thus if a fistula does form after drain removal, it will be between the pancreatic duct and the stomach, rather than the skin. Pancreatic secretions will therefore pass harmlessly into the stomach. Although it is possible to puncture the stomach under US guidance, the greater degree of confidence is given by using CT. Having entered the pseudocyst, a drain is inserted as for a normal collection. However, it should be noted that the fluid from pancreatic collections is often quite thick, and larger drains are often required.

NON-VASCULAR INTERVENTIONAL TECHNIQUES: GASTROINTESTINAL TRACT

Oesophagus

Interventional techniques in the oesophagus are most commonly used in the relief of obstruction which causes dysphagia, although treatment is sometimes required for oesophageal fistulae or perforations. Oesophageal obstruction may be due to benign causes such as peptic strictures caused by chronic reflux oesophagitis, achalasia, radiotherapy or ingestion of caustic substances. Alternatively, the cause may be malignancy, due to oesophageal carcinoma or extrinsic compression from malignant lymph nodes.

Oesophageal dilation

Oesophageal dilation, when performed under fluoroscopy alone, is achieved using balloon dilators. It appears that many endoscopists are also switching to use balloons rather than bougies (a series of flexible dilators of increasing thickness). Dilation alone is suitable only for treating benign lesions of the oesophagus (Fig. 34.8A,B), when dilation is required owing to resection after surgery for malignancy, rather than due to the original malignancy; when used in an attempt to relieve malignant dysphagia the results are usually only very short-lived, and there is up to a 10% incidence of oesophageal perforation.

At the start of the procedure the patient is placed on the fluoroscopic table in the left lateral position. The throat is anaesthetised with xylocaine spray, and the patient is sedated. A suitable catheter and guide wire are used through a per-oral approach to cross the stricture, and the catheter is exchanged for a balloon. The size of balloon used varies according to the type of lesion being treated. Thus fibrotic lesions such as those caused by radiotherapy or ingestion of caustic substances need to be treated initially with small angioplasty balloons, with diameters of 8–10 mm, as there is a high incidence of perforation. Over a number of treatments progressively larger balloons are used, with the aim of reaching a final diameter of 20 mm. Strictures resulting from chronic reflux oesophagitis can normally be treated with 20 mm balloons immediately, whereas in achalasia, where the aim is to tear muscle fibres, larger balloons of 30–40 mm in diameter are required.

Generally, technical success rates of around 95% are quoted.[26-28] These results are as good as if not better than those of bougienage, and avoid the morbidity and mortality associated with surgery. Stricture recurrence can be a problem, but up to 70% of patients remain asymptomatic at 2 years. Recurrent dysphagia can usually be successfully treated with repeat dilation. The main potential complication of oesophageal dilation is perforation. Overall, the perforation rate does appear to be very low, with some workers reporting no incidence of this; when taking consent from patients, quotation of a perforation rate of less than 1% can be supported.[23-25] However, there are important exceptions to this: for example, the perforation rate for dilation of caustic strictures has been quoted as being as high as 25%. One would expect the situation to be similar for strictures induced by radiotherapy.

Oesophageal stent insertion

At the time of presentation a significant proportion of patients with oesophageal carcinoma have lesions that are not amenable to surgical resection. However, they all have or will develop dysphagia that requires palliation. Available treatments include surgery, chemotherapy, radiotherapy, laser therapy, rigid plastic tubes and self-expanding metallic oesophageal stents. There is now wide experience in the use of oesophageal stents, and they form an important part of the palliation of malignant oesophageal obstruction.

The technique of insertion is very similar to that for oesophageal dilation. However, once the stricture has been crossed with a guide wire it is pre-dilated to 15 mm in diameter. Using a balloon of a smaller diameter than the stent diminishes the risk of over-dilating the oesophagus, which would increase the risk of stent migration. Some practitioners do not dilate the oesophagus prior to deploying a stent; however, in some cases this may mean that the stent expands insufficiently to allow removal of the delivery system through it. Once the stent has been deployed the delivery system is removed and contrast medium injected to ensure patency and that there has been no perforation. After the patient has recovered from the sedation they are allowed initially to take sips of fluid, and over the next few hours to take increasing volumes.

The results of oesophageal stenting are generally good, with improvement or complete relief of dysphagia in 83–100% of patients.[29-31] Complications include perforation, for which insertion of a covered stent is the treatment anyway; stent migration; pain; upper gastrointestinal haemorrhage; aspiration pneumonia and fistula formation. The results of stenting are better than those reported for palliative surgery,[32] chemotherapy and radiotherapy,[33,34] in terms of both success in the relief of dysphagia and the complications encountered. Results of a randomised study have in addition shown stent insertion to be superior to the use of laser therapy.[35] Covered stents are also highly successful in sealing leaks and fistulae to the airways caused by malignant tumours[36] (Fig. 34.9A,B).

Stomach and duodenum

The two main interventional radiological procedures undertaken in this anatomical location are percutaneous gastrostomy and stent insertion. Balloon dilation is occasionally undertaken for strictures involving surgical anastomoses or due to pyloric dysfunction after gastric pull-up operations performed for oesophageal carcinoma. However, such balloon dilation differs little from that performed in the oesophagus, and will not be described in further detail here.

Percutaneous gastrostomy

In many hospitals in the UK fluoroscopically guided gastrostomy insertion is only undertaken if the endoscopic approach has failed. Gastrostomy is performed most commonly to provide enteral nutrition if there is an anatomical or functional difficulty in swallowing. It is also sometimes undertaken to decompress the stomach. Over the last few years fewer gastrostomies have been required in cases of oesophageal carcinoma because of the advent of oesophageal stents. One of the commonest reasons, if not the most common, for gastrostomy insertion is stroke causing swallowing difficulties.

Prior to gastrostomy a nasogastric tube needs to be inserted, preferably the day before, to drain gastric contents. A US scan is performed to identify the left lobe of the liver, and this is marked on the skin. In addition, some radiologists advocate the administration of barium the night before to opacify the transverse colon. Both of these are aimed at preventing inadvertent puncture of adjacent organs. The stomach is then fully inflated with air introduced via the nasogastric tube; this displaces the colon inferiorly and brings the anterior gastric wall as close as possible to the anterior abdominal wall. A suitable pathway to the stomach is identified under fluoroscopy and the skin is infiltrated with local anaesthetic. A needle is then passed into the stomach; either the stomach can be fixed to the anterior abdominal wall with 'T' fasteners, or a guide wire can be inserted, followed by proceeding directly to gastrostomy tube insertion.

The technical success of the procedure is reported as being 99–100%.[37-39] Potential complications include reflux of the enteral feed into the oesophagus, with the risk of causing aspiration pneumonia. If such reflux occurs the gastrostomy can be converted to a gastrojejunostomy, which usually solves the problem. Further major complications of the procedure include severe bleeding, peritonitis and sepsis, and have been reported in 1.4–6.0% of cases. Minor complications include peritoneal irritation, local infection and tube migration or displacement.[37-39]

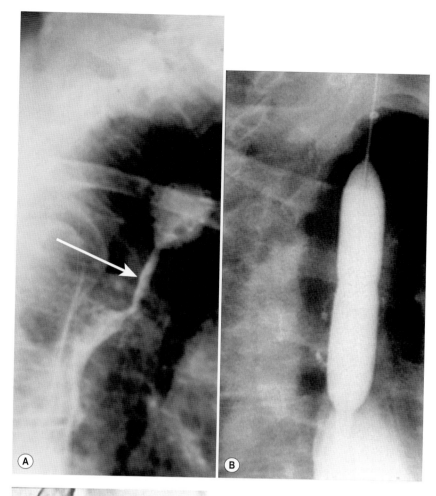

Figure 34.8 (A) Stricture requiring oesophageal dilation – contrast swallow showing a tight stricture at the anastomosis between the upper oesophagus and a gastric pull-up after resection of an oesophageal carcinoma (arrow). (B) Oesophageal dilation – 20 mm oesophageal balloon fully inflated across the stricture.

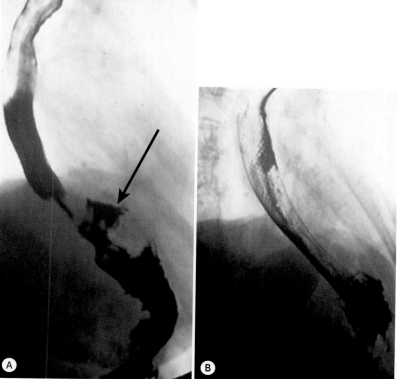

Figure 34.9 (A) Oesophageal malignancy and endoscopic perforation – carcinoma of the oesophagogastric junction causing obstruction and associated with perforation after endoscopy (arrow). (B) Using a covered stent to treat a stricture and seal perforation – the stricture has been successfully treated and the perforation sealed with a covered oesophageal stent.

Gastric and duodenal stenting

In the stomach and duodenum stents are used in the management of strictures, which are usually caused by malignant tumours of the stomach or the pancreas. They are occasionally required for the treatment of pyloric dysfunction after gastric pull-up operations if balloon dilation is unsuccessful.[40] Peptic strictures are becoming increasingly uncommon with improved treatment for peptic ulcer disease. Often insertion of gastric or duodenal stents for malignancy is only requested if patients are considered unfit for surgery. However, as experience grows, it would appear that stents are being used for these indications more commonly as an alternative to surgery in fit patients.

Stent procedures in the stomach and duodenum are technically more complex than those in the oesophagus. The reasons for this are that the large size and distensibility of the stomach allows space for loops of guide wire and catheter to form, and the fact that longer catheters and delivery systems are required, both making manipulation across strictures more difficult. For these reasons many workers advocate the use of endoscopy in conjunction with fluoroscopy; albeit not always required, endoscopic assistance can be very helpful in difficult cases.

Prior to the availability of dedicated stents diameter vascular wall stents were used (Fig. 34.10A,B), as the standard oesophageal stents were not available on a sufficiently long delivery system. However, there are now specific stents available for use in the stomach, duodenum and colon. The procedure is very similar to that for oesophageal stent insertion, apart from the different anatomical location, so it will not be described in any further detail. Success rates of 80–100% have been reported.[41–44] The only reported complication is aspiration of gastric contents into the airways, and this is infrequent. Although perforation of the stomach or the duodenum is a theoretical possibility it has not been reported.

Colon

Colonic stents

Colonic stents were originally intended for temporary use in patients presenting with acute large bowel obstruction secondary to colonic carcinoma. This allows bowel preparation to be given and a primary bowel anastomosis to be formed at the time of tumour resection, rather than having to perform a defunctioning colostomy and return some weeks later to rejoin the bowel loops. However, more recently, colonic stents have been used as the sole treatment for obstruction for patients who will only receive palliative therapy. As such they are used not only in the management of unresectable colon tumours, but also in the management of other extensive pelvic tumours causing colonic obstruction.

A number of stents are available for use in the colon. The technique involves gaining access to the colon via a rectal approach and traversing the stricture with guide wire and catheter techniques (Fig. 34.11A,B). As the colon is tortuous and the haustra can make catheter and guide wire manipulation difficult, it may be helpful to use either a supporting sheath or a colonoscope to provide additional support. Once the stricture has been crossed the stent is deployed; following deployment balloon dilation is occasionally required, though if possible this is to be avoided: rely instead on gradual stent expansion over 24 hours or so in order to minimise the risk of bowel perforation.

Around 70% of colonic carcinomas are on the left side of the large bowel. Clinical success rates of 64–100% are reported, with right-sided lesions being much more difficult to reach and treat.[45–47] In addition, cost reductions of around 28% have been reported when using stents rather than the conventional approach of defunctioning colostomy. Complications of colonic perforation, stent displacement

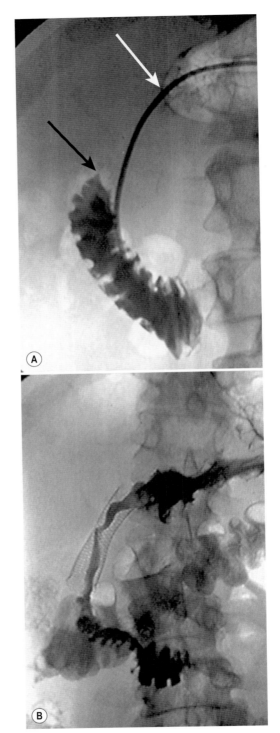

Figure 34.10 (A) Gastric outlet obstruction – this patient had gastric outlet obstruction due to carcinoma of the pancreas. A catheter is positioned across the obstruction, the limits of which are defined by air in the stomach proximally and contrast in the duodenum distally (arrows). (B) Relieving gastric outlet obstruction – a contrast study performed on the day after stent deployment shows full stent expansion and complete relief of gastric outlet obstruction.

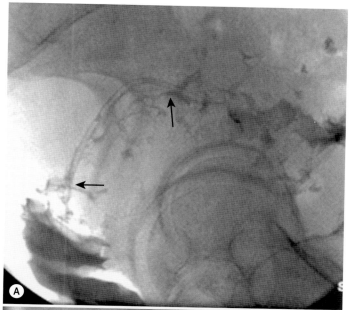

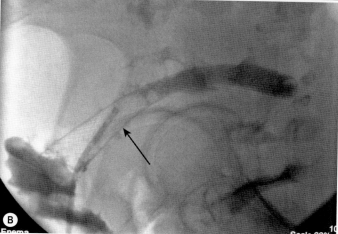

Figure 34.11 (A) Rectal stricture – catheter placed across a fairly long rectal stricture caused by a carcinoma. The approximate limits of the stricture are shown by the arrows. (B) Relieving rectal obstruction – the obstruction has been relieved by deployment of an enteral wall stent.

and obstruction have been reported. More minor complications include rectal bleeding, tenesmus, transient anorectal pain and fecal impaction.[45–47]

NON-VASCULAR INTERVENTIONAL TECHNIQUES: THE BILIARY TREE

It should be noted that the majority of interventions in the biliary tree are undertaken at the time of endoscopic retrograde cholangiopancreatography (ERCP). However, if ERCP fails for any reason the percutaneous approach to the biliary tree is required. The most common procedure undertaken by interventionists in the biliary tree is stent insertion. Biliary drainage is also frequently carried out, usually prior to stenting, and there is occasionally a call to dilate benign biliary

strictures. Biliary drainage will be described first, as access to the biliary tree is an essential component of all of these procedures.

Indications for intervention in the biliary tree include palliation of unresectable primary or metastatic malignancy, benign biliary strictures, sepsis accompanying biliary obstruction, and preoperative decompression. ERCP is also frequently used in the treatment of calculi in the bile ducts, and percutaneous biliary intervention may be required where the bile ducts have been opacified at ERCP but it has not been possible to secure drainage with a stent; if obstructed bile ducts are left undrained in this situation there is a significant risk of cholangitis.

ERCP

In most centres ERCP is now the first line in imaging and intervention for the biliary tree, and technical success rates of 75–98% are reported.[48] The procedure involves using a side-viewing endoscope to visualise and then cannulate the ampulla of Vater in the second part of the duodenum. Contrast is then injected through the cannula, and the biliary tree and pancreatic duct are opacified. Having made a diagnosis, appropriate therapy can often be delivered at the same sitting. Thus, in cases of obstruction a sphincterotomy is first performed; essentially this involves making a cut at the lower end of the common bile duct to allow instruments to pass. If obstruction is being caused by gallstones in the common bile duct, sphincterotomy alone occasionally allows a stone to drop out of the duct; more frequently it proves necessary to trawl the duct with baskets or balloons to extract the calculi. If there is a benign biliary stricture this can be balloon dilated, whereas malignant strictures require stent insertion.

ERCP is also of value if the biliary tree is not dilated. One example of this is in patients who have experienced bile duct trauma at the time of laparoscopic cholecystectomy and have a resultant biliary leak. Placement of a plastic biliary stent for around 6 weeks to divert the flow of bile away from the area of leakage into the duodenum will usually result in sealing of the leak. After 6 weeks the stent can be removed.

A further example is that of primary biliary sclerosis, where there is widespread narrowing of bile ducts. In this situation it is sometimes possible to identify a 'dominant stricture' that can be dilated, with the relief of some or all of the patient's symptoms.

Potential complications of ERCP include death, sepsis, haemorrhage and bile leak. If ERCP is not possible, for example due to previous partial gastrectomy or duodenal stenosis, or if it fails for some other reason, then percutaneous biliary intervention can be attempted. In addition, there are strong arguments for using percutaneous biliary intervention as the primary mode of palliation for malignant hilar strictures, i.e. proximal lesions that involve one or more of the common hepatic duct or right or left hepatic ducts.[49]

Percutaneous biliary drainage

The first step in any percutaneous biliary tract intervention is to gain access to the bile ducts. This is done by first performing a percutaneous transhepatic cholangiogram (PTC). Having ensured that the blood clotting is normal and prophylactic antibiotics have been administered, the patient is placed on the X-ray table in the supine position with their right arm raised above their head. The right upper quadrant is imaged by fluoroscopy and a suitable point for skin puncture is selected. Local anaesthetic is administered along with intravenous sedation and/or analgesia. A thin (22 or 21 G) Chiba needle is advanced into the liver and then gradually withdrawn while contrast is gently injected. Several passes of the Chiba needle may be required in order to access a bile duct, although if the biliary tree is dilated it is rare to fail.

Once the bile ducts have been opacified a suitable guide wire is inserted through the Chiba needle. Occasionally it proves necessary to reposition the needle prior to guide wire insertion. The Chiba needle is exchanged for a coaxial dilator system, allowing insertion of a larger and stiffer guide wire. If biliary drainage alone is to be performed, it is possible at this stage to insert a pigtail drainage catheter over the guide wire into the bile duct, to provide external drainage of bile; this option may be chosen, for example, if there is cholangitis that requires treatment before definitive therapy.

If it is possible to pass the guide wire through the ampulla of Vater, it is possible to use an internal/external biliary drain. This device has drainage holes along a greater length than the standard external drainage catheter such that, when positioned with the pigtail in the duodenum, drainage holes lie above and below the papilla. This allows much of the bile to drain internally, while retaining access to the biliary tree for future intervention. Internal/external biliary drains tend to be more secure, and can be useful for providing internal drainage while making decisions regarding management.

Biliary stenting

Both plastic and metallic stents are available for relief of biliary obstruction. At ERCP the vast majority of stents used are plastic, as they are relatively cheap. However, because they are much smaller in diameter than metallic stents they have a much greater tendency to block. There is evidence that, when stents are being used for the palliation of malignant biliary strictures, metallic stents are in fact more cost-effective than plastic devices because of the lower reintervention rate.[50,51]

When placing stents percutaneously, some consideration needs to be given to the size of the device being placed across the liver parenchyma. At 12 Fr in diameter the plastic stents placed at ERCP are considered by many operators to be too large to be inserted through the liver, so many percutaneously placed stents are only 10 Fr in diameter, with a consequent reduction in lumen size. It is advantageous to use self-expanding metallic stents percutaneously (Fig. 34.12A,B): these not only have the advantage of a small delivery system (6 Fr), they also provide a much larger lumen (up to 10 mm, or the equivalent of 30 Fr).

The other factor in deciding whether to use a metallic or plastic stent is the cause of the biliary stricture. If metallic stents are used in benign strictures, for example those caused by chronic pancreatitis, most will occlude over a period of months owing to the overgrowth of epithelial cells through the stent mesh. As a result, one can face great difficulties in management, and it is better where at all possible to manage such patients by ERCP and regular elective stent changes. In malignant biliary strictures the reduced reintervention rate and delivery system size associated with metallic stents makes a compelling case for their use.

Dilation of benign biliary strictures

There is a wide variety of potential causes for benign biliary strictures. However, in the Western world the majority are iatrogenic, either as a result of trauma to the bile ducts at the time of laparoscopic cholecystectomy or occurring at anastomoses formed between the small bowel and the biliary tree, either at the time of liver transplantation or at biliary bypass for the management of biliary strictures or surgery for pancreatic carcinoma. Benign biliary strictures may also be caused by chronic infection associated with bile duct calculi.

Decision making and management in this patient group can be complex, and requires a multidisciplinary approach. Even relatively mild strictures can cause stone formation, cholangitis and cirrhosis. Surgery has traditionally been used, but ERCP has become

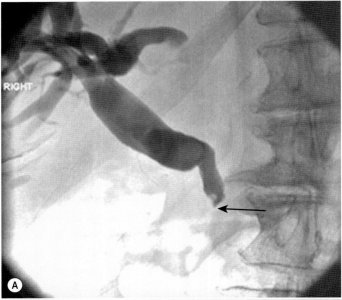

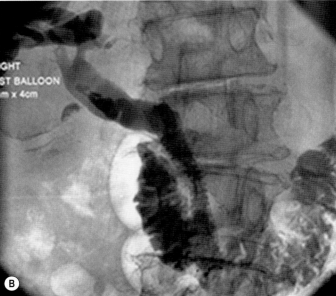

Figure 34.12 (A) Obstructed common bile duct – cholangiogram performed via catheter positioned in the biliary tree. Complete obstruction of the distal common bile duct has been demonstrated (arrow). (B) Stenting bile duct obstruction – the obstruction has been relieved by the deployment of a 10 mm diameter self-expanding metallic stent.

increasingly important in the management of such patients, and good long-term results with plastic stents and repeated stent changes have been reported.[52,53] Where ERCP is not possible, perhaps because of previous surgery, percutaneous treatment may be required. Plastic stents are frequently used, and balloon dilation of strictures is reported as being very successful. However, several treatments may be required in order to achieve a satisfactory result; if percutaneous therapy is to be used this will require long-term placement of a biliary drain, which is inconvenient for the patient.[54]

NON-VASCULAR INTERVENTIONAL TECHNIQUES: UROGENITAL TRACT

The most widely undertaken procedure in the urogenital tract is percutaneous nephrostomy. Having gained access to the urinary tract it is also possible to introduce ureteric stents to relieve obstruction and use balloons to dilate strictures. Percutaneous nephrolithotomy (PCNL) is also used in the treatment of renal calculi. In recent years, increasing numbers of uterine artery embolisations (UAEs) have been performed for the treatment of uterine fibroids.

Percutaneous nephrostomy

Percutaneous nephrostomy is usually performed to relieve urinary tract obstruction. An alternative approach is to place retrograde ureteric double 'J' stents cystoscopically. However, nephrostomy has advantages in certain situations, such as malignant obstruction and if infection is present (pyonephrosis).

The procedure itself can be carried out using either fluoroscopy or US alone or a combination of the two, which may ensure more confidence. The patient is placed prone on the fluoroscopy table with the side to be treated slightly elevated. A US scan is performed to identify the hydronephrotic kidney; it is usually possible to identify calyces and to select one for puncture. Wherever possible one aims to puncture a posterior lower pole calyx, as the arrangement of intrarenal vessels at this site means that the risk of bleeding complications is less with this approach. The skin and deep tissues are infiltrated with local anaesthetic and intravenous sedation and/or analgesia is administered. A suitable needle is then introduced into the collecting system under US guidance.

After the collecting system has been successfully punctured a stiff or superstiff guide wire is introduced; if at all possible the guide wire is directed down the ureter to give the most secure position. It is impossible to see this reliably on US and it is best visualised on fluoroscopy, hence the combined US and fluoroscopic method is most often preferred. Once the operator is satisfied with the guide wire position a suitable nephrostomy catheter (typically 8 Fr in diameter) is introduced, fixed to the skin and attached to a drainage bag.

If the cause of the obstruction is self-limiting, such as a small ureteric calculus, the nephrostomy may only be required for a few days and then removed. Similarly, it may be removed after definitive treatment such as ureteroscopy and stone removal has been carried out. In other situations further intervention may be required, either at the same time as nephrostomy insertion or on another occasion. This will be discussed in the following sections.

Minor complications requiring no additional therapy are fairly common, and virtually every patient will develop transient mild haematuria. Severe bleeding necessitating transfusion or other intervention is reported as occurring in 1–3% of cases.[55]

Ureteric stent insertion

Ureteric obstruction may arise from a variety of causes. Antegrade stenting via a nephrostomy track is only rarely required for temporary causes such as calculi. However, causes such as strictures or obstruction caused by malignancy or radiotherapy can rarely be stented retrogradely, and antegrade ureteric stenting is of immense value in this patient group.[56,57]

The stents used have a pigtail shape at either end and are made of plastic. They need to be changed every few months, although this does not require repeat nephrostomy; once the obstruction has been crossed it is almost always possible to change stents retrogradely.

The principles behind antegrade ureteric stenting are relatively simple. Having gained access to the upper urinary tract by performing a nephrostomy, an angiographic catheter and guide wire are manipulated into the ureter and through the obstruction. The guide wire is exchanged for a stiff guide wire and a suitable size of stent is introduced over it. In order to achieve a suitable angle for stent insertion it may prove necessary to gain access via middle or even upper pole calyx, as attempting to push the stent forwards from a lower pole puncture can lead to a loop forming in the proximal guide wire, which is then pushed into the upper pole region. If stenting from a lower pole puncture, a peel-away sheath advanced into the proximal ureter will normally remedy this problem without having to resort to a further puncture.

Balloon dilation of ureteric strictures

Benign strictures in the native ureters may occur for a variety of reasons, including calculus disease, radiotherapy and surgical trauma. In renal transplants, ureteric strictures may be due to periureteric fibrosis, anastomotic fibrosis or ischaemia. Diffuse strictures caused by chronic rejection or necrosis cannot be successfully dilated with balloons.

The procedure is identical in many respects to that of ureteric stent insertion, except for the fact that a high-pressure balloon is placed across the stricture and dilated, followed by insertion of a stent. The stent is then removed some weeks later. Good long-term results can be anticipated in up to 50% of benign ureteric strictures.[58]

PCNL

PCNL was developed in the mid-1970s and, as it became accepted, largely replaced open surgery for urinary tract stones. Despite the subsequent development of extracorporeal shockwave lithotripsy and ureteroscopic techniques, PCNL is still regularly used for the management of urinary tract stone disease.

PCNL may be carried out either in the operating theatre with a mobile image intensifier, or in the radiology department; in either instance the patient is placed under general anaesthesia. It is important to establish which calyces contain stones on preoperative imaging; the appropriate calyx for puncture is then selected. Initially the urologist performs a cystoscopy and passes a ureteric catheter into the proximal ureter. The patient is then turned prone, and the collecting system is opacified with contrast medium injected through the ureteric catheter. The chosen calyx is then punctured and a guide wire introduced and placed in the ureter.

A peel-away sheath is introduced over the guide wire, which allows the insertion of a second superstiff guide wire. This provides two guide wires, one for dilating the track and the other as a safety guide to prevent access being lost. The track is dilated to 30 Fr in diameter using either coaxial metal dilators or a balloon system, followed by insertion of a 30 Fr working sheath. This allows the introduction of a nephroscope, baskets and mechanical lithotripters for the breaking up and removal of calculi. This part of the procedure is undertaken by the urologists, so teamwork is very important.

After successful stone removal the working sheath is removed and a large nephrostomy tube left in situ for 1–2 days. Success rates for stone removal are high. The mortality rate for such large-bore access to the urinary tract is low (less than 0.3%).[59] Significant bleeding is more likely than with smaller-bore tubes, but can usually be managed by inserting a balloon dilation catheter into the track to provide tamponade. If tamponade over a few days fails, angiography and embolisation may be needed.

UAE for uterine fibroids

Embolisation in general has been described earlier in this chapter. However, UAE for uterine fibroids merits special consideration under genitourinary therapies.

The technique was first described in the mid-1990s and has been taken up enthusiastically by many radiologists and patients alike. It is attractive as an alternative to hysterectomy as it is a day-case procedure, whereas hysterectomy is a major surgical procedure with a prolonged period of recovery often required. There are other clear resource benefits, such as a reduction in hospital bed and nursing care requirements compared to hysterectomy.

The technique involves selective catheterisation of both uterine arteries and embolisation is achieved using polyvinyl alcohol particles. A tightly collimated beam should be used, and where pulsed fluoroscopy is used the slowest pulse rate compatible with adequate visualisation should be employed. If at all possible, formal angiographic runs should be avoided, but where these are necessary they should be kept as short as possible. This is because the patients who undergo this examination are relatively young women, and one wishes to minimise the radiation dose to the pelvis.

Initial reports regarding UAE were very enthusiastic, claiming few if any complications and great success both for reducing the size of the fibroids themselves and in treating the associated symptoms. However, as experience with the technique has grown it has become apparent that it is not without complications. All patients experience pelvic pain of varying severity after the procedure, and many professionals advocate patient-controlled analgesia in the post-procedure period to counter this. Perhaps the most worrying, though thankfully relatively uncommon, complication is sepsis. Although deaths are reported they are rare, and it should not be forgotten that hysterectomy has a significant morbidity and mortality. Randomised data indicates that the two treatments have similar outcomes,[60,61] so there is a strong case for patient choice, in the light of the available evidence, determining which treatment is used.

REFLECTION ON INTERVENTION AND THERAPIES

This chapter illustrates the immense breadth of procedures undertaken by interventional radiologists today. Although there is much commonality between the techniques used, for example the use of catheter and guide wire manipulation, ever-increasing amounts of clinical knowledge are required for the safe application of these techniques. As a result, there has in many cases been a tendency for individuals to subspecialise further within interventional radiology, for example to concentrate on vascular radiology alone. In some cases organ specialists undertake the interventional procedures relevant to them. A good example of this is in musculoskeletal radiology, where specialists often undertake bone biopsy and even vertebroplasty; there is insufficient space to describe all of the available techniques in this chapter, hence their omission.

Another issue facing interventional radiologists is that as techniques become more complex, the clinicians looking after the patient will have less knowledge of them, making subsequent patient care more difficult. This is especially the case where junior staff care for a patient on the ward after the procedure.

There is thus a strong case for greater clinical involvement of interventional radiologists by performing ward rounds and maybe even outpatient clinics, both to assess patients prior to treatment and to follow them up afterwards. Such clinical involvement should also allow for improved quality of patient consent, given the direct communication with the expert in the interventional procedure, rather than a representative from a different specialist area. Although some might argue that this would be appropriate, the unique knowledge of imaging that is brought to these procedures by interventional radiologists should improve the quality of their conduct, although this is difficult to measure.

REFERENCES

1. Van Andel G, et al. Percutaneous transluminal dilatation of the iliac artery: long term results. Radiology 1985;156: 321–3.
2. Wolfe GL, et al. Surgery or PTA for peripheral vascular disease; a randomised controlled trial. Journal of Vascular and Interventional Radiology 1993;4: 639–48.
3. Ballard J. Aortoiliac stent deployment vs. surgical reconstruction. Journal of Vascular Surgery 1998;28:94–103.
4. Lofberg A-M, et al. Percutaneous transluminal angioplasty of the femoropopliteal arteries in limbs with chronic critical lower limb ischaemia. Journal of Vascular Surgery 2001;34: 114–21.
5. Shaw M, et al. The results of subintimal angioplasty in a district general hospital. European Journal of Vascular and Endovascular Surgery 2002;24:524–7.
6. Perkins J, et al. Exercise training versus angioplasty for stable claudication: long and medium term results of a prospective, randomized trial. European Journal of Vascular and Endovascular Surgery 1996;11:409–13.
7. Whyman M, et al. Is intermittent claudication improved by percutaneous transluminal angioplasty? Journal of Vascular Surgery 1997;26:551–7.
8. Brown K, et al. Infrapopliteal angioplasty: long term follow-up. Journal of Vascular and Interventional Radiology 1993;4: 139–44.
9. Tetterooe E, et al. Randomised comparison of primary stent insertion versus primary angioplasty and selective stent insertion in iliac artery occlusive disease. Lancet 1998;351:1153–9.
10. Bosch J, Hunink M. Meta analysis of the results of PTA and stent placement in aortoiliac occlusive disease. Radiology 1997;204:87–96.
11. Bosch J, et al. Iliac arterial disease: cost effectiveness analysis of stent placement versus PTA. Radiology 1998;208: 641–81.
12. Van de Ven P, et al. Arterial stenting and balloon angioplasty in ostial atherosclerotic renovascular disease: a randomised trial. Lancet 1999; 353(9149):282–6.
13. Reidy J, Taylor P. The use of stent grafts in thoracic aortic disease. Cardiovascular and Interventional Radiology 2000;23: 249–51.
14. Faries P, et al. A multicentre experience with the Talent endovascular graft for the treatment of abdominal aortic aneurysms. Journal of Vascular Surgery 2002;35: 1123–8.
15. Fifth report on the registry for endovascular treatment of aneurysms. The Vascular Surgical Society of Great Britain and Ireland and the British Society of Interventional Radiology 2001.
16. Katz D, et al. Operative mortality rates for intact and ruptured abdominal aortic aneurysms. An eleven year state wide experience. Journal of Vascular Surgery 1994;19:804–17.
17. EVAR trial participants. Endovascular aneurysm repair versus open repair in patients with abdominal aortic aneurysm (EVAR trail 1): randomised controlled trial. Lancet 2005;365:2179–86.

18. Prinssen M, et al; Dutch Randomised Endovascular Aneurysm Management (DREAM) Trial Group. A randomised trial comparing conventional and endovascular repair of abdominal aortic aneurysms. New England Journal of Medicine 2004;351:1607–18.

19. http://www.nice.org.uk/nicemedia/pdf/Ultrasound_49_guidance.pdf.

20. Lameris J, et al. Percutaneous placement of Hickman catheters: comparison of sonographic guided and blind techniques. American Journal of Roentgenology 1990;155:1097–9.

21. Girard P, et al. Medical literature and vena cava filters: so far so weak. Chest 2002;122:963–7.

22. Decousus H, et al. A clinical trial of vena caval filters in the prevention of pulmonary embolism in patients with proximal deep vein thrombosis. New England Journal of Medicine 1998;338:409–16.

23. Morice M-C, et al. for the RAVEL study group. A randomized comparison of a Sirolimus-eluting stent with a standard stent for coronary revascularization. New England Journal of Medicine 2002;326:1773–80.

24. Sousa J, et al. Two year angiographic and ultrasound follow-up after implantation of Sirolimus-eluting stents in human coronary arteries. Circulation 2003;107:381–3.

25. Yerly J, et al. A simulation-based analysis of the potential of compressed sensing for accelerating passive mr catheter visualization in endovascular therapy. Magnetic Resonance in Medicine 2010;63:473–83.

26. McLean G, et al. Radiologically guided balloon dilatation of gastrointestinal strictures. Radiology 1987;165:35–43.

27. Starcke E, et al. Esophageal stenosis: treatment with balloon catheters. Radiology 1984;153:637–40.

28. Sabharwal T, et al. Balloon dilation for achalasia of the cardia: experience in 76 patients. Radiology 2002;224:719–24.

29. Cowling M, et al. The use of self-expanding metallic stents in the management of malignant oesophageal strictures. British Journal of Surgery 1998;85:264–6.

30. Cwiekiel W, et al. Malignant esophageal strictures: treatment with a self expanding nitinol stent. Radiology 1993;187:661–5.

31. Saxon R, et al. Treatment of malignant esophageal obstructions with covered metallic Z stents: long term results in 52 patients. Journal of Vascular and Interventional Radiology 1995;6:747–54.

32. Earlam R, Chunha-Melo J. Oesophageal squamous cell carcinoma: 1. A critical review of surgery. British Journal of Surgery 1980;67:381–90.

33. Earlam R, Chunha-Melo J. Oesophageal squamous cell carcinoma: 2. A critical review of radiotherapy. British Journal of Surgery 1980;67:457–61.

34. Herskovic A, et al. Combined chemotherapy and radiotherapy compared to radiotherapy alone in patients with cancer of the oesophagus. New England Journal of Medicine 1992;326:1593–8.

35. Adam A, et al. Palliation of inoperable esophageal carcinoma: a prospective randomized trial of laser therapy and stent placement. Radiology 1997;202:344–8.

36. Morgan R, et al. Malignant esophageal fistulas and perforation: management with plastic-covered metallic endoprostheses. Radiology 1997;204:527–32.

37. Hicks M, et al. Fluoroscopically guided percutaneous gastrostomy: analysis of 158 consecutive cases. American Journal of Roentgenology 1990;154:725–8.

38. Wills J. Percutaneous gastrostomy: applications in gastric carcinoma and gastroplasty stoma dilatation. American Journal of Roentgenology 1986;147:826–7.

39. De Baere T, et al. Percutaneous gastrostomy with fluoroscopic guidance: Single centre experience in 500 consecutive cancer patients. Radiology 1999;210:651–4.

40. Cowling M, et al. Self expanding metallic stents in the treatment of pyloric dysfunction after gastric pull-up operations. European Radiology 1999;9:1123–6.

41. Binkert C, et al. Benign and malignant stenoses of the stomach and duodenum: treatment with self-expanding metallic endoprostheses. Radiology 1996;199:335–8.

42. Feretis C, et al. Palliation of malignant gastric outlet obstruction with self expanding metal stents. Endoscopy 1996;28:225–8.

43. Wong Y, et al. Gastric outlet obstruction secondary to pancreatic cancer: surgical vs endoscopic palliation. Surgical Endoscopy 2002;16:310–2.

44. Yim H, et al. Clinical outcome of the use of enteral stents for palliation of patients with malignant upper GI obstruction. Gastrointestinal Endoscopy 2001;53:329–32.

45. Mainar A, et al. Colorectal obstruction: treatment with metallic stents. Radiology 1996;198:761–4.

46. Dauphine C, et al. Placement of self expanding metal stents for acute malignant large bowel obstruction: a collective review. Annals of Surgical Oncology 2002;9:574–9.

47. Aviv R, et al. Radiological palliation of malignant colonic obstruction. Clinical Radiology 2002;57:347–51.

48. England R, Martin D. Endoscopic and percutaneous intervention in malignant obstructive jaundice. Cardiovascular and Interventional Radiology 1996;19:381–7.

49. Deviere J, et al. Long-term follow-up of patients with hilar malignant stricture treated by endoscopic internal biliary drainage. Gastrointestinal Endoscopy 1988;34:95–101.

50. Prat F, et al. A randomised trial of endoscopic drainage methods for inoperable malignant strictures of the common bile duct. Gastrointestinal Endoscopy 1998;47:1–7.

51. Davids P, et al. Randomised trial of self expanding metal stents versus polyethylene stents for distal malignant biliary obstruction. Lancet 1992;340:1488–92.

52. Draganov P, et al. Long term outcome in patients with benign biliary strictures treated endoscopically with multiple stents. Gastrointestinal Endoscopy 2002;55:680–6.

53. Born P, et al. Long term results of endoscopic and percutaneous transhepatic treatment of benign biliary strictures. Endoscopy 1999;31:725–31.

54. Gabelmann A, et al. Metallic stents in benign biliary strictures: Long term effectiveness and interventional management of stent occlusion. American Journal of Roentgenology 2001;177:813–7.

55. Farrell T, Hicks M. A review of radiologically guided percutaneous nephrostomies in 303 patients. Journal of Vascular Interventional Radiology 1997;8:769–74.

56. Chitale S, et al. The management of ureteric obstruction secondary to malignant pelvic disease. Clinical Radiology 2002;57:1118–21.

57. Sharma S, et al. A review of antegrade stenting in the management of the obstructed kidney. British Journal of Urology 1996;78:511–5.

58. Lucey B, et al. Miscellaneous visceral renal intervention. Seminars in Interventional Radiology 2000;17:367–72.

59. Segura J, et al. Percutaneous removal of kidney stones: review of 1000 cases. Journal of Urology 1985;134:1077–81.

60. Dutton S, et al. A UK multicentre retrospective cohort study comparing hysterectomy and uterine artery embolisation for the treatment of symptomatic uterine fibroids (HOPEFUL study): main results and medium-term safety and efficacy. BJOG 2007;114:1340–51.

61. Hehenkamp WJ, et al. Symptomatic uterine fibroids: treatment with uterine artery embolisation or hysterectomy: Results from the randomised clinical Embolisation versus Hysterectomy (EMMY) trial. Radiology 2008;246:823–32.

Section | 8 |

Additional imaging methods

Chapter | **35** |

Computed tomography

Barry Carver

INTRODUCTION

Radiography produces 2D images of 3D objects; it is important to remember that they are shadow projections (Ex Umbris Eruditio). This inevitably means that structures are superimposed, and the structure that is the object of imaging may be obscured from view. To address this problem focal plane tomography was developed shortly after the First World War, blurring out layers above and below the region of interest to provide an image of the required structure, but again it is 2D and prone to equipment and operating problems. The ideal is a technique that allows for 3D rendition of images.

The advent of X-ray computed tomography (CT) has had a great impact on medical imaging, primarily because CT solves this fundamental limitation of radiography by eliminating the superimposition of imaged structures.

CT uses a rotating X-ray source coupled to a bank of detectors to produce diagnostic images of the body. The basic premise of CT is that the attenuation pattern of the X-rays can be measured during rotation and spatially located; the sum of attenuation at each point can then be calculated and displayed. Since its inception at the beginning of the 1970s CT has now become a major technique in the routine diagnosis of disease, and scanners can be found in almost all district general hospitals (DGHs) in the UK.

Advantages of CT include:

- Axial acquisition of cross-sectional images: with modern isotropic imaging, data can be post processed into multiple planes or rendered volumes, producing 2D or 3D images. Magnetic resonance (MR) is truly multiplanar, as scans are acquired directly in different planes without the need for reconstruction; however, the quality of CT isotropic reconstructions is high.
- Cross-sectional imaging has excellent low-contrast resolution (LCR), which is superior to other imaging methods with the exception of MR, which matches and in some cases exceeds the LCR of CT.
- CT images also show good high-contrast (spatial) resolution and excellent bone detail. MR does not image bone directly owing to the lack of free hydrogen within cortical bone.
- Digital imaging: this enables the manipulation of images, as well as post processing to other planes; the applied algorithm and windows can be adjusted to better visualise specific tissues. The application of filters and digital processing can enhance content, e.g. the use of edge enhancement for looking at bone.
- CT is generally well tolerated by patients, certainly more so than MR, which is less well tolerated owing to noise and claustrophobia. Contraindications for MR due to safety requirements do not apply to CT.
- CT is still more readily available than MRI and radionuclide imaging (RNI), being in situ in the vast majority of DGHs in the UK.

Disadvantages of CT include:

- Ionising radiation dose: CT is undeniably an extremely high-dose technique, many examinations being among the highest, if not the highest doses, in use in medical imaging. Multiple examinations may approach the thresholds for deterministic radiation effects.
- Metallic artefacts cause loss of image detail; on many modern scanners this effect is much reduced by software corrections.
- Soft tissue structures surrounded closely by bone can be difficult to image, e.g. in the posterior fossa, where the soft tissue contrast of MR is superior. This is again a problem largely overcome in the latest generation of scanners.
- Misregistration artefact can be caused by relative movement of the body structures from the acquisition of a single slice to the next, e.g. due to inconsistencies in the patient's respiratory pattern. If misregistration occurs then the reconstruction will be meaningless, as the same portion of anatomy could be portrayed at different positions in the reconstructed image. With the advent of single breath-hold scanning this is now less of a consideration. However, many centres, when scanning two areas such as the chest and upper abdomen, will overlap the two acquisition blocks to ensure no loss of information due to breathing differences between the two acquisitions. The dose implications of this technique are worthy of consideration.

In some quarters there is an attitude that CT can be undertaken by anybody, including non-radiographically qualified staff such as departmental assistants. It can be argued, however, that, along with every other branch of imaging, CT is operator dependent. Image quality is dependent on factors that should be adjusted for each examination, and more importantly, for each patient. In addition, because of the high dose burden all operators of CT equipment should be trained and skilled in optimising CT examinations;[1] indeed, specific additional training requirements are mandatory in some countries, such as the USA;[2] unfortunately, the need for requirements such as this can be only too evident.[3]

EQUIPMENT CHRONOLOGY

1874   Sir William Crookes constructs the cathode discharge tube. During his experiments over the next few years he discovers fogging of photographic plates stored near discharge tubes.

1895   Wilhelm Roentgen discovers X-rays while investigating gas discharge using a Crookes' tube.

1935   Grossman coins the term 'tomography' to describe his apparatus for looking at detail in the lungs.[4]

1951   Godfrey Hounsfield starts work at EMI, initially working on early computers.

1956   Ronald Bracewell uses Fourier transforms to reconstruct solar images. At the same time Alan Cormack starts to work on solving 'line integrals'.

1958   Korenblyum and colleagues in Ukraine work on obtaining thin-section X-ray images using mathematical reconstructions.

1961   William Oldendorf produces an image of the internal structure of a test object using a rotating object. He was unable to make further progress owing to the lack of available equipment to provide the computation that would have been required.

1963   Cormack publishes a paper on mathematical reconstruction methods.

1965   David Kuhl, one of the pioneers of RNI, produces a transmission image using a radioactive source coupled to a detector.[5]

1967   Bracewell produces a mathematical solution for reconstruction with fewer errors and artefact than found with Fourier.

Hounsfield and Ambrose come together to develop CT head scanning. Hounsfield uses an iterative algebraic technique rather than more complex mathematical formulae.

1971   The first clinical CT scanner is installed at Atkinson Morley Hospital under the supervision of James Ambrose. The first patient is scanned on 1 October. The first scanners were somewhat crude and took several minutes to produce each slice, which were of fairly poor quality. However, at the time even these crude images were revolutionary, enabling a first non-invasive glimpse at the soft tissue contents of the skull.

1972   Ambrose and Hounsfield discuss the clinical use of CT at the British Institute of Radiology annual conference.[6] Clinical images are shown at RSNA.

1973   Hounsfield and Ambrose publish papers describing the design and clinical applications of the CT system.[7,8] EMI scanner becomes commercially available.

Hounsfield starts work on the second-generation scanner.

1974   Hounsfield produces abdominal images with a 20-second acquisition time.

1975   EMI CT 1010 second-generation scanner becomes available, soon to be followed by the CT 5005 – the first EMI body scanner.

In the next few years third-generation scanners become available but have problems with artefact, a problem solved by General Electric (GE). Fourth-generation scanners were later introduced to avoid the artefact problems initially suffered by the third-generation machines.

1979   Hounsfield and Cormack are awarded the Nobel prize for medicine.

1983   The first 2-second scanner introduced by GE (CT 9800).

1985   Electron beam CT developed.

1989   Siemens introduce spiral (helical) CT, using slip ring technology to enable the tube to rotate continuously without the need to go back to unwind its cables.

1992   Elscint Twin scans two slices simultaneously, which is a return to a method used by the original EMI scanners.

1998   Multislice CT initially incorporating four slices is introduced; GE, Picker, Siemens and Toshiba displayed systems at RSNA. Since then 8-, 16-, 32-, 40-, 64- and 128-slice machines have become available. Sub-second scan times enable body areas to be scanned in a single breath-hold. Advancements have in many cases had to await the development of computer systems robust enough to cope with the huge quantities of data generated, a problem initially encountered by Oldendorf.

2005   Siemens launch dual-energy scanners, opening the way to characterisation of chemical make-up of materials via simultaneous imaging at different kV values.

2007   Toshiba launch Aquilion One, 320-slice, ending the numbers game? Enables single rotation imaging of entire organs due to 16 cm coverage.

As mentioned above, CT systems have been classified according to the motion of the X-ray tube and detectors during scanning. There have been several generations of CT scanner, which are described here in brief.

First-generation scanner (Fig. 35.1)

The first-generation CT scanner used a single pencil beam of X-rays being measured by a single detector. In order to cover the area of interest, the movement required is a combination of translation and rotation. In the initial position, the tube/detector assembly moves

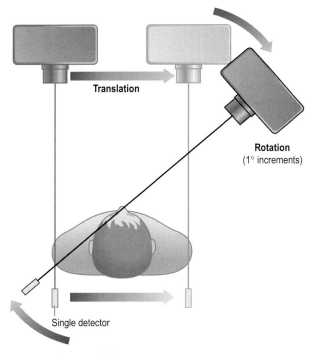

Figure 35.1 Schematic of first-generation scanner.

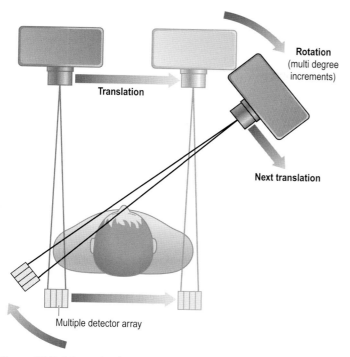

Figure 35.2 Schematic of second-generation scanner.

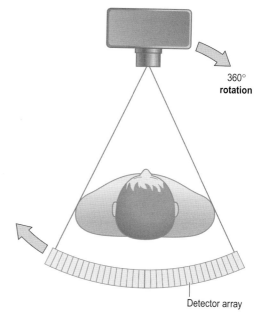

Figure 35.3 Schematic of third-generation scanner.

across the scan field of view (translation) and a series of measurements of transmitted intensity are made. It then rotates 1° to its next position before commencing another translation.

This is a very time-consuming method and typical scan times were of the order of 4–6 minutes per slice acquisition. The early scanners attempted to compensate by having two detectors to perform two slices at once, a technique now resurrected in the latest generation of spiral scanners that offer 'new' multislice acquisition.

- Advantages: it was the first of its kind and offered the first opportunity for axial imaging of the head
- Disadvantages: mechanically complex, slow scans, which were only practical for scanning the head of patients who could be adequately immobilised using a water bag. The water bag was used to reduce the range of information required, as its density is closer to air than to that of tissue

Second-generation scanner (Fig. 35.2)

The second generation used the same principles of movement as the first, i.e. a combination of translation and rotation, but used several new innovations. Instead of a pencil beam a narrow fan beam was now used, being measured by a bank of detectors. The fan beam is still not sufficient to cover the entire area of interest, so translation and then rotation is still required, but because more information is being gathered at each position, multiple degree rotational incrementation is possible.

- Advantages: as several detectors were being used, scanning times were significantly reduced and quality was increased. Typical scan times of the order of 20–80 seconds per slice were achievable. Again, two slices were acquired simultaneously on the EMI 1010 with a fixed slice thickness of 13 mm
- Disadvantages: the maintenance of the translate–rotate movement renders these scanners still mechanically complex

Third-generation scanner (Fig. 35.3)

Also known as a rotate–rotate scanner, this model was the first to do away with the requirement for translation across the patient by using a wide fan beam of X-rays. A large number of detectors (up to 1000) are used to allow for the increased beam width, and the tube and detectors are rigidly coupled and rotate jointly about the patient. Rotation only is required, as the fan beam covers the entire body. It is this configuration that is still the most commonly used, even in the latest multislice equipment.

- Advantages: the greater number of detectors plus the rotation-only movement allows shorter scan times, typically of the order of 2–8 seconds. The width of the fan beam can be adjusted (collimated) to limit the beam to the area under examination. Use of the rotation-only movement renders this type of unit mechanically simpler than its predecessors
- Disadvantages: detectors were expensive, therefore more detectors equals more cost. Also more processing power is required, as more information is gathered at one time. Initially problems were encountered with circular artefacts, but this was overcome by adjusting the detectors

Fourth-generation scanner (Fig. 35.4)

This scanner was similar to the third-generation scanner, again using a wide fan beam but with a complete circle of detectors around the patient. In this case only the tube rotates, the detector ring being stationary.

- Advantages: mechanically simpler owing to having fewer moving parts. Scan times reduced and now taking 1–10 seconds
- Disadvantages: the high number of detectors equals high cost. There were also greater calibration difficulties. As the tube is rotating within the detector ring, the detectors are further away from the patient, leading to a greater penumbral effect

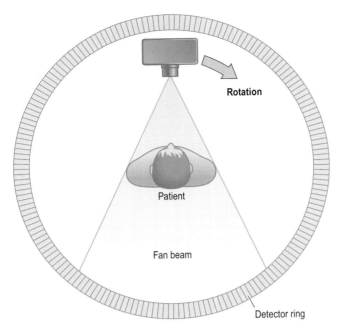

Figure 35.4 Schematic of fourth-generation scanner.

Electron beam computed tomography (EBCT)

A completely different concept, the electron beam is directed to the anode rotating around the patient, and is again linked to a bank of detectors. As mechanical rotational movement is now not used, quick (50 ms) scans are possible. EBCT has been used for gated cardiac studies for some time. For several years this was the only CT technology that could provide high-quality cardiac imaging, but now commonly available multislice and dual-source equipment can match EBCT in cardiac studies.

Spiral/helical CT

Helical scanners are also described as volume acquisition or spiral scanners, so for clarity the term helical will be used throughout this chapter.

In the 1990s 'conventional' CT began to be replaced by helical scanners. Owing to cost, availability and equipment replacement programmes, it was only in the late 1990s that these became the norm in the UK. Ironically, this occurred just as this technology itself was superseded by the introduction of multislice helical scanning.

Helical scanning differs from conventional CT in the method of data acquisition. Instead of a single 360° rotation that produces a single slice followed by an incremental table movement, in helical scanning a volume of data is acquired.

One of the main advantages of this method of continuous data acquisition is its speed. As a large volume of data can be acquired very rapidly, a series of images that would take several minutes to acquire in conventional 'slice by slice' mode can now be obtained in seconds.

This is due to both the use of slip ring technology, enabling continuous rotation of the X-ray tube around the gantry (without the cables, which previously had to be 'unwound' by a return rotation prior to the next slice being obtained), and improvements in the design of the tube and its drive motors enabling sub-second acquisition times.

This rapid data acquisition means that large areas of the patient can be imaged within a single breath-hold, eliminating one of the major problems for image reconstruction and interpretation:

misregistration. Respiratory misregistration can be completely eliminated, and the short scan times make it less likely that patient movement becomes a factor.

Multislice CT

The latest advance in scanner design is the multidetector volume acquisition scanner, ironically a return to one of the features of the original EMI scanner – multiple detector arrays. The difference is that the first EMI scanner had two rows of one detector, whereas the latest multislice scanners have tens of thousands of detector elements. The majority of scanners are of the third-generation type with rotating tube and detector array.

Large volumes can be rapidly imaged with thin slice widths, enhancing the diagnostic capacity of CT. Large numbers of thin slices can be reconstructed to produce high-quality volume rendered images, with the elimination of 'stair step' artefacts and the reduction of partial volume artefacts.

Advantages of multislice include:

- Speed of acquisition – sub-second rotation speeds are now the norm
- Compared to single-slice helical, multislice enables the same acquisition in a shorter time, or larger volumes to be scanned in the same time, or thinner slices to be scanned
- All manufacturers have sub-millimetre scan capabilities. Toshiba have detectors that are 0.5 mm, matching the pixel size to produce a voxel which is the same size in each dimension: termed isotropic (see Fig. 35.10). Isotropic and near isotropic voxels enhance the 2D reformatting ability of the scanner, enabling high-quality multiplanar reconstructions from an axial data set. 3D reformats produced are also excellent, with none of the problems of possible misregistration and information loss inherent in MR owing to its longer scan times.

EQUIPMENT

The X-ray tube

The advent of spiral scanning with its continuous rotation means that huge demands are placed on the X-ray tube used in modern scanners. The tube needs to provide high output while effectively dissipating the heat produced. Air conditioning is generally required to maintain a comfortable temperature in the scan room and to assist with heat dissipation. Large anode discs in metal or ceramic tube envelopes are common, the anode usually being mostly graphite with a tungsten/rhenium target track.

Beam shaping filter

In any CT scanner the X-ray beam produced is in fact heterogeneous, having a range of energies. Filters are applied to the beam on exiting the tube to reduce the range of energies. Filters also shape the beam to produce a more uniform result at the detectors in order to reduce the dynamic range required in the detector electronics.

Collimators

In a single-slice system a pre-patient collimator will limit the beam to the prescribed slice width at the centre of rotation; a post-patient collimator will then limit the beam incident on the detectors to the slice width. For example, pre-patient collimation to 4 mm will result in a 4 mm slice being produced.

In a multislice system the beam is again collimated at the centre of rotation but the result will differ. For example, in a four-slice system the 4 mm collimation given above will result in 4×1 mm slices being obtained.

Table

The table is an important element in CT. They are usually of carbon fibre construction with rise and fall action; this gives strength without interfering with the resultant image, and facilitates patient handling. The table must be able to provide a wide range of movement at various speeds. Accuracy of movement is vital, as any inconsistency would have detrimental effects on the image produced.

Table-tops are generally curved, except for those tables used in radiotherapy planning, where a flat table-top is essential to allow CT simulation. Simulation needs to reproduce accurately the patient's position on the flat treatment table. Consequently, scanners used for both purposes will often have interchangeable table-tops for diagnostic and planning sessions.

Detectors

Modern detectors are of the solid state type, mostly using ultrafast ceramic detector elements. An incident beam causes scintillation; the photon produced is then converted to an electrical signal by a photodiode and sent on to the electronics. The detector array is formed by a series of individual elements, as shown in Figure 35.5.

Different manufacturers have differing approaches to the format of detector arrays, with four-slice machines being available as fixed matrix, adaptive or mixed arrays. Each of the major manufacturers has taken a different approach to 16-slice, and as can be seen in Figure 35.6, the choice of array format affects the minimum slice width available, the number of slices available at minimum width, and the range of slice widths available.

Data acquisition system (DAS)

The DAS 'reads' the measurements from the detector array, converts these analogue signals into digital format, and transmits the digital signal to the computer systems for reconstruction into the presented images.

The DAS needs to be able to deal rapidly with a vast amount of data being generated every second; in current computing technology there is a limit to how much data can be handled at the necessary transfer rates. Development of these systems is advancing rapidly, but they have been a limiting factor to the speed of development of larger multislice arrays.

Computer system

The computer system processes operator input to set scanning parameters, patient information and archiving instructions. It also receives the information from the DAS which is then processed to form the image. A wide range of post-processing options are available on modern scanners which again take place within this system, or alternatively on dedicated workstations. High-speed high-capacity computers are required to perform these tasks at speeds that were unthought of until relatively recently.

Archiving requires some consideration; although archiving systems have increased greatly in capacity (and decreased in cost) in recent years the amount of data generated has followed the same pattern. Only selected reconstructions are generally sent for storage and access on picture archiving and communication systems (PACS); raw data, if stored, is often on high-capacity optical discs.

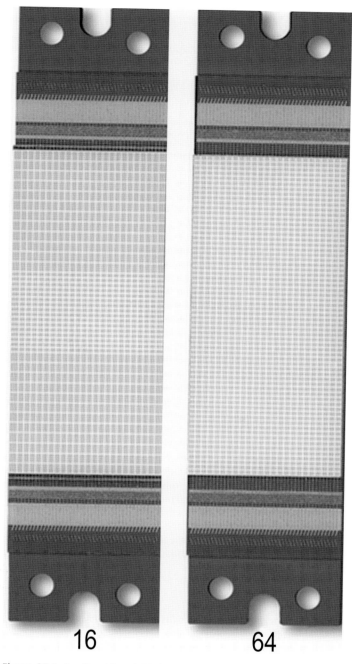

Figure 35.5 Aquilion 16 and 64 detector arrays. Both provide up to 32 mm coverage per rotation. The 16-slice detector has 16×0.5 mm elements centrally, with 12×1 mm elements either side, enabling acquisition of 16×0.5 mm or 16×1 mm or 16×2 mm slices per rotation. The 64-slice detector provides 64×0.5 mm slices per rotation. *Reproduced with permission from Toshiba.*

PHYSICAL PRINCIPLES OF SCANNING

What happens to a homogeneous X-ray beam as it passes through an object? The X-ray photons interact with the material through which they pass and are attenuated by it. If the intensity of the emerging beam is measured, we know the initial intensity and so the attenuation within the object can be measured.

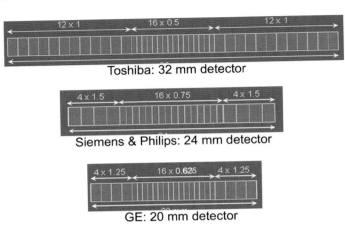

Figure 35.6 Comparison of 16-slice detector arrays.

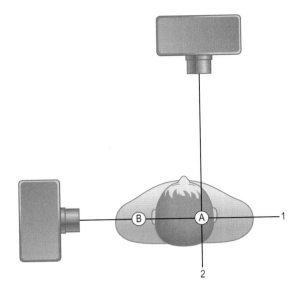

Figure 35.7 Localisation of position.

With the X-ray tube of a CT scanner in one position, a narrow X-ray beam passes through the patient and the attenuation along the line taken by a particular beam through the patient can be calculated from the intensity of the emergent beam measured by a detector. The X-ray intensity transmitted through an object along a particular path contains information about all the material it has passed through, but does not allow the distribution of the material along the path to be discerned.

For the energies used in CT the attenuation of the beam is due to:

- Absorption: photoelectric
- Scattering: Compton (mainly)

Attenuation due to photoelectric absorption is strongly dependent on the atomic number of the material (αZ^3).

Attenuation due to Compton scattering does not depend upon atomic number, but on the number of free electrons present. The number of electrons per gram of an absorber is remarkably constant over a wide range of materials; however, because their density varies considerably, the number of electrons per metre does show variation across a range of biological materials. It is this difference between attenuation processes that enables differentiation of chemical composition in dual-energy equipment.

If we consider the simplistic case of a homogeneous beam passing through the medium, the attenuation in the tissues follows the Lambert–Beer law, which states:

$$I = I_o e^{-\mu x}$$

where μ = linear attenuation coefficient

I_o = original intensity
I = transmitted intensity
x = thickness of material.

In CT we are interested in measuring the linear attenuation coefficient (LAC). Solving the Lambert–Beer equation for LAC, we get:

$$\mu = \frac{1}{x} \cdot \ln\left(\frac{I_o}{I}\right)$$

I is measured by the detectors, I_o and x are known, hence μ can be calculated.

As mentioned earlier, the X-ray beam produced is in fact heterogeneous, having a range of energies. Filters are applied to the beam on exiting the tube to reduce the range of energies incident on the detector array.

Traditionally a narrow beam was required for accurate localisation of the attenuating tissues. Readings are taken from multiple angles to give a series of values of linear attenuation of the beam along

intersecting lines through the patient. For example, in Figure 35.7 a bony object would have the same attenuating effect on 'beam 1' whether at position 'A' or 'B'. However, from 'beam 2' it is possible to localise the structure to position 'B'.

In general, then, the transmitted intensity depends on the sum of the attenuation coefficients for all points along the path of the beam. Thus the log transmission measurement is sometimes referred to as a 'ray sum' or 'line integral' of the attenuation along the path.

A radiograph can be considered to be composed of many such ray sums, produced unidirectionally, hence superimposing all structures encountered by the beam. Because of the differences in transmitted intensity, interfaces between bone, tissue and air are well demonstrated. The differences between adjacent soft tissues are not sufficient for good differentiation and so they are less well demonstrated.

To demonstrate soft tissues we need to eliminate superimposition by taking ray sums from multiple directions; these ray sum measurements can then be mathematically reconstructed to generate an axial image formed by estimating the distribution of the linear attenuation coefficient within the irradiated volume. The image produced can then be digitally manipulated to maximise contrast, enabling adequate visualisation of subtle changes in tissue density. The ability to produce such images is the main strength of CT as an imaging modality.

The information acquired by the detectors is passed to the computer. Once this data is committed to the computer memory it can be manipulated by the resident software to produce an image which is reconstructed on the screen of the viewing console. Reconstruction takes place via the application of a complex mathematical algorithm to the data obtained, usually a filtered back projection. Consideration of the detail of this mathematical process is beyond the scope of this chapter, but is well described in texts such as Seeram.[9]

Image reconstruction in its simplest form consists of recalling the digital information fed to the computer from the detectors via the DAS, and converting this information to an analogue voltage signal that controls the electron sweep within the display monitor.

Helical image reconstruction is more complex: because the table is continuously moving only one ray sum lies in the scan plane; the rest of the 'slice' information is interpolated from the acquired volume. 360° and 180° interpolations are used. As seen in Figure 35.8, a 360° interpolation requires data from two tube rotations for slice reconstruction. 180° interpolation allows smaller slice widths to be accurately reconstructed.

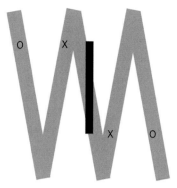

Figure 35.8 Diagrammatic representation of interpolation of helical data. 180° interpolation – X to X; 360° interpolation – 0 to 0.

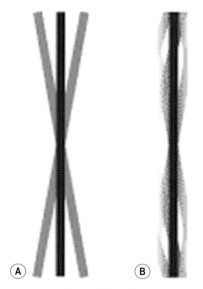

Figure 35.9 Cone beam problem. (A) A wide X-ray beam is required to give full coverage of the detector elements. The beams produced at opposing angle form a cone; the slice profile is sharp at the centre but spatial resolution is lost at the edges due to 'cone beaming'. (B) For example, Toshiba's TCOT algorithm calculates these complex angles to provide a more accurate slice profile.

Multislice is more complex again, as it uses two or more data samples to produce each point within a projection, but the basic principles are the same. There is, however, an additional complication in that the more slices that are scanned, the wider the beam becomes in the z direction (along the patient length), meaning the beam ceases to be a narrow fan as seen in conventional and helical scanners; in multislice, the volume of data is the volume between two cones (Fig. 35.9). Each of the manufacturers has different mathematical methods for 'cone beam' correction; the complexity of the multislice reconstruction process is again beyond the scope of this chapter, but is addressed in specialist texts.[9]

The amount of movement within the data set is governed by the table movement, and is measured as the scan pitch. Helical pitch is defined as:

$$Pitch = table\ travel\ per\ rotation/nominal\ slice\ width$$

There are two definitions for pitch quoted in multislice, each of which provides a different number to represent pitch; it is therefore

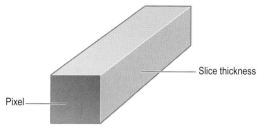

Figure 35.10 Pixel and voxel.

important to know which definition is in use when comparing techniques:

$$Pitch = table\ travel\ per\ rotation/X\text{-}ray\ beam\ width$$

Or

$$Pitch = table\ travel\ per\ rotation/detector\ width$$

The data is stored within the computer as a matrix of intensities. The image produced consists of a matrix of cells with various brightness levels on the display monitor; the brightness of each cell is related to the intensity detected.

Each image square (or PICture ELement) is called a pixel. The value of the number represented in each cell is relative, and is used to define image contrast. In CT the numeric information contained in each pixel is a CT number (or Hounsfield unit: HU) and is expressed relative to the density of water. The detector array is calibrated to give a zero value for water.

Each of these 2D picture elements represents a volume of patient data, the volume element, or voxel, and is equal to the pixel size × slice thickness. If the voxel is the same size in each direction then it is called isotropic. This is the ideal for multiplanar reconstruction as the blocks are effectively the same when viewed from any direction, hence maximising the quality of reconstructions (Fig. 35.10).

The size of image matrix used is determined by the characteristics of the equipment and the storage capacity of the computer. The size of the image matrix is important, as the more squares there are to form the image, the greater will be the image definition.

Measurement of the CT number of an object in an image can be useful for tissue characterisation, as by comparing it to known values such as those in Table 35.1 we can get a feel for the composition of the material (although a definitive tissue diagnosis cannot be made).

Windowing

The displayed image will comprise areas of high X-ray attenuation, shown in white; low attenuation is shown in black. The intervening soft tissues will be shown in various shades of grey according to their individual attenuation properties.

As CT is sensitive to small changes in density, use can be made of the variation in shades of grey represented on the image to give better contrast discrimination. The image can be viewed on a variety of chosen settings to better view the particular structures of interest. This is termed 'windowing'.

The window level is set to the tissue of interest; this will place the tissue of interest in the midpoint of the grey scale. The window width is set to enable the required range of tissues to be viewed, and straddles the window level evenly. For example, a window width of 400 set with a window level of 40 will include tissues with HU values from −60 to 240. Anything below −160 will appear black, and anything above 240 will appear white. The shades of grey on the image will

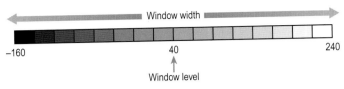

Figure 35.11 Windowing: grey scale.

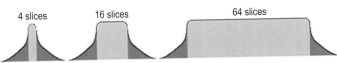

Figure 35.12 Multislice *z* axis dose profiles. In single-slice scanners the X-ray beam is a close match to the imaged width. 'Overbeaming' occurs in multislice scanners as there is a non-uniform beam distribution, but each detector requires equal beam intensity. The 'overbeamed' portion of the dose profile (generally a few mm – dark shading) can be seen for each scanner type. As the number of slices increases the proportion of excess radiation decreases with respect to the total profile, so the greater the number of slices the greater the 'overbeamed' dose efficiency.

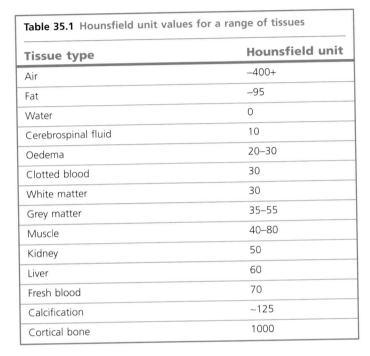

Table 35.1 Hounsfield unit values for a range of tissues

Tissue type	Hounsfield unit
Air	−400+
Fat	−95
Water	0
Cerebrospinal fluid	10
Oedema	20–30
Clotted blood	30
White matter	30
Grey matter	35–55
Muscle	40–80
Kidney	50
Liver	60
Fresh blood	70
Calcification	~125
Cortical bone	1000

divide the 400 units to be demonstrated. A typical monitor displaying 16 grey shades will display these window settings as shown in Figure 35.11.

As window width is increased, each grey scale shade represents a greater number of attenuation values, so more tissues are seen, but with a reduction in image contrast. Thus the image appears flat, i.e. it has an overall grey appearance. Lower window widths enable tissues of closer attenuation values to be discriminated, so small changes in density may be seen. The image will be of high contrast, i.e. it has more black and white. Low widths make the noise inherent in the image appear more apparent.

Introduction of contrast media can raise the attenuation values of soft tissue structures. It is important then to adjust the window level accordingly to ensure the tissues of interest remain in the centre of the grey scale and that structures that need to be visualised remain within the range of the selected window width.

On modern scanners thresholds can be set using specific HU values to produce a range of data sets to provide a variety of image types, e.g. maximum intensity projections (MIPs). Colourised images can also be produced on the workstation to delineate different structures, particularly in 3D, and surface rendered images, for example.

IMAGE QUALITY

It has previously been stated that CT can be considered to be an operator- or user-dependent modality; this is because the user has a direct influence on the quality of the images produced and, as will be

discussed later, the radiation dose administered to the patient. Given the potential for the administration of high doses with CT, adequate training of appropriately qualified staff is essential.

The greatest influence on image quality is the choice of scanning factors, which include mA, scan time, slice thickness and kVp. These parameters essentially determine the number of photons emitted from the X-ray tube and registered on the detector, which in turn determines the noise level, which has a detrimental effect on image quality.

Noise is superimposed over the whole image as a uniform grainy appearance and is dependent on the number of photons reaching the detectors (signal-to-noise ratio). Several factors influence the noise level on the image, the primary ones being slice thickness, patient size and applied mAs. In order to obtain good-quality images, noise should be kept to a minimum. However, there is a trade-off to be made: images can be produced with almost no noise, but at the cost of increased dose as the noise level is related to the applied mAs. Noise varies as $(1/\text{dose})^{1/2}$, and consequently doubling the mAs applied (and therefore patient dose) only reduces noise by a factor of about 1.4.

The influence of slice thickness has changed, particularly with the higher-end scanners (16 or more slices). Conventionally thick slices would be used for general soft tissue use. More photons contribute to image quality, so noise is lower, a larger area is covered more quickly, the dose is reduced and examination time is faster. Thinner slices were reserved for areas where high resolution was required: fewer photons contribute to the image, therefore noise level is higher, and to achieve a similar image quality to the thicker slice, the dose administered needs to be increased to improve the signal-to-noise ratio. More slices are also needed to cover the same area, so dose is increased but resolution improves.

With the more recent multislice units the beam collimation is equivalent to a thick slice on a single-slice unit (Fig. 35.12), so we have the benefits of a thick slice but can reconstruct very thin slices from this irradiation of the patient. For example, if we consider a 16-slice scanner with a detector array of 0.5 mm elements, an 8 mm collimation (thick slice on a standard helical scanner) can yield 16 × 0.5 mm images (very thin slice).

Reconstruction algorithms or filters are applied to the image reconstruction in conjunction with factors such as slice thickness so that optimal image quality is obtained. They too affect the amount of noise and spatial resolution in the final image.

Increasing kVp provides greater penetration, and so this should be considered when scanning areas of higher attenuation; this can be used instead of, or as well as, increases in applied mA, depending on the anatomical area being examined.

Artefacts are patterns on an image that are not on the original object. There are many causes of CT artefact, such as movement, metal, beam hardening, and partial volume effect. Motion artefacts have been greatly reduced owing to the rapid acquisitions available in multislice in particular. The ability to scan whole body areas in a single breath-hold has great advantages.

Some metals absorb X-rays, producing radiation shadows; this results in a streak artefact in the reconstructed CT image. Where practicable, all metal objects such as jewellery, coins and clothing with metal fasteners should be removed in order to prevent this effect. This must, however, be balanced against the psychological needs of the patient. Only if the objects are likely to be situated within the scan field should they be removed. There is no need to change every patient into a hospital gown, and indeed it is better for patient comfort and dignity if they can remain dressed whenever possible.

Beam hardening artefact appears as a streak artefact on the image. As the X-ray beam is heterogeneous on entering an object, particularly if it is high density, the lower-energy photons are absorbed. This increases the effective energy of the beam, so adjacent soft tissues are more easily penetrated. This is also seen in non-circular areas such as the shoulder and pelvis, where the attenuation is greater along the long axis, producing directional noise. This can be addressed by adaptive filters and correction software.

Partial volume artefact is caused by structures being partially included in the scan thickness. Each voxel represents an average attenuation value for the structures in that slice: if a high-attenuation structure (e.g. bone) is partially included in a voxel, that voxel will have an average value higher than its surroundings, producing an error in reconstruction. This is avoided by the use of thinner slices (structures are then less often partially included) or volume artefact reduction software provided by several manufacturers.

CT SAFETY: DOSE

In a little over 40 years, CT has progressed from giving the first glimpse of imaging of cranial contents to the potential to replace planar radiography. However, with all CT examinations the over-riding concern is that of dose to the patient.

In 1989 in the UK it was reported that 20% of the dose from medical examinations was from CT, which at the time accounted for just 2% of examinations.[10] By 2003 this had grown to 47% of the dose and 9% of examinations.[11] By 2000 there were in the region of 34 000 scanners worldwide, accounting for 5% of examinations and 34% of the dose.[12] In the USA even higher figures have been quoted, with CT accounting for up to 17% of examinations and 49% of the collective dose.[13]

The introduction of multislice scanners produced an increase in patient dose, as the first scanners of this type were less dose efficient than single-slice equipment owing largely to 'overbeaming' (Fig. 35.12). With the production of more efficient detectors and increasing numbers of slices creating a greater effective slice width, this dose increase has been reduced.

Concern is warranted as tissue doses resulting from CT are among the highest used in diagnostic imaging. Repeat examinations can produce dose levels that approach and may exceed levels at which an increased incidence of cancer has been observed,[1] hence the arguments put forward regarding hormesis and reduced risk from radiation exposure[14,15] do not apply to CT.

Effective dose equivalent (EDE) is, in many circumstances, the quantity used to describe patient dose, but owing to the complex manner of its calculation it is difficult to assess for individual patients in CT. There is a requirement to record doses; those typically used in CT are the CT dose index (CTDI) and dose length product (DLP), both of which can be used for approximation of EDE.

The first line of approach to dose reduction is to ensure the appropriateness of the examination: CT must be the imaging modality best suited to answer the clinical question. In the UK there is a requirement for all complex examinations, such as CT, to be vetted and justified by a consultant experienced in the imaging modality.[16] Given the greater capabilities of modern scanners, there is a wider variety of examinations and techniques available; multiphase contrast examinations should not be routine and should be used only for those clinical situations for which they are the most appropriate.

The operator can have a significant effect on administered dose, with up to 50% reduction achievable by use of appropriate parameters, including auto-exposure control, reinforcing the case for appropriate training.[1] Automatic exposure controls include mA modulation to match beam quantity to patient body part. This can be achieved in a variety of ways: two scout views can be used to assess the patient size, and then vary the mA slice by slice during the scan. Another alternative is using feedback from the previous rotation to determine the signal received by the detectors and alter the mA accordingly. Despite the availability of these dose-reduction measures, without proper training and awareness it has been reported that often they can be unused.[17]

Patient dose can be increased by failure to alter scan parameters to match the individual patient, especially in *children*, who *should not be scanned using adult protocols*.

COMMON CLINICAL APPLICATIONS

CT is widely used in imaging virtually every anatomical region, and the full range of clinical applications of CT is a text in itself. The following section therefore considers major areas for discussion; it is not intended to be a thorough evaluation of all CT applications. The use of CT in paediatrics is necessarily limited by the radiation burden, which is more significant owing to the greater radiosensitivity of children's tissues. This is a specialist topic that will not be considered in detail in this chapter.

It would be inappropriate to attempt to be prescriptive regarding detailed protocols for examinations. In any case the differences in requirements of single-slice compared to 16-slice, and in turn both of these to 320-slice, are such that this would not be possible.

As CT is a user-dependent modality protocols vary widely, and must take into account local preferences. In view of the high radiation burden associated with CT, any local variations should, however, fall within the framework of accepted best practice, with evidential support, rather than being simply an individual clinician's preference. It was previously reported that differing techniques for the same examination in different institutions have the potential to increase (or reduce) doses by a factor of more than four;[18] this amount of variation is clearly unacceptable. The UK national dose survey in 2003 demonstrated significant reductions in average dose from the 1991 survey, but there are still wide variations in applied techniques, and hence dose.[11]

The objective of the individual examination must always be considered, the objective being to provide the referring clinician with sufficient diagnostic information to enable the appropriate clinical management of the patient. Contrast enhancement is a good example of this: with modern scanning equipment it is possible to perform an initial unenhanced scan followed by multiphasic studies. Initial unenhanced images may not aid the answering of the clinical question and can therefore be omitted; the number of phases of contrast-enhanced scans should then be limited again to those that will address the clinical question for each individual patient, rather than blindly following a 'routine' protocol.

In the evaluation of major trauma modern CT is invaluable, as it facilitates rapid and thorough evaluation of the head, neck, thorax, abdomen and pelvis. This should not, however, be used as a 'routine' screening tool for all trauma: clinical justification for the inclusion of each body area is as essential as in all other circumstances. If used in this way, there is the danger that imaging replaces clinical acumen. Hadley, in a study of a major trauma centre in the USA, has shown that the application of 'routine' imaging involving computed radiography and CT led to 73% of examinations being performed 'unnecessarily'.[19] This has clear implications for over-irradiation of patients and could lead to litigation. However, recent experience in military scenarios, and some trauma studies, have shown that in polytrauma rapid screening with CT does provide potentially life-saving information, shortens time to theatre, and results in significantly better outcomes.[20]

Preparation for the examination

Owing to the association of CT with cancer (*CT – cancer test*) it is important to remember that preparation is both mental and physical. A good explanation of the procedure can allay the patient's nervousness, which may be due not only to fear of the examination but also of its result.

The patient may be changed into a hospital gown, depending on departmental protocol, but if this is not necessary in order to remove artefacts from the scan field then consideration should be given to scanning without the patient having to undress, to avoid depersonalisation.

Any checks required for intravenous (IV) contrast administration should be made as appropriate. Here again there is a wide variety of local practice, particularly regarding administration to asthmatic patients, and to diabetic patients taking metformin.

For abdominal scanning the patient may be starved for several hours prior to the scan to avoid the appearances of food in the stomach, although starving may increase associated anxiety. An oral contrast medium is commonly given to outline the bowel, and is typically administered at least an hour before scanning to allow transit. Increasingly, negative contrast is used, e.g. water, often for looking at the stomach, and this is finding increasing popularity in other abdominal examinations. Water has the advantages of being cheap, readily available and well tolerated by the patient.

'Scout'

For almost all examinations the first image taken is a 'scout' (also called topogram, surview, scanogram). The X-ray beam and detectors are kept stationary as the patient moves through a thin, collimated beam of radiation. Depending on anatomy and equipment, this projection may be performed as an AP (anterposterior), lateral or both.

The scout is used for localisation and scan selection. Gross abnormalities may be demonstrated; the presence of metal or other artefacts may also be seen. The combination of two scouts can be used on some equipment for calculation of mA modulation to reduce dose. This requires some thought on the part of the operator: for example, when performing cranial CT and not using mA modulation, is it appropriate to perform two scouts? The reason for each aspect of every examination needs to be considered so that the 'as low as reasonably achievable' (ALARA) principle is maintained.

Use of IV contrast

The high speed of modern equipment enables contrast enhancement to be viewed in multiple phases: arterial, portal venous, venous and delayed. As previously stated, the selection of the phases to be performed should be dictated by the clinical question to be answered.

Non-ionic media delivered via a pressure injector is the norm; coupled with scanner software, accurate timing of contrast delivery

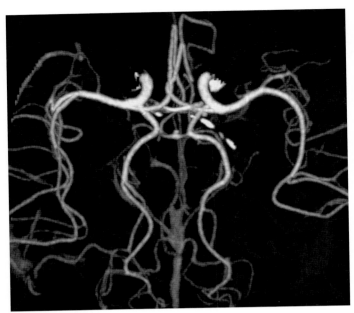

Figure 35.13 CTA – circle of Willis.
Reproduced with permission from Toshiba.

is relatively straightforward. Again, the dose implications of such methods must be considered; for example, if observing contrast build-up in a region of interest, is it necessary to begin observation scans at the same time as starting the injection? Can the interscan delay be made longer to produce fewer of these scans but maintain an optimal start for the diagnostic scan?

CT angiography (CTA) is made possible; multiplanar reconstruction, MIPs, 3D and surface rendered images are easily created on the typical workstation (Fig. 35.13). Large areas of anatomy can be demonstrated in a manner that is less invasive than conventional angiography, using less contrast and providing extra luminal information on the surrounding tissues and organs.

The brain

CT is the investigation of choice in the trauma setting as bony injury and intracranial haemorrhage are more readily demonstrated, and also for the investigation of acute stroke and paranasal sinus disease, although MR should be used for the staging of neoplasia prior to resection. Perfusion imaging is available for the demonstration of blood flow, particularly in the immediate investigation of stroke; as described in Chapter 33, the size of the infarct and the volume of ischaemic but viable brain tissue can be determined.

In head injury CT is the investigation of choice where there is a suspicion of a clinically important brain injury. The Canadian Head CT rule[21] has been adopted by both the National Institute for Health and Clinical Excellence[22] and the Royal College of Radiologists (RCR) for their guidelines.[23]

Patients presenting with acute stroke should be scanned as soon as possible, as per the national clinical guidelines for stroke.[24] The information required for appropriate treatment is whether or not the stroke is haemorrhagic, as this informs treatment options. This guidance postdates the RCR guidelines,[23] and is designed to facilitate swift, appropriate treatment for this group of patients. Research has shown that rapid intervention can have significant results.

It *must* be remembered that:

Stroke is a medical emergency. With active management in the initial hours after stroke onset ischaemic brain may be saved from infarction.[25]

Common indications

- Trauma
- Acute stroke
- Transient ischaemic attack
- Space-occupying lesion
- Acute severe headache (suspected subarachnoid haemorrhage)
- Sinus disease

The use of CT for vascular studies of the head is covered in Chapter 33.

Typical protocol

Lateral scan projection radiograph from the skull base to the vertex is commonly taken and used for planning axial slices/volume. In multiple trauma cases the cervical vertebrae may be included.

In general, thinner slices are acquired through the posterior fossa, which is often not well visualised on CT. MR is superior if posterior fossa pathology is suspected. Although cranial CT is still commonly performed using sequential scans, thin spiral scans can be performed and reformatted into the required slice thickness; 64+ slice in particular demonstrates the posterior fossa well; thin slices are combined for viewing and provide good axial demonstration of this area. Isotropic or near isotropic multiplanar reconstructions are also readily produced.

Patient positioning for cranial CT is the subject of debate. Many centres adopt the 'supraorbital baseline'; slices are planned parallel to a line running between the external auditory meatus (EAM) and the superior orbital ridge. The reasoning for this is to reduce the dose to the lens of the eye by not scanning through the globe. In practice this is often badly performed, as can be seen by the eyes being present on the lowermost images of many scans. This baseline exacerbates the problems of visualising the posterior fossa, which is not well demonstrated.

The commonest alternative is Reed's baseline, which extends from the EAM through the inferior border of the orbit. Although it irradiates the orbit it does better demonstrate the posterior fossa and the path of the optic nerve. This method is in use in several specialist neurocentres. The use of bismuth shields to protect the eyes during scanning, as seen in Figures 35.14 and 35.15, has been suggested and seems worthy of consideration.[26]

Whichever baseline is to be used, thought needs to be given to patient positioning in order to minimise the use of gantry angulation, which is to be avoided because of the potential to increase patient dose.[27]

Cranial CT is usually performed without the addition of contrast media. A second scan after the administration of contrast is useful in some acute circumstances. The exception to this is in scanning for metastases, when a single contrast-enhanced scan is usual; referral for MRI should also be considered subject to availability.

Cranial CT reporting by radiographers is a role development that has been demonstrated to be a feasible way of addressing radiologist shortages and of reducing waiting lists. Studies have shown that high accuracy rates are achievable after suitable training,[28,29] and radiographers have taken on this role in some centres.

With multislice technology in particular there is no longer any requirement for additional direct coronal scanning for paranasal sinuses, as reconstructions can be obtained in any plane. The effect of this when looking at fluid levels does, however, need to be considered.

Spine

CT is of limited application other than in trauma. Its use is mandatory in cases of cervical spine trauma where plain film findings are

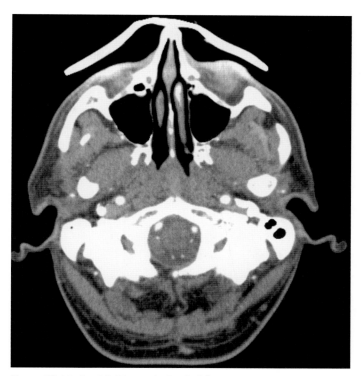

Figure 35.14 Cranial CT – at the level of foramen magnum. Note use of bismuth eye shields and lack of artefact remote from shielding. *Reproduced with permission from Toshiba.*

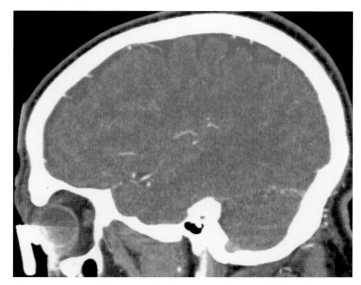

Figure 35.15 Cranial CT – sagittal reconstruction. Again bismuth shielding is seen without artefact affecting visualisation of brain. *Reproduced with permission from Toshiba.*

equivocal or have failed to demonstrate the cervicothoracic junction (see Chapter 11 for further discussion). CT is increasingly replacing plain film imaging, particularly in cases of major trauma and/or when the patient is undergoing cranial CT. In the case of thoracic or lumbar trauma with neurological deficit, CT can be used to demonstrate bony detail.

MRI is the investigation of choice for spinal pathology because of its greater soft tissue resolution and its ability for multiplanar imaging of the cord.

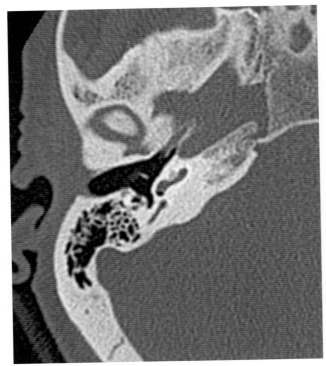

Figure 35.16 Cranial CT – high resolution imaging of the temporal bone.
Reproduced with permission from Toshiba.

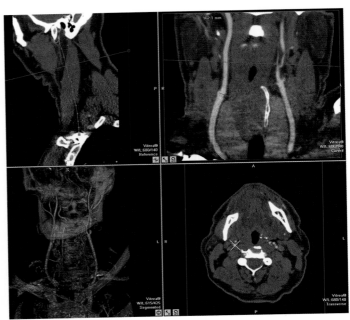

Figure 35.18 Neck CT – workstation images of carotid study.
Reproduced with permission from Toshiba.

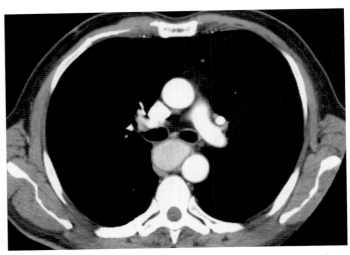

Figure 35.19 CT thorax – axial slice through thorax. Excellent arterial contrast enhancement is seen on this image.
Reproduced with permission from Toshiba.

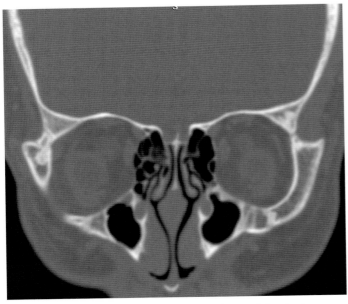

Figure 35.17 Cranial CT – coronal reconstruction used for viewing sinuses or facial bones.
Reproduced with permission from Toshiba.

The neck

CT may be used for the staging of tumours in the neck, but MR is better in this area and should be used where available. Other investigations are generally used for the diagnosis of lesions in the neck, although carotid studies can be performed, as shown in Figure 35.18.

The chest (Figs 35.19, 35.20)

Justification for the CT examination of young women should be particularly robust considering the potential for breast cancer induction.[30] Consideration should be given to the application of breast shielding, which has been shown to achieve a breast dose reduction of more than 50% without compromising the demonstration of the thoracic contents.[31]

Staging of both primary lesions in the chest and metastatic spread from other primary sites in association with chest radiography is a commonly seen use of CT in this body area. Generally the thorax and upper abdomen are scanned; this is to enable assessment of upper abdominal lymphadenopathy and to view the adrenals and liver, particularly for metastatic spread. CT has high accuracy rates and can facilitate biopsy. The introduction of positron emission tomography

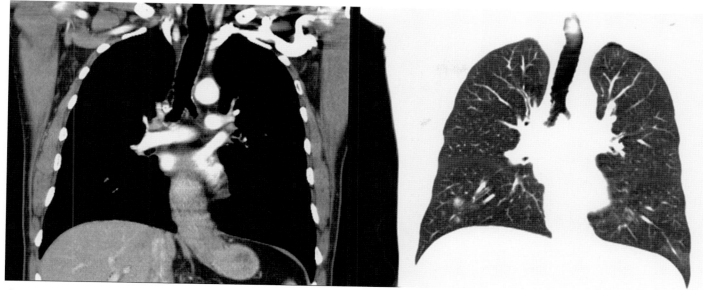

Figure 35.20 CT thorax – coronal reconstructions viewed on 'soft tissue' and 'lung' windows. *Reproduced with permission from Toshiba.*

(PET) will have an impact in this area, particularly when used in conjunction with CT (see Fig. 35.43).

Nodal disease is well visualised. Specific sites in which nodes are often seen are the aortopulmonary window in the subcranial and perihilar regions, and the retrocrural area. Multiplanar reconstructions can be helpful in interpretation, as can the use of varying window settings, and techniques such as the use of MIPs.

High-resolution CT (HRCT) is used for detailed evaluation of the lung parenchyma. When scanning using thin slices on high-end multislice equipment, using lung windows effectively provides 'free' HRCT imaging, which again can be reconstructed into any desired plane.

There is debate on the use of 'low-dose' CT as a screening tool. Whereas CT may increase the detection of early tumours, there is a high rate of detection of nodules that require follow-up with standard-dose HRCT to classify them as benign or otherwise, and prevent interventions[32] (in one large study approximately 23% of screened patients had nodules and 2.7% had a malignancy[33]). The requirement for a second scan with 'normal' dose rates makes such screening costly, both financially and in terms of dose burden, particularly to asymptomatic patients. If patients with benign nodules are then followed up with interval scans the potential for extremely high dose burdens is clear.

It has been suggested that there is no difference in survival rate between patients with solitary lesions of 1 cm or 3 cm on diagnosis.[34] Further evaluation of the utility of CT screening is suggested and would seem appropriate. There are, however, already centres offering a CT screening service for chest and other body areas, even with self-referral, which is of some concern without evidence of benefit, particularly given that multiple examinations will inevitably involve a high cumulative dose and the attendant risks.

Rapid scan times enable visualisation of the entire thorax in a single breath-hold, eliminating the previous problems associated with respiratory misregistration. Using software to optimise the timing of IV contrast injections the area can be scanned in arterial phase, enabling demonstration of vascular structures in the thorax. CT is rapidly becoming the examination of choice for the investigation of pulmonary emboli. High accuracy rates are achieved and the examination can, if required, be coupled with an examination of the upper legs for underlying deep vein thrombosis (Fig. 35.21). Dual-energy scans

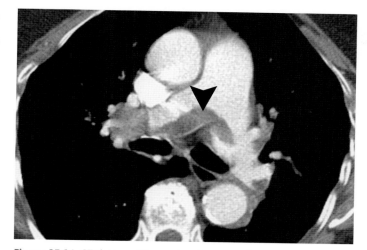

Figure 35.21 CT thorax – PE scanning demonstrating saddle embolus (arrowed).

enable accurate calculation of perfusion defects. Use of lower kVp (80) has been shown to be effective for CT pulmonary angiography, producing dose benefits without loss of image quality.[35]

Cardiac CT

Another use for fast scan times is in imaging of the heart. This has been described as the ultimate goal for multislice CT. Electrocardiography gating techniques enable high-quality imaging of the heart and associated vascular structures in as few as five cardiac cycles. Image quality now matches and in some cases exceeds that of EBCT, and the availability of multislice scanners has certainly become more widespread than EBCT has been. Dual-source systems enable more rapid visualisation, so that temporal resolution can be reduced to 40–80 ms, comparable to that of EBCT (50 ms).[36]

Coronary artery calcium scoring has been in use for some time and is used to provide an indication of the presence and amount of atherosclerotic plaque, enabling the detection of potential disease

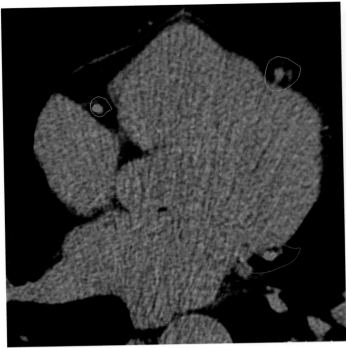

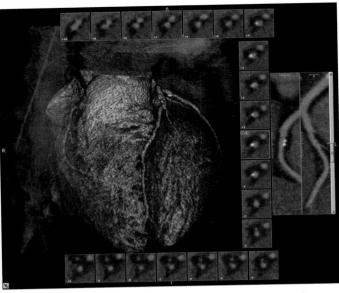

Figure 35.23 Cardiac CT – CTA. High-quality 3D reconstruction from a 32-slice scanner. The sternum and great vessels can be seen semi-transparent on this image. Curved reconstructions demonstrate the selected vessel which can be viewed 'sliced' in any direction.
Reproduced with permission from Toshiba.

Figure 35.22 Cardiac CT – coronary artery calcium scoring. Regions of interest around coronary arteries can be seen.
Reproduced with permission from Toshiba.

prior to the development of symptoms such as angina and dyspnoea. High-resolution non-contrast scans are obtained and volumetric analysis used to produce a calcium score. This score can then be compared with a database of known scores adjusted for age and gender, and appropriate advice given on the risk of coronary artery disease (Fig. 35.22).

The information gained from calcium scoring does not give a direct measure of arterial narrowing, but has good correlation with the severity of underlying disease. It does not rule out the presence of soft non-calcified plaque, but soft plaque evaluation is now becoming available. Although useful for patients with specific risk factors, screening remains impractical because of the dose and cost.[37] Dissection, aneurysm and coarctation of the aorta can also be assessed, as well as the structure of the heart itself. Such structural information can also be obtained using MRI, which should be considered as an alternative where available (Figs 35.23, 35.24).

CTA is in widespread use, and with 320-slice machines now available may even be used in some patients with atrial fibrillation, which has previously been a contraindication.[38]

Gastrointestinal tract

Oesophageal perforation may be demonstrated on a contrast swallow; however, use of CT will enable the additional demonstration of complications in surrounding tissues. CT is also used for staging of oesophageal and stomach tumours: the primary tumour may be visualised and any local or nodal spread demonstrated. Water is useful as a negative oral contrast in this case as it enables visualisation of the stomach wall, which may be partially obscured by the use of positive oral contrast media (Fig. 35.25).

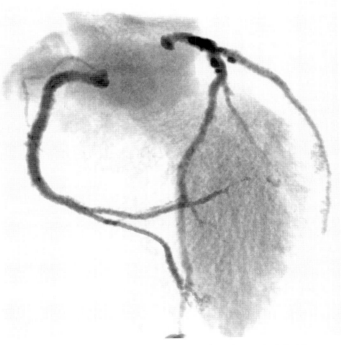

Figure 35.24 Cardiac CT – CTA. The image here is manipulated to provide an 'angiographic' appearance.
Reproduced with permission from Toshiba.

In adults with acute abdominal pain CT may be used to establish the cause and level of obstruction. Colonic lesions are well demonstrated by CT colonoscopy, with full and thorough preparation results compared with direct colonoscopy. The use of reconstruction techniques such as virtual colonoscopy allows for comparable images but with the advantage of visualisation of involvement external to the lumen. CT is the investigation of choice for frail patients, as it may be better tolerated than barium enema or colonoscopy because of its less invasive nature. CT also facilitates staging of lesions during the same examination (Figs 35.26, 35.27, 35.28).

Abdomen

Abdominal CT is a common examination that has a high diagnostic yield, but equally a high radiation dose burden. It is the examination of choice for nodal staging of many malignancies, including lymphoma. Although CT is generally thought to be the 'better' examination in cases of suspected abdominal mass, sepsis or pyrexia of unknown origin, ultrasound (US) should be performed first, as it may yield the required information to answer the clinical question without the high radiation dose associated with abdominal CT. Both imaging methods may be used to facilitate biopsy or drainage.

Liver (Fig. 35.29)

CT is far more sensitive than US and is commonly used for staging prior to resection, although US is again usually the first-line investigation for diagnosis. Three-phase post-contrast techniques are particularly useful for diagnosis and preoperative staging of liver metastases, which are the most frequently occurring malignant tumours of the liver. Many liver lesions look similar before contrast and can look similar at different timings after contrast injection. The use of precontrast scans has been questioned for some time; both its utility and its dose implications must be considered. The soft tissue contrast sensitivity of MR makes it the investigation of choice for staging of primary lesions, and if available, it should be considered for the evaluation of metastases.

CT can also be used in the investigation of cirrhosis, demonstrating fatty infiltration, and also to characterise possible haemangioma. The use of MRI should be considered in these cases.

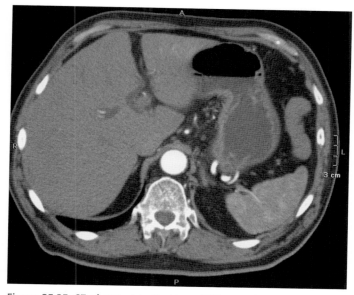

Figure 35.25 CT of gastrointestinal tract (GIT). Use of water as negative contrast enables visualisation of the stomach wall.
Reproduced with permission from Toshiba.

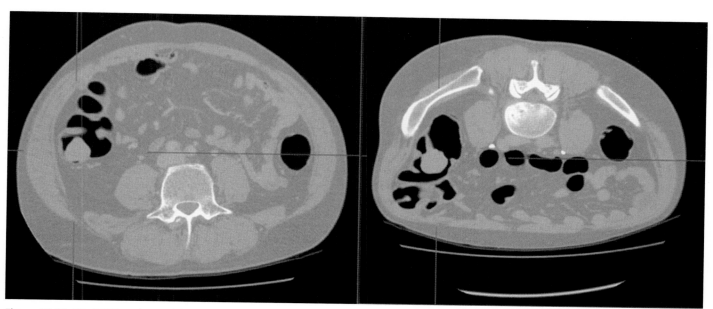

Figure 35.26 CT of GIT – colon. Axial scans can visualise pathology external to the colon. A polyp is seen in the ascending colon. On the prone view the polyp has moved anteriorly under gravity and its stalk can be seen.
Reproduced with permission from Toshiba.

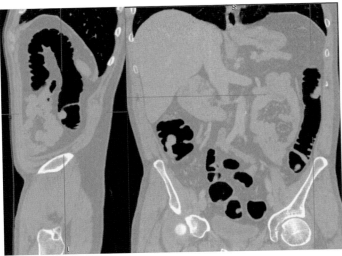

Figure 35.27 CT of GIT – colon. Sagittal and coronal reconstructions from Figure 35.26.
Reproduced with permission from Toshiba.

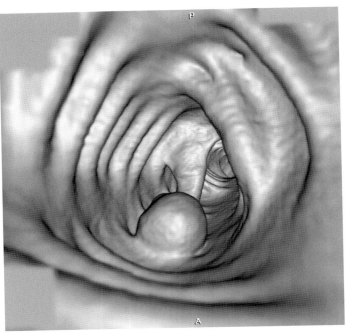

Figure 35.28 CT of GIT – virtual colonoscopy. Prone reconstructions from patient in Figure 35.26, demonstrating the polyp in the bowel, hanging from its stalk.
Reproduced with permission from Toshiba.

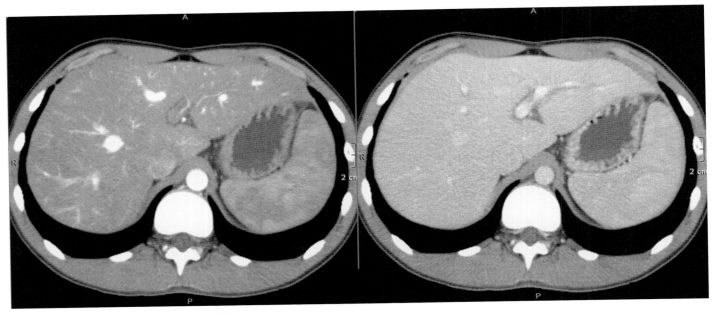

Figure 35.29 CT liver – arterial and venous phases.
Reproduced with permission from Toshiba.

Kidneys and adrenal glands

The adrenals are commonly scanned in association with the thorax for bronchial staging as they are a common site for metastatic spread from a lung primary (Fig. 35.30). There is potential for unenhanced CT of the kidneys, ureter and bladder (KUB) region to replace the intravenous urogram; it is already the investigation of choice for renal colic and detection of calculi. It should be performed with reduced exposure factors as it has been shown that diagnostic accuracy can be maintained with a low dose protocol.[39]

Contrast-enhanced CT is the investigation of choice for renal masses. Again, it is usual for US to be the first-line investigation, but CT can detect smaller lesions. MRI may be used in staging of advanced disease, where it is superior to CT. CT is the examination of choice in renal trauma, in which case a post-contrast two-phase examination is indicated.

Pancreas

US is better in thin patients and CT is better in larger individuals, where the peripancreatic fat is useful for delineation. IV contrast enhancement is used to assess necrosis in the immediate post-acute phase of pancreatitis, and is better than US for follow-up, but owing to the dose implications US should be used for monitoring chronic conditions. For pancreatic tumours, CT is required for staging, but both US and CT may be used to facilitate biopsy (Fig. 35.31).

Musculoskeletal system (Figs 35.32, 35.33)

CT is classified as a specialised examination by the RCR guidelines.[24] It has an important place in musculoskeletal imaging owing to its ability to demonstrate occult and complex fractures, and bone healing. For example, CT can be used to clarify a clinically suspected scaphoid fracture, but MRI is better where it is available. Conventional radiography is still the first-line technique for the detection of fractures and dislocations. RNI is sensitive but not specific for the detection of occult or stress fractures and metastatic disease. US and MRI are the investigations of choice for associated soft tissue injuries.

CT is used for orthopaedic surgical planning, clarification of complex fractures and demonstration of developmental deformities. Areas of particular value are the tibial plateau, calcaneus and pelvic fractures. CT can also be used for leg length measurement and assessment of scoliosis. If scout views are used for measurement they have the advantage of being obtained using a non-divergent beam, rendering measurement more accurate. High-end scans can produce 4D cine-like images, useful to assess musculoskeletal function.

CT angiography (CTA)

CT has long been used to image vascular structures, but the advent of multislice technology has opened up a new range of examinations, which are now achievable owing to increased speed, coverage and

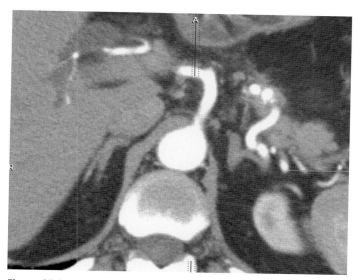

Figure 35.30 CT adrenals.
Reproduced with permission from Toshiba.

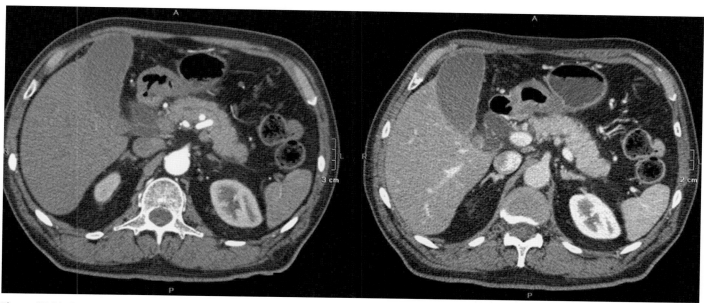

Figure 35.31 CT pancreas – arterial and venous phases.
Reproduced with permission from Toshiba.

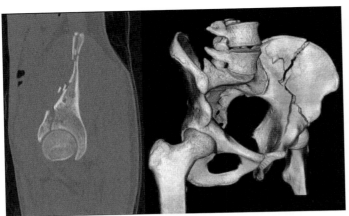

Figure 35.32 CT pelvis. A combination of oblique reconstructions and surface rendered images are used here to clarify a complex fracture. *Reproduced with permission from Toshiba.*

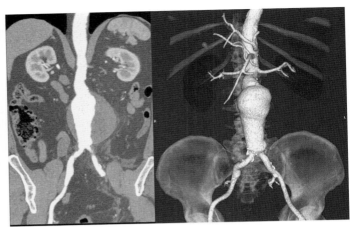

Figure 35.34 CTA – abdominal aortic aneurysm. Curved MIP demonstrating extent and location of aneurysm. 3D image demonstrates non-involvement of renal arteries. *Reproduced with permission from Toshiba.*

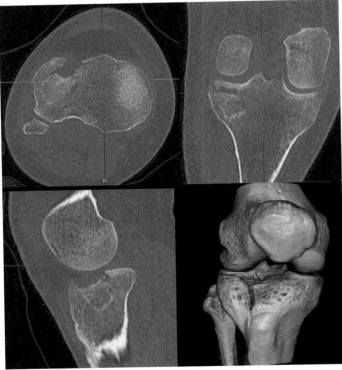

Figure 35.33 CT knee. Tibial plateau fracture, well demonstrated by axial scan, coronal and sagittal reformats, and surface rendered 3D image. *Reproduced with permission from Toshiba.*

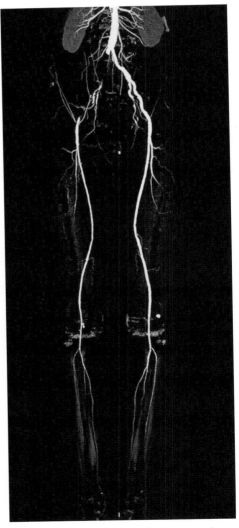

Figure 35.35 CTA – peripheral angiography. Coverage from renal arteries to ankles shown on this MIP. *Reproduced with permission from Toshiba.*

reconstruction techniques. The aorta is commonly scanned for dissection and aneurysmal disease; coronal reconstructions, MIPs, or 3D images can clearly resolve questions, e.g. regarding renal artery involvement (Fig. 35.34).

Peripheral angiography can be performed in a far less invasive manner than traditional angiography (Figs 35.35, 35.36); the dose advantages of magnetic resonance angiography should be considered where this technique is available. This is an area where the ability to scan faster with more slices may be disadvantageous, as it is possible to scan faster than the contrast bolus can travel.

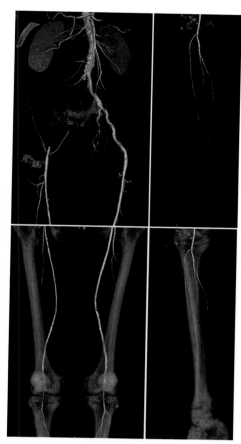

Figure 35.36 CTA – peripheral angiography. Using image reformatting, a single volumetric acquisition can be used to view key areas from different planes/angles, and with or without semi-transparent bone for positional reference.
Reproduced with permission from Toshiba.

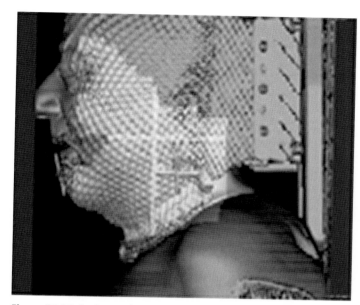

Figure 35.37 ProSoma. Skin surface image reconstructed from CT data set. This demonstrates the radiotherapy light field to aid treatment set up verification.
Reproduced with permission from Oncology Systems Limited and Accuray Incorporated.

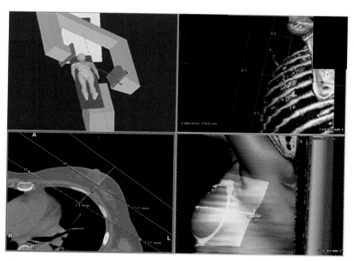

Figure 35.38 ProSoma. CT simulation of radiotherapy for breast cancer.
Reproduced with permission from Oncology Systems Limited and Accuray Incorporated.

THERAPY

CT has many applications in radiotherapy. Tumour staging has already been mentioned, but recent years have seen the growth in the use of CT for treatment planning. CT simulation uses CT data sets to plan the delivery of radiotherapy treatment beams (Fig. 35.37).

The patient is scanned using immobilisation devices on the treatment table, which is flat; consequently, the scan table used for planning must also be flat, as it is vital for planning accuracy that the positions are duplicated exactly (Fig. 35.38).

A recent development is TomoTherapy®,[40] the use of megavoltage CT for the delivery of therapy treatments. The megavoltage beam can be used to image the tumour as it responds to treatment; its size, shape and position may alter, and the megavoltage images obtained can be used to replan treatment, enabling more effective use of the delivered doses (Figs 35.39, 35.40).

FUTURE DEVELOPMENTS

New technology is being launched on a regular basis, and such developments have made CT the most rapidly evolving imaging technology.

No sooner was spiral CT replaced by quad multislice, than it in turn has been replaced by 8-slice and now 320-slice machines. Already it is possible to scan 16 cm volumes in a single rotation; this may be extended by the development of flat plate digital detector systems, raising the possibility of single rotation scanning of a larger body area. This could produce a data set of an anatomical area, e.g. the chest, from which could be reconstructed a chest image plus lateral and obliques as required, as well as slices in any plane, 3D and MIP reconstructions – all from a single rotation. This would have a similar acquisition time to standard chest X-ray.

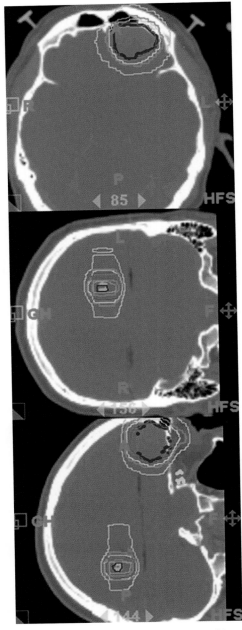

Figure 35.39 TomoTherapy®. Dose distribution for small intracranial stereotactic-type lesion.
Reproduced with permission from Oncology Systems Limited and Accuray Incorporated.

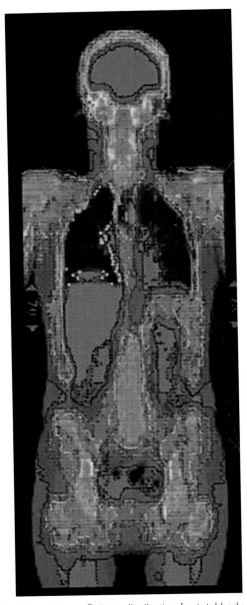

Figure 35.40 TomoTherapy®. Dose distribution for total body irradiation prior to bone marrow transplant.
Reproduced with permission from Oncology Systems Limited and Accuray Incorporated.

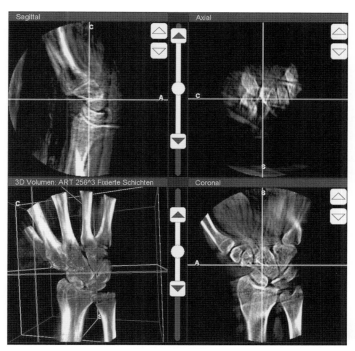

Figure 35.41 Vario 3D. Multiplanar and 3D images reconstructed from images taken during rotation of the C-arm.
Reproduced with permission from Xograph.

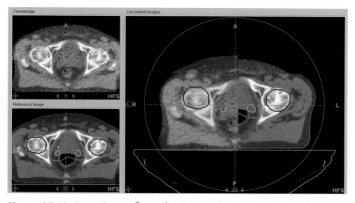

Figure 35.42 TomoTherapy®. Verification CT ('tomoimage' – MV acquisition) fused with planning CT ('reference image' – kV acquisition) at the planning console. These are images the radiographer will use and evaluate on the treatment machine on a daily basis.
Reproduced with permission from Oncology Systems Limited and Accuray Incorporated.

C-arm CT systems have been developed for use in operating theatres and interventional suites. These systems can be used as a standard image intensifier: the CT function is selected and a series of images taken at fixed angles as the intensifier C-arm rotates around a preselected isocentre (Fig. 35.41).

These advances in medical imaging technology are being driven by the rapid advances in computing and associated technologies. Already we can look to the image registration of various cross-sectional studies, for example the registration of CT and MR images may enable bony and soft tissue structures and their relationships to be better demonstrated than is possible with each individual modality.[41] CT and PET images can be combined to provide anatomical and functional information simultaneously. Kilovoltage and megavoltage images are combined in TomoTherapy® (Fig. 35.42).[40]

It continues to be an exciting and challenging time to be working with this dynamic imaging modality. Changes are rapid and new advice is constantly emerging, for example the utility of Bismuth shielding for dose reduction. At the time of writing this was seen to be of potential use,[26,31] however there is recent evidence to suggest that the disadvantages might outweigh the advantages of use, and alternative methods for dose reduction should be considered.[42]

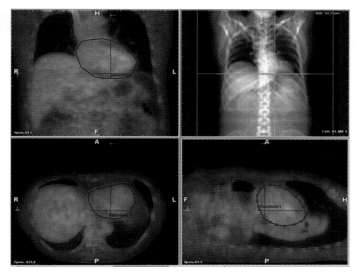

Figure 35.43 ProSoma – CT-PET image fusion. The image fusion aids delineation of tumour volume for radiotherapy.
Reproduced with permission from Oncology Systems Limited and Accuray Incorporated.

REFERENCES

1. ICRP. Managing patient dose in computed tomography. ICRP Publication 87. Elsevier; 2000.
2. American College of Radiology. ACR practice guideline for performing and interpreting diagnostic computed tomography (CT). ACR; 2002.
3. Bogdanich W. Radiation overdoses point up dangers of CT Scans. Bottom of form. October 15, 2009. New York Times. http://www.nytimes.com/2009/10/16/us/16radiation.html.
4. Grossmann G. Lung tomography. British Journal of Radiology 1935;8:733.
5. Kuhl D. Transmission scanning. Radiology 1966;87:278–84.
6. Ambrose J, Hounsfield G. Computerised transverse axial tomography. British Journal of Radiology 1972;46:148.
7. Hounsfield G. Computerised transverse axial scanning (tomography), Part 1: Description of system. British Journal of Radiology 1973;46:1016.
8. Ambrose J, Hounsfield G. Computerised transverse axial scanning (tomography), Part 2: Clinical applications. British

Journal of Radiology 1973;46: 1023.

9. Seeram E. Computed tomography: physical principles, clinical applications, and quality control. 3rd ed. Philadelphia: Saunders; 2009.

10. Shrimpton P, et al. Survey of CT practice in the UK. Part 2: Dosimetric aspects. NRPB-R249. London: HMSO; 1991.

11. Shrimpton P, et al. National survey of doses from CT in the UK: 2003. British Journal of Radiology 2006;79: 968–80.

12. UNSCEAR. Report to the general assembly, Annex D: Medical Radiation Exposures. New York: UN; 2000.

13. Mettler F, et al. Radiologic and nuclear medicine studies in the United States and Worldwide: Frequency, radiation dose, and comparison with other radiation sources: 1950–2007. Radiology 2009;253: 520–31.

14. Cameron J. UKRC 2004 debate: Moderate dose rate ionising radiation increases longevity. British Journal of Radiology 2005;78:11–3.

15. Feinendegen L. UKRC 2004 debate: Evidence for beneficial low level radiation effects and radiation hormesis. British Journal of Radiology 2005;78:3–7.

16. The Ionising Radiation (Medical Exposure) Regulations. Statutory Instruments 2000, no. 1059. London: HMSO; 2000.

17. Freiherr G. Dose-saving technologies proliferate throughout CT: Many hardware and software tools onboard high- and midtier scanners go unused despite availability. Diagnostic Imaging 29 April 2010. http://www.diagnosticimaging.com/focal-points/2010/ct-dose/display/article/113619/1561981.

18. Shrimpton P, et al. Reference doses in computed tomography. Radiation Protection Dosimetry 1998;80:55–9.

19. Hadley J. Over utilization of imaging in the acute trauma setting. In: RSNA scientific assembly and annual meeting program. Oak Brook, IL: RSNA; 2004. p. 372.

20. Huber-Wagner S, et al. Effect of whole body CT during trauma resuscitation on survival: a retrospective, muticentre study. Lancet 2009;373:1455–61.

21. Steill I, et al. The Canadian CT head rule for patients with minor head injury. Lancet 2001;357:1391–6.

22. NICE. Head injury – triage, assessment, investigation and early management of head injury in infants, children and adults. Clinical Guideline 56. September 2007.

23. Royal College of Radiologists working party. Making the best use of a department of clinical radiology: guidelines for doctors. 6th ed. London: Royal College of Radiologists; 2007.

24. Intercollegiate Stroke Working Party. National Clinical Guidelines for Stroke. 3rd ed. London: Royal College of Physicians; July 2008.

25. Intercollegiate Stroke Working Party. National clinical guidelines for stroke. 2nd ed. London: Royal College of Physicians; June 2004.

26. Hopper K, et al. Radioprotection to the eye during CT scanning. American Journal of Neuroradiology 2001;22:1194–8.

27. Murphy U. Dose implications of gantry tilt in cranial computerised tomography. Radiography Ireland 1998;6(3):137–9.

28. Carver B. Meeting service needs: cranial CT reporting by radiographers. In proceedings of UKRC 2004. BIR Congress Series 2004; p. 10.

29. Carver B. Is cranial CT reporting by radiographers a feasible option to assist radiologist workload and provide a route for radiographer role extension? In: RSNA scientific assembly and annual meeting program. Oak Brook, IL: RSNA; 2004. p. 553.

30. Jansen-van der Weide M, et al. Exposure to low-dose radiation and the risk of breast cancer among women with a familial or genetic predisposition: a meta-analysis. European Radiology 2010;20:2547–56.

31. Hopper K, et al. The breast: in plane x-ray protection during diagnostic thoracic CT: shielding with bismuth radioprotective garments. Radiology 1997;205:853–8.

32. Bach P, et al. Computed tomography screening and lung cancer outcomes. JAMA 2007;297(9):953–61.

33. Henschke C, et al. Early lung cancer action project: a summary of the findings on baseline screening. Oncologist 2001;6: 147–52.

34. Patz E, et al. Correlation of tumour size and survival in patients with stage 1A non-small cell lung cancer. Chest 2000;117:1568–71.

35. Zamboni G, et al. Low voltage CTPA for patients with suspected pulmonary embolism. European Journal of Radiology. In Press. Available online 15 July 2011.

36. Flohr T, et al. First performance evaluation of a dual-source CT system. European Radiology 2006;16:256–68.

37. Blankstein R, et al. Predictors of coronary heart disease events among asymptomatic persons with low low-density lipoprotein cholesterol. Journal of the American College of Cardiology 2011;58: 364–74.

38. Xu L, et al. Diagnostic performance of 320-detector CT coronary angiography in patients with atrial fibrillation: preliminary results 2011. European Radiology 2011;21:936–43.

39. Meagher T, et al. Low dose computed tomography in suspected acute renal colic. Clinical Radiology 2001;56:873–6.

40. www.tomotherapy.com/intro/index.html.

41. Panigraphy A, et al. Registration of three-dimensional MR and CT studies of the cervical spine. American Journal of Neuroradiology 2000;21:282–9.

42. AAPM. Use of Bismuth shielding for the purpose of dose reduction in CT scanning. www.aapm.org/publicgeneral/BismuthShielding.pdf, 2012.

Chapter 36

Magnetic resonance imaging

John Talbot

INTRODUCTION

Magnetic resonance imaging (MRI) is still considered a relative new-comer to the field of diagnostic imaging. In fact, it was first identified as a possible imaging modality in 1969 and was developed almost in tandem with computed tomography (CT).

MRI uses a combination of magnetic fields and electromagnetic radiation in the radiofrequency range to produce diagnostic images of the body. The basic premise of MRI is that a radiofrequency pulse is applied to the hydrogen nuclei within the patient's tissues which causes them to change their energy state and net magnetic alignment to an external magnetic field. As the nuclei lose this energy to realign with the field, their transmitted energy can be received, measured and spatially located.

Since its inception at the beginning of the 1980s, MRI has become a first-line technique in the routine diagnosis of disease, and scanners can be found in all major hospitals.

Like CT, MRI is a cross-sectional imaging modality acquiring user-definable slices having variable size (field of view) and thickness. MRI does however have certain advantages over CT:

- MRI uses non-ionising radiation rather than X-rays. To be precise, MRI uses electromagnetic radiation in the radiofrequency range – between 6 and 340 MHz, depending on the magnetic field strength of the scanner. This portion of the electromagnetic spectrum has a longer wavelength than that of X-rays and is correspondingly less energetic and less damaging to tissues.
- MRI has very marked soft tissue contrast. MRI is unique among diagnostic modalities in that the signal that forms the image is generated by the body tissue itself. Radiographs and CT rely on X-rays passing through, and being attenuated by, the area under investigation. Although the user has control over the penetrating power and intensity of the beam, the resulting image is still essentially a shadow of the anatomy. MRI on the other hand has multiple user-definable parameters which exploit the molecular behaviour of the tissues and can dramatically modify tissue contrast in much the same way as nuclear magnetic resonance (NMR) spectroscopy can differentiate between individual elements in a chemical substance.

- MRI acquires images in any given plane without having to change the position of the patient. Although CT data can be post-processed into many different planes and rendered volumes, the acquisition plane is still essentially axial.
- MRI can obtain both structural (morphological) information and *functional* information. Functional MRI (fMRI) exploits the fact that MRI can detect minute changes in the chemical composition of body tissues, such as the amount of haemoglobin versus deoxyhaemoglobin. The principle of fMRI imaging is to rapidly acquire a series of images of the brain and to statistically analyse the images for differences between them. This is usually done after a baseline scan, and the patient is asked to perform a physical or mental task during acquisition.

There is a developing trend for more powerful scanners, operating at higher magnetic field strengths, which can investigate metabolic function[1] and have microscopic resolution. Because of these advantages, the use of MRI has exponentially increased over the last 20 years, not to replace CT but to sit comfortably alongside it.

EQUIPMENT CHRONOLOGY

The chronology of MRI charts the discovery and development of a physical phenomenon known as NMR.

1845 Michael Faraday investigated the magnetic properties of dried blood.

1938 In the 1930s American physicist Isidor Rabi researched methods of observing atomic spectra. During his work he demonstrated that the spin state in a molecular beam can be reoriented in a magnetic field. In 1944 he received the Nobel Prize in physics 'for his resonance method for recording the magnetic properties of atomic nuclei'.[2]

1946 The process of NMR was discovered by the independently operating research teams of Felix Bloch (Stanford University) and Edwin Purcell (Harvard University).

1948 Nicolaas Bloembergen presented his theory of relaxation times, based on experiments in Purcell's laboratory.

1950   Irwin Hahn 'accidentally' discovered spin echoes while working on relaxation experiments. He originally cursed the symmetrical oscilloscope reading as an 'annoying glitch'.

1950s   NMR was used in the field of analytical chemistry.

1960s   NMR spectroscopy revolutionised the non-destructive analysis of the composition of chemical compounds. These techniques tested very small samples that were placed inside high field magnets having a very narrow bore only a few centimetres wide. Paramagnetic reagents were used in NMR spectroscopy and can be thought of as the forerunners of modern MRI contrast media.

1966   Richard Ernst showed that Fourier transform increases the sensitivity of magnetic resonance (MR) spectroscopy.

1969   Dr Raymond Damadian (SUNY Downstate Medical Centre) used NMR spectroscopy in research into sodium and potassium in living cells. This led him to his first experiments with NMR and caused him to first propose the possibility of an NMR body scanner.[3]

1971   Following animal studies on rats, Damadian discovered considerable differences in the NMR signals emitted by healthy tissues and tumours. He authored a paper entitled 'Tumor detection by nuclear magnetic resonance',[4] and although this work was met with scepticism from many quarters Damadian maintained his idea of the MR body scanner.

1972   Damadian filed the first of his patents for an MRI body scanner. The patent described how liquid helium could be used to create a supercooled electromagnet housed within a cylindrical cryostat. The patent also described how the nuclei of hydrogen atoms in the body would react to the resultant magnetic field, and how a 3D spatial localisation method could encode the signals into a scan.

1973   The journal *Nature* published an article written by Professor Paul Lauterbur, Professor of Chemistry at the State University of New York, entitled 'Image formation by induced local interaction: examples employing magnetic resonance'.[5] Lauterbur described a new imaging technique for which he coined the term zeugmatography (from the Greek meaning 'to join together'). This alluded to the principle of his technique, which involved the joining of two magnetic fields in the spatial localisation of two test tubes filled with normal water sitting in a bath of heavy water. Lauterbur used a static main magnetic field over which he applied a weaker gradient field. He then used a back-projection method (as used in CT) to produce an image of the two test tubes (Fig. 36.1).

This landmark imaging experiment was of great importance for two reasons. First, it was the first time that NMR had given spatial information rather than just spectroscopic information. Second, it had never previously been possible to distinguish between heavy water and normal water using analytical techniques.

Ironically, the journal editor nearly declined to publish the paper on the grounds that it was 'not of sufficiently wide significance for inclusion'. Professor Lauterbur received a Nobel Prize for this and other work in the field of MRI in 2003.

1973   In the same year Professor Peter Mansfield was beginning his studies into NMR at the University of Nottingham in the UK. He initially worked on studies of solid objects, such as crystals. However, one year later, Mansfield and collaborator Alan Garroway filed a patent and published a paper on image formation by NMR.[6]

1975   Richard Ernst proposed MRI using phase and frequency encoding, and the Fourier transform. This technique is still the basis of spatial encoding in the modern MRI scanner. Peter Mansfield and another colleague, Andrew Maudsley, who were also working in the field of spatial encoding proposed a technique that could produce in vivo imaging.

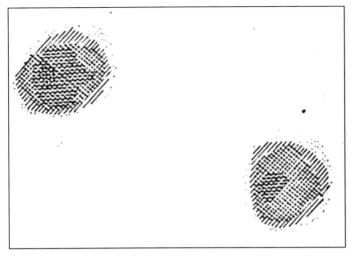

Figure 36.1 The first use of spatial encoding with NMR by Professor Paul Lauterbur. The shaded areas represent the spatial position of two tubes filled with water.[5]
Image reproduced by kind permission of Professor P. Lauterbur and Nature.

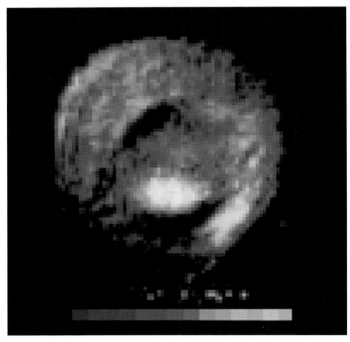

Figure 36.2 First human MRI scan by Mansfield and Maudsley.[7] Axial cross-section through a finger.
Image reproduced by kind permission of Professor Mansfield.

1976   Professor Mansfield et al. began to study ways of fast imaging using NMR and an improved picture display. They produced the first in vivo image of human anatomy, a cross-section through a finger (Fig. 36.2).[7]

1977   Raymond Damadian, aided by graduate students, built a prototype NMR body scanner consisting of a homemade superconducting magnet. The magnet itself was made of nearly 50 km of niobium–titanium wire spun onto a cylinder, a technique still used today. The magnet bore itself was 134 cm in diameter, big enough to allow the positioning of a human body. To ensure superconductivity the magnet was supercooled using liquid helium, but unlike today's systems the boil-off and leakage was so great that refills cost $2000 per week.

The receive coil was constructed from cardboard and copper wire and designed to be worn around the body like a corset, very much like modern phased-array wrap-around body coils. The patient transport system was little more than a wooden tray. After an abortive first attempt to scan Damadian, one of his research assistants, Laurence Minkoff, was placed into the scanner. The receive coil was positioned around his thorax and the scan procedure itself took nearly 5 hours. The result was a rudimentary image, reconstructed from the data acquired using crayons. It showed a 2D view of Minkoff's chest including his heart and lungs.[8] Meanwhile, in the UK, Professor Mansfield et al. published two papers on imaging using NMR and a paper on multiplanar image formation.[9-11]

1978 Following on from earlier images of small body parts, Professor Mansfield presented his first image through the abdomen. He also published animal studies showing how NMR could be used in the diagnosis of tumours.

Professor Paul Lauterbur began work on finding a suitable MRI contrast agent in this year using paramagnetic reagents in an animal study.[12]

1979 The Mansfield team continued their studies into the NMR imaging of tumours, specifically carcinoma of the breast.

1980 In the late 1970s and early 1980s many groups took up the challenge to produce a commercially viable MRI system. This needed to be large enough to scan a human but also to have sufficiently good field homogeneity to produce diagnostic images. These pioneers included the group from the Hammersmith Hospital (Professor R. Steiner and Professor G. Bydder) working in conjunction with Picker Ltd at Wembley (Dr I. Young), two independent groups in Nottingham (Professor P. Mansfield and Dr W. Moore), and in Aberdeen (Professor J. Mallard and Dr J. Hutchinson).

1981 Peter Mansfield and his team introduced the concept of real-time moving images by NMR and presented a paper critically evaluating NMR imaging techniques.[13]

Philips Medical Systems produced their first scanner.

Schering applied for a patent for an MRI contrast agent, gadolinium diethylenetriamine penta-acetic acid (DTPA).

1983 The first commercial MR scanner in Europe (from Picker Ltd) was installed at the Department of Diagnostic Radiology at the University of Manchester Medical School (Professor I. Isherwood and Professor B. Pullen).

1984 MRI contrast agent gadolinium DTPA (Magnevist, Schering) was tested on humans.

1985–1990 In the latter half of the 1980s NMR applications and refinements really began to evolve rapidly and included dynamic imaging, cardiac applications, more efficient shimming methods, echoplanar imaging, active magnetic shielding and surface coil improvements.

Gadolinium DTPA was licensed for use in brain and spine imaging. Approval for use in other body areas followed.

1990–present Since the advent of commercial scanning, MRI equipment has been constantly modified and improved. These improvements have not just been in the physical construction but also in the design of the software used to produce the pulse sequences used in scanning.

Instrumentation and pulse sequence design will be discussed more fully in the following sections, but still in the historical context of MRI it is worth mentioning here some of the advances that have been made in the design of MRI scanners over recent years.

In the field of medical imaging the word 'nuclear' has been dropped from the term 'nuclear magnetic resonance imaging'. This is because the word 'nuclear' is associated by many patients with nuclear power, nuclear war and radioactivity in general. This was felt to be unnecessarily off-putting in the context of a scan that did not use ionising radiation.

Although there are variations such as 'open' magnets, and Fonar's Erect system,[14] most modern scanners still have the same basic design featuring a closed-bore superconducting magnet orientated horizontally, allowing the patient to be positioned supine within the field. There have been many modifications and improvements to the original design since the advent of clinical scanning, and some of these are outlined in the next section.

SCIENCE AND INSTRUMENTATION

MRI scanners can be categorised in terms of field strength. The unit used to measure magnetic flux density is the Tesla (T). 1 T equals 10 000 Gauss; note that the Earth's magnetic field varies from 0.2 to 0.7 Gauss.[15] Clinical scanners are generally described as high-, mid- or low-field systems:

- High-field (1.0 T and above)
- Mid-field (0.5 T)
- Low-field (<0.15 to 0.5 T)

The major manufacturers have been making 3T magnets for research purposes since the 1990s, but such magnets are now used fairly commonly in the clinical setting for the benefits that high-field brings.

Modern research scanners are often of considerably higher strength than clinical scanners and can be as much as 11 T in strength. These machines are typically used for applications such as fMRI and spectroscopy. At the time of writing the most powerful research MRI in the world is the 21 T magnet at the National High Magnetic Field Laboratory, Tallahassee, Florida. The scanner has a vertical bore just 10 cm wide, which is just large enough to perform studies on rats and mice.

MRI scanner design falls into two main categories: closed-bore and so-called open systems.

Open magnet systems

Open systems are configured with a vertical magnetic field. The patient is positioned between the poles of the magnet, usually in a supine position, although some systems allow the patient to sit or stand. Open systems do not completely encircle the patient and therefore allow better access for biopsy etc. They are more patient friendly in terms of claustrophobia, and allow nervous patients or children to stay close to their parent or carer throughout the entire procedure. Their other major advantage is in permitting access for very obese patients, who simply would not fit in a closed-bore scanner. The main trade-off is that open systems tend to have slightly poorer geometric accuracy than closed-bore systems.

Open systems can use permanent magnets, resistive electromagnets and superconducting electromagnets in their design.

Permanent magnets

Permanent magnet systems generally have two opposing magnetic plates constructed from a highly magnetic alloy of metals such as iron and nickel. The patient lies on a couch inside the imaging volume between these plates.

From a cost point of view, these scanners are relatively cheap to run and maintain as they do not require expensive cryogen fills.

The disadvantages of permanent magnet design include the fact that it is difficult to achieve field strengths above 0.7 T, and that permanent magnets are very heavy. Weighing up to 15 tons, they may be difficult to site, requiring deep structural foundations for the magnet room.

Resistive magnets

These machines use an electromagnet to generate a magnetic field. An electromagnet is typically constructed from a coil of wire through which current is passed. Resistive systems are usually of the open configuration, but lighter and smaller in design than permanent magnet systems. They also have the advantage that they may be switched off when not in use.

Because the coil is not supercooled, there are cost implications in having to supply power when in use. This is offset by the fact that they do not require cryogen refills.

The main disadvantage of these systems is that the field strength is limited by the amount of current that can be applied to the coil without causing overheating due to resistivity in the windings. To achieve a high field, the number of windings would have to be increased exponentially, which would result in a rather oversized and heavy system.

Superconducting magnets

Superconducting systems use electromagnets that are supercooled by cryogens. The wire used in the windings of a superconductive system is made from an alloy of niobium and titanium coated in copper. This material is superconductive, which means that at extremely low temperatures the resistance to electrical current drops to virtually zero. The advantage is that a very high current can be applied to the windings without any associated heating, which allows the production of a very powerful magnetic field. The current will also continue to flow indefinitely while the coils are maintained at a low temperature. To achieve this low temperature, the coils are immersed in liquid helium.

To generate the main magnetic field electrical current is applied to the windings, gradually increasing until the magnet is ramped up to the desired field strength. The supply can then be disconnected and the current will continue to flow through the windings for as long as the low temperature is maintained.

Closed-bore magnet systems

The modern closed-bore scanner design resembles a CT scanner, but with the patient aperture having a depth of 70–100 cm. This is a great improvement over early systems, where the patient was totally enclosed by the bore. The MRI scanner itself consists of a large cylindrical supercooled electromagnet mounted inside a covered cryostat.

The major system components, when viewed in transverse cross-section, form concentric circles, as shown in Figure 36.3.

Working from the outermost structure inwards, the important components are the outer cover, cryostat, active shielding, main magnet, shim system, gradient system, radiofrequency (RF) transmitter/receiver and receive coils. These are discussed in more detail below.

Outer cover

This is a plastic or fibreglass shell protecting the scan components from damage and dust.

Cryostat

The cryostat is essentially a large Dewar flask made of non-ferrous metal. Its main function is to contain the cryogen used to maintain the superconductivity of the magnet. The cryogen of choice in modern MRI systems is liquid helium; with a boiling point of −269 °C it

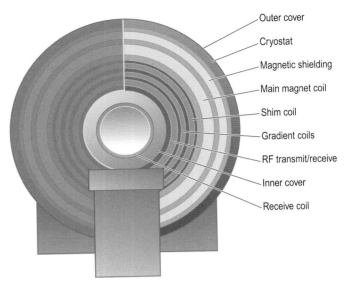

Figure 36.3 The components of a closed-bore MRI scanner in transverse cross-section.

creates the ideal environment for superconductivity. Helium is extracted from natural gas, and is therefore an increasingly rare and finite resource, with only a handful of extraction sites worldwide. At room temperature this expensive material would boil away to nothing in a fairly short time, so the cryostat has some features to reduce helium boil-off. First, the shiny outer wall of the cryostat reflects heat away. Second, there is a vacuum chamber inside the cryostat that prevents heat convection, and finally there is a chiller unit built into the cryostat that keeps the entire metal structure as cool as possible. A combination of these factors coupled with sophisticated helium re-condensing features provides a highly efficient device that never requires topping up.

The cryostat is equipped with a chimney-like vent known as the quench pipe to allow the expulsion of helium gas in the event of a quench. The term *quench* refers to the suppression or stifling of the main magnetic field when the cryogen liquid boils off rapidly to gas – perhaps due to contaminants such as ice particles being inadvertently drawn into the cryostat. One litre of liquid helium produces approximately 750 L of gas,[16] and a full cryostat can liberate around 1 000 000 L of gas in a fairly short explosive burst. This gas must be safely vented away from the patient and other personnel because, although non-toxic, it can quickly displace oxygen in the magnet room and other areas. There has been at least one reported case where suffocation has occurred as a result of cryogen leakage. There is usually a button in the magnet room that can be used to quench the system in the event of an emergency. It should be noted from a safety viewpoint that the magnetic field can take several minutes to reduce.

Magnetic shielding

Early MRI scanners were not shielded and the main magnetic field was therefore not confined to the magnet room itself. The fringe field, as it is known, could even extend beyond the boundaries of the building. This was a safety concern, because certain implanted medical devices, particularly cardiac pacemakers, are adversely affected by a strong magnetic field. To maintain the magnetic field within a reasonable area (or footprint) magnetic shielding was originally achieved by bolting large metal plates around the body of the scanner or within the walls of the magnet room. Modern machines feature an active shielding system that uses electromagnetic coils positioned around each end of the main magnet and producing an equal but opposite effect. This provides for a much smaller and (for the patient) less intimidating equipment design. Both shielding methods are still in use today, passive shielding being required for very high field systems of 7 T or above.

Magnet

Inside the cryostat is the main electromagnet. Superconductive wire is wound around a reel-shaped structure known as the bobbin. At each end of this assembly are the windings that generate the main magnetic field. These are formed by continuous strips of niobium–titanium alloy wire, many kilometers in length. The wire is wound onto the reel evenly and carefully under the control of a technician. This main magnetic field is known as B_0 and is of very high flux density and good homogeneity.

There is an exponential relationship between the number of windings used and the field strength. Keeping all other factors the same, it requires 4× the windings to double the field strength.

At each end of the bobbin, encircling the main coils, there are separate windings that form the active shielding system designed to reduce the size of the fringe field.

Shim system

Moving further towards the centre of the scanner, the next layer consists of the shim system.

As stated previously, MRI demands a homogeneous magnetic field. Homogeneity can be described in terms of parts per million (ppm). Perfect homogeneity is impossible to achieve and the raw magnetic field of the main MRI magnet is homogeneous to approximately 1000 ppm. This can be further improved by a process known as shimming. Shimming is achieved in two ways, known as active and passive.

Passive shimming is performed by placing metal discs (or shims) at strategic positions inside the scanner assembly. This is facilitated by the use of shim trays, non-ferrous metal trays encircling the magnet bore. Each tray can be slid out in turn and has a series of holders along its length designed to house the small ferromagnetic shims. The placement of the shims is calculated by software after scanning a phantom or test object, and is usually only performed once, when the system is first set up for use.

Active shimming uses the *shim coil*, a resistive electromagnet that can be activated every time a pulse sequence is performed, and can therefore correct for any field inhomogeneity caused by the introduction of differently sized patients into the magnet bore.

After shimming the homogeneity of the magnetic field should be better than 10 ppm, which equates to a difference in precessional frequency of <4 Hz over a 22 cm spherical volume. A full explanation of precessional frequency can be found later.

The homogeneous volume of the magnet bore in closed-bore scanners can be described as an imaginary sphere approximately 50 cm diameter, centred at the very midpoint of the bore in all three directions – the point known as the magnetic isocentre.

Gradient system

The main difference between MRI and NMR spectroscopy is the ability to determine the spatial origin of the signal returned by a sample. Spatial encoding is performed by the application of gradients to the main magnetic field. The gradient coils form the next layer in the construction of the MRI scanner and consist of three separate electromagnets orientated inside a cylindrical structure encircling the bore.

Each element of the gradient set can be individually activated by the application of an electrical current sent from the gradient amplifiers. This results in the generation of a secondary field superimposed onto the main magnetic field on either side of the isocentre and producing a linear slope in magnetic field strength from end to end. The orientation of the elements in the gradient coil allows the gradient to be applied in any plane.

In convention with the modern three-dimensional cartesian coordinate system, the three orthogonal planes are given the labels X, Y and Z. There are differences between manufacturers in the way gradient directions are interpreted, but for a majority of closed-bore scanners, with a patient lying in the magnet in the head-first supine position, the X, Y and Z directions are as follows:

- X direction: left to right (horizontal)
- Y direction: posterior to anterior (vertical)
- Z direction: inferior to superior (end-to-end)

Open systems have a vertical magnetic field, and therefore the Z direction is anterior to posterior and the Y direction inferior to superior. Activating the gradient coils in isolation allows the selection of sagittal, coronal and axial slices. Activation of the different gradient elements in tandem can produce imaging planes with any degree of obliquity, i.e. parasagittal, paracoronal or para-axial. These imaging planes are achieved without having to reposition the patient.

When purchasing a scanner, it is worth investigating the various specifications of gradient system offered by the manufacturer. The speed and power of gradients vary, and there is usually a cost implication when purchasing high-speed power gradients because they require better gradient amplification and sometimes require water cooling owing to resistivity effects. This cost is often justified because the increased scan speed will allow higher throughput and increased temporal resolution for dynamic studies. Increased gradient strength will allow better spatial resolution, thinner slices and a smaller minimum field of view. For applications such as fMRI, spectroscopy, perfusion and diffusion imaging, power gradients are strongly recommended.

Gradient strength is usually measured in milliTesla (mT) per metre, i.e. how much the magnetic field strength in mT changes over distance in metres. At the time of writing, power gradients for clinical use deliver around 80 mT/m. The limiting factor for gradient strength in clinical applications is the point at which physical side effects occur. Volunteers undergoing research scans at high gradient power/speed have reported unpleasant temporary side effects, such as flashing visual disturbances known as magnetophosphenes and peripheral nerve stimulation causing tingling sensations in the extremities. These effects are caused by the induction of electrical voltage in nerve fibres and stop when the gradients are switched off.

Another important point to mention about gradient systems is that they are responsible for the noises made during scanning. MRI scans can be very loud, reaching over 100 decibels for some pulse sequences.[17] The reason for this noise is that the gradient coils carry current and are situated in the main magnetic field. Faraday's Law of Electromagnetic Induction states that a conductor lying in a magnetic field will move if unrestricted. The MRI gradient system is subject to a current of rapidly changing polarity and will therefore vibrate vigorously against its mountings. The higher the power and speed of the gradient set, the louder and more unpleasant the noise becomes. This acoustic noise problem has been tackled by the use of ear defenders, music systems and special noise-cancelling headphones.

Radiofrequency (RF) transmitter/receiver

The innermost component consists of an RF transceiver, another electromagnetic coil whose task is to transmit and receive RF pulses. This device is colloquially known as the 'body coil'. The primary purpose of this transmitter is to produce a secondary electromagnetic field (known as B_1) at 90° to the main magnetic field. This is achieved by the use of an RF synthesiser which applies an alternating electric current to the coil at various amplitudes and frequencies. The frequency of this alternating current is matched to the precessional frequency of hydrogen nuclei within the patient, allowing a transfer of energy from the secondary field to the oscillating nuclei, a process known as nuclear magnetic resonance. The very latest generation of scanners from a leading manufacturer uses more than one transmitter, allowing a more homogeneous distribution of RF throughout the imaging volume. This is a particularly desirable feature at high field strengths, where dielectric effects in the patient's tissues can spoil image quality due to a shading artifact.[18] An additional benefit is a reduction in scan time.

Receive coils

Having transmitted an electromagnetic pulse into the patient, the system then has the task of receiving a (comparatively microscopic) amount of returning signal; the mechanism behind this is covered in the next section. Although the body coil is capable of receiving RF, it has inherent image quality problems, primarily a poor signal-to-noise ratio (SNR). The coil is situated quite a distance away from the area under investigation, and when imaging a small region of interest such as the knee, the body coil tends to receive a comparatively high level of random electrical noise compared to useful signal. For this reason, manufacturers provide a wide range of purpose-built receiver coils designed to be positioned in close proximity to the area under investigation, and sized to match the field of view required.

The three main types of receive coils are as follows.

Surface coils

These coils are typically circular or elliptical in shape and consist of a wire antenna encased in a padded protective jacket. Generic surface coils are positioned close to the skin surface over the region of interest, such as the temporomandibular joint or wrist.

Surface coils receive less electrical noise than large volume coils such as the body coil, and because of this, and because of their close proximity to the patient, surface coils have a good inherent SNR. Their main disadvantage is the fact that they can only receive signal from a depth equal to the coil diameter $\times 0.75$, so a 12 cm wide coil will only image structures to a depth of 9 cm below the surface of the skin. Signal falls off dramatically with distance from the coil. For uniform signal reception, a volume coil is needed.

Volume coils

Volume coils are designed to encircle the entire region of interest, usually the head, elbow, wrist, knee, ankle or foot. Their design often resembles a cylinder or cage, and the head coil often incorporates a mirror or prism allowing the patient to see an unrestricted view down the magnet bore. Volume coils detect signal uniformly across the region of interest without the signal fall-off associated with surface coils. This is because their size is matched to the region of interest, meaning that they tend not to detect noise originating elsewhere inside the patient. The head coil is capable of transmitting as well as receiving RF, and on some systems the knee coil may also be a transmit coil.

Phased-array coils

A phased array refers to a number of receive coils ganged together. The signal detected by each element of the array is incorporated into one large field of view. Phased-array coils give the best of both worlds in that they offer the coverage of the body coil but with the good SNR of a surface coil. The elements themselves can be selected or deselected depending upon the anatomical coverage sought. For example, a phased-array spine coil might have five distinct elements, only one of which would be switched on for a cervical study. A cervicothoracic study may require three elements to be activated, and a scan for the whole spinal cord may employ all five elements simultaneously. Currently there are phased-array versions of coils used for most anatomical areas.

Modern phased-array coils have multiple elements, typically up to 32 or more, each detecting signal which is routed through its own channel. This makes for a high SNR, as the noise collected by each element is random and tends to average out in the reconstructed image. Such coils can also be used for parallel imaging, whereby each element contributes to a separate area of the image and speeds up scan time accordingly. This method makes use of a technique known as sensitivity encoding. In modern scanners, where gradients are operating at the maximum speed possible, sensitivity encoding is one way that scan time can still be reduced.

Patient transport system

The patient couch has evolved over the years into a fairly sophisticated mechanism that allows accurate positioning of the region of interest using laser positioning devices.

Table movement and positioning are controlled by the scan computer ensuring that the region under examination is always positioned optimally at the homogeneous isocentre of the magnet for every acquisition. With the advent of phased-array coils it is now possible to position the patient for one examination area and then perform imaging of multiple regions without physically disturbing the patient. An example of this is contrast-enhanced magnetic resonance angiography (CEMRA), where a single injection of contrast agent is imaged in stages as it passes in a bolus through the arterial system from the abdomen to the lower extremities. This kind of scan requires fast acquisition times and also very rapid table movement between areas of interest.

When purchasing a scanner it is well worth investigating the option of a detachable patient table. Detachable tables offer the advantage of a non-ferrous (safe) patient trolley that can quickly remove the patient from the scan room in an emergency, such as a magnet quench or in the event of a cardiac arrest. Having a second detachable table can improve patient throughput by allowing the positioning of non-ambulant patients in readiness for their procedure while the previous patient is still being scanned on the other table.

MRI SAFETY

The scope of MRI safety considerations is very wide and there are books and websites devoted to this complicated topic.[19] This section provides a brief overview, not a complete safety strategy, and practitioners working (or intending to work) in the field of MRI should seek further information before entering the MRI environment. Unit guidelines and hospital health and safety procedures should also be consulted.

RF pulses

From a radiation protection viewpoint, MRI can be said to be a very safe modality. The electromagnetic radiation used is non-ionising and therefore does not present the risk of radiation-induced cancers associated with X-ray exposure. RF applications do, however, deploy energy into the body tissues (measured in watts per kilogram (W/kg)) and this causes a heating effect, particularly at high field strengths. Many of the body systems can be adversely affected by overheating, so the scanner requires information about patient weight to ensure that safe levels are not exceeded.[20]

Magnetic fields

The magnetic fields used in MRI can pose a significant safety risk to staff and patients owing to:

- Projectiles attracted to the main magnetic field
- Damage to implanted devices by the main magnetic field
- Torque applied to implanted devices and foreign bodies by the main magnetic field
- Damage to implanted devices due to gradient magnetic fields
- Nerve stimulation due to gradient magnetic fields
- Damage to implanted devices due to RF magnetic fields
- Heating of tissues or implanted devices due to RF magnetic fields

Projectiles

Projectiles have caused a number of deaths and injuries to patients since 1980. Ferromagnetic objects such as wheelchairs, stretcher poles, floor polishers, oxygen cylinders and ancillary equipment have a strong attraction to the main magnetic field and may be dragged from the floor into the magnet bore. Experimentation by one equipment manufacturer has demonstrated that ferromagnetic objects may reach a speed of up to 40 miles per hour and follow a complex trajectory through the scanner causing serious trauma to a patient (and damage to the equipment, costing hundreds of thousands of pounds to repair).[21]

Implanted devices

Implanted devices such as pacemakers may be adversely affected by a strong magnetic field and cease to function properly. There have been a number of deaths caused by patients entering the proximity of an MRI scanner with a pacemaker in situ. Other non-MRI compatible implanted devices such as artificial heart valves, breast implants and stents may experience violent deflection, causing injury.

The application of rapidly fluctuating gradient magnetic fields and RF pulses can induce voltages in conductive elements of a device, causing damage. Electromagnetic induction can occur in any looped conductor. For this reason it is a good idea to keep any cables away from the patient's skin and to ensure that the patient does not lie in a position where the arms and legs are crossed.[20]

Foreign bodies

Items such as shrapnel and other metal fragments may experience a torque or attraction to the main magnetic field. This could lead to haemorrhage or damage to internal organs. Deflection of intraocular foreign bodies can also cause damage to the interior of the eye.[22]

To prevent patients with contraindications from entering the scan environment it is common policy to administer a screening form on attendance. There is currently no British Standard MRI safety screening form, but the British Association of MR Radiographers offer the following advice:

The MR safety questionnaire should be designed to determine if there is any reason that the patient or individual would undergo an adverse reaction if they were to undergo an MRI investigation.[23]

They suggest that the questionnaire should be designed to obtain information concerning:

- Relevant previous surgery
- Prior injury from metallic foreign bodies
- Pregnancy
- Electrically, magnetically or mechanically activated devices

Further consideration should be given to:

- Permanent colouring techniques
- Body piercing
- Previous reaction to contrast agent
- Breastfeeding
- Last menstrual period

A set of example questions is also available from their website.[23]

It is good practice to inform patients of contraindications at the time of their appointment letter. This will prevent inconvenience to the patient and gaps in workflow if an individual cannot be scanned.

For further safety information on the wide ranging topic of MRI safety visit: http://www.mrisafety.com.

THE PHYSICAL PRINCIPLES OF MRI

As already stated, the basic mechanism of MRI is that a radiofrequency is applied to the hydrogen nuclei in the patient's tissues which causes them to change their energy state and net magnetic alignment to an external magnetic field. As the nuclei lose this energy their magnetic moments realign with the field and their transmitted energy can be measured and spatially located. This technique uses a series of electromagnetic pulses and magnetic field gradient applications, collectively known as a pulse sequence. The timing of the pulse sequence components determines image contrast by exploiting the different molecular behaviours of the various body tissues such as collagen, fat, muscle and free water.

Resonance

Resonance can be defined as the transfer of energy from one oscillating body to another. In NMR this refers to the transfer of energy from an electromagnetic wave (radio wave) to the nucleus of an atom. To understand how this process works, the properties of electromagnetic waves and atomic nuclei must first be considered.

Electromagnetic waves

Electromagnetic waves form a broad spectrum comprising different kinds of radiation. They all travel at the speed of light, but have different wavelengths and therefore occur at different frequencies. This means that if the waveforms are plotted on a graph or oscilloscope, some would have more cycles per second than others. Frequency is measured in Hertz: 1 Hz = 1 cycle per second. The electromagnetic spectrum encompasses waves with frequencies from 10^2 Hz (radio waves) through microwaves and visible light to high-energy waves of the frequency 10^{24} Hz (X-rays and gamma rays). High-energy ionising radiation can damage biological tissue, whereas the lower-energy components of the spectrum such as radio waves are comparatively harmless.

Atomic nuclei

In the traditional Bohr model of the atom (proposed by Niels Bohr in 1913)[24] there is an arrangement of subatomic particles called protons, neutrons and electrons. Protons and neutrons (collectively called nucleons) are bound together to form a nucleus, with the electrons existing in discrete orbits around the nucleus like satellites around a planet. Modern science had modified this model slightly to describe the electron 'cloud' – a roughly spherical area surrounding the nucleus where there is a statistical probability of finding electrons.

All of the subatomic particles can be described in terms of mass, electric charge and movement:

- Electrons have negligible mass, are negatively charged, spin on their own axes in either direction and orbit the nucleus
- Protons have measurable mass, are positively charged and spin on their own axis in either direction
- Neutrons also have mass, have no electrical charge and spin on their own axes in either direction

Nuclei can have different numbers of protons and neutrons, and elements are given a mass number referring to the number of nucleons present and an atomic number that reflects the number of protons present.

If a nucleus has an even number of nucleons (such as helium, which has two protons and two neutrons) the nucleus will have a positive electrical charge (due to the protons), but because the nucleons can spin in either direction the clockwise spins will cancel out the anti-clockwise spins. The nucleus will therefore have a net positive charge but no net spin.

If a nucleus has an odd number of nucleons (as in lithium, which has three protons and four neutrons) there will be a net positive charge and a net spin. This is because there will be an unpaired spinning proton in the nucleus. Whenever there is an electrically charged spinning particle, a magnetic field will be generated by that particle. Nuclei having an odd mass number therefore have an induced magnetic field.

The hydrogen nucleus

The nucleus used in clinical MRI imaging (morphological not spectroscopic) is that of the hydrogen atom. Hydrogen is chosen because its nucleus is a solitary proton with spin, charge, and hence a magnetic moment. Hydrogen is by far the most common element in the universe, accounting for 90% of everything that is known to exist,[25] and forms approximately 60% of the human body.

Quantum theory states that different atomic nuclei exist in one of several possible energy states. The number of possible energy states of an individual nucleus varies depending upon the element in question. The single hydrogen proton can only spin in one of two possible directions; its magnetic field can therefore only be generated in one of two possible orientations, and it exists in one of two energy states.

Normally the orientation of these tiny magnetic vectors is distributed randomly, but when subjected to an external magnetic field such as that found inside an MRI scanner the magnetic vectors of the nuclei will line up with B_0. Approximately half of the nuclei will align with their magnetic vector pointing in the same direction as the main magnetic field (called spin-up) and the other half will align with their magnetic vectors in the opposite direction (spin-down). The nuclei can absorb energy from, and emit energy to, the main magnetic field and therefore flip between the two energy states constantly. However, as it requires less energy to align *with* the external field rather than *against* it, the ratio between spin-up and spin-down nuclei will change, and after a few seconds there will be slightly more spins in the low-energy/spin-up orientation than in the high-energy/spin-down orientation (Figs 36.4, 36.5).

The net magnetic vector (NMV)

In MRI it is the behaviour of the combined magnetism of all the hydrogen nuclei within a sample of tissue that is important. This bulk

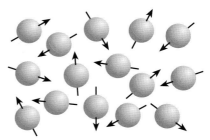

Figure 36.4 Magnetic vectors of hydrogen nuclei in random alignment.

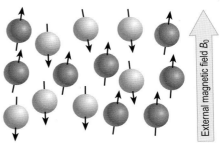

Figure 36.5 Magnetic vectors of hydrogen nuclei in an external magnetic field.

magnetic vector is also known as the net magnetic vector (NMV). As more of the hydrogen nuclei shift their magnetic vector into the parallel orientation, the NMV becomes aligned with B_0. This is because, at the outset, the populations of spin-up and spin-down nuclei are equal and their magnetic fields cancel out. Over time, more spins attain the spin-up orientation and the NMV becomes aligned accordingly. The resulting magnetisation is said to be 'longitudinal' or in the +Z direction. The time taken for the NMV to make this shift is known as T1[26] and is an important factor in image contrast (to be absolutely precise, T1 is defined as the time taken for 63% of the longitudinal magnetisation to orientate into the +Z direction).

The actual ratio between spin-up and spin-down nuclei is very small: in approximately every million spins there are only three extra spin-up nuclei. This does not sound like many, but when you remember that there are some 7 000 000 000 000 000 000 000 000 000 atoms in the human body, this still equates to billions of extra spin-up nuclei in a tissue sample, and it is these nuclei that provide the signal and contrast on an MRI scan. For the rest of this chapter, these important surplus nuclei will simply be referred to as the 'spins'.

One final important point to note is that the surfeit of spin-up nuclei increases with field strength. This is because more energy is required to oppose a strong field than a weak field, and the spin-up and spin-down populations will reflect this. High-field scanners therefore have an inherently better SNR than low-field systems.

Precession

When describing motion in the atom earlier, the terms *spinning* and *orbiting* were mentioned. There is also another important kind of motion involved in NMR, known as precession. When the nuclei are subjected to an external magnetic field they not only spin on their axes but they also wobble slightly. This is often described as being analogous to a spinning top. Consider a gyroscope spinning on a table-top: it will spin at hundreds of revolutions per minute but will also be seen to wobble at a much slower rate. Imagine a line drawn through the vertical axis of the gyroscope: as the gyroscope wobbles this imaginary line will prescribe a cone shape. This movement is known as precession and is due to gravity. The *speed* at which the gyroscope wobbles is also related to gravity: on the moon, with less gravity, the gyroscope would precess more slowly (fewer wobbles per minute) than on the Earth.

The spinning hydrogen nuclei also precess, not because of gravity but owing to the presence of the external magnetic field. If the field strength is increased, the nuclei will precess at a faster rate; if the external field is reduced they will precess more slowly.

Phase and frequency

The precessional speed and orientation of a spinning nucleus can be described in terms of frequency and phase.

The frequency of precession (i.e. how many wobbles per minute) can be calculated by an equation first published by mathematician Joseph Larmor (1857–1942), and it is the only equation used in this chapter.

The Larmor equation states that

$$\omega = \gamma B_0$$

where ω is the angular precessional frequency of the proton
γ is the gyromagnetic ratio of the nucleus
B_0 is the external field strength.

Every nucleus has its own fixed gyromagnetic ratio expressed in Hertz/Tesla. For hydrogen this is 42.6 MHz/T, so at a field strength of 1 T the hydrogen nuclei will be precessing at a frequency of 42.6 MHz (at 1.5 T it will be 63.9 MHz and so on).

Knowledge of the precessional frequency for hydrogen at a particular field strength is important because in order to resonate the nuclei it is necessary to apply an electromagnetic wave at a matching frequency, and this will differ depending upon the field strength of the scanner being used.

Phase is a term that can be used to describe the angular orientation of the magnetic vector of a nucleus compared to other nuclei nearby. The gyroscope analogy can be expanded to explain phase. It was stated earlier that the vertical axis of a precessing gyroscope (or nucleus) prescribes a cone shape. If the gyroscope is viewed from above, the top of the gyroscope can be seen to move in a circular path as it wobbles about its axis. That is to say, its orientation goes from a 12 o'clock position round to 3 o'clock, 6 o'clock, 9 o'clock and finally ends up back at 12 o'clock. If a number of gyroscopes were set spinning at the same time, it is unlikely that they would all precess in synchrony. Even though they might be spinning at the same speed (frequency), one gyroscope might be at the 12 o'clock position while its neighbour is at 6 o'clock. This is analogous to the spins being out of phase with each other.

At equilibrium the nuclei are all precessing at the same frequency because they are all in the same magnetic field strength, but they are out of synchrony when it comes to the orientation of their vectors. The orientation of a single vector around its cone-shaped path is known as its phase position, and at equilibrium the spins can be said to be out of phase. (Figs 36.6, 36.7).

Signal

To construct an image it is necessary to receive signal from the region of interest and spatially encode it. MRI signal is in the form of a weak electromagnetic wave created by the oscillating net magnetic vector of the spins following excitation by an RF pulse.

Faraday's law of electromagnetic induction states that:

> ***The induced electromotive force or EMF in any closed circuit is equal to the time rate of change of the magnetic flux through the circuit.***[27]

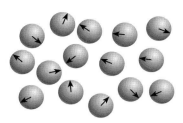

Figure 36.6 The magnetic vectors of hydrogen nuclei, out of phase. (These spins are depicted as being viewed from 'above', i.e. we are looking from a direction parallel to the main magnetic field.) Dephased magnetic vectors cancel out, resulting in a loss of signal.

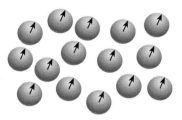

Figure 36.7 The magnetic vectors of hydrogen nuclei, in phase. The combined magnetic effect of all these spins is known as the net magnetic vector (NMV).

In the case of the MRI signal, the NMV is a moving magnetic field that will induce a voltage in an antenna (or conductive loop) placed in proximity to the region of interest. The maximum signal is generated when the NMV is 90° to B_0 and the contributing individual vectors are in phase.

At equilibrium the NMV is aligned in the same direction as B_0 and the spins are out of phase. There is no coherent transverse magnetisation to be detected by the receiver coil. To generate signal an RF pulse at the Larmor frequency transfers energy to the nuclei in the sample. This process of resonance has two important effects:

1. First, the surfeit of nuclei in the low-energy spin-up direction will absorb energy and become high-energy spin-down nuclei. If the right amount of RF is used the populations of spin-up and spin-down nuclei will become equal. (The scanner determines the critical amount of RF required to do this during the prescan.) The effect of having equal populations of spin-up and spin-down nuclei is that the NMV will change orientation. Instead of being aligned with the main magnetic field, the NMV will rotate (or more accurately nutate) to precess at 90° to B_0. In this orientation it can be detected using a suitable antenna (receive coil). This magnetisation is said to be in the transverse plane, i.e. the RF pulse has converted longitudinal magnetisation into transverse magnetisation. Because it has changed the angle of the NMV by 90° the pulse used is known as a 90° RF pulse (Fig. 36.8).

2. The second effect of the RF pulse is that it forces the magnetic vectors of the spins to process in phase. This is important, as the signal from out-of-phase spins cancels out and cannot be detected by the receive coil. In-phase spins result in an NMV that precesses at the Larmor frequency at 90° to B_0 and produces maximum signal in the receive coil.

The spins do not stay in phase for very long, for two reasons. The main cause of dephasing is field inhomogeneity. Even with a field homogeneous to 4 ppm there will be a fluctuation in field strength across the imaging volume. The secondary cause of dephasing is the fact that the nuclei themselves have magnetic fields, and these fields

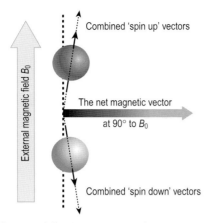

Figure 36.8 The NMV following a 90° RF pulse.

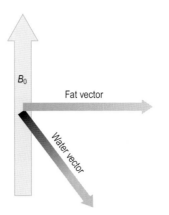

Figure 36.9 Fat and water vectors during rapid TR. Fat vector is repeatedly flipped to 90° but water is flipped to beyond 90° and the signal becomes saturated.

interact over time, attracting and repelling each other, a process known as spin–spin interaction. The important point to note here is that dephasing due to inhomogeneity is undesirable, as it causes signal loss indiscriminately, whereas spin–spin interactions are desirable because they provide a powerful contrast mechanism. Fortunately, the dephasing caused by inhomogeneity can be reversed by the use of a 180° RF pulse. The signal that would otherwise be lost reappears briefly as the spins come back into phase; this is known as a spin echo.

The time taken for the spins to lose (63% of) their phase coherence due to spin–spin interactions is known as T2, and it is this that can be exploited as a contrast mechanism.

Contrast

So far it has been stated that signal from hydrogen nuclei can be generated in a tissue sample and detected by a receive coil. In order to make a diagnostic image, however, it is necessary to create contrast between different structures/tissues/pathologies.

There are various factors affecting contrast on an MRI image, but the three most important are:

- T1 recovery
- T2 decay
- Proton density (PD)

T1

It was mentioned earlier that when a 90° RF pulse is applied to the sample, any longitudinal magnetisation is converted into transverse magnetisation. It is also true to say that any (residual) transverse magnetisation will be tipped into the longitudinal plane. The reason that this factor can be used to produce contrast on the image is that different tissues have different rates of T1 recovery.

As an example, there is a marked difference between the recovery rates of fat and pure water. Following a 90° RF pulse, fat recovers its longitudinal magnetisation quickly. This is because it has large molecules with relatively slow brownian motion that can dissipate energy fairly readily. This means that, in fat, the spin population loses the absorbed energy quickly and the fat vector regains its low-energy spin-up orientation.

Pure water, on the other hand, has high-energy molecules with rapid brownian motion that cannot dissipate energy readily. Pure water nuclei therefore retain the absorbed energy and the magnetic vector associated with pure water remains in the transverse plane for longer than that of fat.

If a second 90° RF pulse is rapidly applied to the sample, the fully recovered NMV from fat will once again be flipped into the transverse plane, giving maximum signal, but the partially recovered water vector will be flipped back into the longitudinal plane in the −Z direction. With little transverse magnetisation to be detected by the coil, water will subsequently return only a limited signal (Fig. 36.9).

If more time was allowed between RF pulses, fat and water vectors would each have time to recover their longitudinal magnetisation and would both be flipped 90° by successive RF pulses, reducing T1 contrast.

The time between RF applications is known as the TR (time to repetition); a T1-weighted image uses a short TR (e.g. 300 ms) and will exhibit bright fat and dark fluid.

A T1-weighted sequence tends to demonstrate morphology clearly because it has a short echo time that yields high SNR and is therefore suited to displaying anatomical detail.

T1 weighting is the contrast of choice when using gadolinium enhancement, as gadolinium is a T1-shortening agent. Such scans are usually performed before and after administration of contrast agent to ensure that any hyperintensity on the image is due to enhancement rather than being an inherently T1-bright structure, such as fat or haemorrhage.

The fact that fat is bright on T1 weighting makes this sequence sensitive to changes in bone marrow, including metastasis and avascular necrosis. If the fat content of bone marrow is replaced, the signal level will fall and the affected area will appear relatively hypointense on T1 weighting.

T2

Following the removal of the 90° RF pulse, the spins dephase rapidly.

The reason that T2 dephasing provides an image contrast mechanism is that different tissues lose phase coherence at different rates. The most marked difference here is between solids and pure water molecules. Following the removal of the 90° RF pulse, the magnetic vectors of slow-tumbling tightly packed nuclei in solid structures such as collagen have a marked effect upon each other and dephase readily and quickly. In water molecules the comparatively rapid tumbling rate ensures that molecules are affected by the north and south poles of neighbouring dipoles in equal measure. This averaging-out causes their magnetic vectors to stay in phase for longer.

Contrast is therefore obtained by waiting for a certain time after the application of the 90° RF pulse before sampling the returning signal. Any tissues that have lost phase coherence (e.g. collagen) will appear darker than tissues whose spins are still in phase (e.g. water).

The time between the 90° RF pulse and the collection of the signal is known as the TE (time to echo); a T2-weighted image uses a long TE (e.g. 100 ms or above) and will exhibit plenty of signal from water, but very reduced signal from solids.

Proton density (PD)

The term proton density (PD) refers to the number of hydrogen nuclei present in a given volume of tissue. To compare extremes, think of air and water. There are more hydrogen nuclei in the fluid-filled ventricles of the brain than in the nearby air-filled paranasal sinuses. A PD weighted image will therefore have varying degrees of signal from different tissues. A PD image is obtained by using parameters that reduce T1 and T2 contrast, i.e. a long TR to reduce T1 effects and a short TE to reduce T2 effects. When the effects of these contrast mechanisms are diminished, an image remains where the signal intensity of the various anatomical structures is determined principally by the concentration of hydrogen within those tissues. PD images can be said to be the most anatomically accurate, in some cases looking very much like monochrome postmortem photographs.

Weighting

When describing the contrast of an MRI image the term 'weighting' is used to indicate that the contrast is weighted or heavily influenced by one of the above parameters. Image contrast never results purely from one of these parameters alone, as all images are affected to some degree by T1, T2 and PD. For example, the air-filled sinuses may appear as hypointense as a melanoma metastasis on a T2-weighted scan, but the lack of signal from the sinuses has nothing to do with T2 contrast and everything to do with PD.

Spatial encoding

Having generated signal and determined the contrast required, the final stage of the procedure is to spatially encode the signal so that it can be reconstructed into a diagnostic image. Spatial encoding using gradient magnetic fields was first proposed by Lauterbur in 1973[5] and a variation of his technique is still used in scanning today. The principle is that spins across the imaging volume can be assigned a particular spatial location depending on their frequency of precession or phase position. Spatial encoding for a 2D slice is achieved by the use of three gradients that perform the following functions:

* Determining the slice position
* Encoding the position of the spins in the horizontal axis of the image
* Encoding the position of the spins in the vertical axis of the image

Slice position

Determining the slice position is the first part of spatial encoding. As mentioned in an earlier section, resonance can only occur if the energy source exhibits the resonant frequency of the target. An example of this would be to obtain two tuning-forks both tuned to the same note, place one of them in a stand and strike the second against an object to start it vibrating. If the vibrating fork is held in close proximity to the silent fork the transfer of energy between the two will induce vibration in the silent fork, even though there had been no physical contact. The critical factor is that they must be tuned to exactly the same note (frequency). This experiment would not work if a tuning fork playing the note A was held close to a tuning fork tuned to the note B.

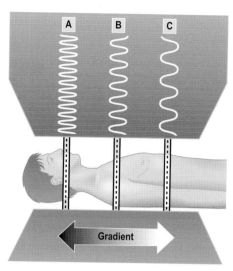

Figure 36.10 Applied RF pulses at different frequencies resonate different slice positions along a magnetic field gradient. Radiofrequency A only resonates spins having the precessional frequency corresponding to the position of the topmost slice. Radiofrequency B is at the centre frequency and only resonates spins at the isocentre. Radiofrequency C only resonates spins having the precessional frequency corresponding to the position of the lowermost slice.

The aim of slice selection is to resonate a thin section of tissue rather than the entire patient: consider a single slice through an abdomen on a patient who is lying supine and head first in the scanner.

The resonant frequency of the hydrogen nuclei can be calculated using the Larmor equation, and similarly if a gradient is applied at a known strength, the precessional frequencies of the spins along the length of the gradient can also be calculated. If a gradient is applied over a certain volume (centred at the magnetic isocentre), the mid-part of the gradient will remain at the centre frequency while spins at the ends of the gradient will exhibit either a slightly lower or a slightly higher frequency. If an RF pulse were applied at the centre frequency it would only resonate the spins at the isocentre. The spins elsewhere along the slope would not be affected, as their induced frequencies would not match the transmitted frequency. If an RF pulsed at a slightly higher frequency it would only resonate spins at a spatial location towards the higher end of the gradient (Fig. 36.10). To achieve an axial slice it is therefore necessary to apply a gradient in the Z direction during transmission of the 90° RF pulse.

In reality it is not quite that simple, because slices must have a finite thickness, so a range of frequencies must be applied to excite a narrow band of spins along the corresponding part of the gradient. This range of frequencies is known as the *transmit bandwidth*.

Phase encoding

Having selected the slice position, it is now necessary to locate the signal returning from within that field of view. First, consider the signal originating from the horizontal axis of the image (left to right on a supine patient). To encode this signal, another magnetic field gradient application is performed. This time the gradient coils are used to apply a slope in the X direction across the magnet bore from left to right. This causes the precession of the spins to speed up or slow down depending on their location. Importantly, the gradient is then turned off. In the absence of the gradient the spins return to the centre frequency, but because of the time spent inside the gradient their *phase* positions will have shifted along this axis. Spins at the isocentre were still at the centre frequency during the gradient application, so their

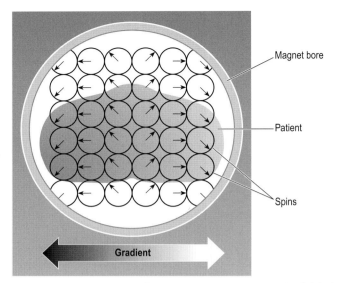

Figure 36.11 The application of a secondary gradient across the field of view changes the precessional frequencies of the spins. When it is turned off, the phase positions of some columns of spins will be advanced or retarded compared to the spins that remained at the centre frequency (isocentre).

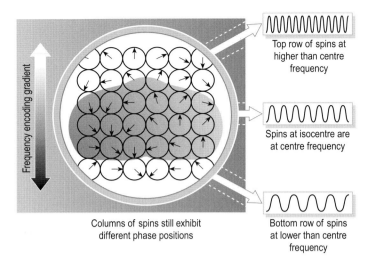

Figure 36.12 Another gradient application at 90° changes the precessional frequency of the spins. Some rows of spins will be precessing more quickly or more slowly than those remaining at the centre frequency (isocentre).

phase position will be unchanged – say at 12 o'clock (or 0°). Spins that were briefly precessing more rapidly than those at isocentre might have an advanced phase position of 5 o'clock (or 150°). Spins that were situated at the lower-than-centre frequency portion of the slope might have a phase position of 7 o'clock (−150°) (Fig. 36.11).

This *phase encoding* gradient is applied many times during the pulse sequence at gradually changing amplitudes, causing a different amount of phase shift across the field of view each time (repetition). The key point to note is that the phase position of the signal from a discrete point along the phase encoding axis will change its phase position incrementally each TR (e.g. TR 01 – 0°, TR 01 – 10°, TR 01 – 20°, TR 01 – 30°, and so forth). Mapped over time this gives the appearance of a frequency, i.e. a waveform having cycles. The spatial resolution in the phase direction is determined by the number of phase encodings performed, typically 128, 256, 512, 1024 or 2048 pixels. A 512 matrix will therefore require 512 RF applications (512 repetitions), and because the TR is of fixed length, a scan having a matrix of 512 will take twice as long to perform as a scan having a matrix of 256.

Frequency encoding

Having applied the previous two gradients, the slice position has been determined and data collected enabling spatial location and resolution along the horizontal axis of the image. The signal originating from the vertical axis of the image is encoded by a third gradient application.

This gradient is applied during the echo, at the same time as the signal is collected. This causes the returning signal to exhibit a range of different precessional frequencies from the spins along the horizontal axis of the region of interest. The gradient is therefore known as either the *frequency encoding* gradient or the *readout* gradient. Once again the spins at isocentre will remain at the centre frequency, but the spins at each end of the gradient will either precess more quickly or more slowly depending on the magnetic field slope. The net effect of this is that the receive coil detects a range of frequencies at time TE (Fig. 36.12).

Having acquired the signal, the system computer uses a mathematical calculation on the collected data known as the Fourier transform (devised by Jean Baptiste Joseph Fourier, 1768–1830) which essentially isolates the individual frequencies and their intensities. Because the applied gradient is linear in nature, each intensity measured will be in a linear arrangement corresponding to its spatial position of origin.

A useful analogy is to imagine playing the note 'middle C' on a piano and asking a concert pianist to name the note. Middle C is the central note on the keyboard, and on hearing the sound they would hopefully be able to identify it as such. They have received a frequency (261.63 Hz) and have assigned it a spatial location (the middle). Middle C can be thought of as the central frequency in MRI, with all of the other white notes representing the range of frequencies along the gradient axis. If a pianist were to play a chord by pressing down on several piano keys at once, the Fourier transform would be able to identify the separate notes (frequencies) – and how hard each key had been pressed (signal intensities).

In terms of spatial encoding, the data collected by the application of the phase and frequency encoding gradients is more or less identical for each, the difference being temporal. All of the frequencies in a single spin echo are collected in 20 ms or less; the data used to reconstruct the equivalent waveforms in the phase direction take the entire duration of the scan to acquire.

Pulse sequences

The succession of RF pulses and gradient applications used in spatial encoding is known as a pulse sequence. Pulse sequences can be divided into two main categories, known as spin echo and gradient echo (GE). The main difference between the two is that spin echo pulse sequences use a 180° RF pulse to rephase the signal that would otherwise be lost due to field inhomogeneity. GE uses a magnetic field gradient to produce an echo but does not correct for field inhomogeneity dephasing. GE is typically faster than spin echo but is prone to artefactual appearances. Figure 36.13 shows the order of events in a typical spin echo and GE pulse sequence.

These basic pulse sequences have been enhanced and developed to include new contrast mechanisms and methods of rapid acquisition; these include inversion recovery sequences, fast spin echo (FSE),

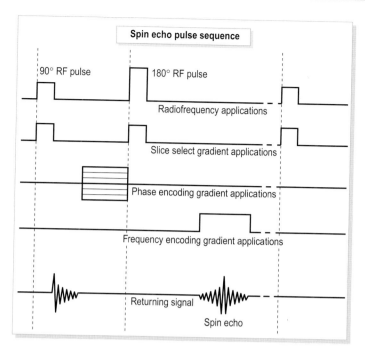

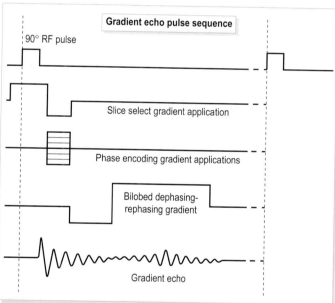

Figure 36.13 Simplified spin echo and gradient echo (GE) pulse sequence diagrams. Note that the GE uses another magnetic field gradient application to produce an echo of signal rather than a 180° RF pulse.

driven equilibrium, single-shot imaging and echo-planar imaging. Further description of MRI pulse sequences can be found in the clinical applications section of this chapter.

Contrast media

Despite the excellent soft tissue capabilities of MRI and its inherently good contrast-to-noise ratio, the development of contrast media for MRI began in tandem with the first scans in 1978. MRI contrast media can be broadly classified into two main categories, positive and negative.

Positive contrast media – T1 agents

Positive contrast agents produce an increase in signal intensity in affected tissues. In MRI the principal positive agents contain gadolinium as their active ingredient. In its native state gadolinium is a silver metal named after a Finnish chemist, Gadolin. Like many other metals, gadolinium is mined for use in industry and its medical application forms only a small percentage of its global use. It is a lanthanide element at number 64 in the periodic table. At room temperature gadolinium is paramagnetic. This is to say that it aligns to and adds to an external magnetic field. Gadolinium is toxic and therefore is attached to a chelate or ligand to produce a contrast agent.

Its mechanism as a contrast agent relies on the fact that it causes T1 shortening at fairly low doses. This ability is due to the presence of seven unpaired electrons that form dipolar bonds with hydrogen nuclei in the tissues (blood). The result of this is that the molecular tumbling rate of water is reduced, allowing a more efficient energy exchange. With a rapid TR, water is able to recover much of its longitudinal magnetisation between RF pulses; this results in more magnetisation available to be flipped into the transverse plane. The outcome is that water combined with gadolinium chelate behaves more like fat, and is therefore hyperintense on a T1-weighted image.

Negative contrast media – T2 agents

Negative contrast agents have now largely fallen from favour, but their action produces a decrease in signal intensity in affected tissues. In MRI the principal negative agents contain iron oxide as their active ingredient. These compounds consist of microcrystalline magnetite cores coated with dextranes or siloxanes. This impervious coating prevents the iron from binding with the body tissues.

The mechanism of a negative contrast agent relies on the fact that it causes T2 shortening at fairly low doses. The signal loss seen in areas of uptake is due to magnetic susceptibility effects. Spins in cells containing the superparamagnetic iron will have a slightly higher precessional frequency than those surrounding them. This results in dephasing at the boundaries of these microscopic areas and a net loss of signal. This is because transverse magnetisation must be coherent (i.e. in phase) to produce maximum signal, and effects that cause dephasing will reduce the signal intensity.

Use of MRI contrast media

Although MRI has the inherent ability to distinguish between types of soft tissue, there are times when the use of contrast media is unavoidable.

Lesion conspicuity

The use of contrast media can greatly increase the conspicuity of certain lesions. This is of particular importance where the presence of lesions would radically alter the treatment plan. As an example, a patient diagnosed with a single cerebral metastasis might be considered a candidate for surgery. If, by increasing conspicuity, gadolinium enhancement demonstrated the presence of multiple smaller lesions, it is unlikely that surgery would be considered.[28]

Lesion characterisation

Certain lesions are difficult to characterise using the inherent contrast parameters of MRI. For example, a neurofibroma returns a high signal on T2 weighting and a low to intermediate signal on T1. Other lesions, such as proteinaceous cysts, would also have similar contrast characteristics. Cystic lesions, however, do not tend to enhance, whereas a neurofibroma does.

Lesion extent

On unenhanced T1-weighted images the boundaries of some lesions are not clearly defined. T2 weighting demonstrates pathology very well, but there is often a lot of associated oedema affecting the surrounding tissues that can distort the appearance of a lesion. The true size, shape and position of a lesion are usually better appreciated on a T1-weighted contrast-enhanced image.

Contrast-enhanced MRA (CEMRA)

Blood vessels can be imaged by MRI using flow-dependent techniques that do not require the use of an exogenous contrast agent. Such studies produce contrast that relies on the flow of spins relative to their surroundings. These techniques suffer from certain shortcomings, such as artefactual exaggeration of stenoses, the ability to only image flow in a particular direction, and small fields of view.

The use of gadolinium has reduced most of these problems. CEMRA allows a larger field of view, gives a more anatomical picture of the anatomy, more accurately reproduces the size of stenoses and shortens acquisition time to a matter of seconds.

Other considerations when deciding whether to use contrast include:

- *Throughput:* on low field systems having longer acquisition times or only having conventional spin echo (CSE) rather than FSE, it may be quicker to make a diagnosis using contrast where the alternative would be to perform a number of more time-consuming sequences to make the same diagnosis. An example might be acoustic neuroma, T1 pre and post gadolinium (10 minutes) vs a high-resolution T2-weighted scan (20 minutes)
- *Dynamic studies:* in some body areas such as the liver and breast, where different kinds of lesion may exhibit different rates of contrast uptake, a diagnosis is more readily made by dynamic scanning. This uses a series of short sequences performed after injection of gadolinium chelate and studies the uptake curve and appearance of lesions in the arterial, venous and delayed stages post injection. This can give more information than a simple pre- and post-contrast scan

COMMON CLINICAL APPLICATIONS

MRI is now used in imaging virtually every anatomical region, and the full range of clinical applications of MRI is therefore well beyond the scope of this chapter. The following section will cover only the most commonly requested examinations, and it is intended that the protocols suggested will act as a basic guide. MRI protocols vary widely and must take into account the preferences of the reporting radiologist, the time available, the compliance of the patient, and the field strength and capabilities of the scanner hardware/software. Please do not alter your scan protocols without consulting other users or backing up the originals! The recommended pulse sequences are generic and are commonly found on equipment from all manufacturers.

Pulse sequences

The pulse sequences referred to in the protocols in the next section of this chapter are described in more detail here.

Spin echo and fast (turbo) spin echo sequences

Conventional spin echo (CSE) sequences use a 180° RF pulse to help eliminate undesirable dephasing due to field inhomogeneity. The result is a sequence that offers high-quality images which are relatively artefact free. The main trade-off is that the scan time can be relatively long compared to FSE or GE techniques. Attempts to reduce scan time, for example by reducing the phase matrix, the TR and the number of signal averages, always result in a deterioration of image quality in terms of resolution, weighting and SNR, respectively.

It is possible to use more than one 180° pulse in a spin echo sequence and therefore collect multiple echoes each having different TE values during the same acquisition. Multiple echo sequences result in more than one set of images, each set of slices having identical anatomical locations but different contrast characteristics. A common example is a dual echo sequence providing one set of T2-weighted images and a second set of PD-weighted images.

Dual (multiple) echo can also be used in a technique known as T2 relaxometry, where there are a number of echoes at different TE values, allowing regions of interest to be drawn and T2 relaxation curves produced for various tissues.

For T1 weighting CSE is a perfectly acceptable sequence choice because T1 contrast relies on a short repetition time, which inherently shortens scan time.

T1-weighted FSE sequences are also available but have some associated trade-offs in terms of weighting and maximum available slice number without offering a significant time saving over CSE T1-weighted images.

FSE sequences, introduced in 1990, shorten scan time by collecting more data per repetition. This is facilitated by the use of numerous 180° RF pulses within each TR period which, in turn, yield a whole train of echoes rather than just one echo per repetition. The echo train length is a user-definable parameter and shortens the scan time proportionally, so an echo train of 8 would reduce an 8 minute scan to a 1 minute scan. The longest echo train at the time of writing is 728, allowing the acquisition of an entire high-resolution image in a single shot.

FSE is usually the sequence of choice for T2-weighted studies because scan factors would make a CSE T2-weighted sequence impracticably slow (the TR must be long to reduce T1 effects). As an example, CSE T2-weighted sequences can take up to 30 minutes to acquire, compared to just a couple of minutes (or less) for FSE.

The trade-offs with FSE include a higher RF deposition to the patient (heating) and a slight change in weighting (brighter fat on T2 compared to CSE). If it is thought that hyperintense fat might reduce the conspicuity of fluid-filled lesions, it is possible to select a fat saturation pulse as an additional imaging option. This technique applies an additional RF pulse to the region of interest, the frequency of which is finely tuned to match only the resonant frequency of fat nuclei. Because fat receives more RF than the other tissues the signal is saturated, essentially removed from the resulting images.

Single shot (SSFSE)

Single-shot techniques have greatly speeded up acquisition times in MRI. These sequences take FSE to the extreme, in that they apply numerous 180° pulses allowing collection of all of the signal for a slice within a single TR. This allows imaging while the patient is free-breathing. The snapshot effect of the scan typically freezes motion in areas of the body where movement can otherwise cause artefactual problems. Uses therefore include abdominal imaging and imaging on non-compliant children. Note that the images are taken one slice at a time, and although motion is frozen on each slice, the anatomy may appear at very different positions on each slice if the patient has moved significantly between each slice acquisition. For the same reason, an abdominal data set may not be perfectly contiguous if the patient is asked to hold their breath for each slice.

Inversion recovery

The term 'inversion recovery' refers to the fact that an additional RF pulse is applied at the beginning of the pulse sequence that tips the NMV by 180° into the −Z direction. Following the application of a 180° pulse, the magnetic vectors of the tissues recover their longitudinal magnetisation to a degree before the application of a 90° RF pulse. The time interval between the 180° and the 90° pulses provides a powerful contrast parameter, known as the tau or 'time from inversion'. Different tissues recover their longitudinal magnetisation at different rates and by changing the timing of the 90° RF pulse, the image contrast can be altered dramatically. Signal can even be nulled (eliminated) from selected tissues if required. The mechanism depends entirely upon the manipulation of the longitudinal and transverse components of magnetisation in various tissues, each having their own rate of recovery. The timing of the 90° pulse is chosen to occur at a time when signal from the desired tissue has recovered to be exactly at 90° to the main magnetic field and is therefore flipped back into complete inversion (90° + 90° = 180°).

Inversion recovery sequences can be very valuable when imaging at very low or very high field strengths. T1-weighted spin echo sequences suffer from poor contrast at these extremes, but inversion recovery provides a method of achieving images having bright fat and dark fluid.

Like spin-echo, inversion recovery sequences can also be speeded up with the addition of an echo train.

STIR (short tau inversion recovery)

In STIR the timing of the 90° RF pulse is set to eliminate any signal from fat. Because the mechanism of STIR relies on longitudinal magnetisation changes rather than precessional frequency, STIR is a robust method of fat suppression that is effective even in the presence of poor field homogeneity. Field inhomogeneity causes a drift in precessional frequency across the imaging volume, and this is a factor that can often spoil spectral fat saturation methods. STIR sequences are very sensitive to pathology and are starting to be used in whole body MRI screening protocols. STIR is also sensitive to bone marrow changes and trabecular microfracture (bone bruising).

FLAIR (fluid-attenuated inversion recovery)

FLAIR is a commonly used inversion recovery technique whereby the timing is chosen to remove any signal from fluid such as CSF. Proteinaceous fluid such as that found in pathology will still appear bright, making this an ideal technique for assessing periventricular disease in the brain or increasing the conspicuity of the cranial nerves.

Gradient echo (GE)

GE sequences were developed primarily to reduce acquisition times. A gradient application is used to dephase and rephase the spins, rather than a 180° RF pulse. Contrast is achieved by the use of variable flip angles (i.e. not just 90°) combined with the TR, the TE, and whether or not residual transverse magnetisation is allowed to contribute to image contrast. Shortened TR and TE makes for a faster sequence, but with some trade-offs.

GE sequences are more affected by susceptibility artefact than spin echo, a fact that is exploited in the diagnosis of haemorrhage. The iron content of haemoglobin causes susceptibility artefact and is therefore more readily demonstrated on GE sequences than with on spin echo. Susceptibility artefact can be a problem, however, when there is metal close to the region of interest, such as dental fixings. In these areas spin echo or FSE may be required to reduce the artefact.

T2*-weighted GE is also sensitive to flow, causing flowing spins to appear hyperintense on the images (NB: * indicates that field inhomogeneity effects have contributed to the dephasing time of the spins: in GE this is because there has been no 180° pulse used). This feature, coupled with a short minimum TE and TR, is exploited in flow-dependent MRA sequences. The use of flow compensation makes GE the sequence of choice where flow may cause image degradation. This includes the spine (CSF flow) and the joints (blood flow in the region of interest).

Another feature of GE is the ability to use echo times that exploit the precessional frequency difference of fat and water. At 1.5 T the magnetic vectors of fat nuclei precess 220 Hz more slowly than those of water. This means that they will drift in and out of phase with each other over time. Fat and water nuclei will be in phase approximately every 4.2 ms at 1.5 T. If the TE is set at a multiple of this factor, signal will be generated from voxels containing fat and water components. If a TE is chosen when fat and water vectors are out of phase there will be a corresponding loss of signal. This is useful in characterising disease where there is a change in the fat to water ratio (such as fatty infiltration of the liver), or lesions where there is a known fat/water content (such as adenoma).

3D volume scans

Volume imaging typically uses GE sequences with an additional phase encoding gradient applied in the slice selection plane. This allows the acquisition of very thin contiguous sections. 2D techniques require a gap between slices of 10–20% of the slice thickness to avoid an artefact known as cross-excitation. Volume imaging does not require a slice gap and is therefore recommended in 3D reconstruction and volume measurement techniques, where a gap between slices would cause distortion and inaccuracy. Because the slice (partition) thickness can be reduced in comparison to a 2D scan it is possible to achieve isotropic voxels (having the same dimensions of width, depth and height). This is also useful in image reconstruction, as the resolution will be the same in every plane (including the slice select direction). This is also one of the reasons why 3D sequences are used in flow-dependent MRA.

Inflow angiography (also called time-of-flight)

Inflow angiography is a flow-dependent method of imaging the vasculature. It relies on the use of GE sequences having a rapid TR causing saturation of signal from tissues within the imaging volume but allowing spins entering the imaging volume to emit signal briefly before becoming saturated themselves. This is known as the *entry slice phenomenon*. The term *time-of-flight* (TOF) is not a particularly apt name for this technique, as TOF can also cause flow to *lack* signal if the flowing nuclei are moving at high speed.

This *high-velocity signal loss* – whereby spins inside an imaging volume flow out of the slice before rephasing occurs – is kept to a minimum by the use of a short echo time. The base data therefore demonstrate bright flow against a saturated noisy background. The images are created using a post-processing technique called maximum intensity projection (MIP). This process reconstructs the data from different apparent points of view and constructs an anatomical-looking representation of the vasculature. The reconstructed images can over-exaggerate the size of stenoses and underestimate the true lumen size of vessels, and in reporting inflow MRA procedures it is recommended that the base data are also taken into consideration.

Another shortcoming of this sequence is that it is sensitive to tissues having high signal on T1 weighting. This includes fat and some stages of haemorrhage (methaemoglobin) that may obscure the vessels on an MIP.

Phase contrast angiography (PCA)

PCA uses a subtraction method to differentiate between flowing and stationary spins. The pulse sequence used is GE with an additional gradient application known as the velocity encoding gradient or VENC. The steepness of this additional gradient is a user-definable parameter used to differentiate between differing flow velocities (e.g. between arterial and venous flow). The principle of this technique is that two acquisitions are performed to encode flow along a particular direction.

The first acquisition uses a VENC that results in the flowing nuclei acquiring an advanced phase position compared to the stationary background spins. The second acquisition uses a flow compensating gradient such as that used in artefact reduction techniques. This gradient causes both stationary and moving spins to retain the *same* phase position. When the data from the two acquisitions are digitally subtracted the resulting images show only the difference, i.e. the flowing spins. This technique can be time-consuming, as the VENC may need to be applied in all three orthogonal planes (X, Y and Z) if flow is tortuous. The advantages are in the excellent background suppression and the fact that flow can be shown as black or white, depending on direction. The subtraction technique means that, unlike TOF images, phase contrast images are not obscured by tissues having short T1 times.

Contrast-enhanced MRA (CEMRA)

As outlined above, phase contrast and inflow angiograms have certain image quality and artefact issues. Most of these problems can be resolved by the use of positive contrast media. In CEMRA, a bolus of gadolinium-based contrast media is injected into a vein, usually in the antecubital fossa. When the bolus reaches the region of interest, a T1-weighted 3D volume GE sequence is performed while the patient holds their breath/keeps perfectly still. This technique has the following advantages:

- Shorter RF pulses may be used
- Shorter TR and thinner sections may be obtained under 1 mm
- Large 3D data volumes may be collected in a 6–20 second breath hold
- Larger fields of view are possible than with inflow MRA and PCA because in-plane flow may be imaged; as an example, the aorta can be imaged with coronal slices rather than axial

The rationale behind the technique is that paramagnetic contrast agents shorten the T1 time of blood. This makes it possible to acquire an MRA in which image contrast is due to the differences in the T1 relaxation times between blood and surrounding tissues. This is an advantage because it results in a more anatomical image. Flow-dependent methods such as inflow MRA and PCA only yield signal from moving blood. Vessels containing very slow flow or stationary flow cannot be visualised. Using CEMRA it is (theoretically) possible to image vessels containing stationary blood, provided there is contrast agent present. This means that CEMRA does not tend to suffer from flow-related artefacts such as over-estimation of stenosis, incorrect representation of lumen diameter and saturation signal loss due to in-plane flow.

Ideally, the dose of contrast agent used must be sufficient to shorten the T1 time of blood compared to the background tissues. A short TR can then be used which saturates signal from all structures apart from blood. The background tissue having the shortest T1 is fat, 270 ms at 1.5 T, so enough gadolinium must be injected per bolus to shorten the blood T1 to under 270 ms.

It is of vital importance in CEMRA that the acquisition is timed so that data are collected during the short time in which the bolus of contrast is present within the imaging volume.

To simplify the procedure and reduce the likelihood of human error, modern scanners have protocols that feature sequences of such high temporal resolution that the operator can inject the entire contrast bolus using a syringe pump and witness its arrival in the vessel of interest in real time. This permits the user to initiate the main data acquisition when the contrast is in exactly the required area.

Moving table-top studies allow the bolus to be chased into the extremities in much the same way as in early iodine-enhanced radiographic arteriography.[29]

To sum up the main advantages of this technique:

- CEMRA is capable of imaging of in-plane flow (i.e. it is not restricted to perpendicular flow like inflow MRA).
- Because CEMRA can image in-plane flow, a wider field of view can be achieved in a short timeframe. This is because, for example, the aorta can be imaged using relatively few coronal slices, whereas with inflow techniques it would require many axial slices.
- Signal is not dependent upon flow (i.e. flow of any speed will yield high signal).

In patients where gadolinium is contraindicated there are other non-contrast methods of blood-vessel imaging, such as so-called 'fresh-blood' imaging where data are collected in systolic and asystolic phases of the cardiac cycle and subtracted to leave just the vessels on the image.

Diffusion techniques

MRI scanners are capable of differentiating between moving and relatively stationary spins. The mechanism behind this was covered in an earlier section on phase contrast angiography. Modern systems with very powerful gradients can take this principle to a microscopic level and can differentiate between the molecular diffusion rates in different tissue environments. This is facilitated by the fact that the random thermal motion of water molecules causes a net flow along an unrestricted pathway, resulting in a loss of signal. Any adjacent area where flow is restricted due to pathology (such as stroke) will not experience as much signal loss and will appear comparatively bright.

Perfusion imaging

Perfusion studies use dynamic contrast enhancement combined with a high temporal resolution scan technique. As the contrast perfuses through the region of interest it will cause either an increase in signal intensity on T1-weighted sequences or a drop in signal intensity when T2* weighting is employed. The high temporal resolution allows rapid re-acquisition of the same slice or block of slices over time. The T2* technique is often used as part of a stroke protocol where the healthy tissue experiences a signal drop due to susceptibility effects of the gadolinium leaving the poorly perfusing pathology comparatively hyperintense.

SUGGESTED MRI PROTOCOLS BY BODY AREA

The brain

MRI of the brain can be used to assess structure, pathology and brain function.

MRI has surpassed CT for imaging of the brain owing to its superior sensitivity and soft tissue contrast; for example, MRI can detect demyelination even in early inflammatory lesions where CT studies have shown no abnormality.

The posterior fossa is well demonstrated on MRI images as MRI does not suffer from the beam hardening artefacts associated with CT scans of this region. Aneurysms and vascular anomalies may be demonstrated using flow-dependent imaging techniques that can demonstrate vasculature without the need for iodinated contrast media. These techniques have additional advantages in that they are comparatively cheap, very quick to perform, have no risk of contrast agent-related side effects, use no ionising radiation, and are more comfortable for the patient than a catheter study.

The multiplanar capabilities of MRI mean that slices can be acquired in non-orthogonal angles. This allows imaging along structures such as the trigeminal nerve and optic nerve as well as sagittal imaging of the pituitary fossa and coronal imaging of the hippocampus.

The functional capabilities of MRI are still being investigated and developed; fMRI is a technique that uses MR imaging to measure the metabolic changes that take place in the cortex of the brain during activation. The areas of the brain responsible for speech, sight, hearing and motor function can vary slightly between individuals. fMRI can be used to assess these areas prior to surgery, allowing the resection of tumours without damaging nearby structures that are critical to the patient. fMRI research is currently looking at applications in the fields of stroke, pain, and the seat of language and memory.

MRI does have some disadvantages in comparison with CT in that it has poorer geometric accuracy, particularly in open scanners, and is much less able to assess bone structure. MRI is not ideal for the trauma patient because of projectile hazards due to incomplete safety screening and attached monitors, etc. CT provides a more immediate solution and can assess bony head injury more readily.

Common indications

- Haemorrhage
- Infection
- Inflammatory processes/multiple sclerosis
- Ischaemia
- Neurodegenerative disease
- Seizures
- Tumours
- Vascular abnormalities

Equipment needed

Quadrature volume head coil or quadrature phased-array head coil

Routine protocol

The routine protocol may include the sequences shown in the following table and in Figures 36.14, 36.15 and 36.16.

	Weighting	Orientation	Pulse sequence
1	T1	Three planes	GE (localiser)
2	T1	Sagittal	CSE
3	T2 or T2/PD	Axial or coronal	FSE (TSE)
4	T2	Axial/coronal/sagittal	FLAIR

It is important to standardise the imaging planes used for every patient. This is because each individual will lie with the head tilted to

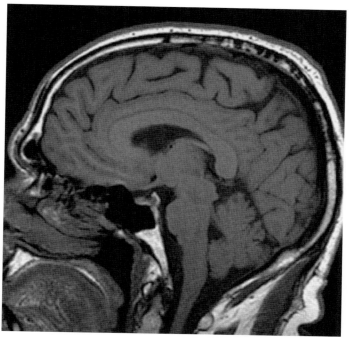

Figure 36.14 T1-weighted, sagittal brain.
Reproduced with permission from Philips Medical Systems.

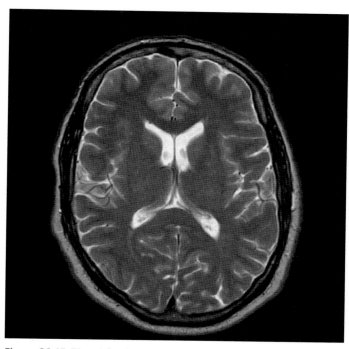

Figure 36.15 T2-weighted, FSE, axial brain.
Reproduced with permission from Philips Medical Systems.

a different extent (chin up or chin down). The sagittal localiser will allow the operator to use a common landmark for the prescription of all axial images. This can be along the hard palate or the line joining the anterior to posterior commissures. Slices should be positioned to cover the foramen magnum to vertex.

Additional sequences may be added to the protocol as follows.

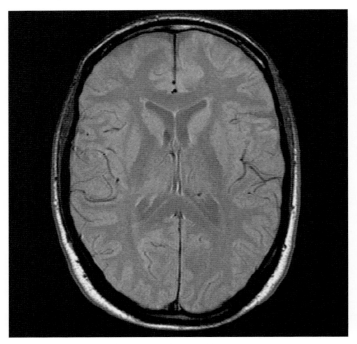

Figure 36.16 PD-weighted spin echo, axial brain.
Reproduced with permission from Philips Medical Systems.

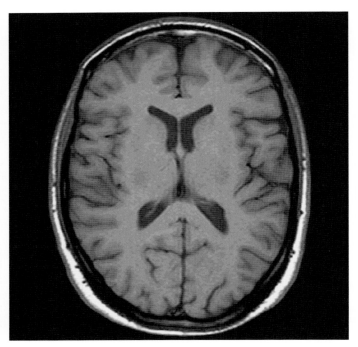

Figure 36.17 T1-weighted, spin echo, axial brain.
Reproduced with permission from Philips Medical Systems.

Tumour or infection (Fig. 36.17)

	Weighting	Orientation	Pulse sequence
1	T1 (+/− gadolinium)	Axial/sagittal/coronal	CSE

T1-weighted images are used with positive contrast enhancement. Positive extracellular contrast media are able to cross any disruption of the blood–brain barrier. This results in the positive enhancement of brain tumours, infection, and other lesions such as active multiple sclerosis plaques.

Multiple sclerosis

	Weighting	Orientation	Pulse sequence
1	T2	Axial/coronal/sagittal	FLAIR

Fluid-attenuated inversion recovery (FLAIR) uses inversion recovery to suppress signal from the CSF in the ventricles, but not the signal from proteinaceous fluid in areas of demyelination. This is useful in defining the extent of periventricular disease (Fig. 36.18).

Epilepsy (Figs 36.19, 36.20)

The protocol may include some of the sequences shown in the following table.

	Weighting	Orientation	Pulse sequence
1	T2	Axial	FSE (TSE)
2	T1	Sagittal	CSE/FSE
3	T1	Coronal (thin slices)	Fast inversion recovery
4	T2	Coronal (thin slices)	FSE (TSE)
5	T1	Coronal 3D volume	GE
6	T2	Coronal 3D volume	FLAIR

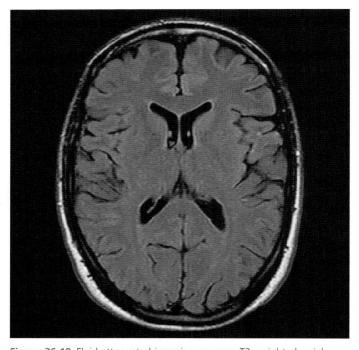

Figure 36.18 Fluid-attenuated inversion recovery T2-weighted, axial brain. Note that an inversion time has been selected to null signal from water so the ventricles appear hypointense despite the T2 weighting.
Reproduced with permission from Philips Medical Systems.

High-resolution T2-weighted scans orientated at 90° to the long axis of the temporal lobe can be useful in assessing hippocampal disease (sclerosis) and structure.

A *3D volume* acquisition will allow the measurement of hippocampal or frontal lobe volumes, as there is no slice gap.

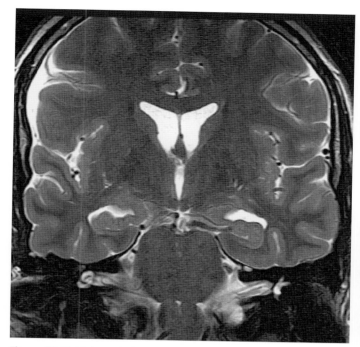

Figure 36.19 High-resolution T2-weighted, FSE, coronal – brain.
Reproduced with permission from Philips Medical Systems.

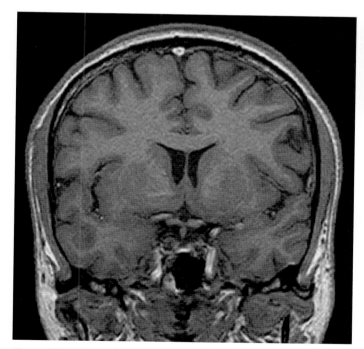

Figure 36.20 T1-weighted incoherent GE, 3D volume – brain.
Reproduced with permission from Philips Medical Systems.

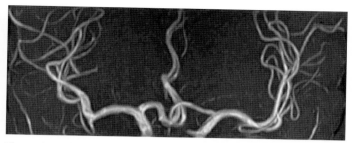

Figure 36.21 3D TOF (post maximum intensity projection) – cerebral angiogram.
Reproduced with permission from Philips Medical Systems.

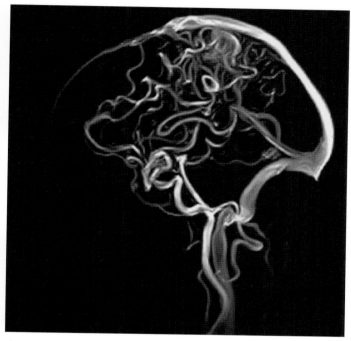

Figure 36.22 PCA – cranial vessels.
Reproduced with permission from Philips Medical Systems.

Vascular abnormalities and presence of flow (Fig. 36.21)

	Vessels	Orientation	Pulse sequence
1	Arteries/aneurysms	Axial	3D inflow MRA
2	Veins	Sagittal oblique	2D inflow MRA
3	Veins	Axial	3D phase contrast MRA

3D TOF gives a high-resolution image having isotropic voxels. This allows MIPs having the same resolution along every axis. The field of view (slab thickness) is limited owing to saturation effects.

2D TOF can be acquired one slice at a time and therefore allows wider coverage than 3D acquisition. Individual 2D slices are not thick enough to cause saturation of slow-moving inflowing spins and therefore can be used for venography. Non-isotropic voxels result in lower resolution of the MIP images.

Phase contrast studies allow the encoding of flow in any direction, not just perpendicular flow. The VENC can be selected for arterial or venous flow (Figs 36.22, 36.23).

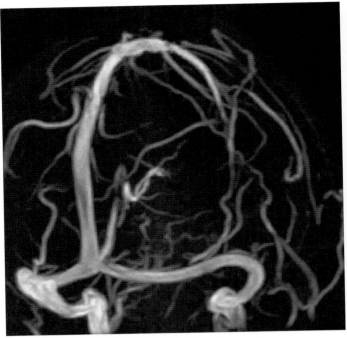

Figure 36.23 Phase contrast venography of the brain.
Reproduced with permission from Philips Medical Systems.

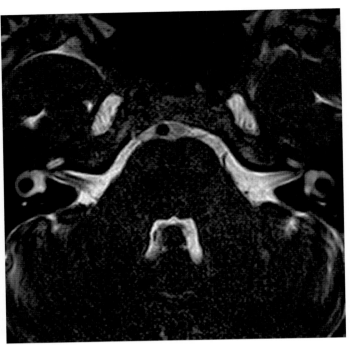

Figure 36.24 High-resolution T2-weighted FSE, axial – internal auditory meati.
Reproduced with permission from Philips Medical Systems.

Assessment of the internal auditory meati or trigeminal nerves (Fig. 36.24)

	Weighting	Orientation	Pulse sequence
1	T2/T2*	Axial (thin slices)/3D volume	FSE (TSE)/balanced GE

or

	Weighting	Orientation	Pulse sequence
1	T1 (pre/post gadolinium)	Axial/coronal (thin slices)	CSE

Thin slices 2–3 mm give high-resolution images of the acoustic nerves to exclude acoustic neuroma etc. A *3D volume* acquisition has the additional advantage of requiring no slice gap. T1-weighted pre- and post-contrast studies can demonstrate lesions within the trigeminal nerve and reveal vascular abnormalities in adjacent vessels which may be causing symptoms due to compression and pulsatile irritation.

Note that balanced GE can be used as an alternative to T2 weighted FSE, as it has the advantage of reducing CSF flow motion artefacts.

Pituitary fossa (Figs 36.25, 36.26)

	Weighting	Orientation	Pulse sequence
1	T1 (pre/post gadolinium)	Sagittal/coronal (thin slices)	CSE

The absence of a blood–brain barrier in the pituitary gland and stalk results in homogeneous enhancement after gadolinium chelate injection. A focal hypointense area within the gland immediately after Gd-DTPA is abnormal and is the most common appearance of an adenoma.

Orbits (Figs 36.27, 36.28)

	Weighting	Orientation	Pulse sequence
1	T2 (fat suppression)	Axial/coronal (thin slices)	STIR/FSE (TSE)
2	T1 (pre/post gadolinium)	Axial/coronal/sagittal (thin slices)	CSE

STIR and T2 fat-suppressed sequences reduce the signal from orbit fat, improving contrast in assessing the optic nerves. If fat suppression is required on the T1-weighted images chemical fat saturation may be used. Appropriately angled parasagittal projections can be used to demonstrate the optic nerve along its full length to the optic chiasm. Note that this protocol may also be used in imaging the other cranial nerves.

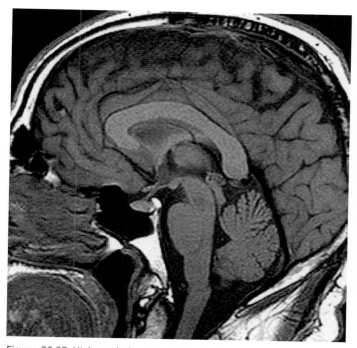

Figure 36.25 High-resolution T1-weighted spin echo, sagittal – pituitary fossa.
Reproduced with permission from Philips Medical Systems.

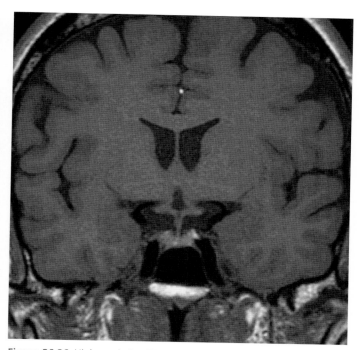

Figure 36.26 High-resolution T1-weighted spin echo, coronal – pituitary fossa.
Reproduced with permission from Philips Medical Systems.

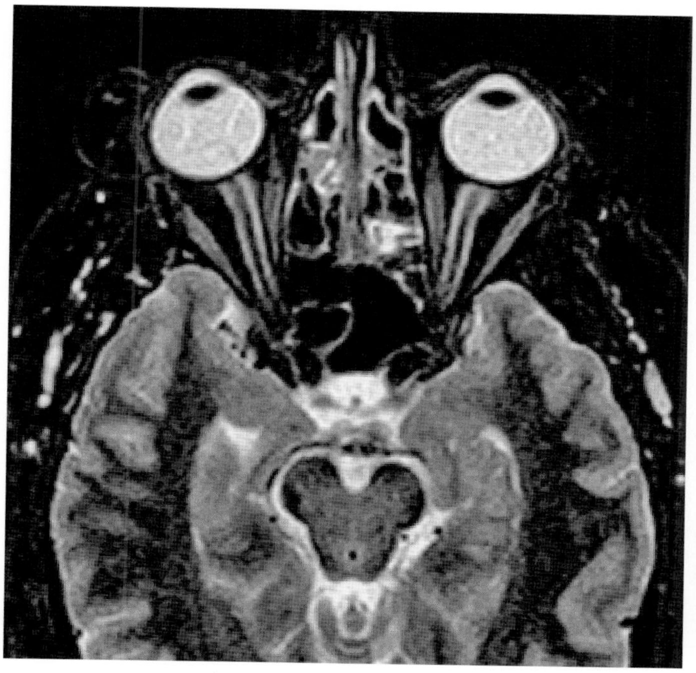

Figure 36.27 STIR, axial – orbits.
Reproduced with permission from Philips Medical Systems.

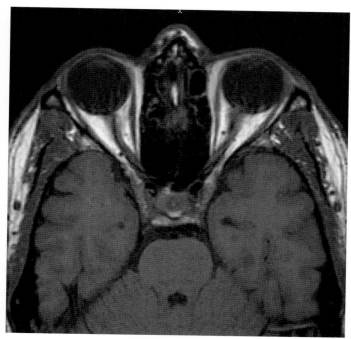

Figure 36.28 T1-weighted spin echo, axial – orbits.
Reproduced with permission from Philips Medical Systems.

Spine

The spine is an anatomical area that is inherently suited to MRI. The area is relatively immobile, has good PD and excellent contrast-to-noise ratio. Artefactual appearances can occur due to the movement of nearby structures such as the throat, anterior body wall, heart and bowel, but these can usually be reduced by using a saturation pulse. A saturation pulse is a user-defined region that is subjected to additional RF pulses to suppress all signal. If a region is not emitting signal then it cannot cause artefactual appearances on the image.

In many cases MRI is replacing conventional radiography of the spine because of the wealth of additional information it provides and because of its non-ionising nature.

Common indications

- Congenital abnormalities
- Cord atrophy
- Cord compression
- Degenerative disease
- Demyelination
- Disc disease (new and recurrent following surgery)
- Epidural fibrosis (following surgery)
- Haemorrhage
- Infarction
- Infection
- Metastatic disease
- Tumour
- Vascular malformations

The soft tissue capabilities of MRI make it particularly suited to the demonstration of congenital abnormalities such as Chiari malformation, spina bifida, cord tethering, dysraphisms and diastematomyelia.

Changes in bone marrow are also well demonstrated and make MRI a useful tool in the assessment of metastatic disease. Bone marrow is usually of intermediate signal on T1 weighting because of its fat content. Metastatic infiltration has a higher water content and therefore reduces the signal in affected areas.

MRI has a unique sensitivity to demyelinating conditions; T2-weighted sagittal images of the cord are therefore valuable in demonstrating lesions of multiple sclerosis. CT rarely shows such lesions, although areas may enhance on delayed scanning after a double dose of iodinated contrast medium in advanced cases of disease.

Tumours are well demonstrated on MRI, usually causing a widening of the cord, high signal on T2 weighting and possible enhancement on T1-weighted images. There are several classifications of cord tumour that can be differentiated by close inspection of MRI images in many cases.

The contrast-to-noise ratio generated on T2 weighting between CSF and cord allows MRI to replace conventional myelography in most cases. Disc disease, cord compression and spinal stenosis will cause indentation of the theca.

Haemorrhage can be detected using GE sequences owing to increased susceptibility effects.

Cervical spine

Equipment needed

Volume neck coil, quadrature phased-array neurovascular coil, quadrature spine coil or quadrature phased-array spine coil

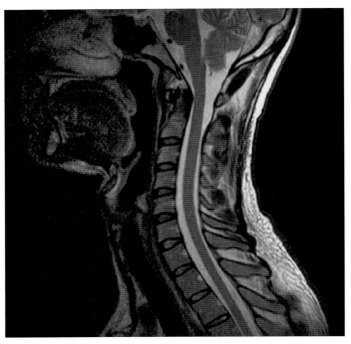

Figure 36.29 T2-weighted FSE, sagittal – cervical spine. *Reproduced with permission from Philips Medical Systems.*

Routine protocol

The routine protocol may include the sequences shown in the following table and in Figures 36.29, 36.30, 36.31, 36.32 and 36.33.

	Weighting	Orientation	Pulse sequence
1	T1	Three planes	GE (localiser)
2	T2	Sagittal	FSE (TSE)
3	T1	Sagittal	CSE/FSE
4	T2/T2*	Axial/3D volume	FSE (TSE)/GE
5	T1	Axial	CSE/FSE

The coronal localiser will allow the operator to orientate the sagittal sections. The field of view should include the posterior fossa to the second thoracic vertebra. The sagittal localiser allows the operator to prescribe the axial slices. Axial slices should cover the intervertebral discs.

Additional sequences may be added to the protocol as follows.

Syringomyelia or tumour (Fig. 36.34)

	Weighting	Orientation	Pulse sequence
1	T2	Sagittal	STIR
2	T1 (pre/post gadolinium)	Sagittal/axial	CSE/FSE

T1 weighting is used with positive contrast enhancement. STIR images are useful to demonstrate intrinsic signal change within the cord and bone marrow. If fat suppression is required on the T1-weighted images chemical fat saturation may be used. In cases of syringomyelia, the full length of the lesion must be demonstrated. This may include separate scans of the thoracic and lumbar regions.

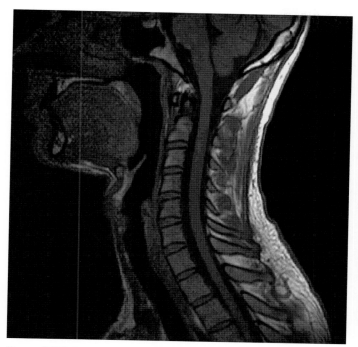

Figure 36.30 T1-weighted spin echo, sagittal – cervical spine.
Reproduced with permission from Philips Medical Systems.

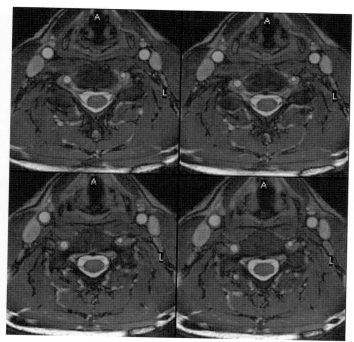

Figure 36.31 T2*-weighted GE, axial – cervical spine.
Reproduced with permission from Philips Medical Systems.

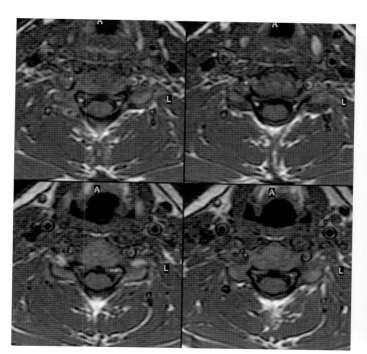

Figure 36.32 T1-weighted spin echo, axial – cervical spine.
Reproduced with permission from Philips Medical Systems.

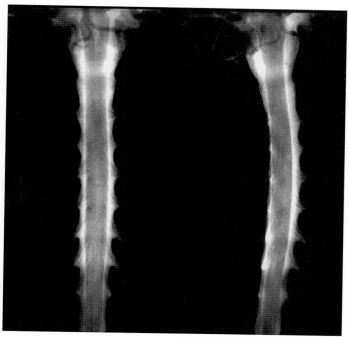

Figure 36.33 Long T2-weighted 'myelographic' maximum intensity projection, cervical spine.
Reproduced with permission from Philips Medical Systems.

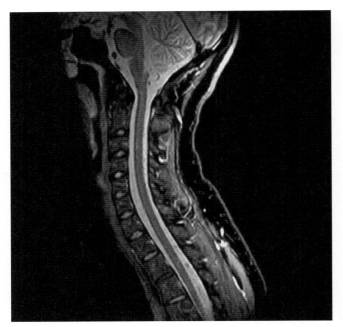

Figure 36.34 Short tau inversion recovery, sagittal – cervical spine. *Reproduced with permission from Philips Medical Systems.*

Brachial plexus

	Weighting	Orientation	Pulse sequence
1	T2	Coronal	FSE (TSE)/ STIR
2	T1	Coronal/axial	CSE/FSE
3	T2	Axial	FSE (TSE)

Slices prescribed from the angle of the mandible to the lung apices. Coronal sections are not usually very useful in routine spine imaging but are very useful when looking for lesions such as neurofibroma. The coronal plane demonstrates the classic dumbbell shape of the lesion which may not be appreciated on sagittal views.

Thoracic spine

Equipment needed

Quadrature spine coil or quadrature phased-array spine coil

Routine protocol

The routine protocol may include the sequences shown in the following table and in Figures 36.35 and 36.36.

	Weighting	Orientation	Pulse sequence
1	T1	Three planes	GE (localiser)
2	T2	Sagittal	FSE (TSE)
3	T1	Sagittal	CSE/FSE
4	T2/T2*	Axial/3D volume	FSE (TSE)/GE
5	T1	Axial	CSE/FSE

The coronal localiser will allow the operator to orientate the sagittal sections. The field of view should include the seventh cervical vertebra

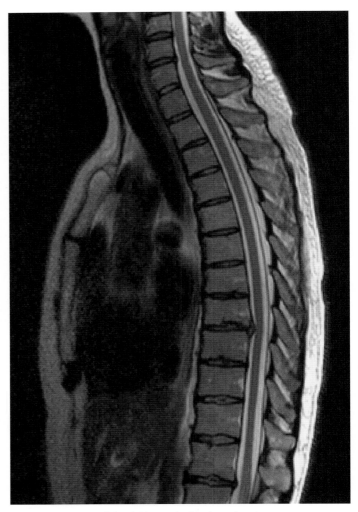

Figure 36.35 T2-weighted FSE, sagittal – thoracic spine. *Reproduced with permission from Philips Medical Systems.*

to the first lumbar vertebra. Identification of vertebral level can be facilitated by including the second cervical vertebra on at least one sequence (such as the localiser). The sagittal localiser allows the operator to prescribe the axial slices. Axial slices should cover any relevant intervertebral discs.

Additional sequences may be added to the protocol as follows.

Syringomyelia or tumour

	Weighting	Orientation	Pulse sequence
1	T2	Sagittal	STIR
2	T1 (pre/post gadolinium)	Sagittal	CSE/FSE
3	T1 (pre/post gadolinium)	Axial	CSE/FSE

T1 weighting is used with positive contrast enhancement. STIR images are useful to demonstrate intrinsic signal change within the cord and bone marrow. If fat suppression is required on the T1-weighted images chemical fat saturation may be used. In cases of syringomyelia, the full length of the lesion must be demonstrated. This may include separate scans of the cervical and lumbar regions.

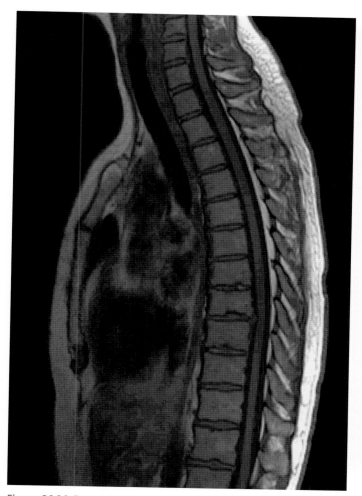

Figure 36.36 T1-weighted spin echo, sagittal – thoracic spine.
Reproduced with permission from Philips Medical Systems.

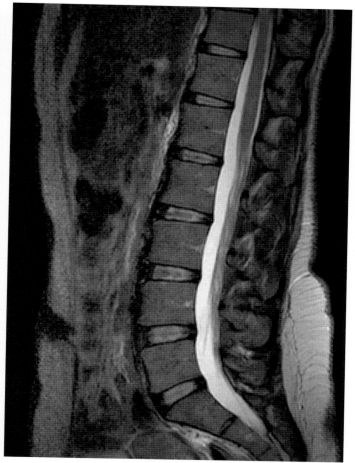

Figure 36.37 T2-weighted FSE, sagittal – lumbar sacral spine.
Reproduced with permission from Philips Medical Systems.

Scoliosis

	Weighting	Orientation	Pulse sequence
1	T1 or T2	Coronal	CSE/FSE

Scoliosis causes the spine to curve out of the sagittal plane and therefore a coronal data set will provide better coverage and more readily understandable anatomical information.

Lumbar–sacral spine

Equipment needed

Quadrature spine coil or quadrature phased-array spine coil

Routine protocol

The routine protocol may include the sequences shown in the following table and in Figures 36.37, 36.38 and 36.39.

	Weighting	Orientation	Pulse sequence
1	T1	Three planes	GE (localiser)
2	T2	Sagittal	FSE (TSE) or STIR
3	T1	Sagittal	CSE/FSE
4	T2	Axial	FSE (TSE)
5	T1	Axial	CSE/FSE

The coronal localiser will allow the operator to orientate the sagittal sections. The field of view should include the 12th thoracic vertebra to the tip of the coccyx. The sagittal localiser allows the operator to prescribe the axial slices. Axial slices should cover any relevant intervertebral discs.

STIR may be used instead of T2 sagittal images, particularly if the examination is limited replacement for radiographic evaluation. STIR is often described as a 'search and destroy' sequence due to its sensitivity to pathology.

Additional sequences may be added to the protocol as follows.

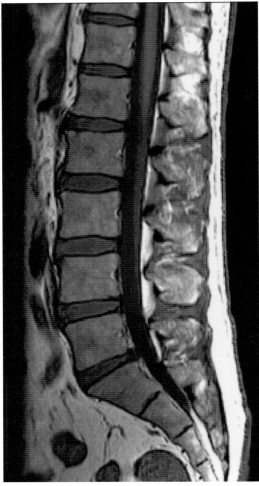

Figure 36.38 T1-weighted spin echo, sagittal – lumbar sacral spine.
Reproduced with permission from Philips Medical Systems.

Syringomyelia or tumour

	Weighting	Orientation	Pulse sequence
1	T2	Sagittal	STIR
2	T1 (pre/post gadolinium)	Sagittal	CSE/FSE
3	T1 (pre/post gadolinium)	Axial	CSE/FSE

T1 weighting is used with positive contrast enhancement. STIR images are useful to demonstrate intrinsic signal change within the cord and bone marrow. If fat suppression is required on the T1-weighted images chemical fat saturation may be used. In cases of syringomyelia, the full length of the lesion must be demonstrated. This may include separate scans of the cervical and thoracic regions.

Some MR systems have software capabilities that enable image fusion from separately acquired data sets so that a reconstructed whole spine can be visualised. This both speeds up the acquisition of data as re-centering/patient re-positioning for each area becomes unnecessary, and is useful in ascertaining the correct vertebral level of any lesions demonstrated.

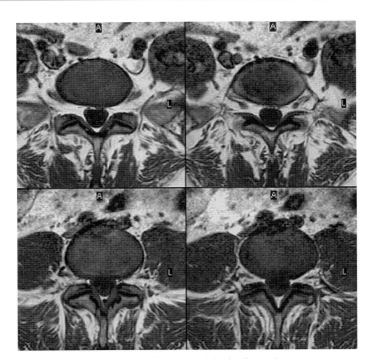

Figure 36.39 T1-weighted spin echo, axial – lumbar spine.
Reproduced with permission from Philips Medical Systems.

Musculoskeletal system

MRI has an important role in the diagnosis and treatment of musculoskeletal disorders. MRI accurately depicts soft tissue injuries such as muscle, ligament and meniscal tears as well as cartilage and bone injuries. Muscle has an intermediate to slightly long T1 relaxation time and a short T2 relaxation time. It appears relatively hypointense on both T1- and T2-weighted sequences, particularly FSE T2.

The fat planes allow identification of individual muscles owing to fat's hyperintensity on T1 weighting. Injured muscles have associated oedema and haemorrhage, which prolong the T1 and T2 relaxation times of the injured tissue, so T2-weighted images with fat suppression (or STIR images) demonstrate tears. Water-bearing oedematous tissue is hyperintense compared to the relatively hypointense muscle and saturated signal of fat.

T1-weighted imaging may be useful in providing information about haemorrhage, which has changing intensity with time owing to the altering state of the haemoglobin component (oxyhaemoglobin, deoxyhaemoglobin, intracellular methaemoglobin, extracellular methaemoglobin and haemosiderin).

PD-weighted images have an inherently high SNR and have been found to be well suited to the visualisation of the internal structures of joints such as the knee. Fat-saturated PD-weighted images have increased water sensitivity and are useful in the detection of bone marrow oedema, and in demonstrating hyaline cartilage surface injuries or irregularities.[30]

This knowledge is invaluable in formulating the optimum treatment plan for a patient. The sensitivity of MRI is such that it can detect injuries such as rotator cuff tendonitis and bone bruising. These injuries are ideally treated conservatively, so an MRI scan can spare the patient unnecessary surgery. MRI is also an ideal modality to diagnose bone and soft tissue tumours, infection and avascular necrosis of bone.

MRI studies may now also include MR arthrography. This technique involves the injection of a dilute solution of gadolinium chelate (1 in

100 dilution) into the joint capsule followed by T1 fat-saturated images. The joint capsule is distended by the high-signal gadolinium and allows better visualisation of the intra-articular structures.

Shoulder

The shoulder joint allows a wide range of movement at the cost of having a shallow socket. It is therefore susceptible to a range of soft tissue injury involving the ligaments and tendons of the rotator cuff.

Common indications

- Rotator cuff disease
- Labral injury
- Biceps tendon disruption

Equipment needed

Dedicated phased-array shoulder coil, phased-array flex coil, surface coil or wrap around coil

Routine protocol

The routine protocol may include the sequences shown in the following table and in Figures 36.40, 36.41 and 36.42.

	Weighting	Orientation	Pulse sequence
1	T1	Three planes	GE (localiser)
2	T1/T2/PD (fat suppression)	Sagittal	CSE/FSE
3	T1	Coronal	CSE
4	T2/PD (fat suppression)	Coronal	FSE (TSE)
5	T2*/PD (fat suppression)	Axial	GE/FSE (TSE)
6	T1	Axial	FSE/CSE

The axial localiser will allow the operator to orientate the coronal sections parallel to the supraspinatus muscle. The field of view should include the entire joint and rotator cuff.

The parasagittal sections may be prescribed from the paracoronal data to ensure perpendicular orientation. MR arthrography may be performed in examinations of the shoulder joint.

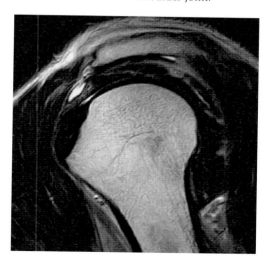

Figure 36.40 T2-weighted FSE, sagittal – shoulder joint. *Reproduced with permission from Philips Medical Systems.*

Elbow

The elbow is a very stable joint but elbow dislocations and fractures are common.

Complex elbow injuries involve related fractures and/or neurovascular injuries. MRI is not particularly useful in acute trauma where conventional radiography can be used to assess bony injury. In the subacute setting, however, MRI is invaluable in assessing soft tissue damage.

From a practical viewpoint the elbow can be difficult to image owing to its lateral position. Comfortable patient positioning is therefore of great importance.

Common indications

- Ligament and tendon injury
- Articular cartilage injury
- Occult fractures
- Assessment of neurovascular structures

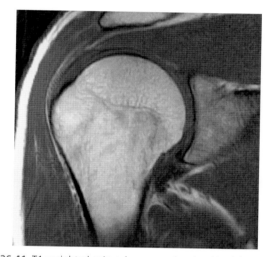

Figure 36.41 T1-weighted spin echo, coronal – shoulder joint. *Reproduced with permission from Philips Medical Systems.*

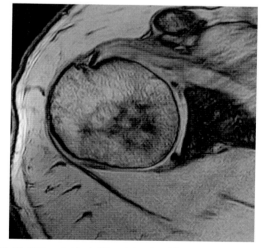

Figure 36.42 T2*-weighted GE, axial – shoulder joint. *Reproduced with permission from Philips Medical Systems.*

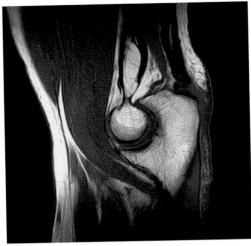

Figure 36.43 T1-weighted spin echo, sagittal – elbow joint. *Reproduced with permission from Philips Medical Systems.*

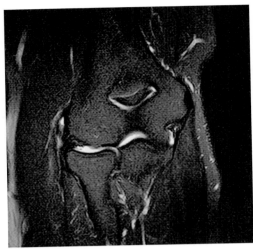

Figure 36.44 T2-weighted FSE with fat saturation, coronal – elbow joint. *Reproduced with permission from Philips Medical Systems.*

Equipment needed

Dedicated phased-array elbow (extremity) coil, phased-array flex coil, surface coil or wrap around coil

Routine protocol

The routine protocol may include the sequences shown in the following table and in Figures 36.43, 36.44 and 36.45.

	Weighting	Orientation	Pulse sequence
1	T1	Three planes	GE (localiser)
2	T1	Sagittal (thin slices)	CSE
3	T1	Coronal (thin slices)	CSE
4	T1	Axial (thin slices)	CSE
5	T2 (fat suppression)	Axial (thin slices)	FSE (TSE)
6	PD or T2 (fat suppression)	Coronal (thin slices)	FSE (TSE)
7	T2*	Sagittal 3D volume	GE

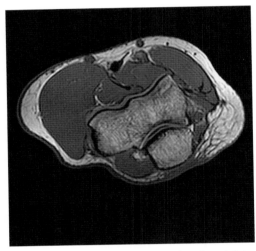

Figure 36.45 T1-weighted incoherent GE, axial – elbow joint. *Reproduced with permission from Philips Medical Systems.*

The axial localiser will allow the operator to orientate the sagittal and coronal sections. The field of view should include the entire joint, the distal humerus and the proximal radius and ulna.

MR arthrography may be performed for examination of the elbow joint.

Wrist

In the wrist, dislocations and fractures are common.

MRI is not particularly useful in acute trauma where conventional radiography can be used to assess bony injury. In the subacute setting, however, MRI is invaluable in assessing soft tissue damage and instability due to ligament damage. As an anatomical area, the wrist is not particularly amenable to MRI. Bone and ligaments have low PD and there is a fair amount of flow from veins and arteries.

Common indications

- Ganglia
- Carpal tunnel syndrome
- Occult fractures
- Assessment of ligaments
- General pain/repetitive strain injury
- Synovitis
- Rheumatoid disease

Equipment needed

Dedicated phased-array wrist (extremity) coil, phased-array flex coil, surface coil or wrap around coil

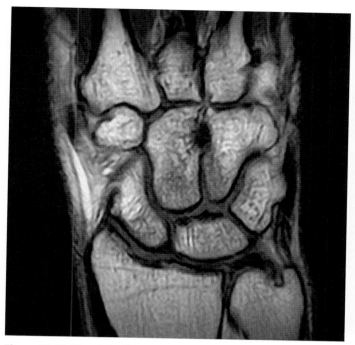

Figure 36.46 T1-weighted spin echo, coronal – wrist joint.
Reproduced with permission from Philips Medical Systems.

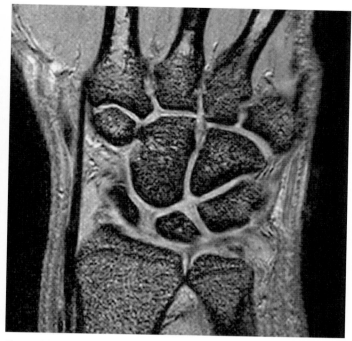

Figure 36.47 T2*-weighted coherent GE, coronal – wrist joint.
Reproduced with permission from Philips Medical Systems.

Routine protocol

The routine protocol may include the sequences shown in the following table and in Figures 36.46, 36.47 and 36.48.

	Weighting	Orientation	Pulse sequence
1	T1	Three planes	GE (localiser)
2	T1	Axial/coronal (thin slices)	CSE
3	T2*	Coronal 3D volume	GE
4	PD (fat suppression)	Coronal (thin slices)	FSE (TSE)
5	T2 (fat suppression)	Axial (thin slices)	FSE (TSE)
6	T2	Coronal (thin slices)	STIR

The sagittal localiser will allow the operator to orientate the coronal and axial sections. The field of view should include the entire joint, carpal bones and distal ulna and radius. Sagittal imaging is occasionally used as it can help demonstrate carpal dislocations.

MR arthrography may be performed for examination of the wrist joint.

Hip

Hip pain is a very common clinical problem and can have a wide number of causes, some musculoskeletal and some not related to the joint itself (e.g. sciatica, hernia or aneurysm).

As an anatomical area the hip is very amenable to MRI as it has a high PD and is easily immobilised.

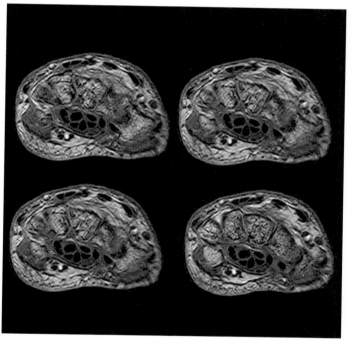

Figure 36.48 T2*-weighted coherent GE 3D volume – wrist joint.
Reproduced with permission from Philips Medical Systems.

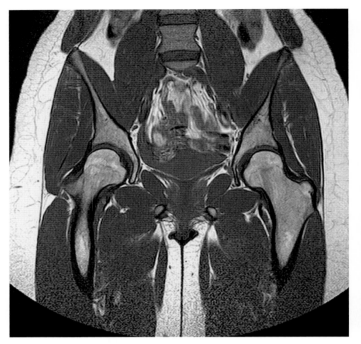

Figure 36.49 T1-weighted coronal – hip joints.
Reproduced with permission from Philips Medical Systems.

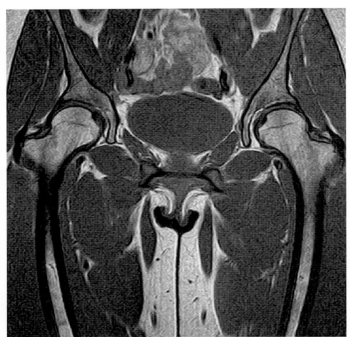

Figure 36.50 PD-weighted, coronal – hip joints.
Reproduced with permission from Philips Medical Systems.

Common indications

- Avascular necrosis
- Bone marrow disorders
- Occult fractures
- Neoplasm
- Osteomyelitis

Equipment needed

Phased-array torso coil

Routine protocol

The routine protocol may be bilateral or unilateral (having a reduced field of view). It may include the sequences shown in the following table and in Figures 36.49 and 36.50.

	Weighting	Orientation	Pulse sequence
1	T1	Three planes	GE (localiser)
2	T1	Coronal	CSE
3	T2 or PD (fat suppression)	Coronal	STIR/FSE (TSE)
4	T1/T2 (fat suppression)	Axial	CSE/FSE

The field of view should cover the area from above the acetabulum to below the lesser trochanter.

Knee

The knee joint is the most commonly imaged joint in the body. Plain radiography of the knee is of little value unless there has been a direct trauma to the joint causing bone fracture. MRI can accurately demonstrate the soft tissue structures of the knee and detect quite subtle damage to these components.

Common indications

- Arthritis
- Bone bruising (trabecular microfracture)
- Cartilage injury chondromalacia
- Cruciate ligament damage
- Evaluation of knee pain
- Infection
- Neoplasm
- Patellar disorders/maltracking

Equipment needed

Dedicated quadrature volume knee coil or phased-array knee coil

Routine protocol

The routine protocol may include the sequences shown in the following table and in Figures 36.51, 36.52, 36.53, 36.54, 36.55 and 36.56.

	Weighting	Orientation	Pulse sequence
1	T1	Three planes	GE (localiser)
2	PD (+/– fat suppression)	Sagittal	FSE (TSE)
3	T1	Sagittal	CSE
4	T2/PD (fat suppression)	Coronal	FSE (TSE)
5	T1	Coronal	CSE
6	T2/PD (fat suppression)	Axial	FSE (TSE)
7	T2*	Sagittal/volume	GE

The field of view should cover the entire joint and should include the skin surfaces laterally and medially.

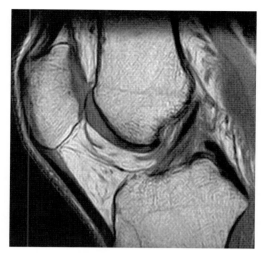

Figure 36.51 PD-weighted, sagittal – knee joint.
Reproduced with permission from Philips Medical Systems.

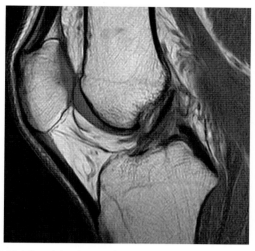

Figure 36.52 T1-weighted sagittal – knee joint.
Reproduced with permission from Philips Medical Systems.

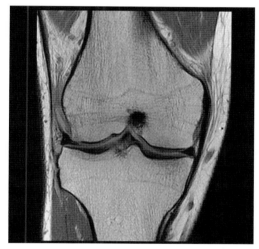

Figure 36.53 PD-weighted, coronal – knee joint.
Reproduced with permission from Philips Medical Systems.

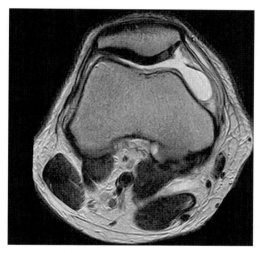

Figure 36.54 T2-weighted FSE, axial – knee joint.
Reproduced with permission from Philips Medical Systems.

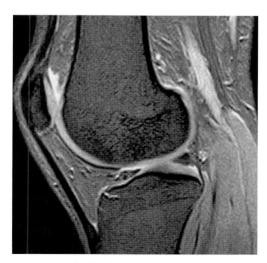

Figure 36.55 T2*-weighted coherent GE, sagittal – knee joint.
Reproduced with permission from Philips Medical Systems.

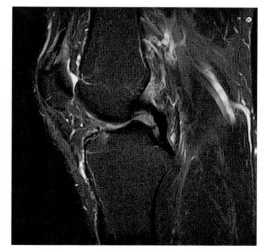

Figure 36.56 STIR, sagittal – knee joint.
Reproduced with permission from Philips Medical Systems.

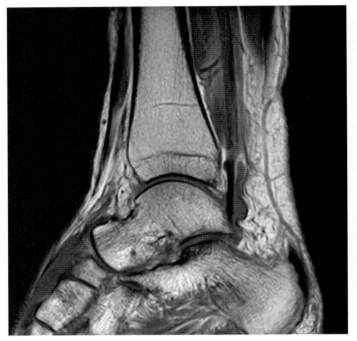

Figure 36.57 T1-weighted sagittal – ankle joint.
Reproduced with permission from Philips Medical Systems.

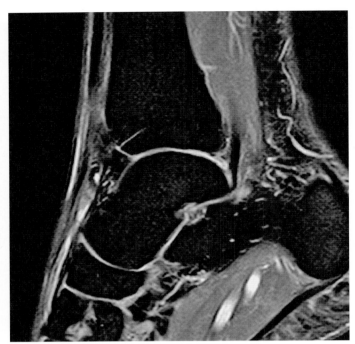

Figure 36.58 STIR, sagittal – ankle joint.
Reproduced with permission from Philips Medical Systems.

Ankle

Plain X-rays of the ankle are of use when ruling out fracture or joint instability.

MRI can demonstrate the soft tissue components of the joint. MR arthrography can be performed in the ankle joint to demonstrate ligament tears and intra-articular lesions.

Common indications

- Arthritis
- Bone bruising (trabecular microfracture)
- Cartilage injury chondromalacia
- Ligament damage
- Infection
- Neoplasm

Equipment needed

Phased-array extremity coil or quadrature volume knee coil

Routine protocol

The routine protocol may include the sequences shown in the following table and in Figures 36.57 and 36.58.

	Weighting	Orientation	Pulse sequence
1	T1	Three planes	GE (localiser)
2	T1	Coronal	CSE
3	T2/PD (fat suppression)	Coronal	STIR/FSE (TSE)
4	T1	Sagittal	CSE
5	T2	Sagittal	FSE (TSE)
6	T2/PD (fat suppression)	Sagittal	STIR/FSE (TSE)
7	T2 (fat suppression)	Axial	FSE (TSE)
8	T1	Axial	CSE

BREAST

MRI is very sensitive at detecting breast lesions and unlike mammography is not limited by dense tissue. Specificity is variable, however, and MRI is therefore used in combination with clinical examination, mammography, ultrasound and biopsy to obtain an accurate diagnosis.

Focal lesions within the breast usually enhance after the administration of gadolinium contrast, and T1-weighted 3D volume imaging data are collected dynamically. The technique should feature both high spatial and temporal resolution for accurate analysis. Enhancement curves are produced for regions of interest. Lesions can then be characterised by the pattern and rate of enhancement, malignant lesions tending to have rapid bright enhancement with rapid wash-out.[31]

Common indications

- Screening high-risk groups
- Guided biopsy
- Staging extent of known disease
- Diagnosing recurrent disease
- Lesion characterisation after equivocal ultrasound/mammography results
- Neoadjuvant radiotherapy response
- Implant integrity/rupture

Equipment needed

Dedicated phased-array breast coil or phased-array torso coil with breast support

Routine protocol

The routine protocol may include the sequences shown in the following table

	Weighting	Orientation	Pulse sequence
1	T1	Three planes	GE (localiser)
2	T2	Coronal	SSFSE[a]
3	T2 (+/– fat suppression)	Axial	SSFSE /STIR
4	T1 (dynamic) (+ gadolinium) (+/– fat suppression)	Axial/sagittal/ coronal volume	GE
5	T1 (post gadolinium)	Sagittal of each breast	FSE (TSE)/GE
6	T2 (+/-water suppression)	Axial/sagittal	STIR, FLAIR

[a]If single shot is not available/preferred, FSE may be used. T1 3D dynamic volume with fat suppression negates the need for subtraction images.

ABDOMEN

The commonly imaged areas in abdominal MRI include the liver, the pancreas, the kidneys and adrenal glands and the reproductive system. With the advent of new hardware and pulse sequences the trend seems to be towards breath-hold and free breathing scans. T2 weighting can be achieved using SSFSE, T1 weighting by GE.

Liver

Liver MRI is commonly used for the detection and characterisation of focal liver lesions, especially tumours. On a T1-weighted sequence the signal intensity of normal liver is greater than that of muscle or spleen, less than that of subcutaneous fat and approximately the same as that of the pancreas. On T2-weighted sequences normal liver tissue is of relatively low signal owing to short T2 relaxation time, and is less intense than spleen. Focal lesions in the liver generally enhance after the administration of Gd-DTPA.

The liver is a common site for metastatic disease, and so imaging of metastases is a very common indication for liver MRI. Metastases generally appear at a lower signal intensity than normal liver tissue on T1-weighted images, but owing to the presence of oedema they are usually hyperintense on T2-weighted sequences. They can also have haemorrhagic components, which appear as inhomogeneous areas at varying intensities depending upon the age of the haemorrhage and the weighting used.

Imaging usually involves dynamic contrast-enhanced studies where diagnosis is based on the rate and pattern of enhancement of any lesions present.

Several manufacturers also offer hepatobiliary gadolinium-based agents. Healthy liver cells enhance and their contrast enhancement accumulates over time. The focal lesions remain low in signal on post-contrast T1-weighted fat-suppressed images owing to nil or poor uptake of contrast by abnormal cells.

Common indications

- Characterisation of benign/malignant lesions
- Assessment of diffuse liver disease, e.g. fatty liver, haemochromatosis
- Visualisation of biliary tree in obstructive jaundice

Equipment needed

Phased-array torso coil
Respiratory compensation/triggering

Routine protocol

The routine protocol may include the sequences shown in the following table and in Figures 36.59, 36.60 and 36.61.

	Weighting	Orientation	Pulse sequence
1	T1	Three planes	GE (localiser)
2	T1 (pre gadolinium)	Axial/3D volume (breath hold)	GE
3	T1 (dynamic) (+ gadolinium) (fat suppression)	Axial/3D volume (breath hold)	GE
4	T2 (fat suppression)	Axial (breath hold)	SSFSE[a]
5	T1	Axial/coronal (breath hold)	GE
6	T2/T2*	Axial/coronal (free breathing)	SSFSE[a] (triggered)/ balanced GE
7	T1	Axial (breath hold)	GE, fat and water in phase
8	T1	Axial (breath hold)	GE, fat and water out of phase

[a]If single shot is not available/preferred, FSE with respiratory gating may be used.

Free-breathing SSFSE is usually performed with respiratory gating to ensure that each slice is acquired at the same point in the respiratory cycle.

Balanced gradient sequences can be used as an alternative to T2-weighted FSE as they also reduce circulatory/biliary flow artefacts.

In- and out-of-phase imaging (either run separately or as one dual acquisition) can help to diagnose fatty liver, as voxels containing fat and water will decrease in signal intensity on the out-of-phase image (Fig. 36.61).

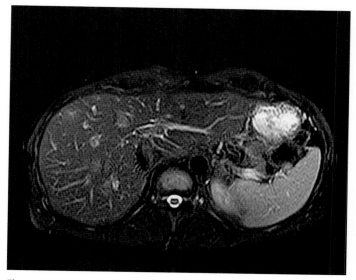

Figure 36.59 T2-weighted single-shot – liver (patient free breathing). *Reproduced with permission from Philips Medical Systems.*

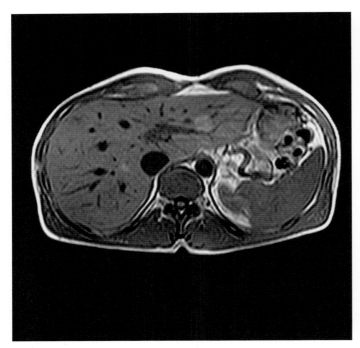

Figure 36.60 T1-weighted GE – liver (breath holding).
Reproduced with permission from Philips Medical Systems.

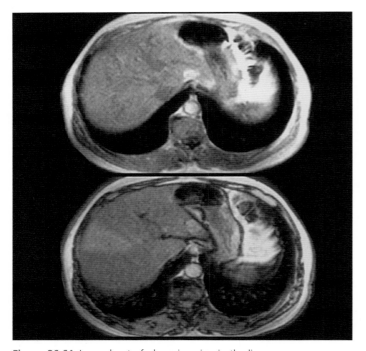

Figure 36.61 In- and out-of-phase imaging in the liver.
Reproduced with permission from Philips Medical Systems.

Dynamic scanning can help to differentiate between enhancing liver lesions. These studies are performed after positive contrast agent injection, typically in the arterial, portal, venous and delayed phases. Fat suppression may be used following contrast injection to help improve the contrast-to-noise ratio.

Multiple echo T2-weighted sequences may be useful in characterising haemangiomas as these lesions remain hyperintense on late echoes.

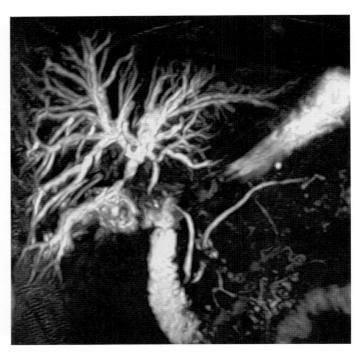

Figure 36.62 Heavy T2 weighting and maximum intensity projection – biliary tree.
Reproduced with permission from Philips Medical Systems.

The biliary tree may be imaged using T2-weighted sequences having very long echo times (Fig. 36.62). This provides an image resembling an endoscopic retrograde cholangiopancreatogram, but without the need for any intervention or contrast media. This technique is often referred to as a magnetic resonance cholangiopancreatogram (MRCP). A very long echo time (perhaps up to 400 ms) results in an image where only water spins are still in phase. If a 3D volume technique is used the data can also be post-processed using MIP to give multi-projectional images.

Pancreas

The pancreas can be seen on a Tl-weighted image as a medium signal intensity structure with an intensity similar to that of the liver, surrounded by hyperintense fat. With increased age the homogeneity of the pancreas decreases due to parenchymal atrophy. The margins of the gland may be smooth or lobulated, and the pancreatic duct is shown as a low signal intensity structure on Tl-weighted images. Narrow slice thickness is required to show the duct as it is less than 2 mm across. Fat-suppression imaging leaves the pancreas as a homogenous high-signal structure which has a greater signal intensity than any of the surrounding structures. The pancreatic duct may also be demonstrated on MRCP.

Common indications

- Evaluation of pancreatitis
- Neoplasms
- Trauma

Equipment needed

Phased-array torso coil
Respiratory compensation/triggering

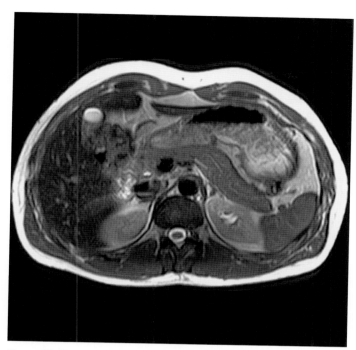

Figure 36.63 T2-weighted axial – pancreas.
Reproduced with permission from Philips Medical Systems.

Routine protocol

The routine protocol may include the sequences shown in the following table and in Figure 36.63.

	Weighting	Orientation	Pulse sequence
1	T1	Three planes	GE (localiser)
2	T1 (+/– fat suppression)	Axial (thin slices) or 3D volume (breath-hold)	GE
3	T1	Axial (breath-hold) respiratory compensation	FSE (TSE)/GE
4	T2 /T2*	Axial (breath-hold)	SSFSE[a]/balanced GE
5	T1	Axial (breath-hold)	GE fat and water in phase
6	T1	Axial (breath-hold)	GE fat and water out of phase

[a]If single shot is not available/preferred, FSE with respiratory gating may be used.

On T1-weighted images the normal pancreas has higher signal intensity than any other abdominal organ.

Fat-saturated T1-weighted sequences are useful for distinguishing normal from abnormal pancreatic parenchyma because distracting bright signal from intra-abdominal fat is removed. For patients unable to hold their breath, respiratory compensated spin echo sequences may be performed.

Breath-holding, in- and out-of-phase, T1-weighted GE images display similar anatomical information as spin echo sequences but with the additional bonus of signal suppression due to fat and water phase opposition. This technique, which is also used in the liver, can help in distinguishing between some common lesions and tumours in this anatomical area. These include adenoma (in the adrenal area), focal fatty change in the pancreas and renal cell carcinoma metastasis in the pancreas.[32–37]

Kidneys

The diagnosis of malignant renal masses requires visualisation of the mass and usually positive enhancement with gadolinium-based contrast media. Typically, T1-weighted GE sequences are used.

For renal transplant assessment, T2-weighted sequences and contrast-enhanced 3D GE sequences give anatomical information about causes of graft dysfunction. These may be supplemented by dynamic contrast renography and MRA. MRA is also frequently used for renal artery stenosis as a non-ionising radiation alternative to CT.

MR urography is a technique which is gaining popularity as information can be acquired from either *static-fluid* imaging using T2-weighted images with long echo times or *excretory* imaging using delayed, contrast-enhanced, T1-weighted fat-suppressed 3D GE sequences to assess kidney function. These can be performed pre, and post contrast to provide subtraction data.[38]

Common indications

- Adrenal gland assessment
- Neoplasms
- Renal transplant

Equipment needed

Phased-array torso coil
Respiratory compensation/gating

Routine protocol

The routine protocol may include the sequences shown in the following table and in Figures 36.64, 36.65 and 36.66.

	Weighting	Orientation	Pulse sequence
1	T1	Three planes	GE (localiser)
2	T1	Coronal	CSE/FSE/GE
3	T1	Axial	CSE/FSE/GE
4	T2, (+/-fat suppression)/T2*	Coronal/axial (breath-hold)	SSFSE[a]/balanced GE
5	T1	Axial (breath-hold)	GE fat and water in phase
6	T1	Axial (breath-hold)	GE fat and water out of phase

[a]If single shot is not available/preferred, FSE with respiratory gating may be utilised.

If renal angiography is needed (Fig. 36.67)

	Weighting	Orientation	Pulse sequence
1	T1	Coronal 3D volume	GE

Pelvis

The pelvis presents an ideal area for MRI imaging. It has a high PD, good inherent contrast-to-noise ratio, and is easily immobilised using compression.

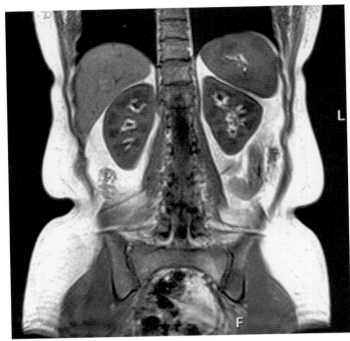

Figure 36.64 T1-weighted coronal – kidneys.
Reproduced with permission from Philips Medical Systems.

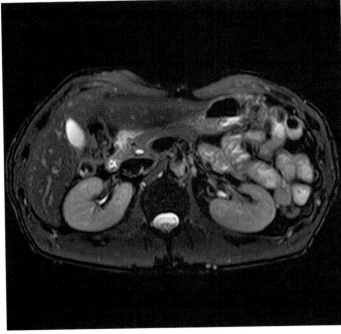

Figure 36.65 T2-weighted (fat suppression), axial – kidneys.
Reproduced with permission from Philips Medical Systems.

Common indications

- Anal fistulae
- Assessment of prostate gland (male)
- Fibroids (female)
- Location of undescended testis (male)
- Neoplasms (prostate, cervix, uterus, ovaries, bladder, rectum)

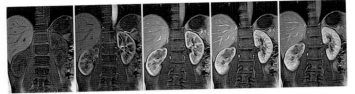

Figure 36.66 T1-weighted dynamic study, coronal – kidneys.
Reproduced with permission from Philips Medical Systems.

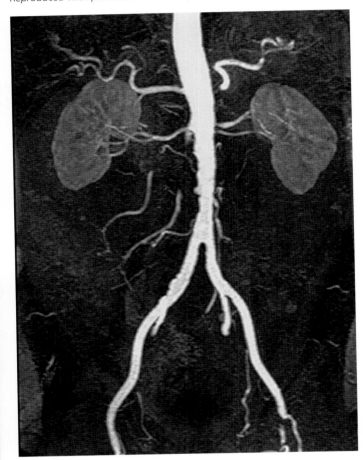

Figure 36.67 Renal contrast-enhanced MRA.
Reproduced with permission from Philips Medical Systems.

Equipment needed

Phased-array torso coil, compression band

Routine protocol

The routine protocol may include the sequences shown in the following table and in Figures 36.68, 36.69 and 36.70.

	Weighting	Orientation	Pulse sequence
1	T1	Three planes	GE (localiser)
2	T1	Axial	FSE (TSE)
3	T2	Axial	FSE/SSFSE[a]
4	T2	Coronal	FSE/SSFSE[a]
5	T2	Sagittal	FSE/SSFSE[a]

[a]If single shot is not available/preferred, FSE with respiratory gating may be utilised.

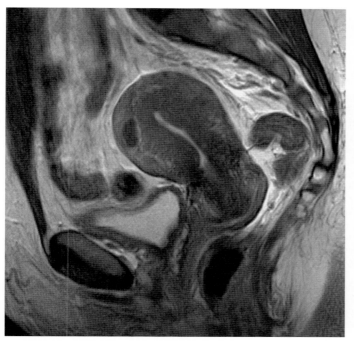

Figure 36.68 T2-weighted sagittal – female pelvis.
Reproduced with permission from Philips Medical Systems.

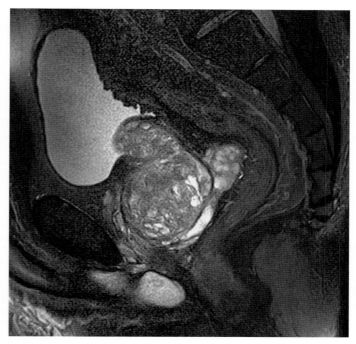

Figure 36.69 T2-weighted (fat suppression), sagittal – male pelvis.
Reproduced with permission from Philips Medical Systems.

For anal fistulae

	Weighting	Orientation	Pulse sequence
1	PD/T2 (fat suppression)	Coronal	FSE (TSE)
2	T2 (+/-fat suppression)	Sagittal	FSE (TSE)
3	T2 (+/-fat suppression)	Axial	FSE (TSE)
4	T1	Axial	FSE (TSE)
STIR may be used instead of FSE.			

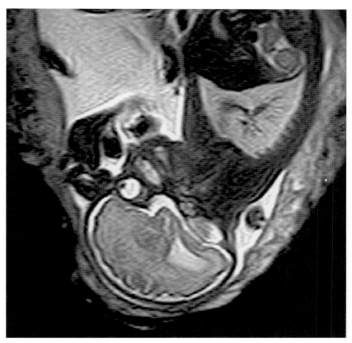

Figure 36.70 T2-weighted sagittal – fetus.
Reproduced with permission from Philips Medical Systems.

REFERENCES

1. Chang G, et al. 3D Na MRI of human skeletal muscle at 7 Tesla: initial experience. European Radiology 2010 Aug;20(8):2039–46.

2. http://nobelprize.org/physics/laureates/1944/.

3. Wakefield J. The 'Indomitable' MRI. Smithsonian magazine. June 2000. http://www.smithsonianmag.com/smithsonian/issues00/jun00/object_jun00.html.

4. Damadian R. Tumor detection by nuclear magnetic resonance. Science 1971;171(976):1151–3.

5. Lauterbur P. Image formation by induced local interaction; examples employing magnetic resonance. Nature 1973;242(5394):190–1.

6. Garroway P, et al. Image formation in NMR by a selective irradiative process. Journal of Physics C (solid state physics) 1974;7:457.

7. Mansfield P, Maudsley A. Medical imaging by NMR. British Journal of Radiology 1977;50:188.

8. Damadian R, et al. FONAR image of the live human body. Physiological Chemistry and Physics 1977;9:97–100.

9. Mansfield P, Maudsley A. Planar spin imaging by NMR. Journal of Physics C (solid state physics) 1976;9:L409–411.

10. Mansfield P, Maudsley A. Line scan proton spin imaging in biological structures by NMR. Physics in Medicine and Biology 1976;21:847–52.

11. Mansfield P. Multi-planar image formation using NMR spin echoes. Journal of Physics C (solid state physics) 1977;10(3):L55–L58.

12. Lauterbur P, et al. Augmentation of tissue water proton spin-lattice relaxation rates by in vivo addition of paramagnetic ions. In: Dutton P, et al., editors. Frontiers of biological energetics. New York: Academic Press; 1978. p. 752–9.

13. Ordidge R, et al. Rapid biomedical imaging by NMR. British Journal of Radiology 1981;54:850–5.

14. http://www.fonar.com/standup.htm.

15. Philips. Basic principles of MR imaging. Philips Medical Systems.

16. Baker G. The Science and Technology Facilities Council, Safety in the Handling and Use of Cryogenic Liquids. 2008. Available at: http://www.shepublic.stfc.ac.uk/Codes/STFC/SC02 Cryogenic/SC2 Cryogenic.aspx, Accessed 25/3/10.

17. Ezzeddine B. Active noise cancellation system for magnetic resonance imaging. Neuroscience Directions. 1,1 p3. Wallace-Kettering Neuroscience Institute. http://www.wkni.org/directions/dv01i01.pdf.

18. Imai Y. 2009 New MultiTransmit Technology Advances 3T Imaging. Fieldstrength Magazine Issue 38, Best, Philips Medical Systems.

19. http://www.mrisafety.com.

20. Shellock F. Reference manual for MRI safety, implants and devices. Los Angeles: Biomedical Research Publishing Group; 2007.

21. Chaljub G, et al. Projectile cylinder accidents resulting from the presence of ferromagnetic nitrous oxide or oxygen tanks in the MR suite. American Journal of Roentgenology 2001;177:27–30. Baltimore: Williams and Wilkins.

22. Vote B, Simpson AJ. X-ray turns a blind eye to ferrous metal. Clinical and Experimental Ophthalmology 2001;29:262–4.

23. http://www.bamrr.org.uk.

24. Graham D, et al. 2007. Principles of radiological physics. 5th ed. Edinburgh: Elsevier.

25. Singh S. Big bang. London: Harper Collins; 2005.

26. Hashemi R, Bradley W. The basics of MRI. Baltimore: Williams and Wilkins; 1997.

27. Sadiku MNO. Elements of electromagnetics. 4th ed. Oxford: Oxford University Press; 2007.

28. Anslow P. in Talbot J, et al. Somerset MRI Course CD ROM Volume 2. MRI Education Company; 2001.

29. Meaney J. Magnetic resonance angiography of the peripheral arteries: current status. European Radiology 2003;13(4):836–52.

30. Lal NR, et al. Evaluation of bone contusions with fat-saturated fast spin-echo proton-density magnetic resonance imaging. Canadian Association of Radiologists Journal 2000;51:182–5

31. Shinil K, et al. Current role of magnetic resonance imaging in breast imaging: a primer for the primary care physician. Journal of the American Board of Family Medicine 2005;18:6.

32. Mitchell D, et al. Benign adrenocortical masses: diagnosis with chemical shift MR imaging. Radiology 1992;185:345–51.

33. Outwater E, et al. Distinction between benign and malignant adrenal masses: value of T1-weighted chemical-shift MR imaging. American Journal of Roentgenology 1995;165:579–83.

34. Jacobs J, et al. Pancreatic sparing of focal fatty infiltration. Radiology 1994;190:437–9.

35. Isserow J, et al. Focal fatty infiltration of the pancreas: MR characterization with chemical shift imaging. American Journal of Roentgenology 1999;173:1263–5.

36. Outwater E, et al. Lipid in renal clear cell carcinoma: detection on opposed-phase gradient-echo MR images. Radiology 1997;205:103–7.

37. Carucci L, et al. Pancreatic metastasis from clear cell renal carcinoma: diagnosis with chemical shift MRI. Journal of Computer Assisted Tomography 1999;23:934–6.

38. Leyendecker J, et al. MR Urography: techniques and clinical applications. RadioGraphics 2008;28:1.

Chapter 37

Nuclear medicine imaging

David Wyn Jones, Julian MacDonald, Peter Hogg

INTRODUCTION

Nuclear medicine has three distinct practice areas: in-vitro laboratory-based diagnostics; unsealed source radionuclide therapy; and diagnostic radionuclide imaging. In all three areas the power of nuclear medicine is its ability to diagnose and/or treat disease at a physiological or molecular level.

In-vitro nuclear medicine is often performed remote from the imaging unit, in laboratories. Radioactive substances are used on human tissue and/or fluid samples to diagnose a wide range of pathologies. Examples of diagnostic tests include: analysis of renal function (glomerular filtration rate) using radiolabelled chromium (^{51}Cr); assessment of vitamin B_{12} absorption using radiolabelled cobalt (^{57}Co); and evaluation of thyroid function using radio-labelled iodine (^{125}I). Surprisingly, in-vitro nuclear medicine is performed at many more hospitals than is nuclear medicine imaging.

Unsealed source therapy is used to treat and/or palliate benign and malignant disease. The intention is to deliver an appropriate radiation dose to the offending tissue in order to cause cell death. Consequently, radioactive substances that emit particles (notably beta) are commonly used. Radionuclide therapy for malignant disease is generally performed in oncology units, not least because the radiation protection restrictions are stringent and expensive to implement. A wide range of malignant diseases can be treated in this fashion, an example being thyroid cancer using iodine (^{131}I). The most common benign disease to be treated is thyrotoxicosis, again using ^{131}I, but at a much lower dosage.

When radioactive substances are administered to patients, whether for diagnostic or therapeutic purposes, they are collectively referred to as radiopharmaceuticals. For diagnostic imaging these radiopharmaceuticals provide a way of visualising patterns of growth and biological activity in the organs of interest. This is achieved by imaging the distribution of radiopharmaceuticals which are selected based on their ability to be taken up in the area of interest. Abnormalities, trauma, or the effects of pathogenic invasion can be identified. The great advantage of nuclear medicine imaging is that, except in the case of trauma, physiological changes usually precede anatomical changes.[1]

The modality is highly reliant on the skills of a multidisciplinary team; a suspected clinical condition needs to be matched to an appropriate nuclear medicine investigation, which usually involves complex medical and scientific decisions. The most obvious decision is whether to proceed, in terms of net benefit from the radiation dose received, and if so, which radiopharmaceutical and which imaging technique to use.

EQUIPMENT CHRONOLOGY

1896   Henri Becquerel discovers radioactivity.

1930s   Cyclotron invented: providing means to produce usable quantities of radionuclides. Technetium-99m (^{99m}Tc) first produced in the late 1930s.

1940s   Radionuclides become available for medical use.

Early 1950s   Cassen et al. produced a scintillation detector mounted in an automatic scanning gantry, which was probably the first incarnation of the rectilinear scanner.[2]

1953   First study involving the imaging positron emitters published.[3] As cyclotrons became more available, development accelerated due to the availability of positron-emitting radionuclides that could be labelled as clinically useful molecules. Even so, positron emission tomography (PET) remained only a research tool until the late 1970s.

Late 1950s   Commercial machines available: these devices allowed the acquisition of an image by tracing a collimated scintillation detector in a rectilinear pattern over the area of interest. Rectilinear scanners, however, were very slow and could not produce images of dynamic processes.

Hal Anger developed a scintillation detector, which has since become known as the gamma camera.[4] This device is kept stationary and collects gamma rays over the field of view, resulting in much more rapid image acquisition than the rectilinear scanner and allowing dynamic imaging.

1960   Developed at the Brookhaven National laboratory the ^{99}Mo/^{99m}Tc generator became commercially available. One of the earliest reported uses of ^{99m}Tc was for brain scanning.[5]

1963   First single photon emission tomography study published.[6]

This technique acquires data at a series of angular positions around the patient allowing the production of multiplanar images.

By 1964 Commercial Anger gamma camera systems available. 1967 Hounsfield develops computer algorithms for image production. These algorithms accounted for attenuation and scatter and converted the emission tomography technique to single photon emission computed tomography (SPECT). At this time reconstruction of data took several hours; however, owing to advances in computing, the same processes today take a few seconds.

1970s Radiopharmaceuticals developed allowing imaging of most organs in the body.

mid 1970s Rotating gantries developed to allow automatic SPECT acquisitions.

Late 1970s Clinical PET systems started to become commercially available.

1980s Cardiac radiopharmaceuticals became available.

Since the 1980s, systems for planar, dynamic and SPECT acquisition, have been commercially available and have been further developed and refined.

1990s Rectangular camera heads replaced circular ones to allow imaging of greater areas.

Late 1990s PET started to become routinely used as a clinical tool in the USA. A proliferation of literature started to appear to indicate that PET had a value in the diagnosis and management of certain malignant conditions, and it was not long before it was realised that PET imaging was an essential component in the management of certain cancers. The American healthcare economy then drove the PET market, and as a consequence PET scanning systems and cyclotrons became more available and at a lower cost. The increased clinical use of PET encouraged more research to be conducted into its potential applications and presently a large number of dedicated PET centres exist purely for research purposes.

SCIENCE AND INSTRUMENTATION

Radioactivity

The atoms of some substances are unstable owing to an imbalance in the number of protons and neutrons in the nucleus. Such substances emit radiation spontaneously and are said to be radioactive. Radiation is emitted from a radioactive atom when it undergoes disintegration, i.e. a transformation or decay to another atom. The radioactivity of a substance is defined as the number of disintegrations per second. The unit of radioactivity is the Becquerel (Bq): 1 Bq = 1 disintegration per second.

As atoms decay over time, the amount of radioactivity of a substance reduces. The time taken for the radioactivity to reduce to a half of its original value is called the half-life of the radionuclide. The radiation emitted by a radioactive substance can be of several types, e.g. alpha particles, beta particles, gamma rays, positrons. For imaging purposes, only penetrating radiation, such as gamma radiation, is of use.

Radionuclides

Table 37.1 gives the ideal radionuclide requirements for use in nuclear medicine imaging.

The physical characteristics of ^{99m}Tc (half-life and gamma-ray emission) are ideal for gamma camera imaging in humans, not only because the gamma-ray energy is well suited to gamma camera detection, but also there is no particulate emission (reducing potential patient dose). Although its short half-life (approximately 6 hours) could be considered self-limiting in terms of geographical availability, the invention of the molybdenum (^{99}Mo) generator allowed for a

Table 37.1 Ideal radionuclide requirements for use in nuclear medicine imaging

Property	Ideal requirements
Radiation emitted	Detection relies on radiation being emitted from the body and thus requires a penetrating form of radiation, i.e. gamma rays
Energy	The gamma rays must possess sufficient energy to escape the body but, conversely, their energy must be low enough to allow them to be efficiently stopped within the detector
Half-life	The radioactivity must be sufficient to allow good image quality throughout the duration of the imaging period. The half-life must therefore be long enough to allow this. Conversely, if the half-life is much longer than the period of imaging, this may result in a higher exposure to the patient than is necessary
Cost and availability	The ideal radiopharmaceutical will be cheap and readily available

ready supply of ^{99m}Tc in most hospital locations. ^{99}Mo decays to ^{99m}Tc, and using the generator principle this process can be capitalised on through daily or twice-daily elution (elution is a method of removing ^{99m}Tc from ^{99}Mo in a sterile solution).

^{99m}Tc can be chemically bound to an extensive range of non-radioactive chemical compounds, which can remain chemically stable for quite long times after introduction into the patient, allowing imaging to take place. Examples of uses of ^{99m}Tc include phosphate labelled to ^{99m}Tc, which permits bone imaging, and ^{99m}Tc labelled to a chelate (e.g. diethylenediaminetetra-acetic acid) for renal imaging. Other commonly used radionuclides, and their uses in nuclear medicine imaging, are given in Table 37.2.

Radiopharmaceuticals for PET comprise radionuclides that emit positrons. The positrons lose energy in a short distance in the body and annihilate with atomic electrons to produce two 511 keV gamma-ray photons (180° apart) that allow coincidental detection of the tracer. PET radionuclides have to be produced by cyclotron. If the cyclotron is offsite, the half-life of the radionuclide must be sufficiently long to allow it to be transported to the imaging centre while enough activity remains. The most commonly used PET radionuclide is fluorine-18 (^{18}F), which has a half-life of 1.8 hours.

Chemical component

The chemical component attached to the radionuclide determines where the radiopharmaceutical travels in the body. There are several ways in which a desirable distribution can be achieved, including:

- Using a chemical found physiologically in the organ of interest, e.g. iodine for imaging the thyroid.
- Using an analogue. This is a chemical that simulates one found physiologically, for instance thallium is a potassium analogue and thus can be used to image muscle. Similarly, fluorodeoxyglucose (FDG) is a glucose analogue and can be labelled with ^{18}F for PET imaging to illustrate areas of high glucose metabolism, which has several clinical uses.
- Labelling cells that fight disease, thereby targeting the areas of disease, e.g. white blood cells or antibodies.

Radiopharmaceuticals are normally administered intravenously but are occasionally given subcutaneously, orally or via inhalation. Once incorporated, the radiopharmaceutical remains in the body for a

Table 37.2 Other commonly used radionuclides

Radionuclide	Production method	Principal photon energy (keV)	Used to image
^{99m}Tc	Generator (parent: reactor)	140.5	Skeleton, heart, lung perfusion, kidneys, brain, thyroid
^{201}Tl	Cyclotron	78	Heart, parathyroid
^{123}I	Cyclotron	160	Phaeochromocytoma, thyroid, brain
^{67}Ga	Cyclotron	93,185,300	Inflammation and infection
^{131}I	Reactor	364	Thyroid
^{81m}Kr	Generator (parent: cyclotron)	191	Lung ventilation

period determined by the chemical form, the half-life of the radionuclide and the physiology of the patient. The patient will receive a radiation dose that will depend on the radioactivity administered and the residence time (i.e. the time during which the radionuclide is present in the body). The effective dose, which allows comparison with other imaging modalities using ionising radiation, is determined from the weighted sum of the absorbed doses to each organ. The weighting factors are organ dependent owing to their different radiosensitivities.

The gamma camera

Until the introduction of the gamma camera, imaging was performed on rectilinear scanners using a limited range of radiopharmaceuticals. These scanners tended to produce poor-quality low-resolution images. The gamma camera changed this, resulting in massively improved image quality, thereby increasing the diagnostic value of this modality. The basic principles of operation of the gamma camera have remained largely unchanged from its inception until today, and it continues to be used extensively.

The most fundamental part of any imaging system is the detector. In the case of a gamma camera the detector is a large crystal, normally rectangular, of a scintillation material that produces a weak flash of light when radiation is absorbed, due to excitation. Flashes of light are produced when gamma rays emitted by a patient, previously administered with a radiopharmaceutical, fall on the detector (Fig. 37.1).

The light formed in the crystal is detected by photomultiplier tubes (PMTs) which convert the light to electronic signals whose magnitude is determined by the intensity of light reaching the PMT. There are, in fact, many PMTs packed into the space of the scintillator crystal, and those around the point of light emission will detect some amount of light, depending on their distance from that point. Those closest will detect more light and, in turn, produce a greater electronic pulse, whereas those further away will produce proportionally smaller pulses. The relative magnitude of these pulses can then be used to determine the point of light emission. The pixel count value in a corresponding location in a digital matrix can then be allocated, allowing the accumulation of an image (Fig. 37.2).

However, the system so far described does not provide a method of tracing the point of light emission in the detector back to the point of origin of the gamma ray within the patient, which is critical to producing a meaningful image. This is the function of the collimator.

A collimator is essentially a block of attenuating material with a network of holes and is attached to the gamma camera between the detector crystal and the patient. The holes allow gamma rays travelling

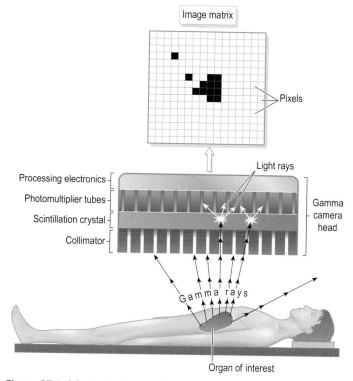

Figure 37.1 Schematic diagram of a gamma camera showing the gamma rays emitted by the patient, the collimator allowing only those aligned with the collimator holes to pass through to the scintillation crystal. Light rays produced by the crystal are detected and quantified to obtain energy and positional information used to assign a count to the correct pixel location in the image matrix.

in a certain direction to pass through to the crystal and be detected. Gamma rays travelling in different directions are attenuated, and so the collimator effectively acts as a filter, allowing only gamma rays travelling in a known direction to contribute to the image. In this way there is a direct one-to-one mapping between the origin of the gamma ray and the position of the pixel within the image matrix. A flow diagram illustrating the process of nuclear medicine image formation is shown in Figure 37.3.

The scintillation material used is sodium iodide, which contains a small amount of thallium impurity [NaI(Tl)]. The thallium impurity significantly increases the amount of light produced. The properties of the detector affect many aspects of the image, as detailed below:

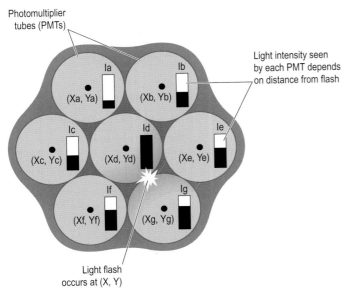

Photomultiplier tubes (PMTs)

Light intensity seen by each PMT depends on distance from flash

Light flash occurs at (X, Y)

Figure 37.2 The intensity of light detected depends on the distance of the PMT from the position within the crystal where the gamma ray was absorbed and the light flash occurred. These relative intensities are used to reduce a weighted average of the PMT positions (Xa, Ya), (Xb, Yb) etc. to determine the origin of the light flash.

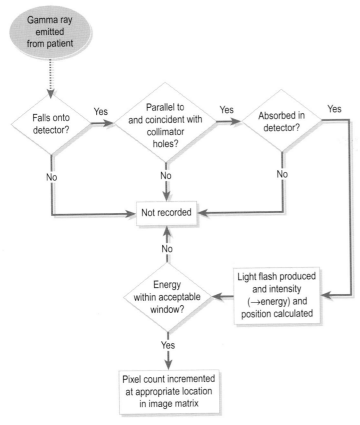

Figure 37.3 The imaging process.

- *Thickness.* The thicker the crystal, the more likely the radiation will be absorbed, thereby improving efficiency. However, if the crystal is too thick there will be an increase in the drift of the light photons, adding to the uncertainty in the calculated point of interaction and hence a worsening in the spatial resolution, i.e. blurring.

- *Light output.* Different scintillator materials produce different amounts of light per interaction and release the light at different rates. The latter affects the duration of the processing required to assign the event to a position within the image matrix, a period known as the *dead-time.* Ideally a large amount of light is required in a short time. It is also essential that the light intensity produced is proportional to the energy of the radiation absorbed. This allows energy discrimination and hence the ability to disregard gamma rays outside a certain energy range, which is used to reduce scatter.

- *Transparency.* This factor affects the amount of light lost as it passes through the crystal before being detected by the PMTs. The more light photons that pass through the crystal and are detected by the PMTs, the more accurate the calculated point of interaction will be.

Collimators vary with regard to their thickness and the number, direction and diameter of the holes. The most common type of collimator used is the parallel hole collimator, in which the holes, as well as being parallel with each other, are perpendicular to the camera face. The number of holes, and hence the thickness of the attenuating material between them, known as the *septa*, is altered to allow imaging for different energies. For example when imaging ^{131}I gamma rays of 364 keV, a collimator with fewer holes and correspondingly thicker septa is essential to prevent penetration of the radiation through the septa. High-resolution high-sensitivity collimators are also generally available and feature variations in collimator thickness and hence hole length. There is a trade-off between resolution and sensitivity such that a high-resolution collimator will have lower sensitivity and therefore take longer to obtain the same number of counts than a high-sensitivity collimator, and vice versa.

Other geometric arrangements of holes are also available. The holes of a diverging hole collimator fan outwards and allow demagnification of the object, which is useful for large objects. Converging hole or fan beam collimators fan inwards, providing magnification of the object, and are commonly used in brain imaging. Pinhole collimators have a single aperture at the end of a lead shield that allows magnification of objects near the collimator and demagnification further away. The magnitude of the effect of all these collimators depends on the distance from the collimator, and hence distortions in the image will occur. This is particularly the case with the pinhole collimator, which can really only be used with thin objects. Nonetheless, the pinhole collimator is a very useful way of providing magnified images of, for example, the thyroid gland or small bone joints in children.

Multiheaded gamma cameras

Gamma cameras can be purchased with one, two or three detector heads, each consisting of scintillation crystal, collimator and associated electronics. In most common use are the dual-headed systems, and many of the available systems can offer flexibility in the position and orientation of the heads. The advantage of multihead gamma cameras is basically that of speed. Dual-headed cameras can be used for whole-body scanning systems: one head can acquire data anteriorly and the other posteriorly simultaneously. For SPECT imaging, multiheaded cameras allow each head to acquire data from part of the complete revolution, thereby speeding up acquisition by a factor equal to the number of detector heads. Three-headed systems are most commonly used for dedicated brain SPECT imaging.

Single photon emission computed tomography (SPECT)

The majority of nuclear medicine studies require the acquisition of static or dynamic planar images, which are acquired with the gamma camera in a fixed position against the patient for the duration of imaging. SPECT imaging, on the other hand, acquires a series of images as the gamma camera rotates around the patient. These images, or *projections*, can then be mathematically reconstructed to form a 3D dataset from which slices through the body or 3D visualisations can be formed, in a similar way to X-ray CT. Reconstruction techniques are beyond the scope of this chapter, but are based on back-projection or iterative algorithms.

This imaging technique allows much greater contrast owing to the effective removal of overlying structures present in planar imaging. Some common applications are in assessing myocardial perfusion, brain functionality and bone lesions.

SPECT-CT systems

It is becoming increasingly common for gamma cameras and CT scanners to be housed on the same system to give what are termed SPECT-CT systems. The CT scanners for this purpose range from low-dose non-diagnostic CT to fully fledged multislice diagnostic CT systems, depending on their intended use.

The CT component provides two advantages:

1. *Attenuation correction.* Gamma rays emitted from within the patient are attenuated by various anatomical structures before they leave the patient and are detected by the gamma camera. The amount of attenuation varies depending on the path the gamma ray travels along from its point of origin, i.e. which anatomical structures the rays have to pass through, and this will vary with the orientation of the camera during a SPECT acquisition.

   The number of gamma rays detected may not actually represent the distribution of the radiopharmaceutical in the body: for example, during myocardial perfusion imaging on large-breasted female patients there is more attenuation from the front than from the side, and this gives rise to artificially low counts in the anterior wall of the heart when the data are reconstructed.

   To obtain an accurate image of the actual distribution, it is necessary to know the attenuation of the various anatomical structures so that the attenuation differences at different angles can be corrected for. This is achieved by acquiring a transmission image via CT. If X-rays of similar energy as the gamma rays are used, the resulting CT image will effectively be an attenuation map and can be used as a correction in the reconstruction process. The resolution of the CT images for this purpose need not be particularly high, and it is therefore possible to use a low-dose CT protocol. Some systems acquire the CT over a relatively long time period compared to conventional CT examinations, which are normally performed during a breath-hold. This has the advantage that the CT images are more consistent with the relatively long SPECT acquisition, making the attenuation map a better match than one obtained from a breath-hold.

2. *Image fusion.* The limited spatial resolution of nuclear medicine imaging, together with the efficient targeting of some radiopharmaceuticals, can result in specific uptake which is difficult to localise. On the other hand, a CT image provides good anatomical detail without the functional information. By overlaying the nuclear medicine SPECT images onto the corresponding CT image, the best of both modalities can be obtained. It is possible, for example, to see exactly which bone is affected in infection or trauma of complex areas such as the hand or foot. Hybrid systems are calibrated such that the CT and SPECT images can be accurately and consistently co-registered, and this must be checked as part of routine quality control.

Dedicated specialised systems

As well as three-headed gamma cameras for dedicated brain SPECT imaging, other dedicated systems have been developed, particularly for myocardial perfusion imaging. These include systems based on traditional gamma camera technology but with fixed head positions and smaller fields of view, with patient chairs designed to maximise comfort and minimise movement. Other systems are based on different detector technology, i.e. solid-state detectors such as cadmium zinc telluride (CZT); a number of individual CZT detectors may be used to scan the heart volume, producing similar resolution images in a significantly reduced time compared to conventional SPECT imaging.

Positron emission tomography (PET)

PET scanning is gaining popularity in the UK and is becoming part of a routine nuclear medicine service. PET imaging is desirable because positron emitting radionuclides are relatively simple to label to biologically active organic molecules. By far the most common PET radiopharmaceutical is ^{18}F-FDG, which provides an image of glucose metabolism that is useful in oncology, cardiology and neurology.

The basic principle of PET imaging is shown in Figure 37.4A,B. PET tracers emit positrons that annihilate with electrons to form two

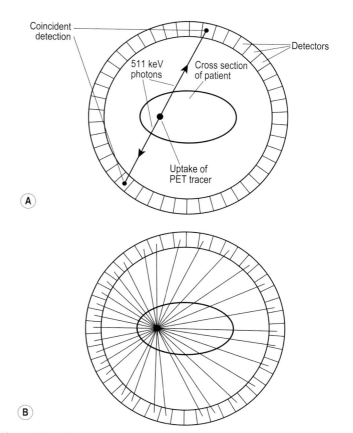

Figure 37.4 The principle of operation of a PET scanner.

511 keV photons which are emitted in opposite directions. PET scanners consist of a ring of detectors in which the two photons are detected coincidentally. The point of emission in the patient must then be somewhere along a line between the two detection events. When sufficient coincident events have been accumulated, the distribution in the body is indicated by a superimposition of these lines. Reconstruction of the data produces a 3D dataset, which can be used to obtain slices through the area of interest.

Modern PET systems commonly include CT scanners, which provide a means of attenuation correction and image fusion similar to that discussed for SPECT.

Image acquisition

The image information leaving the gamma camera head(s) in the form of the X, Y and Z signal is stored in digital form and can be manipulated later to provide image and quantitative data. The final data output is highly dependent on radiographic technique. Once the patient has been correctly prepared and given the appropriate radiopharmaceutical, the appropriate imaging acquisition factors need to be selected and the patient correctly positioned at the predetermined time.

Most gamma cameras can acquire images in many different ways for a variety of purposes. There are usually a number of predetermined imaging frames, and the act of collecting each frame is conventionally referred to as an acquisition. Some of these operator-dependent parameters are described below.

- *Image matrix.* The data are acquired into a predefined image matrix, which affects the spatial resolution, 'counts per pixel' obtained (noise) and number of frames acquired (owing to memory constraints). The matrix is the division of the field of view (FOV) of the gamma camera into predefined pixels. A common example is a 256×256 matrix used for planar imaging.
- *Planar imaging*
    - Static. The most basic acquisition is a static planar image. In this mode of operation the gamma camera head is simply positioned over the area of interest and an image acquired for a specified period or a number of counts (detected photons).
    - *Dynamic.* Dynamic planar imaging allows a succession of images (frames) to be acquired over a specified period. The operator will have control over the duration of each frame, and most systems allow several phases to be defined to acquire, e.g. a rapid succession of frames initially, followed by a series of longer duration frames. This mode of operation is commonly used to image initial blood flow to an area or the excretion of an organ over time. Subsequent processing of such studies can yield curves showing variations in uptake over time (time–activity curves).
- *Whole body scanning.* Most commercially available gamma cameras nowadays offer a scanning feature. This essentially allows data to be acquired over an area greater than the area of the detector head. Typically, data acquired over this extended length is processed to produce a whole-body image of the distribution of the radiopharmaceutical. This is achieved in one of two ways:
    - '*Step and shoot' mode.* Several automatically programmed distinct detector positions are used to acquire individual images, which are subsequently 'knitted' together.
    - *Continuous scanning mode.* Either the gamma camera gantry or the patient couch is moved slowly during acquisition to build up the whole body image.

- *Dual-energy acquisition.* The ability of the gamma camera to discriminate incident energies is exploited to produce two simultaneous frames of separate data representing differing images of the distribution of more than one administered radionuclide. An example would be with 190 keV gamma rays of ^{81m}Kr gas during a lung ventilation scan being stored in one frame and the 140 keV gamma rays from the technetium lung perfusion image being simultaneously stored in another frame.
- *Gated acquisition.* The initiation of collection of data into individual frames is controlled by a physiological 'switching' process, for example by connecting electrocardiograph (ECG) electrodes to the patient and using 'R' wave pulses to initiate and terminate a sequence of frames: e.g. 'gated' SPECT in myocardial perfusion imaging or gated cardiac ventriculography (multiple gated cardiac acquisition). The data can then be used for motion studies of the heart and calculating physiological information.
- *SPECT.* Multiple frames of data are acquired at predefined locations around a central axis within the patient. This can be in a 'step and shoot' mode, where the camera head(s) rotates a fixed number of degrees, stops, acquires a frame of image data for a predefined period, and then moves on to acquire the next frame. A 'continuous' mode allows the head(s) to rotate continually while acquiring data at the required angles. The final data can be reconstructed into three orthogonal planes.
- *Body contouring.* Spatial resolution is related to the distance between the detector and the patient. The closer the detector is to the patient, the sharper the images are. For static imaging, it is fairly straightforward for the operator to position the gamma camera heads as close to the patient as possible. However, for whole-body scanning or SPECT acquisition the detectors are constantly moving, making it difficult for the operator to optimise the position manually during the scan. To overcome this, some systems have methods of achieving this optimisation automatically. There are two basic methods:
    - '*Learn mode'.* The operator programs the position of the camera heads at certain positions of the scan individually to fit the patient; the system will then move the camera heads during the scan to those predefined positions.
    - *Body surface detector.* For example, an infra-red beam, or capacitive sensors, mounted on the surface of the camera head determines how far to move the camera head towards the patient during the scan.

    The latter method has the advantage that it can adjust in real time, e.g. if the patient has moved during the course of the scan.

Annotation and orientation for viewing

Nuclear medicine images need to be correctly orientated for viewing and marked with the appropriate anatomical side. It is common practice to use a cobalt (^{57}Co) marker to identify the correct orientation during imaging, and for later viewing. Another point of note is that, contrary to the practice in radiography of denoting a projection by the 'entry' and 'exit' route of the incident radiation (anteroposterior (AP), posteroanterior (PA)), it is correct in nuclear medicine practice to denote the body part directly adjacent to the surface of the collimator, e.g. anterior image or posterior image – not AP or PA. Also, images at 90°, e.g. 'lateral knee', would be correctly annotated as being 'lateral aspect' if the lateral aspect of the knee were adjacent to the collimator. Finally, a study should always have the radiopharmaceutical used and delay time to imaging or frame times marked on the images. Correct annotation is vital for effective image evaluation.

Image quality

The quality of an image produced by any imaging modality is affected by the amount of noise. In nuclear medicine, contributions to noise come from:

- *Insufficient counts in the image.* Statistical noise arises from uncertainties in the number of counts in each pixel of the image. As radioactive decay is a random process, acquired counts follow a Poisson distribution. This means that the uncertainty, measured as the standard deviation of the mean, is equal to the square root of the number of counts. For a pixel with 100 counts the standard deviation is 10, which is 10% of the mean. Similarly, a pixel count of 10 000 has a standard deviation of 1%.

  The higher the number of counts, the lower the relative uncertainty or noise. Doubling the number of counts improves the noise by a factor of the square root of 2 (1.4). The pixel size has an important impact on this, as larger pixels will collect more counts and thus will inherently have less noise.

- *Scatter.* This occurs both within the patient and in the detector. Scatter of gamma rays in the patient causes them to change direction. In some cases a gamma ray may be scattered towards the gamma camera and, if detected, would result in a count being assigned to a wrong pixel within the image matrix, thereby adding to the noise. In many cases the collimator would filter out such scattered gamma rays but, if the new direction of the gamma ray was parallel to the collimator holes, it would reach the crystal and be detected. This is where the energy discrimination ability is used. The gamma ray will have lost some energy as a result of the scattering interaction. Because the light intensity produced by the scintillator detector is proportional to the energy absorbed, the system can distinguish such scattered gamma rays and disregard them. Unfortunately, however, the various processes involved in the detection process carry their own uncertainties, which means that even unscattered gamma rays may appear to have energies slightly above or below the expected energy (photopeak). This means that there has to be a range (energy window) of acceptable energies applied, which in turn results in some scatter being included. In modern systems, with improved and more stable components, the detection uncertainties have reduced, allowing the window of acceptable energies to be narrowed and hence more noise to be eliminated, with a consequent improvement in image quality.

Quality control

As with any other imaging modality, regular assessment of equipment performance is essential. Some of the parameters assessed routinely for a gamma camera are given below:

- *Uniformity.* The gamma camera has a large field of view and the count-rate observed over its surface for a uniform source should be constant. This is tested either by placing a large uniform source of radioactivity on the collimated camera or by using a small volume source at a distance from the uncollimated detector. An image is acquired in each case and assessed visually and quantitatively for non-uniformity.

- *Energy resolution.* The range of apparent energies erroneously assigned to unscattered gamma rays due to the uncertainties involved in the detection process has been mentioned previously. Energy resolution is essentially a measure of this. A uniform source of radiation is used and data are acquired in the form of a plot of 'the number of gamma rays being assigned a particular energy' against 'energy'. The result is a gaussian curve centred on the photopeak, and the energy resolution is defined as the full width half maximum (FWHM) of that curve. The smaller the value the better, as this means that the energy acceptance window can be narrowed, thereby reducing image noise.

- *Spatial resolution.* The test consists of imaging a narrow line source and then producing a curve profile through the resulting image. The profile will be a gaussian curve and the spatial resolution is defined as the FWHM of the curve. The smaller the value the better, as this means that the camera can resolve objects that are closer together.

SAFETY

Radiation protection in nuclear medicine has always been complex and highly regulated. This was brought about through the use of unsealed radioactive sources which present as highly hazardous because they can lead to contamination, from which people may receive internal and external radiation doses. The scenario became more complex when X-ray machines were attached to radionuclide scanners, creating PET-CT and SPECT-CT. Such hybrid systems have associated X-ray energies (continuous spectra) together with positron (annihilation radiation: 511 keV), or single photon gamma radionuclides (typically between 100 and 300 keV).

The use of radioisotopes demands particular department design characteristics. These are highly evident in laboratory and clinical areas in which radionuclides are prepared and given to patients. Examples include the need for non-absorbent surfaces, splash guards and physical shielding. Also, because patient urine can be radioactive, designated toilets have to be provided. Physical radiation shields (typically lead) are used for both positron and single photon gamma radionuclides, but positron emitters, because of their higher energy, require thicker shields.

To minimise extremity dose to healthcare staff, remote handling devices such as tongs and syringe radiation shields should be used in all instances. Additionally, time (speed of working) and distance are allies of radiation protection, but must not be at the expense of sloppy practice. At regular intervals, and in a systematic fashion, the nuclear imaging department should be monitored for contamination, using a calibrated contamination meter. X-radiation protection would be the same as for anywhere else within a medical imaging facility.

In relation to radionuclide and X-ray exposures, the patient should be afforded the least amount of radiation consistent with attaining a diagnosis. This philosophy is articulated in international guidance and national regulations. In many countries specific upper levels are set for particular diagnostic procedures, and these should be adhered to. The radiation exposure of those professionals who work in nuclear medicine imaging departments should be monitored, in accordance with legal requirements.

Supply of unsealed sources for imaging

It is necessary to have a radiopharmacy facility 'on site' or within a relatively short distance of the gamma camera suite, in order to provide an effective nuclear medicine imaging service. Those without 'on-site' radiopharmacy facilities usually have a radiopharmaceutical dispensary from which daily deliveries can be made.

The radiopharmacy is sited in a 'clean' room where the air is 'ultra-filtered' and has a positive pressure. This, together with protective laminar flow cabinets and clothing, ensures the microbial sterility of the manufactured radiopharmaceuticals. Quality tests are undertaken on the eluate from the ^{99m}Tc generator to check for microbial sterility, and purity (in that it is free of the parent nuclide, ^{99}Mo) and structural alumina from within the generator. Dispensed radiopharmaceuticals are measured according to volume and radioactivity required at a reference time. Calculations are made to account for the physical half-life of the particular radionuclide used and a larger volume is dispensed, to allow for the decay time until administration later in the day at the required activity. Clearly this indicates that the patient's actual attendance time must be in concordance with the allocated appointment and administration time, and this, again, underlines the importance of good advance preparation. In addition to patient explanation, this should include careful explanation to ward personnel if the patient is attending from a ward area rather than from home.

The radioactivity administered to the patient is checked in a calibrator before leaving the radiopharmacy, and it is good practice to double-check the intended activity directly before patient administration. Any patient administration must be within agreed diagnostic reference levels to give results consistent with the minimum amount of radioactivity necessary. It is also obligatory to scale down adult activities for administration to children. Schemes for fractional reduction usually try to maintain similar image acquisition times as that of the equivalent adult scan. Most departments follow their national professional and regulatory bodies' advice in terms of administered activity, but there is usually scope for local variation.

CLINICAL APPLICATIONS

Fundamentals of nuclear medicine technique

The basic principles of nuclear medicine instrumentation necessitate careful radiographic technique to ensure optimal image quality. Conventional radiographic positioning principles lend themselves to positioning in nuclear medicine. Care must be taken to avoid simulating or masking disease by poor positioning of the patient in relation to the gamma camera, misuse of radioactive anatomical markers or incorrect use of imaging equipment and technical parameters.

Optimal patient preparation is paramount for a successful outcome from nuclear medicine investigations. Many procedures can be ruined by incorrect advice or poor patient compliance prior to the investigation. This can partly be remedied by having clear written protocols for each investigation type and by providing the patient with unambiguous written instructions on how to prepare for the investigation. The advice can include the cessation of certain drugs, avoidance of particular foods, or avoiding food intake altogether for certain procedures. This sometimes involves dialogue with the referring clinician regarding interactions, and carefully relaying advice to the patient. An example of a failed procedure would be the patient who has consumed caffeine on the day of a pharmacological myocardial perfusion stress study. Caffeine has a deleterious action on the effectiveness of some pharmacological stressing agents, giving a dubious result when using dipyridamole or adenosine. The examination might need to be repeated in this scenario, clearly with associated additional risks from the repeated test.

It is necessary to have a thorough knowledge of human physiology and anatomy to fully understand the complexities of nuclear medicine imaging investigations. An understanding of how various radiopharmaceuticals are 'handled' by the body (pharmacokinetics) is necessary in order to undertake the appropriate investigation for the clinical question being asked, and to interpret the image appearance correctly. Some image appearances can also represent technical defects in terms of radiopharmaceutical quality or equipment failure.

COMMON NUCLEAR MEDICINE INVESTIGATIONS

Nuclear medicine has many techniques for imaging organs and systems of the human body. The focus here is on some common investigations, to illustrate the rationale involved for imaging, and to suggest their usefulness in the clinical setting.

Skeletal scintigraphy

The bone scan still represents a significant part of the workload of most nuclear medicine departments. This examination is highly sensitive: it can image bone pathology and trauma at a cellular level. More recently the increasing capability of magnetic resonance scanners to image the whole skeleton has shown promising results and, subject to cost and availability, it could become a suitable alternative for some traditional skeletal scintigraphy indications in the future.

For some pathologies isotope bone scanning has been shown to be a highly sensitive method of imaging bone disease, and it can show abnormal areas much sooner than that shown on radiographs, with an increase of up to 50% of calcium in affected areas being required to show changes on a radiograph.[7] Indeed, Alazraki[8] reported that less than 5% of bone scans are normal when radiographs show abnormalities, thus demonstrating the high sensitivity of the imaging modality.

Common indications would include screening for metastatic bone disease; isolating primary bone tumours; confirming occult fractures; identifying potential areas of bone infection or osteomyelitis; differentiating infection from loosening orthopaedic hardware; and investigating metabolic bone diseases, e.g. Paget's disease or microfractures in cases of osteoporosis.

Limitations include its lack of specificity in characterising disease of bone. In many instances there is a need for scan results to be interpreted with clinical history and relevant radiographs in order to make a definitive diagnosis. However, the recognition of particular radiopharmaceutical distribution patterns can allow for a more accurate provisional diagnosis, by understanding the characteristic patterns of uptake of ^{99m}Tc-MDP (methylene diphosphonate), for example:[9]

- *Metastases*: often with multiple lesions with random distribution in the skeleton (Fig. 37.5)
- *Rib fractures*: where the focal increase in uptake is linear along the rib cage (Fig. 37.6)
- *Osteomyelitis*: with intense increased uptake on a three-phase bone scan

Given that there are some instances where a bone scan can be interpreted fairly safely on its own, Sharp confirms the general non-specificity of the technique by quoting some examples of non-specific abnormal uptake, which need further investigation to clarify their aetiology.[7]

Examples of appearances with *non-specific* interpretation:

- *Osteomalacia with associated pseudo fractures*: can be mistaken for multiple metastases in the skeleton or vice versa
- *Simple collapsed vertebrae showing linear increase uptake in spine*: can be mistaken for discitis or vice versa
- *A solitary spinal lesion can be interpreted as a metastasis*: could alternatively be due to fracture of the pars interarticularis; osteoid osteoma; active arthropathy, or primary tumour such as chondrosarcoma

Symmetry is of prime importance in the determination of a normal whole-body bone scan, and it is important that the two halves of the skeleton should be mirror images of each other. There should be

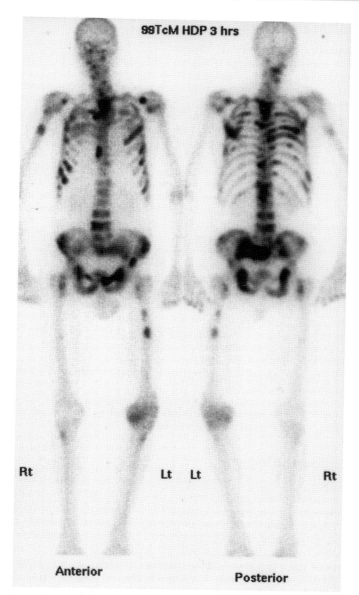

Figure 37.5 Metastatic deposits. This bone scan shows multiple areas of increased uptake of ⁹⁹ᵐTc-HDP at 3 hours, indicating multiple metastatic deposits in the skeleton. The pattern of uptake suggests a definitive diagnosis.

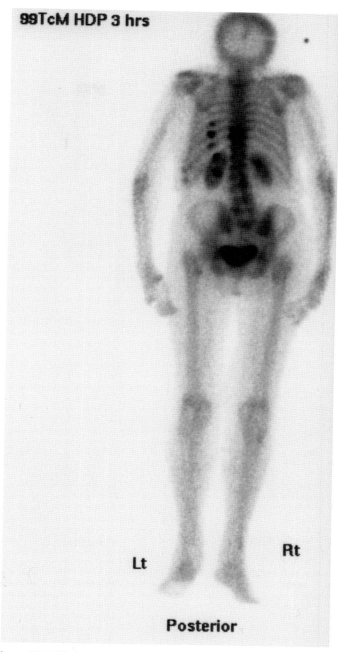

Figure 37.6 Rib fractures. This bone scan shows the typical appearances of rib fractures with the characteristic uptake showing a linear pattern across the left lower posterior ribs.

uniform uptake of the radiotracer in the skeleton, and uptake in organs such as the kidneys and bladder is to be expected. Uptake in the soft tissues of the body can also be an indicator of disease, and should be considered to be a normal area of concern during the interpretation of such an investigation; care needs to be used when 'windowing' these areas (Fig. 37.7).[9]

It is important not only to recognise increased uptake of radiopharmaceutical due to abnormal malignant osteoblastic activity, but also to be aware of a false negative scan, as in the case of multiple myeloma or renal cell carcinoma.[9] Here the characteristic interpretative sign is that of a 'cold' lesion where there is little or no radio-emission from bone. This is of prime importance when justifying the examination, and, once undertaken, must be considered in relation to the clinical history provided.

In cases where systemic disease is concerned the whole skeleton should be imaged. Localised disease present on planar images can sometimes be related to a systemic problem, and so a whole-body bone scan can help to characterise the disease. An example of this would be the multifocal appearance seen with many arthropathies.[7] Given that the nature of this examination only requires one radiopharmaceutical injection, then additional imaging carries no increased radiation burden.

Practical considerations

⁹⁹ᵐTc-MDP and ⁹⁹ᵐTc-HDP (hydroxymethylene diphosphonate) are both commonly used. They are adsorbed onto the surface of bone by incorporation into the hydroxyapatite crystal formed by osteoblastic

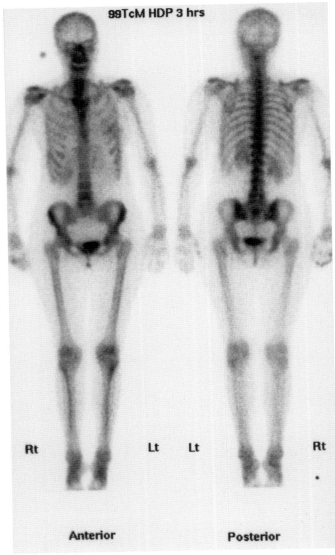

99TcM HDP 3 hrs

Rt   Lt   Lt   Rt

Anterior   **Posterior**

Figure 37.7 Normal bone scan showing symmetrical uptake throughout the skeleton, with soft tissue visible, and the expected activity in the kidneys, ureters, and bladder.

activity. Radiopharmaceutical uptake in bone is related to blood flow and osteoblastic activity. There is no appreciable difference in image quality between the two radiopharmaceuticals, although it has been suggested that there is higher skeletal uptake with HDP.[10] Peak uptake in bone is shown to be at approximately 1 hour[11] and the usual delay to imaging of 3 hours is related to soft tissue clearance by the kidneys of background activity resulting from non-adsorbed phosphonate. Less than 10% of administered activity is present in the blood compartment at 1 hour, and this drops to 2% at 4 hours.[12] It is normal to visualise renal drainage of the tracer and bladder filling, which needs to be emptied prior to imaging. Increased hydration has been conventionally used to improve the object-to-background ratio of radiotracer to improve image quality; however, Klemenz et al.[13] showed that increased hydration had little effect on image quality, and that quality is more related to time delay to imaging and deteriorates with increasing patient age. Increased hydration is, however, recommended to reduce the radiation burden to the bladder wall.[13]

Pulmonary emboli

Ventilation–perfusion (V/Q) lung scanning remains a useful method of diagnosing pulmonary embolism (PE), although CT pulmonary angiography (CTPA) continues to be the imaging method of choice. CTPA elicits controversy when imaging young or pregnant women owing to the relatively high absorbed dose of X-rays in the breast tissue; however, this may be offset by the use of breast shielding as discussed in Chapter 35. Fetal dose remains low enough with V/Q scanning to justify the technique in this scenario. Also, as CT scanners are usually in high demand it might be that patients could be stratified according to presentation and risk of PE. The V/Q scan is recommended, and remains sensitive to PE, when the chest X-ray is normal and the patient's symptoms are consistent with PE. V/Q scanning also has value in evaluating lung function prior to surgery, with its ability to quantify uptake and give functional ratios.

^{99m}Tc-MAA (macro-aggregated albumin) is trapped in the capillaries of the lungs to show normal perfusion, and any occlusion gives rise to a hypoperfused area appearing as a defect on the image. In order to increase the accuracy of diagnosis a ventilation scan is also required, where a radioactive gas (^{81m}Kr) or particulate inhalation (Technegas) is used to image the patent airways (dual-energy acquisition is possible with ^{81m}Kr). This technique relies on a mismatch to suggest the presence of a PE, with the likelihood being greatest when the ventilation scan appears to be normal, thereby effectively eliminating other pathological processes in the lung (Fig. 37.8A,B).

Ventilation agents can be expensive, difficult to obtain, and the examination may be difficult to perform on the very ill patient. It is rare for departments to offer a daily facility with the gold standard of using ^{81m}Kr gas; however, alternatives can often be used to achieve similar results with technetium aerosols.

Endocrinology

Sodium pertechnetate (^{99m}Tc-NaTcO$_4^-$), the raw eluate of the molybdenum/technetium generator, is readily available and can be used to image the thyroid gland. A delay of 20 minutes after intravenous administration shows trapping of the pertechnetate ions in the gland. Abnormal tissue can be highlighted as cold hypofunctioning nodules, or hot hyperfunctioning nodules. ^{123}I is also used for imaging the thyroid gland but gives a higher radiation burden,[14] as it is trapped and taken up by the gland. ^{123}I has an advantage in imaging metastatic thyroid deposits in the skeleton, and the theoretical improved detection of retrosternal extension of the thyroid gland, owing to its higher emissive energy and lower background activity.

MR, CT and ultrasound are all useful in the anatomical evaluation of the thyroid gland, but nuclear medicine imaging provides the necessary functional information together with characteristic uptake in various tumours.[15] Although ultrasound can determine whether a nodule is solid or cystic, the value of nuclear medicine imaging is that of characterisation of the function of the nodule. It has been shown that 99% of 'hot' nodules are benign, whereas 10–20% of palpable cold nodules are malignant.[15]

Thyroid scintigraphy is also useful in the evaluation of thyroiditis in its various forms, and the characteristic uptake of radiopharmaceutical can help evaluate the stages of the disease. Thyroid uptake measurements are possible in nuclear medicine imaging, where a figure can be quoted of the percentage uptake in the gland at a certain time after administration. This is then useful for comparison with the norm, and helps differentiate Graves' disease from other causes of hyperthyroidism, e.g. subacute thyroiditis; and it has a role in the estimation of radioiodine required in thyroid ablation therapy.[15]

Congenital hypothyroidism in neonates can have a devastating effect on mental development if left undiagnosed. Most centres now

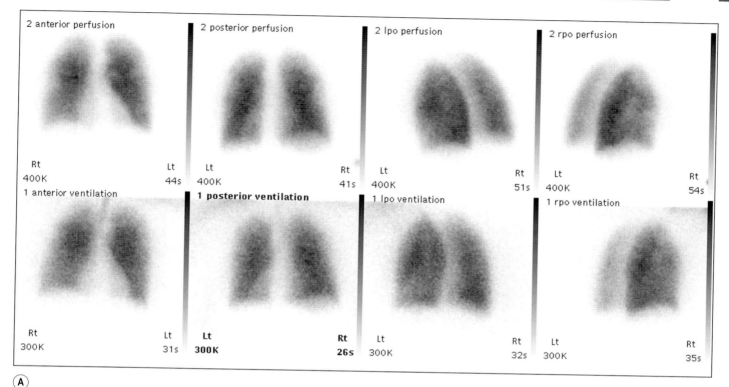

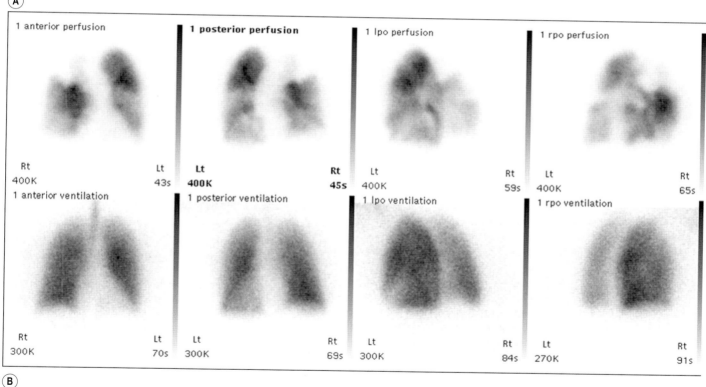

Figure 37.8 (A) A normal ventilation and perfusion scan where the radioactive gas and MAA particles are free to flow around the normal lung. (B) Multiple areas of photopenia. The MAA has not been able to circulate freely around the lung when impeded by pulmonary emboli; however, the lung ventilation with radioactive gas is free to fill the lung unimpeded, as emboli affect the blood circulation and not the aeration. This is a classic mismatch, giving a high confidence of pulmonary emboli.

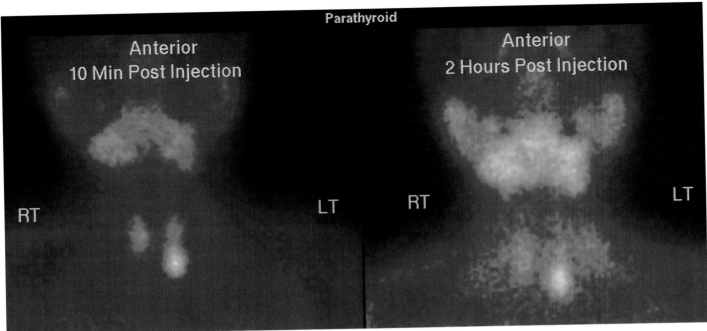

Figure 37.9 ^{99m}Tc-sestamibi parathyroid scan. Showing early 'wash-in' of the tracer with early evidence of a lower left parathyroid adenoma, and the characteristic increased uptake in the tumour in relation to the thyroid on the delayed 'wash-out' image.

screen for this condition soon after birth. Should blood tests show an abnormally low level of thyroid hormones then a technetium thyroid scan is urgently indicated to show the location and function of any thyroid tissue.

In the case of hyperparathyroidism, conventional practice was to image abnormal parathyroid glands with ^{99m}Tc/^{201}Tl subtraction techniques, where normal thyroid tissue would be highlighted by technetium and thallium, and abnormal parathyroid tissue highlighted by the digital subtraction of the normal uptake to leave abnormal thallium activity in the parathyroid gland. This is a useful technique but difficult to perform, requiring the use of expensive and poorly available thallium, not to mention absolute patient compliance, and results in a high radiation dose (>18 mSv).[14]

Technetium sestamibi has more recently been successfully used in highlighting abnormal parathyroid tissue. It is localised in parathyroid adenomas by concentration in the mitochondria-rich tumour, which is related to blood flow.[15] Images are acquired at 15 minutes and 2 hours following administration, as it has been shown that some tumours are more apparent at an early stage (Fig. 37.9). Theory dictates that the tracer concentrates in the tumour within 2 hours and the rest 'washes out' of the normal tissue by then.[15]

Parathyroid glands can be ectopic in the neck or mediastinum and are difficult to localise surgically.[16] The radionuclide technique has advantages over other imaging modalities with respect to imaging ectopic tissue, as it can image the whole area concerned, giving high sensitivity in the detection of adenomas. Sensitivity has been quoted from as high as 86% for planar studies to 90.5% with SPECT.[17] By performing SPECT/CT fusion, anatomical information is readily available for the surgeon to limit the incision size necessary and minimise the operating time (Fig. 37.10).

Renal tract

There are many radiopharmaceuticals available for imaging the renal parenchyma and drainage system; the two most commonly used are discussed here.

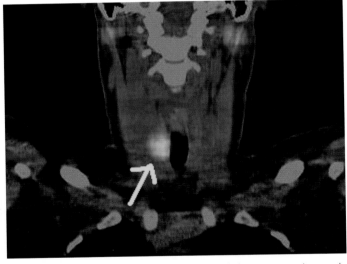

Figure 37.10 The adenoma (arrowed) can clearly be seen superimposed on the anatomical structures of the CT image.

^{99m}Tc-MAG3 (mercaptoacetyl triglycine) is routinely used to image the kidneys, collecting system and bladder. Following intravenous administration it is rapidly removed from the blood circulation by glomerular filtration and tubular secretion, thus effectively representing true renal function. Renal function can thus be imaged with rapid dynamic frames over 30 minutes' duration, and a diuretic can be used to differentiate between true obstructive uropathy or non-obstructed dilatation of the renal pelvis.[18] Data analysis can produce time–activity curves, which have diagnostic value in themselves, and a figure is usually quoted for relative renal uptake at 2–3 minutes (Fig. 37.11). Patients with suspected vesicoureteric reflux can have further imaging while voiding, which will show as an activity peak in the ureter. This

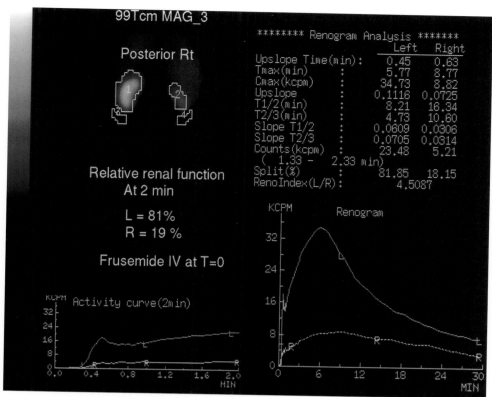

Figure 37.11 ^{99m}Tc-MAG3 dynamic renogram showing the processed data from the dynamic frames of a 30-minute scan. Normal uptake and excretion can be seen on the curve for the left kidney, compared to the poor function of the right kidney. Here the relative renal function at 2 minutes can be seen to be 81% for the left kidney and 19% for the right.

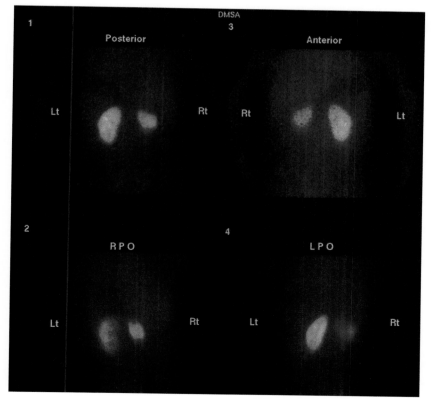

Figure 37.12 ^{99m}Tc-DMSA static renal scan. These images represent renal function and any scarring will be demonstrated, as in the right kidney here. This represents areas of parenchyma without normal function.

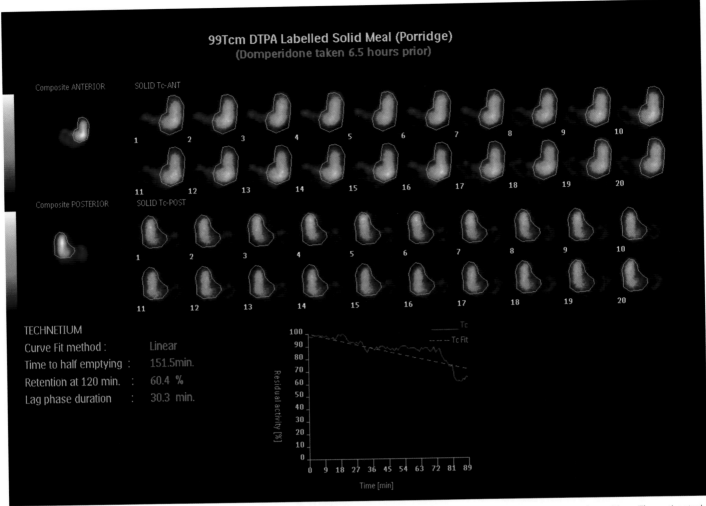

Figure 37.13 Demonstrating gastroparesis: food remains in the stomach for an extended period, causing chronic nausea and vomiting. The estimated half-time in this case is 151 minutes.

technique is less traumatic for paediatric patients as direct catheterisation is not necessary as in the conventional radiological method.

In contrast, ^{99m}Tc-DMSA (dimercaptosuccinic acid) is used to image the renal parenchyma, where the radiopharmaceutical is absorbed in the proximal convoluted tubules, thus being highly representative of functioning tissue. Its value is in being able to delineate areas of scarring (non-function) caused by infection, and localising ectopic kidneys which may have been absent on an ultrasound scan. Owing to its complete binding to the tubules there is no pelvirenal activity to denigrate the images, and it is especially useful in providing quantisation of relative renal function (Fig. 37.12).[18]

Gastrointestinal (GI) imaging

Radiolabelled food is used to image gastric motility. Technetium can be a recipe ingredient for scrambled eggs or porridge, enabling the gamma camera to visualise stomach and intestinal food transit. Abnormal motility is seen in patients with previous gastric surgery, and has many undesirable symptoms. By exploiting the quantitative abilities of nuclear medicine, a 'half-time' can be quoted for emptying gastric contents. The approximate normal half-time is quoted at 40 minutes for a solid meal[19] (Fig. 37.13).

Other problems associated with the GI tract are those of haemorrhage. Bleeding into the bowel can be imaged with technetium-labelled colloid or labelled red cells, where the 'pooling' of activity is representative of a GI bleed. Meckels' diverticuli can be a source of bleeding, where acid produced by ectopic gastric mucosa damages the bowel wall. As sodium pertechnetate is naturally taken up by gastric mucosa, this phenomenon can be used to advantage by highlighting suspect areas of ectopic gastric tissue within the whole abdomen. This enables confirmation of presence and location for subsequent surgical intervention.[20]

Nuclear cardiology

Conventional coronary angiography and CT angiography (CTA) are used to image the patency and location of coronary vessels. Nuclear medicine imaging has the ability to demonstrate functioning and non-functioning areas of the myocardium. Radiopharmaceuticals can be used to perfuse the left ventricular wall: underperfusion of a region of the left ventricle under exercise conditions will be indicative of a narrowing of the related diseased coronary artery or suggest previous damage from ischaemic events. A repeat examination some days later at rest will indicate whether the diseased area has perfused normally

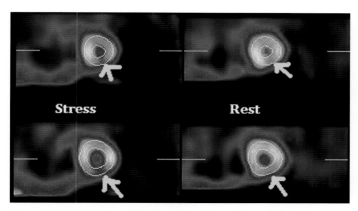

Figure 37.14 Axial slice of left ventricle with perfusion defect at 'stress' which perfuses normally on the 'rest' scan, confirming exercise-induced ischaemia.

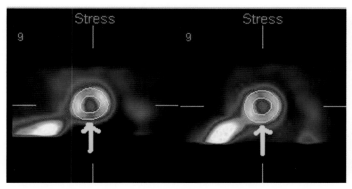

Figure 37.15 Effect of attenuation correction. Soft tissue attenuation 'losses' in signal in the image are compensated by the CT system, which corrects the image thus preventing a false positive result.

when not under stress conditions and is hence more likely to respond to revascularisation surgery; or if it remains unperfused, suggesting irreversible disease best managed medically (Fig. 37.14).

The stress test is now usually done pharmacologically, as it allows for better patient compliance and is more reproducible than dynamic exercise using a treadmill. Adenosine and dipyridamole are potent coronary artery vasodilators that increase coronary blood flow to levels similar to those achieved with maximal physical exercise. The relative ventricular perfusion between 'stress' and 'rest' is useful in differentiating reversible from non-reversible ischaemia in this scenario. Pharmacological stressing techniques allow the cardiac vessels to be imaged at maximum dilatation, highlighting decreased perfusion due to narrowing caused by arteriosclerosis, or indeed lack of myocardial uptake indicative of permanent damage.

Until recently some false positive results were inevitable owing to the attenuation of gamma rays during SPECT data acquisition. Modern SPECT-CT systems create an attenuation map of the patient which is then used to correct the original gamma ray image, to minimise error and improve diagnostic reliability (Fig. 37.15).

During the imaging procedure it is possible to also use the electrical signal from the beating heart to electronically 'gate' the SPECT acquisition. This allows the myocardium to be viewed as a beating entity to illustrate ventricular motion; left ventricular ejection fraction can also be estimated using this technique.

^{99m}Tc-MIBI (2-methoxyisobutylisonitrile) or ^{99m}Tc-tetrofosmin injected intravenously at peak stress, and at rest (on another occasion), will be trapped in the myocardium and will be representative of myocardial perfusion, with minimal redistribution prior to imaging. SPECT imaging then allows tomographic reconstruction in three planes, delineating areas of decreased perfusion due to ischaemia or infarction.

Ischaemic myocardium is sometimes stunned into inactivity functionally, which can seem to be non-viable on a stress and rest study. Evidence shows that stunned (or 'hibernating') myocardium can be successfully reperfused surgically, with a subsequent improvement in myocardial function in some cases.

^{201}Tl has the relative disadvantage of 'redistribution' over a short time period, which is undesirable for stress/rest imaging; however, this feature has been exploited in imaging the hibernating myocardium, as it diffuses into viable but apparently dysfunctional myocardium over a delay of 4 hours. Thus it is possible to delineate areas of suspected hibernating myocardium, to inform subsequent treatment and possible revascularisation.

Infection imaging

Radiolabelled white cells, mouse antibodies, ^{99m}Tc-HIG (human immunoglobulin) and ^{67}Ga can be used for imaging infection. The choice of radiopharmaceutical is usually made in the light of the medical history, and each has its own merit. The basic principle, however, is that the injected radiopharmaceutical will pool in an area of infection, and is especially useful in imaging infected orthopaedic hardware and pyrexia of unknown origin, where the whole body may be imaged.

Biliary system

Ultrasound and CT have largely taken over the role of imaging the liver, but ^{99m}Tc-HIDA (hepatobiliary iminodiacetic acid) continues to be the method of choice for imaging the biliary tree with suspected cholecystitis or biliary leakages postoperatively. Ultrasound is used for imaging calculi in the biliary system, but is not as consistent and specific as HIDA in the diagnosis of acute cholecystitis. The radiographic cholecystogram in this respect should be considered obsolete.[20] HIDA is also useful in imaging biliary reflux, and in the confirmation of biliary leakage following surgery.

Lymphatics

Technetium-labelled colloids can be used to image the lymphatic drainage. The technique is much easier to perform than a conventional lymphangiogram, and satisfactorily delineates areas of stasis (Fig. 37.16).

Another widely used lymphatic imaging method is in the localisation of the sentinel lymph node, which drains lymphatic fluid away from breast tumours and skin melanoma. If the sentinel node is localised and shown to be disease free, then clinicians can be fairly confident that the tumour has not spread via the lymphatics. As the node becomes radioactive surgeons can localise the small nodule using radiation-sensitive 'gamma probes' operatively, and remove it with minimal access required.

Neurology

^{123}I-labelled DATSCAN can be used to confirm Parkinson's disease in difficult cases: some individuals suffer from 'essential tremor', which mimics Parkinson's disease and can be misdiagnosed and treated inappropriately. DATSCAN has an affinity for dopamine transporters in the brain, with little uptake in the associated tissue, representing a confirmation of Parkinson's disease (Fig. 37.17A,B).

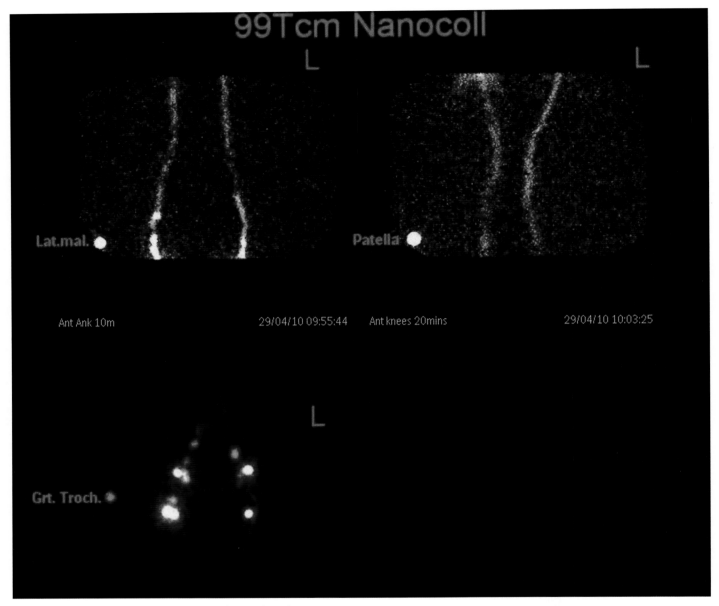

Figure 37.16 Normal free drainage from the feet to the pelvic area.

CLINICAL USES OF IMAGE FUSION IN SPECT-CT

There are many clinical uses for hybrid SPECT-CT imaging. A good example would be the use of ^{111}In-octreotide to target neuroendocrine tumours, which can occupy numerous sites in the body and are difficult to characterise with other imaging modalities such as CT or MR (Fig. 37.18A,B). Other examples would be to pinpoint a fracture of the wrist (Fig. 37.19), or relating cerebral blood flow on a brain scan to areas of normal anatomy, or clarifying apparent areas of hypoperfusion on the physiological image given by nuclear medicine with its corresponding CT slice showing, perhaps, atrophy due to age (Fig. 37.20).

PET AND PET-CT

PET imaging started several decades ago, using expensive dedicated imaging technology and requiring a nearby supply of specialist radio-pharmaceuticals from a particle accelerator (cyclotron). Because positron-emitting radiopharmaceuticals have quite short half-lives 'cyclotron–PET scanner' proximity became essential, and this often added to the cost of establishing a PET service. Cost restrictions and failure to show a clear value of PET imaging to the clinical routine meant its development was inhibited for many years.

On entering the 21st century PET started to become an essential tool for assessing tumour metabolic activity, so a more informed judge-ment could be made about treatment regimes. This drove the need for

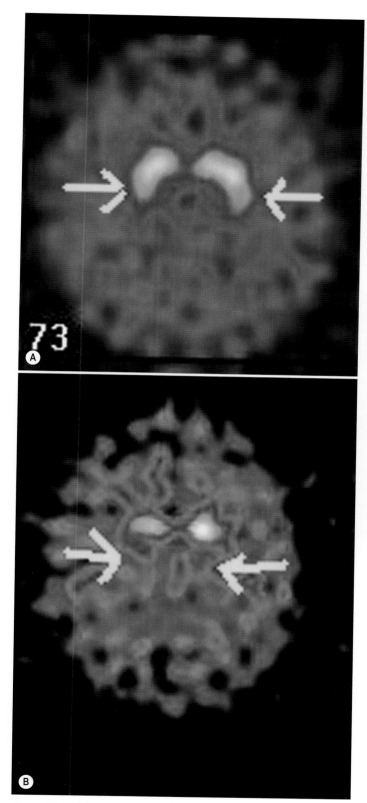

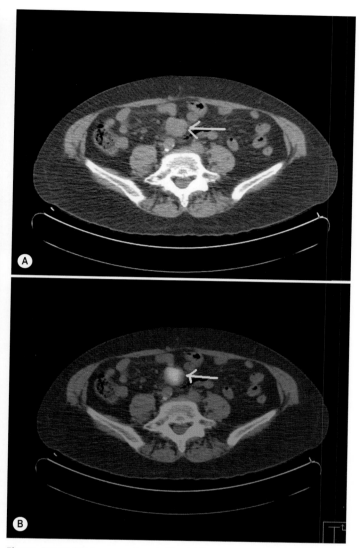

Figure 37.18 (A) A conventional CT axial image of the abdomen with a suspected 'carcinoid tumour'; (B) the fused ^{111}In octreotide image clearly characterising the lesion.

Figure 37.17 (A) Normal uptake of DATSCAN in the brain in an area associated with dopamine transporters; (B) reduced uptake associated with Parkinson's disease.

more accurate analyses of PET radiopharmaceutical uptake (quantification), and in this context the limitations of PET became apparent. In many cases mathematical models for accurate estimation of radiopharmaceutical absolute uptake proved unreliable for the required error levels, and so external radiation transmission sources were considered in order to generate attenuation maps to help correct for lost counts from deep within the patient. This eventually culminated in the creation of bespoke attenuation maps through CT machines which were physically attached to PET scanners. This fusion of two imaging modalities onto a single gantry is termed hybrid technology, and when used clinically it is commonly referred to as hybrid imaging. Today PET-CT is standard: a PET scanner simply cannot be bought without an integral CT system.

There are two types of CT machine for use in PET: low dose for attenuation correction, and diagnostic quality (the same as a standard CT machine located in an X-ray department). Of course the diagnostic-quality CT can also be used for attenuation correction. In terms of diagnostic-quality CT machines, these permit high-quality CT images to be generated and then fused directly to PET images. This process allows for the precise localisation of PET radiopharmaceutical uptake;

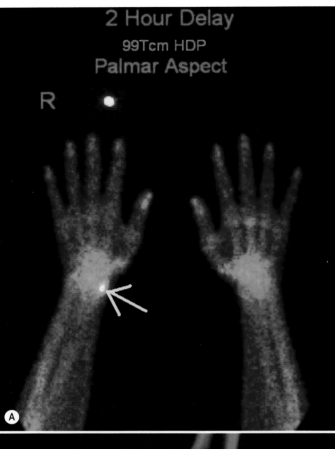

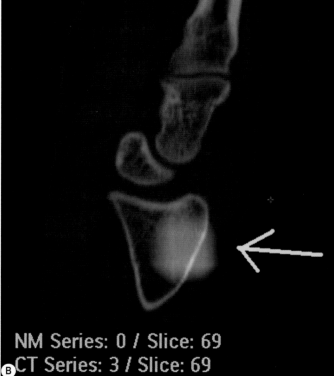

Figure 37.19 A suspected scaphoid fracture is hard to localise on the planar nuclear medicine image (A); however, fusion onto a CT scan clearly shows the fracture associated with the distal radius and not the scaphoid as thought (B).

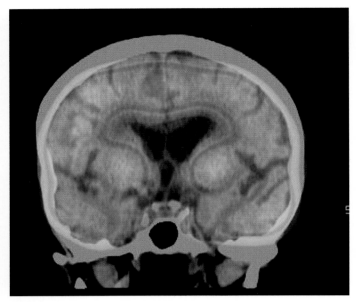

Figure 37.20 Normal cerebral perfusion with the underlying corresponding CT anatomical slice.

also when the diagnostic-quality CT image is viewed there is a chance to add into the PET report a CT report about the architecture and probable nature of any detected lesion. Not surprisingly, the combination of anatomical and physiological imaging is starting to provide a powerful tool in the diagnostic process.

The value and use of PET-CT imaging is evolving at a tremendous rate and there has been a proliferation of articles in the literature about its value. More recent literature surrounds its use in molecular imaging. There is the potential to detect preclinical disease (i.e. the patient has no signs or symptoms); when this is combined with molecular therapy (which might be radionuclide based) it presents as a powerful mechanism for the detection and treatment of disease.

In the UK, as a direct consequence of a government initiative, there has been steady growth in PET-CT imaging facilities. Because of their cost and the requirement for geographical accessibility for patients, in the first instance a high proportion of these clinical PET-CT services were provided on mobile scanners. Finance, clinical value and clinical demand will no doubt determine whether fixed rather than mobile PET-CT sites will increase in number.

SUMMARY

At present nuclear medicine imaging comprises a complex mixture of imaging systems, radiopharmaceuticals and protocols. Imaging systems have evolved significantly since the initial (static) gamma camera. Advances in camera technology and associated software have resulted in improved resolution (image quality), and in some instances a reduction in imaging time. Overall, this has provided the potential for improved diagnostic accuracy and increased patient throughput. To counterbalance this complexity and increasing clinical demand there has been a proliferation of multicamera departments. Generally speaking, year on year, there has been a steady increase in gamma camera studies, albeit with the introduction of complementary imaging modalities there has been a reduction in some specific imaging procedures at various junctures. A notable example of this is that gamma camera brain imaging went into decline when the CT scanner became a standard X-ray department feature.

In recent years the notion of using CT technology integrally with SPECT gamma camera technology has gained popularity. This was a direct consequence of the advances and discoveries made in PET-CT. SPECT gamma cameras can now be purchased with or without CT systems, and, like PET-CT, the CT scanners can be low dose (for attenuation correction) or diagnostic quality. In the UK there are currently around 100 such systems installed.

The final advancement in nuclear medicine imaging worthy of note is PET-MR – this represents the latest evolution in hybrid technology. Simultaneous acquisition of MR and PET data is achievable, and the ability to be used as a standalone MR scanner removes issues concerning productivity.[21] This hybrid technology is currently in its infancy, but commercial systems are already on the market. It is being used in research contexts, and it is likely that as with PET-CT and SPECT-CT there could be a growth in these scanners as robust research evidence emerges and finances permit.

Significant advances continue to be made in radiopharmaceutical design, for both therapy and diagnosis. A major challenge is presented to the nuclear medicine imaging community, and beyond, as to how to make effective use of the imaging tools. It has become evident that the personnel who operate the technology and interpret the images need to evolve too. Not so long ago imaging technologies tended to be discrete and isolated; more recently, PACS (picture archiving and communication systems) has permitted better proximity of different modalities in terms of image viewing and manipulation. With hybrid imaging now a reality, both at the point of acquisition and on subsequent viewing, there is a growing requirement for healthcare workers to have broader competencies, or at the very least to work in multiskilled interdependent clinical teams. Those professionals who support the clinical professionals need to consider their skill base and how the demands of these developing technologies can best be met.

REFERENCES

1. Bailey D, Adamson K. Nuclear medicine: from photons to physiology. Current Pharmaceutical Design 2003;9:903–16.

2. Cassen B, et al. Instrumentation for I-131 use in medical studies. Nucleonics 1951;9:46–50.

3. Brownell GL, Sweet WL. Localization of brain tumors with positron emitters. Nucleonics 1953;11:40–5.

4. Anger HO. Scintillation camera. Review of Scientific Instruments 1958;29:27–33.

5. Kuhl DE, Edwards RQ. Cylindrical and section radioisotope scanning of the liver and brain. Radiology 1964;83:926–35.

6. Kuhl DE, Edwards RQ. Image separation radioisotope scanning. Radiology 1963;80:653–61.

7. Sharp PF, et al, editors. Practical nuclear medicine. 3rd ed. London: Springer; 2005.

8. Alazraki NA. In: Resnick WB, editor. Bone and joint imaging – radionuclide techniques. 2nd ed. London: Saunders; 1996.

9. Ryan, PJ, Fogelman I. Musculoskeletal section. In: Maisey MN, et al, editors.

Clinical nuclear medicine. 3rd ed. London: Chapman & Hall; 1998.

10. Brown M, et al. Technical aspects of bone scintigraphy. Radiologic Clinics of North America 1993;31(4):721–30.

11. Mallinckrodt Medical BV. Summary of product characteristics 1996.

12. McKillop J, Fogelman I. Benign and malignant bone disease. Clinician's Guide to Nuclear Medicine Series (British Nuclear Medicine Society). Edinburgh: Churchill Livingstone; 1991.

13. Klemenz B, et al. The influence of differences in hydration on bone-to-soft tissue ratios and image quality in bone scintigraphy. Clinical Nuclear Medicine 1999;24(7):483–7.

14. Administration of Radioactive Substances Advisory Committee. Notes for guidance on the clinical administration of radiopharmaceuticals and use of sealed radioactive sources 2006.

15. Martin W, et al. In: Sharp P, et al., editors. Practical nuclear medicine. 3rd ed. London: Springer; 2005.

16. Coakley A, Wells C. In: Maisey M, et al, editors. Clinical nuclear medicine. 3rd ed. London: Chapman & Hall; 1998. p. 331–81.

17. Billotey C, et al. Advantages of SPECT in technetium-99-m-sestamibi parathyroid scintigraphy. Journal of Nuclear Medicine 1996;37:1773–8.

18. Testa H, Prescott M. A clinician's guide to nuclear medicine – nephrourology. Amersham: British Nuclear Medicine Society; 1996.

19. Harding L, Notghi A. In: Sharp P, et al, editors. Practical nuclear medicine. 3rd ed. London: Springer; 2005.

20. Harding L, Robinson P. Clinician's guide to nuclear medicine – gastroenterology. London: British Nuclear Medicine Society; 1990.

21. Siemens Healthcare. 2011. http://www.siemens.com/innovation/apps/pof_microsite/_pof-spring-2011/_html_en/biograph-mmr.html.

Chapter 38

Ultrasound

Rita Phillips, Julie Burnage, Barry Carver

INTRODUCTION

Since the introduction of ultrasound to medical imaging in the 1960s its popularity has grown and applications widened into numerous subspecialties of medicine. Excluding plain radiography, ultrasound scans are the most commonly undertaken diagnostic imaging examinations in England. Figures from the Department of Health show that the numbers of ultrasound scans (including obstetric and non-obstetric) more than doubled from 1996 to 2010.[1] In fact, there were more ultrasound examinations performed than computed tomography (CT), magnetic resonance imaging (MRI), fluoroscopy and radio-isotope examinations combined.

Historically the use of ultrasound was confined to the radiology department, but advances in ultrasound technology made this modality more accessible to other healthcare professionals, resulting in a widening of its application across all fields of medicine: for example, obstetrics and gynaecology, general medicine, urology, orthopaedics, vascular studies, anaesthesia, paediatrics, etc.[2-5] Sonography is not currently recognised in the UK as a profession in its own right and there is potential for this imaging modality to be misused. The use of ultrasound in diagnosis is highly operator dependent, and the greatest danger to a patient is the risk of diagnostic misinterpretation by an inadequately trained healthcare professional or the failure of the trained professional to maintain competencies. Not all sonographers are currently required/able to register with a regulatory body such as the Health Professions Council (HPC). However, the majority of practising sonographers are registered under their primary profession, for example radiographer, midwife, nurse or clinical scientist. The postgraduate training of these non-medical healthcare professionals in the UK has long since been standardised, with courses ratified by CASE (the Consortium for the Accreditation of Sonographic Education). In 2005 the Royal College of Radiologists (RCR) also published 'Ultrasound training recommendations for medical and surgical specialties' which set out the minimum standards to be achieved by non-radiological medical staff undertaking ultrasound scans as part of their working practice.[6]

EQUIPMENT CHRONOLOGY

1790   Spallanzani found that bats manoeuvre using hearing rather than sight.

1801   Young's work on light shows that waves can be combined to become stronger or cancel each other out.

1826   Colladon determines the speed of sound through water.

1880   Pierre Curie discovers the piezoelectric effect in crystalline materials.

1917   Langevin invents the hydrophone. The device was able to send and receive low-frequency sound waves through water, and was used to detect submarines in World War I.

1936   Siemens launch the Sonostat, a therapeutic ultrasound machine that used the heating effects on tissue.[7]

Early 1940s   Growth of use of A-mode ultrasound materials testing.

1942   Dussik publishes his work on transmission ultrasound of the brain; the first medical ultrasound publication?

Late 1940s   Ludwig studies the difference in sound waves as they travel through various tissues in animals, later applying these findings to human subjects.

1949   Wild assesses the thickness of bowel tissue and pioneers early developments in ultrasound.[8]

1951   Donald produces static, black and white B-mode scanning.

1954   Edler and Hertz publish their work on measuring cardiac movement.[9]

1958   Donald's equipment now able to demonstrate pathology in live volunteers. Publishes 'Investigation of abdominal masses by pulsed ultrasound'.[10]

1962   First contact B-mode scanner developed, commercially launched in 1963.

1965   Advances in materials technology enable improvements in equipment and the development of real-time images.

1972   First linear array scanners available.

1973   Grey-scale B-mode available; developing computer technologies make ultrasound faster, with improving images.

1974   Duplex pulsed Doppler.

1980s   Fast real-time scanners become widespread, enabling wider range of hospital-based clinical applications.
1984   First 3D fetal ultrasound.
1985   Real-time colour flow Doppler.[11]
1990s   Digital processing enables high-resolution imaging using broadband transducers. Image quality and improvements in accuracy further increase the role of ultrasound, particularly in breast imaging and cancer detection.
2000s   3D and 4D fetal and cardiac imaging becomes widespread; equipment featuring advanced system performance now widespread.

PHYSICAL PRINCIPLES

Sound is transmitted as series of longitudinal waves, vibrating the molecules within the medium through which it passes. The audible range of sound in humans is 20 Hz to 20 kHz; the waves used in ultrasound have a far greater frequency, typically >1 MHz, hence much greater frequency than audible sound.

As with sound and other wave propagation, the properties of an ultrasound wave are governed by the equation

$$v = f\lambda$$

where v is the speed of sound. This is dependent upon the transmitting medium: in the case of ultrasound this will depend upon tissue density and the compressibility of its structure. In soft tissues v has a relatively constant value of 1540 m/s, and this value tends to be assumed for all tissue.

f is the frequency. In ultrasound the frequency is determined by the transducer used, subject to some limited variation. In general higher frequency produces better resolution but reduced penetration.

λ is wavelength. In ultrasound penetration is proportional to wavelength, and wavelength is a determining factor for image resolution.

Production of the ultrasound wave

Curie demonstrated the piezoelectric effect in crystals such as quartz. When an alternating electric current is applied to the crystal it changes shape, and the resulting expansion and contractions generate a sound wave. This also applies in reverse: when a returning wave arrives at the crystal the resulting contraction and expansion generates an electric current, which can be read as a signal used to generate an image. The crystal in an ultrasound transducer is thus used both to transmit the wave and to receive the returning echoes.

Modern transducers use ceramic elements, in various configurations, to control the direction and depth of focus of the wave. It is undesirable for there to be a reflective interface between the transducer surface and the skin, as this would hamper penetration by the wave and the return of its echoes. To minimise this, the surface of the transducer has a coating sonically matched to skin; the application of ultrasound gel also assists in the elimination of this reflection.

Ultrasound wave interactions

As the ultrasound wave travels through the patient it will interact with layers between different tissues. These interactions will cause the wave to be attenuated, i.e. energy is lost as the generated wave traverses the patient. There are several mechanisms by which the wave is attenuated.

- *Absorption.* As the wave passes through the patient some of its energy is lost in the tissues through which it passes. The rate of absorption is dependent upon the tissue type and the frequency of the wave. The tissues are vibrated by the wave, producing heat. It is this heat that is used to advantage in therapeutic applications of ultrasound. In diagnostic applications the induced rise in temperature is a potential hazard.
- *Reflection.* The wave is reflected at tissue interfaces; some of these reflected echoes will return to the transducer, where they will induce an electric signal, forming the basis for the ultrasound image. The degree of reflection is dependent on the acoustic impedance mismatch at the tissue interface.
- *Acoustic impedance mismatch.* The acoustic impedance (Z) is a measure of how the wave traverses a particular tissue: $Z = v\rho$ where v is the speed of sound in the tissue and ρ is the tissue density.
  - The difference between the acoustic impedances at a tissue interface is termed the acoustic impedance mismatch. Minimising the mismatch (e.g. at the skin–tranducer interface) minimises reflection and maximises transmission. A large mismatch creates a lot of reflection with little transmission; the mismatch between soft tissue and air is such that this interface is almost impenetrable by the wave.
- *Refraction.* The wave may undergo refraction (change of direction) at a tissue interface if the wave front is not perpendicular to the interface. This phenomenon can cause misregistration and measurement artefacts.
- *Diffraction.* As the wave travels further from the transducer it becomes divergent, spreading the wave energy over a greater area and hence reducing its effective intensity.

Image formation

As the wave passes through the patient a proportion of it will be reflected back to the transducer. The vibrations caused when the reflected wave is incident on the transducer induce an electric signal, which can be used to form the image. The time taken for the echo to arrive indicates the depth of the tissue interface, and the size of the signal indicates the amount of reflection at the interface. This data is stored by the computer ready for processing.

When the signal is processed, many of the processing functions can be controlled by the sonographer to produce the required image. The quality of the image on screen is dependent on a competent practitioner manipulating the equipment controls and adapting their technique. However, the sonographer cannot influence the depth or the properties of the tissue that the waves must travel through, i.e. the characteristics of the patient, so there is usually a trade-off in the use of the best possible settings to optimise the image.

There are basic controls which can be used to optimise the ultrasound image. These include:

- *Transducer frequency selection.* A variety of transducers are available; on modern equipment they may be multifrequency. The higher the frequency of a transducer, the better the resolution, but at the expense of the depth of penetration.
  - The choice of transducer will depend on the case mix: high-frequency probes with a small footprint are required for small parts, cardiac, vascular and musculoskeletal applications (as these are superficial structures/organs); lower-frequency probes with a wider footprint are used for abdominal/pelvic assessments. An intracavity probe will be required for gynaecological or transrectal scans (Fig. 38.1).
- *Time gain compensation.* Amplifies signals that take longer to return (from deep interfaces) than those (from shallower interfaces) that return faster; this helps to counter the other

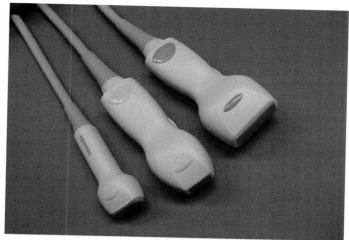

Figure 38.1 Image of transducers.
Reproduced with permission from Toshiba Medical Systems Ltd.

effects of attenuation, which reduce the signal more from a more distant reflection.

- *Overall gain.* Amplifies all returning signals to provide a signal sufficient for display.
- *Scan range/field of view*
- *Focus.* Can be used to provide improved resolution of particular structures
- *Dynamic range.* Can be used to improve image contrast by manipulation of the displayed grey scale
- *Magnification*
- *Zoom*

EQUIPMENT AND TECHNOLOGY

There are a wide variety of ultrasound machines available commercially, from small handheld pieces to laptop-sized portable machines and on to the larger, static departmental machines (Fig. 38.2). It is essential that the correct machine is available to practitioners based on the case mix to be scanned, the throughput of patients expected and the location. It would be inappropriate to expect a sonographer to use a handheld device to scan a list of 20 patients on a machine not much bigger than a mobile phone, but these are ideal for use in 'point of care' situations where a large static machine would be impractical. Whenever machines are to be purchased, it is essential that sonographers are consulted to ensure that the most suitable equipment is acquired.

Room requirements and ancillary equipment

Because of its portability, ultrasound scanning is frequently undertaken away from the imaging department. In the imaging department the requirements for a fixed room are: an appropriately sized and accessible lockable room with dimmable lighting (no natural light); air conditioning; a rise and fall couch; chair; saddle seat; desk; computer with PACS (picture archiving and communication system) connectivity/archiving facilities; wash basin; and adjacent toilet facilities.

A supply of appropriate consumables must be easily accessible: gel (to act as a coupling agent and enable the probe to slide across the skin), paper couch roll, gloves and condoms (including latex free), sterile gel for internal examinations, infection control consumables

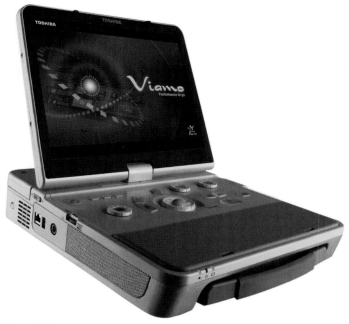

Figure 38.2 Image of portable ultrasound machine.
Reproduced with permission from Toshiba Medical Systems Ltd.

(probe wipes, general disinfectant wipes, hand sanitiser), and waste disposable facilities (for general and contaminated waste).

Where obstetric studies are undertaken a slave monitor is necessary to enable the parents to see the baby on screen without the sonographer having to scan in awkward positions, which has been shown to contribute to work-related upper limb disorder (WRULD) in the sonographer population.[12]

Imaging methods

Several different imaging methods are used in ultrasound imaging.

A-mode

Amplitude (A) mode was the first type of ultrasound to be used, but is rarely employed in imaging now. The received echoes are plotted with the x axis representing depth and the y axis the intensity of the reflected wave.

B-mode

In brightness (B) mode ultrasound the intensity of the reflected wave is represented on a monitor by the brightness of an individual pixel, rather than height on the y axis. An array of transducers simultaneously scanning a plane can be used to produce a 2D image of the scanned plane. Coupling this information with the position of the transducer enables real-time imaging to be produced. This is a dynamic process whereby images are updated at a fast rate to allow visualisation of movement. This is the most commonly used ultrasound technique. Real-time B-mode imaging gives information such as size, volume, shape, wall outline, internal architecture of organs and masses, relationship to adjoining structures, movement of organs and presence of fluid.

M-mode

Motion (M) mode is a variation in which rapidly generated pulses are imaged in succession: as interfaces move relative to the probe their velocities can be calculated. This mode is still used in echocardiography for assessing valve motion and timing.

Doppler mode

The Doppler principle is applied to evaluate blood flow in arteries and veins, and perfusion within an organ of interest. There are several types of Doppler ultrasound techniques in common use:

- *Continuous wave (CW) Doppler*. Electronically, the more basic CW Doppler involves using a transducer with two crystals in a simutanoeus transmission and reception of ultrasound waves; the difference between the transmitted and received frequencies is measured. This dual function can present a disadvantage as there is no information regarding the depth of the vessel being examined or the velocity of the blood flow, and may cause some difficulties in the interpretation of the results, particularly if the ultrasound beam encounters more than one blood vessel along its path. Typical examples of CW Doppler applications are fetal heart monitoring and echocardiography.
- *Pulsed wave (PW) Doppler*. PW is used to measure the velocity and direction of flow. PW uses a transducer that detects the shift in frequency between transmission and reception that results from the moving targets. The degree of frequency shift depends on the velocity and direction of flow relative to the transducer, the transmitted frequency, and the speed of sound of the tissue investigated. The main advantage of a PW transducer is that the operator can select a specific vessel, usually from a grey-scale image of a colour Doppler, to be investigated, called the sample volume, thus returning echoes from vessels outside this chosen sample volume are eliminated.
- *Colour Doppler imaging*. Generally used when additional information is required, such as a pattern of flow within a conventional B-mode image, e.g. perfusion of a specific organ, neovascularity, the direction of blood flow, or to highlight regions of interest such as jets and stenoses. A colour box (sample volume) is placed over the region of interest, the resultant flow is colour coded and is calculated by positive Doppler shift, shown as red for flow towards the transducer, and negative Doppler shift shown as blue for flow away from the transducer. There may also be shades of orange and yellow, either where there is turbulent flow or the Doppler settings on the ultrasound equipment are not set correctly. The transducer alternates between B-mode and colour Doppler imaging, updating each image. This is also known as duplex imaging.
- *Power Doppler*. Power Doppler maps the magnitude of the Doppler signal rather than the Doppler shift. Duplex imaging is used to superimpose a colour box onto a B-mode image, similar to colour Doppler. The resultant colour image is in shades of yellow, orange and red, depending on the strength of the Doppler signal (Fig. 38.3). This imaging mode is sensitive and therefore useful in detecting slow flow and flow through smaller vessels; however, unlike colour Doppler imaging there is no information on the direction of blood flow, and because of its sensitivity it is prone to motion artefacts.

Harmonic mode

In this mode a broad bandwidth transducer (i.e. a transducer capable of receiving a relatively wide range of frequencies) is used. A wave is transmitted at an initial, fundamental frequency, and interactions within the deeper tissues cause frequency shifts to harmonic frequencies. Harmonic frequencies are a multiple of the fundamental frequency. In harmonic imaging the information from the fundamental frequency is filtered out, therefore only the higher harmonic

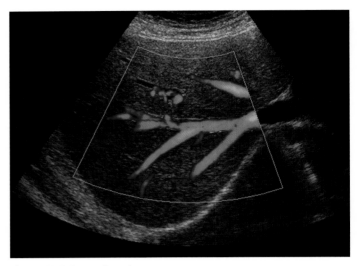

Figure 38.3 Power Doppler.

frequencies are used for image formation. Harmonic imaging offers several advantages over conventional imaging, including improved contrast resolution, reduced noise and clutter, improved lateral resolution, reduced slice thickness, reduced artefacts and improved signal-to-noise ratio (Fig. 38.4A,B). In general, harmonic imaging is useful when examining deeper structures and obese patients.[13,14]

Compound imaging

Real-time spatial and frequency compound imaging uses electronic beam steering to interrogate a structure from different viewing angles and at different frequencies. Several overlapping scans of the structure under investigation are obtained and averaged to form a multiangle compound image that is constantly updated in real time. Compound imaging improves image quality by reducing acoustic artefacts such as 'speckle', caused by coherent wave interference, and 'clutter', which can result from side lobes and reverberations. Applications include imaging of the breast, peripheral blood vessels and musculoskeletal injuries.[14,15]

Extended field of view (EFOV)

The advantage of EFOV is that larger organs or pathology can be seen in one single panoramic image. A real-time transducer is slowly swept along the area of interest, and successive images are interpreted and processed relative to the probe movement. It is most useful for superficial organs such as thyroid or breast, and for musculoskeletal imaging, where the entire length of a muscle and surrounding organs can be visualised (Fig. 38.5). Unfortunately, EFOV imaging is limited when there are other movements present apart from the transducer, e.g. fetal movements.[15]

Very high-frequency imaging and intracavity transducers

With the development of very high-frequency imaging the current imaging frequency range of between 1 and 15 MHz is increased by miniature transducers that will offer very high-resolution imaging at frequencies ranging from 20 to 100 MHz. These transducers can be placed within cavities to give high-resolution images of structures close to the cavity walls; examples of applications include transurethral, transoesophageal and intravascular scanning.[14,15]

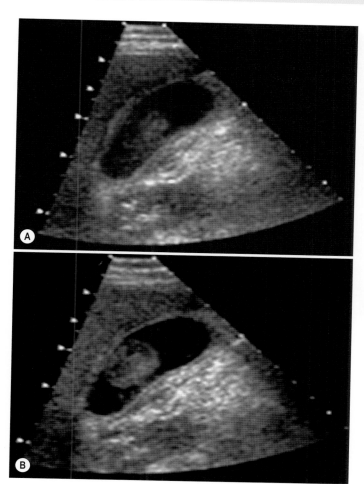

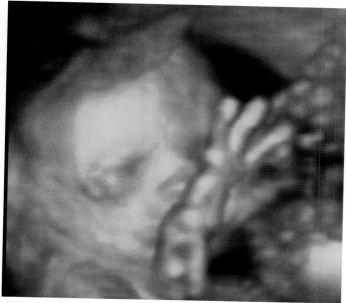

Figure 38.6 3D ultrasound.
Reproduced with permission from Ultrasound Now Limited.

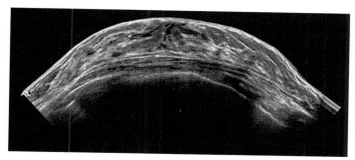

Figure 38.4 Harmonic imaging demonstrating improvement in image of the gallbladder. (A) Image without harmonic imaging; (B) image with harmonic imaging applied.

Figure 38.5 EFOV – scan of breast.
Reproduced with permission from Philips Medical Systems.

Sonoelastography

Sonoelastography is an ultrasound technique for imaging the relative elastic properties of soft tissue and, in particular, for differentiating between benign and malignant tumours. Low-frequency (100–500 Hz) low-amplitude shear waves (a transverse wave that occurs when tissue is subjected to a change in shape without a change in volume) are transmitted into tissue and the resultant vibration is detected using colour Doppler. When a discrete hard mass, such as a tumour, is present in a region of soft tissue, a decrease in the vibration amplitude will occur at its location.[14,15]

3D and 4D ultrasound imaging

3D ultrasound uses a dataset that contains a large number of B-mode 2D planes. Once the volume data is obtained it is possible to optimise the ultrasound image of the area of interest by rotating, reconstructing and rendering, allowing viewing in different planes and angles without further exposure of the patient to ultrasound, thereby reducing scanning times. Unwanted information can be 'sliced' out and the stored data can then be recalled and manipulated after the ultrasound examination.[16]

4D ultrasound is also known as 'real-time 3D ultrasound'. The basic concept is that the ultrasound equipment can acquire and display the 3D datasets with their multiplanar reformations and renderings in real time. However, 3D or 4D can only build on the 2D B-mode images, therefore the limitations and artefacts that affect B-mode imaging, such as presence of gas and overlying structures, will also affect the quality of the 3D and 4D imaging. The main advantage of 3D/4D is that this technique gives better visualisation of spatial relationships by multiplanar imaging, which is useful for therapeutic and follow-up examinations, and rendering abilities to convey information in a different manner (Fig. 38.6). Quantitative volume estimations can also be calculated more accurately than with conventional 2D scans. Despite these advantages, 3D and 4D ultrasound imaging is still considered a complementary tool rather than a replacement for 2D B-mode imaging.

Contrast-enhanced ultrasound (CEUS)

As in MRI, CT and conventional X-ray, the use of contrast media has enhanced the performance of ultrasound imaging. Ultrasound microbubble contrast agents are smaller than the mean diameter of a red blood cell, non-toxic, injectable intravenously, capable of crossing the pulmonary capillary bed after a peripheral injection, and stable enough to achieve enhancement for the duration of the examination. It is evident that CEUS facilitates improvement for the characterisation of focal liver lesions, detection of liver malignancy, guidance for interventional procedures and evaluation of treatment response after local therapies. However, the applications of CEUS have now expanded to other structures such as gallbladder, bile duct, pancreas, kidney, spleen, breast, thyroid, prostate and heart.

Ultrasound contrast agents are not only effective in ultrasonic imaging but are also important tools for the delivery of drug or gene therapy.[17,18] Furthermore, when the use of CEUS is combined with Doppler and harmonic imaging, sensitivity is greatly increased. The application of CEUS is continuously evolving; however, it should be noted that the insonation of gas-filled microbubbles has the potential to cause a number of biological effects, for example the induction of a physiological response to cardiac exposures (premature ventricular contractions), and damage at a microvascular level (microvascular rupture and subcutaneous haemorrhage).[19,20] The effect of insonation depends on the mechanical index (see section below on safety), the contrast agent used and the ultrasound imaging method. Although there is no proven evidence of harm resulting from clinical use of these agents, caution is recommended when contrast-enhanced imaging is undertaken.

SAFETY

It is important to highlight that although there is currently no absolute evidence that ultrasound imaging is harmful in humans, research has been carried out in laboratories and animal studies to investigate the effect of using high-intensity ultrasound.[21] These studies have found that two main changes occur in body tissues:

- *Thermal effect*. There can be a localised rise in tissue temperature owing to the ultrasound energy being absorbed and converted into heat. This effect is displayed on the ultrasound monitor as a thermal index (TI). For example a TI of 1 indicates a temperature rise of $1\,^{\circ}$C. This is particularly important in obstetric scanning during development of the embryo and fetus. Three forms of the TI may be displayed:
  - The thermal index for soft tissue: this is used when ultrasound only insonates soft tissue, as, for example, during obstetric scanning up to 10 weeks after the last menstrual period (LMP)
  - The thermal index for bone: this is used when the ultrasound beam impinges on bone at or near its focal region, as, for example, in any fetal scan more than 10 weeks after LMP
  - The thermal index for cranial bone: this is used when the ultrasound transducer is very close to bone, as, for example, during transcranial scanning of the neonatal skull
- *Cavitation effect*. This can occur in the presence of very high ultrasound pressures, causing oscillation of microbubbles which can result in biological damage to tissue cells. The likelihood of cavitation occurring is related to the peak pressure and is referred to as the mechanical index (MI)

For all ultrasound imaging techniques, prudent use is advised. Comprehensive guidelines on the safe use of ultrasound have been developed by the Safety Group of the British Medical Ultrasound Society;[22] these provide detailed advice on safe working levels for TI and MI. Adherence to these published guidelines and keeping exposure time 'as low as reasonably achievable' to produce an adequate image for interpretation and diagnosis will ensure that sonographers practise ultrasound imaging safely.

It is also important for the sonographer to assess the risk/benefit of not only the ultrasound examination, but also the imaging mode used, to minimise the unnecessary exposure of patients to ultrasound. For example, pulsed Doppler and colour Doppler imaging, with a narrow sample volume, carry a higher risk of thermal effects than a conventional B-mode examination, and the use of contrast agents can increase the potential for cavitation.

Health and safety of sonographers

The popularity of ultrasound and the reported increased prevalence of obese patients have affected the ultrasound workforce. The average time for sonographers to practise before experiencing work-related pain is 5 years.[5] Inadequate equipment, environment and workload planning all have a considerable impact on the potential occupational hazard to the sonographer, especially in WRULD and musculoskeletal injuries to the associated muscles, tendons and ligaments caused by continuous movements of a repetitive, forceful or awkward nature. In addition, regular use of visual display units, such as the ultrasound monitor and reporting workstations, increases the potential for vision fatigue.

Guidelines have been developed by professional bodies[5,23,24] after consultation with manufacturers, employers and sonographers to ensure appropriate working conditions and practices.

CLINICAL APPLICATIONS

Ultrasound is generally non-invasive and readily accepted by patients. It is relatively inexpensive, quick and convenient, and the absence of ionising radiation, or any other clinically significant biological effects, makes it an ideal modality to monitor changes over a period of time, e.g. in tumour growth or a progressive disease. It can be seen in real time, which is essential for dynamic studies, and it is especially useful during drainage and biopsy procedures. The ability to view several sections in one gentle sweep allows organs to be seen distinct from one another, and thus pathologies can be sited with accuracy. Structures can be seen in different planes, such as sagittal, transverse and coronal, and measured directly and accurately using linear, volume and circumferential measurements as well as measuring angles. It is also very suitable as a screening tool in applications such as antenatal screening and abdominal aortic aneurysm screening.

Ultrasound cannot be used for examining areas of the body containing gas or bone, making it of limited use in diagnosing gastrointestinal or skeletal problems, such as bowel pathology, lung lesions, fractures and adult brains. Ultrasound is not specific in diagnosing all pathology, therefore it is important to mention differential diagnoses; the previous and current medical history of the patient is vital to facilitate accurate interpretation. Images are also dependent on the characteristics of the patient: it is not always possible to obtain diagnostic images from patients with a high body mass index.

Technique

All sonographers will develop their own way of obtaining the information needed from a scan to enable interpretation and a clear and succinct report of findings to be written. What is essential is that the method is systematic and thorough.

The patient's identity is checked to ensure that the right patient is examined, as per local protocol. The sonographer must check that the patient has adhered to any requirements for the scan; for example, prior to an upper abdomen scan appointment the patient may be required to fast for 4–6 hours, and for gynaecological and renal tract scans they may be required to fill the bladder. The sonographer must explain the procedure in a manner which the patient can understand, and must state the limitations as well as the capabilities of the examination. Based on the information given, the patient should be asked whether they understand the procedure and if they are happy to proceed: this is the basis of informed consent.

The patient's clothes are protected either by asking them to change into a hospital gown or by the use of paper towels. The area to be examined is exposed and coupling gel applied. The sonographer must chose the appropriate transducer and then adjust the controls to optimise the image. The settings will be adjusted continually throughout the scan, based on the patient's body habitus and the emerging ultrasound findings, including normal variants and pathology. Depending on the area under examination, the patient may be required to move into different positions, such as left or right decubitus, prone, or sitting/standing upright.

Organs are not scanned in isolation, although there may be a request from a referring clinician; a good practitioner will take a clinical history before and during the scan, which will greatly assist them with their final report. There are minimum standards and guidelines for the archiving of images relating to specific scans. Although the images archived cannot prove that organs have been imaged in their entirety, a retrospective assessment of those images should enable a reviewer to determine that a scan has been undertaken with due care and diligence.

Upper abdomen

Ultrasound is often the first line of investigation for the diagnosis of upper abdominal pathology. For many patients an ultrasound scan will lead to a diagnosis, but a normal report may be just as useful to the referring clinician because the ability to exclude a large number of pathological conditions means that onward referral is made in a more appropriate and hence cost-effective manner.

A typical upper abdominal scan will include assessment of the liver, gallbladder, bile ducts, pancreas, kidneys, spleen, and the associated vasculature, and abdominal aorta.

Common clinical indications include:

- RUQ (right upper quadrant) pain
- Abnormal LFTs (liver function tests)
- Confirm/exclude gallstones/renal calculi/organomegaly
- Abdominal aortic aneurysm (AAA), haematuria and investigations into nature of palpable masses

The minimum images to be recorded should include:

- Left lobe of liver: sagittal section (SS) and transverse section (TS)
- Pancreas (ideally demonstrating head, body and tail): TS
- Abdominal aorta: SS/TS
- Right lobe of liver: SS/TS. The size of the liver is based on a measurement from the right hemi-diaphragm to inferior border in the midclavicular line
- Right lobe of liver: through the porta hepatis
- Gallbladder: SS/TS
- Common bile duct: measurement at widest point
- Both kidneys: SS/TS
- Spleen: SS/TS

Common pathology

The liver parenchyma is normally homogeneous and of a similar reflectivity to the renal cortex. Focal lesions can be readily identified, measured, and their blood flow assessed using Doppler. Diffuse pathology such as cirrhosis and fat infiltration, and focal lesions such as simple cysts, haemangiomas and metastases, can usually be confirmed or excluded (Fig. 38.7A,B).

Ultrasound should be the initial investigation for suspected focal pathology. It can demonstrate metastases with varying ultrasonic appearances, but despite there being some correlation between

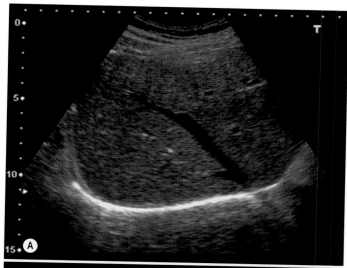
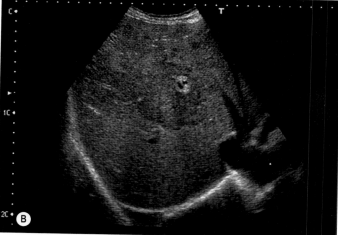

Figure 38.7 (A) Normal liver showing right hepatic vein; (B) liver with tumour demonstrated.
Reproduced with permission from Toshiba Medical Systems Ltd.

appearances and the primary site (such as highly reflective lesions possibly arising from a gastrointestinal primary), there are many differential appearances. Some metastases can show the same reflectivity (isoechoic) as normal hepatic parenchyma and may be missed.

In cases of jaundice, ultrasound can confirm surgical jaundice by the presence of dilated intra- and extrahepatic ducts, as distinct from medical jaundice which appears essentially normal. The level of obstruction can often be clearly demonstrated by the level at which the ducts or gallbladder are seen to be normal. For example, a dilated common hepatic duct and intrahepatic ducts with a normal or small gallbladder and common bile duct would demonstrate a high obstruction of the cystic duct or above, while a fully dilated biliary system would indicate an obstruction at the lower end of the bile duct. If the pancreatic duct was dilated as well, an ampullary/head of pancreas obstruction may be indicated. However, in early cases of obstruction changes to duct calibre may be subtle.

The common bile duct can be seen and assessed for normality, but the distal portion is often quite difficult to see owing to the gas-filled duodenum. As a consequence, calculi and other pathology in this section of the common bile duct are difficult to detect. Endoscopic ultrasound (EUS) can improve detection where distal pathology is suspected.

Ultrasound is an excellent tool to accurately and safely guide a biopsy needle to the area of tissue required for sampling. The needle tip is scanned as it enters the body, and can be seen in real time as it approaches the lesion or tissue required. Careful technique is required, but continual monitoring of the needle tip can avoid the unnecessary penetration of vessels or organs during the procedure.

Gallbladder

Ultrasound is the method of choice in the initial investigation of the biliary system and has long replaced the oral cholecystogram. Preparation for a hepatobiliary ultrasound scan involves the patient fasting for 4–6 hours in order to fully dilate the gallbladder. Gallbladder volume can be calculated using a formula based on three measurements, although most machines have built-in volume calculations. In addition, variations in shape (Phrygian cap, septate, double), position (intrahepatic, low lying), wall thickness and relevant pathology, such as gallstones, biliary sludge, polyps and tumours, can all be observed.

If the examination is urgent and there has been no time for fasting, a scan of the biliary system can still take place, albeit with the caveat that a contracted gallbladder can occur as a result of eating recently as well as because of pathology.

The flexibility of ultrasound allows patients to be scanned in different positions according to need, not least to image the organs but also to confirm or exclude the adherence of a mass to the inner wall of the gallbladder (calculi move freely within the gallbladder lumen unless impacted; polyps and tumours adhere to the lumen). The ability to turn the patient during the scan can help to stretch the neck of the gallbladder and allow better visualisation of that area in order to exclude impacted calculi. Unlike plain radiography, which will only show about 10% of gallstones unless outlined by contrast media as in the oral cholecystogram, ultrasound sees all calculi as being similar, irrespective of composition. Higher frequencies and accurate setting of focusing zones will demonstrate smaller calculi and their characteristic posterior shadowing, although the shadow will not be seen if the calculus is only partially scanned in the beam thickness (Fig. 38.8).

In 95% of cases of acute cholecystitis there is a calculus impacted in the neck of the gallbladder. The gallbladder can necrose and perforate if not treated with antibiotics to control inflammation. However, in acute cholecystitis after surgery, extensive burns, major trauma and parenteral nutrition there can be an absence of calculi; therefore, the absence of calculi on an ultrasound scan is insufficient to exclude acute cholecystitis. Radionuclide imaging is more sensitive here.

Cancer of the gallbladder is the fifth most common gastrointestinal malignancy and is associated in many instances with the presence of gallstones. Ultrasound has the ability to identify concomitant gallstones and the irregular wall thickening of a malignancy or bulky polypoidal mass. Colour flow Doppler and B-mode imaging can be used to investigate invasion and obstruction of biliary/portal vessels by tumour and spread to the liver.

Pancreas

Ultrasound can discern a normal pancreas, especially in normal-sized patients, and can evaluate the lower end of the bile duct through the head of the pancreas. The pancreatic duct can be measured and dilatation excluded or confirmed, dilatation implying distal obstruction. Acute and chronic inflammatory conditions, calcification and pseudocyst formation can be seen, as can tumours in the head and body of the pancreas. Tumours in the tail of the pancreas, albeit significantly less common, are more difficult to see owing to gas in the stomach. In some cases the patient can be asked to drink water to fill the stomach so as to create an acoustic window through which the pancreatic tail can be visualised. CT and MRI are useful in cases of necrotic and severe pancreatitis. MRCP (magnetic resonance cholangiopancreatography) is less invasive than ERCP (endoscopic retrograde cholangiopancreatography) and is excellent at assessing patients in whom pancreatitis is suspected.

The pancreas is harder to see in patients with more adipose tissue, and in these cases CT will show the anatomy more clearly. CT will also show calcification in the pancreas more clearly in chronic pancreatitis, although EUS has excellent sensitivity for detecting biliary microlithiasis. EUS is good for detecting pancreatic tumours, although MRI is best for staging tumours. However, EUS is good at staging many upper gastrointestinal malignancies, e.g. in the oesophagus, stomach, duodenum, duodenal ampulla and bile ducts. In addition, EUS can allow safe fine needle aspiration (FNA) under ultrasound control. Spiral CT and EUS have similar accuracy in staging pancreatic cancer.

Urinary system

In any examination of the urinary system ultrasound can be used to confirm the presence of two kidneys, their size and location. Variations in kidney shape and size can be observed, from the absent kidney on one side with a corresponding hypertrophy of the contralateral one, to cross-fusion anomalies, of which the horseshoe kidney is the most common. Differences of 15% or more between the kidneys can be significant. Renal volume can be calculated, normal parenchymal thickness can be observed and measured, and normal contours confirmed (Figs 38.9, 38.10).

In cases of haematuria, ultrasound with a plain abdominal X-ray is used as the first-line investigation of the urinary tract; the source of the blood can be from a renal, bladder or prostate tumour, or less clinically serious conditions such as renal calculi.

Ultrasound is able to see hydronephrosis and its severity as it has 95% sensitivity, which can help in assessing the level of obstruction. The use of colour Doppler can exclude a pseudohydronephrosis, caused by prominent renal vessels seen on B-mode. Renal calculi can be seen on ultrasound, especially when the kidney is scanned slowly and carefully; if the calculi are not too small they are identified by their highly reflective appearance and posterior acoustic shadowing. They can be clearly seen in the renal pelvis when outlined by urine, but are less obvious when situated in the calyceal system without urine around them, as both structures are highly reflective and the calculi

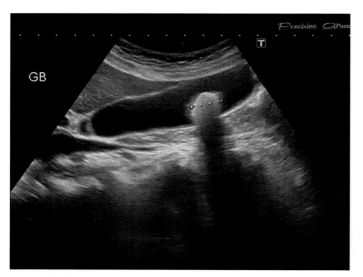

Figure 38.8 Gallbladder demonstrating calculus.

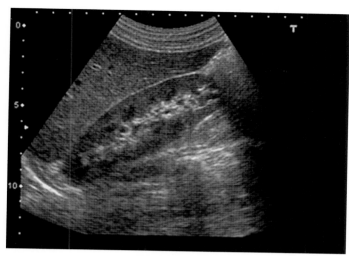

Figure 38.9 Longitudinal view of right kidney.
Reproduced with permission from Toshiba Medical Systems Ltd.

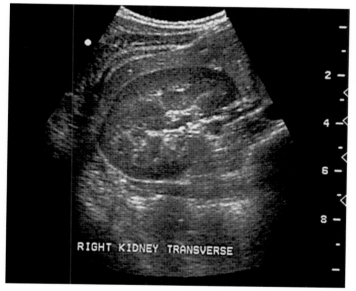

Figure 38.10 Transverse view of right kidney.
Reproduced with permission from Philips Medical Systems.

are often indiscernible. The sensitivity of ultrasound in detecting renal calculi is higher than that of abdominal radiography but lower than of CT.

Ureteric calculi, a common cause of obstruction, are rarely seen on ultrasound as the ureters can only normally be seen when leaving the renal pelvis and on their insertion into the bladder, owing to overlying intestinal gas obscuring the mid-ureters. Patency of the ureters can usually be implied by the presence of ureteric jets, the appearance of the passage of urine into the bladder seen at their insertion at the base of the bladder by grey-scale or colour Doppler. Colour Doppler can be useful in scanning the renal vascular system and is used to image, with spectral Doppler to analyse, the renal arteries in 80–90% of cases. Obesity and overlying stomach and bowel gas sometimes prevent imaging of the renal vessels, particularly on the left. Colour Doppler is helpful in diagnosing renal vein thrombosis and is the accepted first line of investigation for renal artery stenosis.

Renal lesions can often be demonstrated, the most common being simple cysts, which are seen in 50% of patients over 50 years of age

and are frequently asymptomatic. Ultrasound is used to screen those in patients with adult polycystic disease. CT and MRI are useful for staging and assessing more complex solid and cystic lesions initially seen by ultrasound.

In suspected renal cell carcinoma ultrasound is usually the primary imaging modality to confirm tumour presence and size. Colour or power Doppler is used to assess renal vein and inferior vena cava (IVC) tumour involvement. CT/MRI is used subsequently for staging and treatment planning. Small tumours are increasingly being detected incidentally at an early stage on ultrasound, and subsequent venous invasion is less commonly seen.

If it persists for more than 72 hours, infection of the renal system is investigated by ultrasound to exclude any complications such as abscess or obstruction.

Transplant kidneys can be monitored with a higher frequency because of their superficial position, meaning that less depth penetration is necessary to visualise them. B-mode real-time scanning is useful in excluding obstruction caused by impinging postoperative haematomas or lymphocoeles, and demonstrating fluid collections such as urinomas. Renal vein thrombosis or stenosis can be excluded with colour Doppler ultrasound.

Contrast-enhanced CT is superior to ultrasound in determining the extent of post-traumatic abnormalities, although ultrasound is often used to assess the kidneys along with other organs in the trauma situation.

Adequate hydration is essential preparation for demonstrating the bladder. For adults, drinking 0.5–0.75 L of water 1 hour before the due time of the scan allows the bladder to be distended. Ultrasound can clearly demonstrate the bladder wall and any pathology inside, such as tumours (fixed irregular masses), calculi or foreign bodies (normally seen with associated posterior shadowing). Ultrasound is useful in being able to measure the bladder wall thickness when distended and when empty, and can demonstrate residual volume after micturition. Transitional cell carcinomas (the most common bladder tumour) can be detected along the posterior wall near the trigone. Bladder diverticula can also be assessed easily with ultrasound and any contents of the diverticula imaged. Ureterocoeles are easily detected by ultrasound and are seen as dilated ends of the distal ureters protruding into the bladder at the region of the trigone.

Prostate

Any enlargement of the prostate, a common cause of bladder distension in older men, can be seen transabdominally by scanning in a caudal direction at the base of the bladder. Scanning in this way will only give an indication of the size of the prostate; it can be measured and translated into a volume and subsequently into a weight. Outline and reflectivity and whether calcification can be seen are almost the limit of transabdominal prostate scanning.

Transrectal sonography of the prostate, requiring a specially designed intracavitary probe, gives more detail of the prostate gland, but despite hopes of it becoming a screening tool for detecting prostate carcinoma its sensitivity is still only in the region of 60%. In addition, it is not specific enough to assume that any focal lesion is malignant, so the transrectal scan usually accompanies a prostatic biopsy for accurate sampling. 70% of cancers are darker (hypoechoic) and 30% are brighter (hyperechoic) than the normal part of the gland; 75% are situated in the peripheral zone. Classically, a prostatic cancer should be hypoechoic and in the peripheral zone, but only 20–30% of lesions here are actually cancers; the rest are inflammatory patches, atrophy, fibrosis and benign prostatic hyperplasia. Digital examination and prostate-specific antigen tests in addition to biopsy are more common methods of assessing a problematic prostate than imaging alone. CT/MRI is used for subsequent follow-up of confirmed prostatic cancer in order to stage and treat the disease.

Spleen

The spleen is usually scanned as part of the whole upper abdominal examination in conjunction with the liver in portal hypertension, left upper quadrant pain, suspected splenic infection, and when an enlarged spleen is found at clinical examination. It is also useful as an acoustic window in order to see the tail of the pancreas and upper half of the left kidney. Ultrasound can be used to measure the length of the spleen from the left hemidiaphragm to the inferior border: 13 cm is usually used as an upper limit of normal. In cases of trauma, ultrasound is invaluable for detecting haematoma; it can detect splenic lacerations and ruptures, but is less accurate than contrast-enhanced CT. However, there is the advantage of being able to bring ultrasound to the patient in unstable cases.

Ultrasound is useful in detecting cysts; these are usually the result of trauma and haematoma formation. In Hodgkin's or non-Hodgkin's lymphoma 25–33% of patients have splenic involvement. Appearances can be diffuse, focal or multifocal, most of which are of low reflectivity. Splenomegaly is usually present in about two-thirds of these patients. In lymphoma patients up to one-third of enlarged spleens are benign in nature. Biopsy of the spleen can be performed to differentiate between a lymphoma and a metastatic lesion, or to diagnose an infective process such as candida or tuberculosis; but given the highly vascular nature of the spleen biopsy is not commonly performed, as the risk of haemorrhage is high.

Lymph nodes

Ultrasound is able to detect lymph node enlargement, depending on location and size. Enlarged lymph nodes are often seen in the upper abdomen, para-aortic region, neck and axilla. In cases of mesenteric lymph node enlargement, ultrasound is useful in differentiating nodes from bowel loops by observing normal peristaltic movements. Enlarged lymph nodes are often the cause of a 'palpable lump', and taking a history from the patient is useful in these instances.

Aorta and inferior vena cava (IVC)

Ultrasound is used to scan both the great vessels in the abdomen. The IVC is examined with ultrasound and colour Doppler in cases of newly found renal tumours and suspected IVC thrombosis. However, it is the aorta that is examined in far greater numbers. Ultrasound is useful for the detection and monitoring of abdominal aortic aneurysms (AAA) and for measuring their diameter and length. Extension of the aneurysm to the common iliac arteries can also be seen if present. Siting of the aneurysm relative to the renal arteries is also possible by ultrasound, but is more accurate by CT and MRI, especially in larger patients. Thrombus can be seen clearly (Fig. 38.11).

Doppler can sometimes be used to assess leakage after endovascular stent grafting, showing as areas of blood flow outside the lumen of the graft but inside the walls of the aneurysm. Colour Doppler can image aortic dissections by demonstrating flow in both channels: these are sometimes seen on an initial B-mode ultrasound examination, but it is not the modality of choice as intimal flaps are difficult to demonstrate. Aortic rupture is difficult to image owing to overlying bowel gas, although in a patient whose blood pressure is dropping and with fluid in the peritoneal cavity seen on ultrasound there is a high likelihood of rupture. CT is the modality of choice for detecting a ruptured aorta, but the emergency situation often precludes the use of CT and the patient is taken to theatre on clinical evidence alone, although as point of care ultrasound is undertaken in many A&E

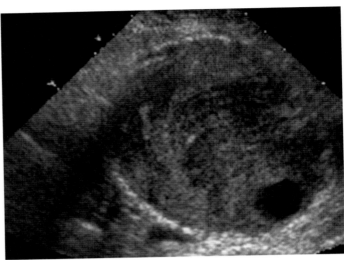

Figure 38.11 Transverse section of abdominal aortic aneurysm (AAA).

departments there is less time wasted in trying to get the patient to the imaging department.

In April 2009 the roll-out of a national screening programme for AAA began, its aim being to reduce deaths from AAA by early detection. The programme aims to invite all men for screening in the year they turn 65, offering either treatment or monitoring, depending on the size of any aneurysm found:[25]

- The aorta has a diameter of less than 3 cm: No aneurysm has been detected. The patient is informed of the result and will not require any further scans.
- The aorta has a diameter of between 3 and 5.4 cm: Patients with a small aneurysm do not need treatment but are invited to have follow-up scans at specific times to monitor the aneurysm.
- The aorta has a diameter of 5.5 cm or more: The patient is referred to a vascular surgeon.

AAA screening is undertaken by technicians whose training takes 3–6 months; they are supported and mentored by qualified sonographers and/or vascular technologists.

Alimentary canal

Although ultrasound is historically not the imaging modality of choice for bowel examinations the resolution of modern systems and their safety and accessibility means that it does play an important part in the diagnosis and monitoring of certain inflammatory bowel conditions such as Crohn's and colitis. The sensitivity and specificity will obviously depend on the location of the disease, as some parts of the bowel are more accessible to ultrasound: the terminal ileum and left colon are easier to visualise than the rectum or upper small intestine, for example.

Ultrasound is used in the diagnosis of suspected appendicitis with an overall sensitivity of 94% and a specificity of 91%.[26] A threshold of 6 mm and larger diameter of the appendix under compression is the most accurate ultrasound finding for appendicitis. It can be used in cases of intussusception and in the evaluation of pyloric stenosis.

Ultrasound has the advantage of being able to differentiate between gynaecological and bowel masses. The ability to see peristalsis, assess blood flow in the wall, lumen diameter and bowel wall thickening contributes to the successful integration of ultrasound in bowel imaging. Endoscopic ultrasound is used in the detection and staging of upper gastrointestinal malignancies, including in the oesophagus, stomach, duodenum, extrahepatic bile ducts and pancreas. Biopsies

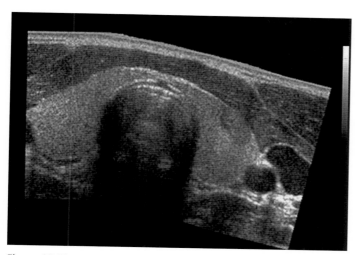

Figure 38.12 Image of thyroid.
Reproduced with permission from Philips Medical Systems.

and FNA can be undertaken accurately during an EUS scan because of the proximity to the structures under investigation. EUS is more accurate than CT or MRI in the staging of oesophageal cancer.[27]

Superficial organs: 'small parts'

High-frequency transducers in the region of 7–12 MHz are generally used for small parts imaging, as these structures lie superficially and therefore there is no requirement for increased penetration.

Thyroid

Ultrasound can visualise the lobes, isthmus, anterior and posterior muscles and main vessels (common carotid artery and internal jugular vein) during a scan of the thyroid gland. Common indications are: abnormal TFTs (thyroid function tests), enlarged thyroid, confirm/exclude multinodular goitre.

As the probe used has a small footprint it is not always possible to see both lobes on one image, and in those situations having a machine with EFOV capability is useful. The ultrasound appearances of benign and malignant disease are not always clear; however, the generally accepted rule is that the characteristics of benign disease are of a hypoechoic/isoechoic nodule with cystic elements, whereas malignant disease is characterised by solid, hypoechoic lesions with microcalcifications and cervical lymphadenopathy. Microcalcifications seen on ultrasound show the highest accuracy, specificity and positive predictive value for malignancy as a single sign.[28] The use of ultrasound-guided FNA greatly increases the accuracy of diagnosis. CT and MRI are used to assess the local extent of spread of malignant disease (Fig. 38.12).

Neonatal head

Ultrasound, being mobile, can be used to scan an infant in a special care baby unit either in or out of an incubator. With a high-frequency probe the infant brain can be scanned through the anterior fontanelle until between approximately 9 and 15 months, when the fontanelle closes.

Immediately after birth, or for the first 4 days in premature babies, the germinal matrix can haemorrhage owing to its rich vascular supply being disrupted by change in blood pressure. In skilled hands ultrasound can detect intraventricular haemorrhage, hydrocephalus and some parenchymal bleeds. Monitoring the appearances can detect the occurrence of periventricular ischaemia and periventricular leukomalacia. Fast MRI scans are used when more complex anomalies are investigated.

Neonatal hip

Using a 5.0–7.5 MHz linear probe, developmental dysplasia of the hip can be confirmed between 3 and 6 weeks according to appearances and measurements taken of the acetabulum, femoral head and ileum. Dynamic studies can be performed by real-time ultrasound to demonstrate instability while the hip is manipulated. Partial or complete dislocation can be demonstrated.

Radiographs have the obvious inherent problem of ionising radiation, and are difficult to interpret until the infant is 6–12 weeks old as it is difficult to see the cartilaginous head. A radiograph also is only a record of the hip joint at one time with the infant supine; an ultrasound scan, as a dynamic physical examination, is a far more comprehensive assessment of the hip during a range of movements. Ultrasound can also detect hip effusions and be used to guide a needle into the joint space to drain fluid if required.

Breast

The use of ultrasound in breast imaging is discussed in Chapter 26.

Testes

Ultrasound is the primary modality for the investigation of the scrotum. As with all superficial structures a linear-array high-frequency probe is required; however, in cases where there is a large scrotal mass, one or both testes may be displaced and it may be necessary to use a lower-frequency probe to find the testicle, which may have been displaced out of the FOV of the higher-frequency transducer. Common clinical indications are a palpable lump, pain, trauma, testicular/scrotal enlargement and varicocoeles.

Tumours are well seen as they are of a different reflectivity from the main body of the testis. Comparison with the unaffected side should always be made, because some tumours can infiltrate the whole testis and so there would be no difference in echotexture visible unless comparison was made with the contralateral side.

Epididymal cysts are the most common cause of scrotal lumps in patients presenting for ultrasound, and the patient can be reassured that these are not life-threatening.

Testicular microlithiasis can be seen and has a high association with malignancy. Where microlithiasis is demonstrated, the importance of regular review should be stressed to the patient. Ultrasound can be used to detect an undescended testis, which is important because of the markedly increased incidence of testicular cancer in such cases. The missing testis is usually found in the inguinal canal, although it can also be sited in the abdomen. If it is not demonstrated then consideration must be given to surgery to locate it, because of the high risk of testicular cancer.

Musculoskeletal

Ultrasound is increasingly used in the diagnosis of musculoskeletal disorders as higher-resolution equipment can give excellent detail of muscle, fat, ligaments, tendons and cartilage, and detect soft tissue masses. Using EFOV a muscle can be visualised in its entirety. Ultrasound can be used to image most joints, the shoulder (rotator cuff injuries), wrist, elbow and knee being the most common. Modern equipment provides better spatial resolution than MRI and has the benefit of being able to scan during a dynamic movement.[29]

Ultrasound can demonstrate complete tendon and muscle tears, but is less accurate in cases of partial tears. It can also demonstrate inflammation, differentiate solid/cystic/complex masses and determine whether the mass shows vascularity. It can help to locate foreign bodies in the extremities and identify fluid collections. The use of ultrasound in drainage procedures and joint injections is well documented.

Vascular

Vascular ultrasound is a subspecialty of ultrasound imaging and is largely performed by sonographers who are accredited by the Society for Vascular Technology of Great Britain and Ireland. Vascular ultrasound is performed to assess the blood flow to organs and tissues, locate and identify stenoses and abnormalities such as plaque or emboli, detect thrombi in the legs or arms, and assess the suitability of patients for procedures such as angioplasty. Follow-up scans can be performed to evaluate the success of procedures such as grafts or blood vessel bypass. Vascular screening programmes include carotid artery stenosis, aortic aneurysm and peripheral arterial disease.

Echocardiography

The majority of echocardiography examinations are performed by cardiac technicians rather than generic sonographers. The British Society of Echocardiographers provides accreditation for those undertaking cardiac scans.

Ultrasound is used to image the heart and surrounding structures. It is helpful in establishing diagnoses and the severity of various acquired and congenital cardiac diseases. Information can be obtained about the size of chambers, cavity volumes and wall thickness. Mass lesions in the heart and outside, as well as the accumulation of pericardial and pleural fluid, can also be easily detected. Applying Doppler principles, further evaluation regarding heart function, for example the pumping power-ejection fraction and heart valve movements, can also be made under stress conditions. Ultrasound imaging includes the use of M-mode, B-mode and 3D imaging. Techniques to acquire diagnostic images include transthoracic, transoesophageal, intravascular and intracardiac approaches. Contrast echocardiography with the injection of microbubbles can be used as an adjunct to conventional techniques.

To facilitate imaging of the heart through a narrow acoustic window to avoid attenuating structures such as ribs and lungs, dedicated cardiac transducers with small footprints are usually used.

EMERGENCY ULTRASOUND

Advances in equipment development have seen portable ultrasound equipment with excellent imaging capabilities, which means that ultrasound can easily be used away from the imaging department. Focused abdominal sonography for trauma (FAST) scanning, when performed by suitably qualified staff, can facilitate timely diagnosis in potentially life-threatening cases, such as patients who are haemodynamically unstable and have intra-abdominal haemorrhage, or to assess for pericardial effusions in cases of potential cardiac problems. Immediate decisions can be made for further patient management.

FAST looks at four areas for the presence of free intraperitoneal fluid and cardiac tamponade:

- Perihepatic and hepatorenal space
- Perisplenic
- Pericardium
- Pelvis

In addition to focused scanning in blunt abdominal trauma, ultrasound contributes to other aspects of emergency care, such as AAA, foreign body localisation, abscess location and gynaecological emergencies.

Emergency ultrasound in gynaecology

Gynaecology patients presenting to the A&E department usually do so with acute pelvic pain or vaginal bleeding. The first line of investigation is clinical palpation and a pregnancy test for women of childbearing age, usually to exclude/confirm a pregnancy, followed by a pelvic ultrasound scan.

In the case of a non-pregnant patient, acute pain can be the result of ovarian torsion, torted cyst, ruptured ovarian cyst, torted pedunculated fibroid or appendiceal abscesses. This results in haemorrhage and/or the presence of free fluid in the pelvis, especially in the pouch of Douglas (rectouterine pouch) or surrounding an ovary. These can be useful ultrasound indicators.

In some cases there may be echoes within the free fluid that represent blood or pyogenic material, as may be in the case of pelvic inflammatory disease (PID). Patients usually complain of bilateral low abdominal pain. Ultrasound findings include free fluid in the pouch of Douglas along with a hydrosalpinx or pyosalpinx, and tubo-ovarian abscess.

In the pregnant woman the role is primarily to exclude an ectopic pregnancy by the identification of intrauterine implantation, and secondly in the detection of an extrauterine gestation sac or ruptured ectopic pregnancy, when pelvic free fluid from a ruptured corpus luteus cyst or ectopic pregnancy may be demonstrated. In equivocal findings, quantitative serum beta human chorionic gonadotrophin (beta-hCG) assays and subsequent ultrasound scans are vital for patient assessment and management.

GYNAECOLOGY

Gynaecological ultrasound is used in the assessment of the uterus, endometrium, ovaries and fallopian tubes. Other structures can also be visualised during a pelvic scan, such as the vagina, cervix, bowel, pelvic vessels and musculature, and the urinary bladder. It is also used to locate intrauterine contraceptive devices and to exclude postoperative complications such as pelvic haematoma and abscesses. One-stop gynaecology clinics with ultrasound as a first-line investigation have made patient management more streamlined and effective. The use of ultrasound is also invaluable in infertility studies.

Different ultrasound techniques are used for obstetric and gynaecological scans; these include transabdominal, transvaginal, transrectal, intraoperative, transperineal/labial examinations, as well as spectral and colour flow Doppler.

The endometrium and ovaries are dynamic organs that undergo changes throughout a woman's life, and on a day-to-day basis in cases of women of childbearing age. Therefore, before any interpretations and diagnosis can be made, it is imperative that the sonographer is aware of factors such as:

- Patient's history: age and menstrual status, i.e. prepubertal, premenopausal, menopausal and recent cycle history
- Clinical indications: abdominal distension; palpable pelvic mass; abnormal vaginal bleeding; pelvic pain; dyspareunia, amenorrhoea, dysfunctional menstrual bleeding and postmenopausal bleeding
- Gynaecological history: including any previous gynaecological surgery that must be known, as must medication such as the oral contraceptive pill, hormone replacement therapy (HRT) and

tamoxifen, which may have an influence on the appearances of the ovaries and the endometrium

In women of childbearing age the results of a recent pregnancy test should always be sought to rule out the possibility of pregnancy-related complications, such as an ectopic pregnancy.

Technique

The two main approaches to pelvic ultrasound examinations are transabdominal and transvaginal. The decision as to which one to use must be evaluated according to the clinical indications, the information required and the suitability of the patient. As a general rule, both methods are advised to give a comprehensive approach to the scan in terms of gross pelvic anatomy, position of the ovaries, presence of large pelvic/abdominal masses, and detailed assessment of the uterus, endometrium, ovaries and any tubal pathology. 3D techniques are useful in the diagnosis of uterine anomalies, the assessment of tubal patency, and in detecting intrauterine, endometrial and ovarian pathology.[30]

In cases of significant pelvic pathology such as large pelvic masses or suspected malignancy, distant associated pathology should also be excluded. These include hydronephrosis, lymphadenopathy, and the presence of ascites. The combination of these two approaches can also aid in the detection of non-gynaecological pathology such as appendicitis, diverticular disease, inflammatory bowel disease, e.g. Crohn's disease, and pathology such as ureteric calculi and bladder tumours in the case of the urinary tract.

The main pitfalls in gynaecological ultrasound are inadequate patient preparation, such as an empty or overdistended bladder in the case of transabdominal scans, or a full or partially full bladder in the case of a transvaginal scan, resulting in artefacts such as reverberations or loss of visualisation due to increased distance between the pelvic organs and the transducer. Inadequate history taking can also lead to misdiagnosis or overdiagnosis.

Bowel shadowing can be problematic in not only obscuring the relevant organs but also in mimicking some pathology. In these cases patience is required to observe the peristalsis in the bowel, or gentle abdominal pressure should be applied to the area of interest to disperse gas in the bowel. Indeed, in some cases the opposite may occur and pathology can mimic bowel; this is common in the case of dermoid cysts owing to the heterogeneous echo pattern resulting from the contents of the cyst. Previous adhesions resulting from surgical interventions, PID or the presence of non-ultrasound detectable endometriotic deposits can be problematic in the assessment of pelvic organs owing to their resultant immobility.

Transabdominal scans (TAS)

This mode of scanning offers a wide field of view, but to visualise the uterus and ovaries adequately a full bladder is required to displace the overlying bowel gas and lift organs out of the pelvic cavity. It also straightens the uterine long axis so that it can lie perpendicular to the transducer ultrasound beam. A TAS uses frequencies in the range of 3–5 MHz, depending on the subject characteristics. This can result in a poorer resolution than with TVS, especially in obese patients and has also the potential to miss small pathologies. Recent advances in transducer technology have allowed an EFOV so that large pathology can be related to other anatomical landmarks.

Transvaginal scans (TVS)

Owing to the proximity of the organs to the transducer a higher frequency can be used, ranging from 6 to 8 MHz. This gives an increased resolution, which is essential when evaluating endometrial thickness or assessing ovarian architecture. The need for a full bladder is eliminated, making the examination more comfortable for the patient. Superior images are gained, especially in obese patients and those with retroverted uterus. However, this examination is not always appropriate, as some patients can perceive it as invading their privacy, and informed consent must be sought because of its intimate nature. Therefore, it may not be suitable for minors, women who are not sexually active, and individuals who are not able to give informed consent. It also has an added disadvantage in that the narrow FOV makes it difficult to image high and lateral organs and to distinguish the absolute margins of a large pelvic mass.

Assessment of the uterus

The uterus can be assessed for its size, shape and outline as it undergoes normal physiological changes with age. Ultrasound is useful in diagnosing uterine congenital abnormalities, such as bicornuate uterus, didelphic (double uterus), unicornuate and septate uterus; it can indicate the presence of serous or intramural fibroids. Changes in the myometrium can be demonstrated, but adenomyosis – the presence of endometriotic deposits within the myometrium – is at times difficult to detect except in the classic cases of an enlarged uterus with low reflective deposits located within the myometrium (Fig. 38.13A,B).

Endometrial assessment

The endometrium is best visualised with a high-resolution TVS. It should be assessed with the knowledge of the patient's menstrual history: this is particularly important in the presence of abnormal vaginal bleeding. In a menstruating woman the endometrial thickness and echo pattern vary according to the menstrual cycle: the upper limit of normal varies with different studies, but is in the region of 14–20 mm. Vaginal bleeding in a postmenopausal woman can be a cause for concern, as there is a higher incidence of endometrial malignancy (Fig. 38.14); however, in the majority of these women there will be a benign cause for the bleeding, such as hyperplasia or polyps. The upper limit of normal for a postmenopausal woman varies with different studies, but is reported to be in the region of 4–5 mm. Measurements below this limit will reliably exclude any significant endometrial pathology, although in the presence of HRT this value is more like 8 mm, and 10 mm in the case of tamoxifen therapy.

Whereas transvaginal ultrasound demonstrates the morphological characteristics of the endometrium (thickness, integrity, presence of intracavitary masses, fluid), transvaginal colour Doppler enables the assessment of blood flow velocity and vascular impedance in cases of endometrial carcinoma, and of vascular resistance in the uterine arteries and its branches. It also has the ability to provide additional information, such as abnormal endometrial perfusion. The accuracy of TVS will be further increased with new technological advances such as 3D sonography, allowing endometrial volume assessment.

Infertility

Ultrasound is used to exclude the presence of pathology that may be the cause of infertility. Conditions such as endometriosis, chronic PID and multiple fibroids, and endometrial pathology such as polyps, may all play a part in the prevention of successful implantation of the embryo. Ovulatory disorders resulting from ovarian dysfunction can also be assessed; these include polycystic ovaries (Fig. 38.15) and failed luteal-phase follicular rupture. It is important to remember that ultrasound is not specific in these cases.

Contrast studies such as hysterosalpingo-contrast sonography have been successful in replacing the conventional hysterosalpingogram in the assessment of tubal patency and the uterine cavity. An obvious

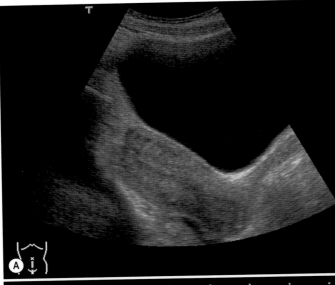

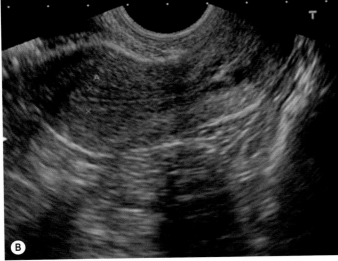

Figure 38.13 (A) Longitudinal TAS – uterus; (B) longitudinal TVS – uterus.

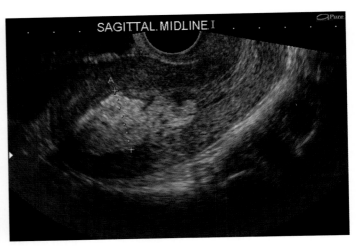

Figure 38.14 Endometrial carcinoma.

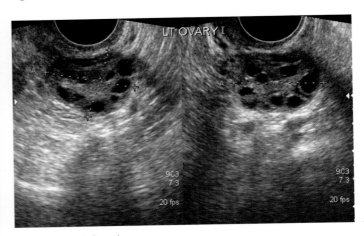

Figure 38.15 Polycystic ovary.

advantage is that it is safe, as it uses non-ionising radiation. Saline can be introduced into the endometrial cavity to outline any pathology, such as polyps, submucosal fibroids or adhesions, and contrast medium can be introduced into the uterine cavity and observed to determine tubal patency.

Ultrasound is a useful tool in monitoring the development of ovarian follicles following stimulation by drug inducement. It can determine the size and number of follicles, the timing of ovulation, and assess endometrial response. These observations, along with serum hormone monitoring, also help prevent ovarian hyperstimulation and avoid the possibility of multiple pregnancies of a large order.

In IVF studies ultrasound is primarily used as a guide in the process of aspiration of the mature follicles. After successful conceptions/implantations, ultrasound can be used to determine the number of gestational sacs and embryos and to exclude ectopic pregnancies.

Ovarian assessment

The size and texture of the ovaries depend on the reproductive status of the patient: for example, in the prepubescent patient immature follicles can be visualised within the ovaries. After menarche these follicles can be visualised maturing, with the development of a dominant follicle measuring between 2.0 and 2.5 cm in diameter before ovulation. In the postmenopausal patient the ovaries appear atrophied, with no evidence of follicular activity.

Ultrasound is sensitive in detecting ovarian pathology; however, further features, such as wall thickness, echogenicity, posterior enhancement/shadowing and internal architecture, all aid in deriving differential diagnoses such as dermoid cysts (Fig. 38.16), endometrioma, Brenner cysts, cystadenomas and cystadenocarcinomas. Sonomorphologic scoring systems have been derived when looking at these features to assess ovarian tumours.[31]

Occasionally, pathology not related to the ovaries can be detected, such as paraovarian cysts, pedunculated fibroids and broad ligament cysts. Further assessment of adnexal and tubal masses can be improved using Doppler and 3D.

Screening for gynaecological malignancy

Screening for early ovarian cancer in asymptomatic and high-risk women using ultrasound and CA125 have been evaluated in the last decade; currently there is no conclusive evidence to suggest an impact on survival rates.[32] Similarly, with endometrial assessment there is no evidence to date to support endometrial screening.[33]

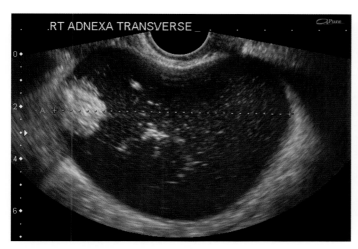

Figure 38.16 Ovarian dermoid.

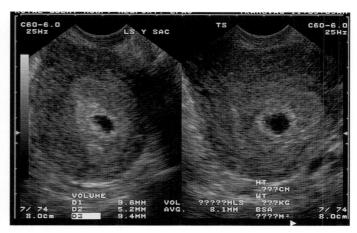

Figure 38.17 Gestational sac measurements in three planes. *Reproduced with permission from Toshiba Medical Systems Ltd.*

OBSTETRICS

The scope of prenatal scanning has undergone a significant change since its introduction in the 1980s. Its primary use then was to reduce obstetric risk to the mother and fetus by correctly estimating gestational age, placental localisation, and excluding multiple pregnancies; and to effectively manage pregnancy by monitoring fetal growth and wellbeing in the presence of abnormal clinical findings and maternal disease such as diabetes and hypertension.

As imaging technology has evolved there has been an increased focus on its use as a screening modality in terms of structural and chromosomal abnormalities through anomaly and nuchal translucency (NT) scans. This has created additional requirements for training and expertise, particularly with regard to ethical concerns and prenatal counselling. The UK National Screening Committee has recommended minimum standards for the provision of antenatal screening that all pregnant women should be offered, and these are set out in the 'model of best practice'.[34]

Overview of fetal biometrics

Evaluating large groups of fetuses with normal growth patterns has led to the development of standard tables and curves of fetal measurements. These can be used as a reference to assess fetal gestational age and growth patterns.[35]

Gestational sac

This is the first measurement of early pregnancy. The gestational sac is measured in three planes and a mean sac diameter (MSD) calculated. This measurement is useful between 5 and 8 weeks' gestation with an accuracy of ±0.5 week, and is usually performed in the absence of an ultrasonically demonstrable fetal pole (Fig. 38.17). Later on, as well as a fetal pole, other structures such as the yolk sac and amnion can also be recognised.

Crown–rump length (CRL)

NICE guidelines have advocated the use of this method of dating a pregnancy, as it is more accurate than the traditional Naegele's rule of calculations from the first day of the LMP. Specific criteria have been developed for the measurement of CRL, in order to improve

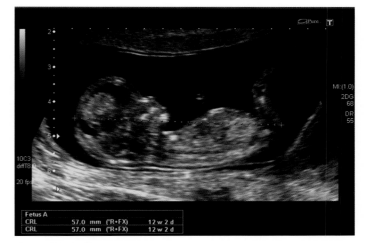

Figure 38.18 CRL measurement.

the accuracy of this method, thereby contributing to the effective management of preterm and post-term pregnancies, as both these conditions are associated with higher rates of perinatal morbidity and mortality than pregnancies delivering at term.

CRL is performed by measuring the longest axis of the fetus in the sagittal plane with the fetus in a neutral position, gestational age accuracy being ±3–5 days (Fig. 38.18). The main pitfall is including the yolk sac in the measurement during early pregnancy, resulting in overestimation of the gestational age. There is also the potential to under- or overestimate the CRL owing to the flexion or extension of the fetal spine, therefore this measurement is not advised after 14 weeks.

Fetal head measurements: biparietal diameter (BPD) and head circumference (HC)

These measurements are taken at the widest diameter of the fetal head, transversely across the parietal bones, and are used to determine gestational age after 14 weeks. The presence of identifiable landmarks such as the cerebral hemispheres, cavum septum pellucidum and lateral ventricles makes these robust measurements for repeatability, although the accuracy decreases with increasing gestational age (14-week accuracy is ±1 week; 30 weeks is ±3–4 weeks).

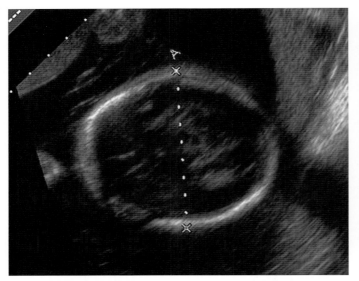

Figure 38.19 BPD measurement.
Reproduced with permission from Toshiba Medical Systems Ltd.

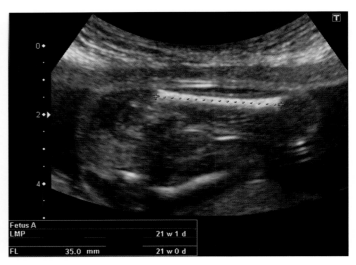

Figure 38.21 FL measurement.

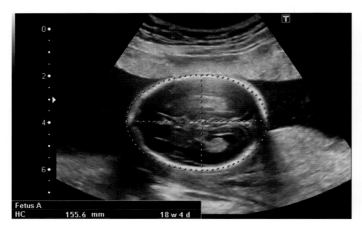

Figure 38.20 HC measurement.

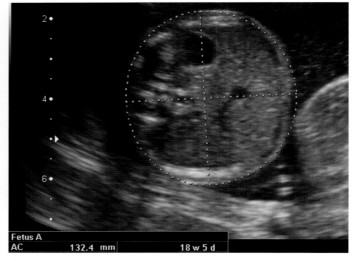

Figure 38.22 AC measurement.

As head size is dependent largely on fetal brain development, these measurements are less affected by conditions such as placental insufficiency and are often spared in fetal growth restriction. When there is evidence of fetal head growth restriction it is usually associated with symmetrical growth retardation as a result of genetic, toxic or infectious factors, or microcephaly.

The accuracy of BPD measurement is dependent on the shape of the fetal head, and can result in under- or over-estimation in the presence of fetal head moulding (Fig. 38.19). The fetal HC is therefore a more reliable measurement, as it allows for variations in fetal head shape (Fig. 38.20).

Femoral length (FL)

This has the same accuracy as a BPD measurement and is reliable in the second trimester if an HC measurement is not possible. It can be affected by skeletal dysplasias, but on the whole, as with fetal head measurement, inconsistencies are usually associated with intrinsic fetal problems (Fig. 38.21).

Abdominal circumference (AC)

This measurement is obtained through the fetal liver, at the level of the left portal vein and stomach (Fig. 38.22). It is crucial in the assessment of fetal growth and wellbeing. Deficiencies in nutrient storage, such as subcutaneous fat and liver glycogen, will reduce this measurement in the setting of maternal/placental insufficiencies, resulting in a 'starved' fetus. The opposite occurs in conditions such as maternal/gestational diabetes, where elevated blood glucose levels result in increased metabolic storage and increased fetal subcutaneous fat, causing macrosomia.

In the presence of such abnormalities serial AC measurements are required to monitor the fetal growth pattern; this is also the case for multiple pregnancies for growth patterns and concordancy, in order to plan pregnancy management.

The ratio of head measurement and abdominal measurement is also used to identify symmetrical/asymmetrical growth patterns.

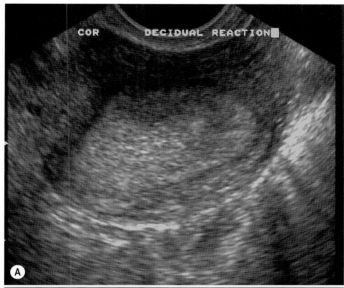

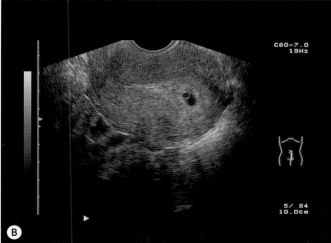

Figure 38.23 (A) Decidual reaction in the uterus; (B) 5-week gestational scan with yolk sac.
Reproduced with permission from Toshiba Medical Systems Ltd.

First trimester

The main aims of a first trimester scan are:

- to exclude an ectopic pregnancy
- to confirm ongoing pregnancy, especially in the setting of vaginal bleeding and pain
- to date the pregnancy accurately by establishing gestational age and estimated date of delivery when menstrual history is inadequate. Factors such as infertility treatment and use of oral contraceptives are important in establishing gestational age and vital for post-term pregnancy management

Decidual reaction can be visible within the uterus as early as 4 weeks, with the presence of a gestation sac at 5 weeks. The gestation sac should be eccentrically placed, with the presence of a yolk sac and amnion within the sac (Fig. 38.23A,B). This observation can help distinguish between the pseudosac of an ectopic pregnancy or fluid collection in the cavity and a true gestation sac.

An early dating scan can also exclude a multiple pregnancy, or determine the amnionicity and chorionicity of multiple pregnancies

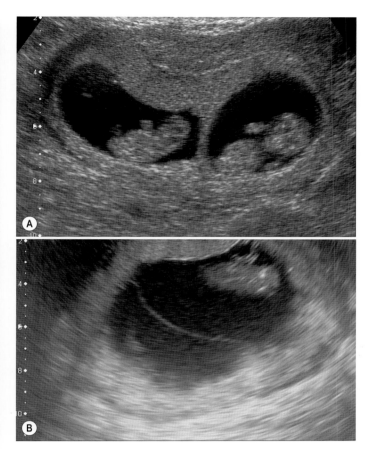

Figure 38.24 (A) Lambda sign, dichorionic; (B) T sign, monochorionic.

in order to aid appropriate management. This is important, as monochorionic twins are at higher risk of fetal structural anomalies and of developing complications such as twin-to-twin transfusion sydrome and intrauterine growth restriction. Sonographic criteria used in the diagnosis of chorionicity are the Lambda sign, which is present when there is placental tissue between the amniotic membranes; the T sign, where there is no placental tissue between the amniotic membranes, suggesting that there is a single placenta; and the thickness of the inter-twin membrane (Fig. 38.24A,B).

Early pregnancy assessment

Early pregnancy assessment can be performed in one-stop clinics designed to streamline the service and select appropriate patient management, thereby eliminating the need for unnecessary admission. These units provide an outpatient service aimed at women who have experienced bleeding in the first trimester. The role of ultrasound is to confirm an ongoing intrauterine pregnancy, or diagnose a failed pregnancy such as missed miscarriage or incomplete miscarriage. Follow-up studies for women presenting with bleeding in the first trimester have shown that 17% of these women had a subsequent miscarriage, but when there was a yolk sac and fetal heart activity 95% of pregnancies proceeded to term.[36]

Gestational sac volumes and MSD can be calculated to aid estimation of gestational age before a fetal pole can be demonstrated. These measurements are also useful in the diagnosis of an anembryonic pregnancy (blighted ovum), where there is an absence of fetal pole or embryonic parts. Once a fetal pole is visualised, fetal heart pulsations should be demonstrated and recorded with M-mode scanning. A CRL is measured to establish gestational age.

Early pregnancy assessment guidelines for diagnosing an early pregnancy failure are MSD of 20 mm or more without evidence of embryonic parts; an empty amnion sign; CRL of >6 mm with no heart activity; or an absence of growth of the gestational sac or fetal pole after a 7–10-day interval.[37,38] Recent studies advocate the use of conservative management in the case of early pregnancy failures, and report a decrease in the incidence of dilatation and curettage induced infection, and the prevention of adhesions and Asherman's disease, which can complicate future pregnancies.[39,40]

Trophoblastic disease, such as complete hydatidiform moles and partial moles, can also be detected with ultrasound in the first trimester. These women present with an enlarged uterus, elevated levels of beta-hCG, vaginal bleeding and hyperemesis. Typically on ultrasound the uterine cavity is filled with trophoblastic tissue with swollen villi presenting as cystic areas. There may or may not be a fetal pole, depending on whether there is a complete or a partial mole.

Occasionally, fluid collections around the gestational sac are detected during the ultrasound scan. These can be for reasons such as implantation bleeds, subchorionic, chorioamniotic and intra-amniotic haematoma, and can be a cause of bleeding in the first trimester. However, the presence of these does not necessarily affect prognosis, although further or prolonged bleeding is experienced in the presence of these findings.

Screening for chromosomal abnormalities

Between the CRL measurements of 45 and 84 mm (11–14 weeks ±1 day) the NT is a reliable screening parameter for chromosomal deviations, namely trisomy 21, trisomy 18 and trisomy 13.[41] NT is defined as the maximum thickness of the subcutaneous area between the skin and the soft tissues overlying the cervical spine (Fig. 38.25).

The UK National Screening Committee (NSC) suggest that a detection rate in the region of 90% with a false positive rate of <2% can be achieved when screening for Down's syndrome.[42] This can be achieved with a three-phase test, but up to 80% can be successfully screened in the first trimester by a combined test where the risk is calculated by combining the NT measurements with biochemical markers in the maternal blood, such as beta-hCG and PAPP A (pregnancy-associated plasma protein A), maternal age, previous obstetric history and fetal gestational age. The advantage of this test is that the results are available before 14 weeks' gestation, which allows for early decision making by the parents.

To enhance detection rates, the combined test can be integrated in the second trimester with a further four markers: alpha-fetoprotein, total hCG, unconjugated oestriol and inhibin-A. However, this test requires the woman to attend twice and the final result will only be available after the second attendance. The 'model of best practice'[34] recommends that the first trimester combined test should be preferred for Down's screening, with the quadruple test for women who present late for booking after 14 weeks.

There have been some further developments that involve looking at the cell free fetal DNA in the pregnant mother's blood to identify genetic disorders in the developing fetus, e.g. fetal mesenchymal stem cells. These non-invasive prenatal diagnosis (NIPD) tests are very much in the early stages of development, and more research is needed to explore the effectiveness and feasibility of NIPD before incorporating them into routine practice.[43]

Increased NT is also associated with other non-chromosomal conditions such as cardiac defects, diaphragmatic hernias and skeletal dysplasia.[41] Further research has identified other useful markers to improve the detection rate for trisomies 21, 18 and 13, for example absence of or hypoplastic fetal nasal bone, tricuspid regurgitation, ductus venosus, and fetal heart rate.[44]

In multiple gestations NT measurements are also useful. In dichorionic gestations discordance for NT thickness is a useful marker for chromosomal and other abnormalities. In monochorionic gestations

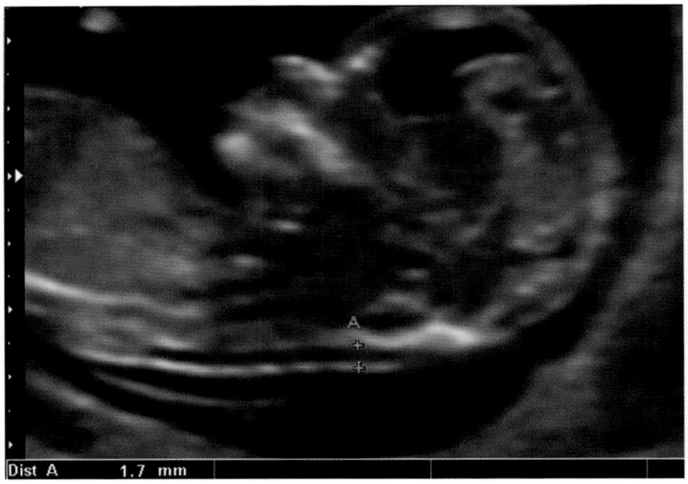

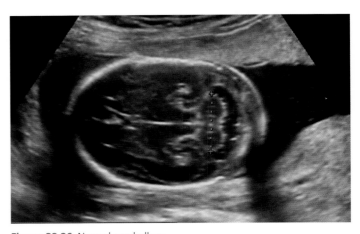

Figure 38.26 Normal cerebellum.

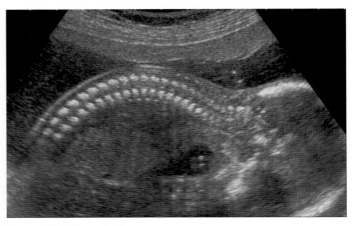

Figure 38.27 Normal spine.

Dist A   1.7 mm

Figure 38.25 NT measurement.

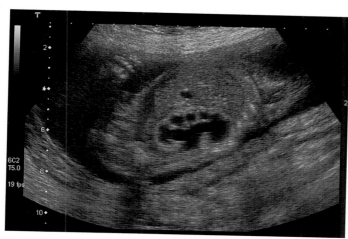

Figure 38.28 Hydronephrotic kidney.
Reproduced with permission from Toshiba Medical Systems Ltd.

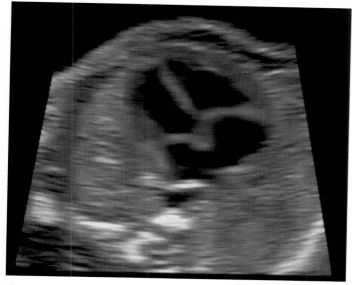

Figure 38.29 Four-chamber view of the heart.

it appears to be a useful marker for potential complication of twin-to-twin transfusion syndrome. With increased image resolution, TVS are also reported to be effective in screening for structural anomalies in the first trimester. These include anencephaly, cystic hygroma, hydrops, renal anomalies, anterior wall defects and skeletal dysplasias.

Second trimester

Routine prenatal screening for structural abnormalities in the second trimester is now accepted as a normal procedure. The timing of the second trimester scan is usually taken as being between 18 and 20 weeks + 6 days. The majority of the screening population will have an apparently normal scan, given that the prevalence of major structural abnormalities in the UK is in the region of 1–2%. Some of these abnormalities will not be detected by ultrasound alone. Women invited for a scan should be made aware from the outset of the main purpose of the scan. Bearing in mind advances in technology and knowledge, additional information regarding the detection rate and the limitations of the scan should also be explained and informed

consent obtained. All women capable of giving consent can accept or refuse any or all of the tests offered. Whatever the reason for an individual choosing or declining a test, the aim should be for each woman to have autonomy and support in the decision she makes for her pregnancy.

The equipment to identify fetal abnormality needs to be of a higher specification than that commonly used in more general ultrasound testing in pregnancy. A range of transducer frequencies of between 3 and 6 MHz and transvaginal transducers in the range of 5–8 MHz are essential. Equipment should be no more than 5 years old unless electronic hardware and software upgrades are available, in which case the most recent relevant upgrade should be no more than 5 years old. A quality assurance programme should regularly monitor equipment performance. The equipment should also have colour flow Doppler capability for the diagnosis of complex cardiac abnormalities.

A second trimester scan can identify normal development of fetal structures such as fetal head and brain structures (Fig. 38.26), fetal spine (Fig. 38.27), and fetal heart chambers and outflow tracks (Fig. 38.29). However, a normal scan result does not completely exclude abnormality in the fetus: it simply means that the operator observed no abnormality at the time of the scan. Apart from technical factors, suboptimal scan images may in part be related to maternal and pregnancy factors: for example, it is difficult to obtain optimum images if the mother is overweight, the fetus is in an awkward position, or if there is too little fluid around the fetus.

The commonest malformations detected are those affecting the central nervous system, urinary tract (Fig. 38.28), gastrointestinal system, skeletal system, and to a lesser degree the heart. If a single malformation is identified it is important to examine closely all other systems for evidence of any associated anomalies. In some pregnancies multiple malformations are detected initially by ultrasound; detailed diagnostic scanning should then be undertaken at a fetal medicine unit. Doppler studies and fetal karyotyping techniques, such as amniocentesis, chorionic villus sampling (CVS) and fetal blood sampling, may then be performed to give a more definite diagnosis. If the parents opt to continue with the pregnancy, adequate provision must be made for ongoing care at a specialist antenatal clinic and contacts established with neonatologists and paediatricians.

Doppler studies can provide the sonographer with additional information to differentiate between normal and abnormal fetal morphology, especially in the case of fetal echocardiography, where duplex Doppler and colour Doppler can enhance the visualisation of the cardiac chambers and major vessels, and with the aid of Doppler spectral analysis give more information on fetal cardiac haemodynamics. By delineating fetal or cord vessels, certain conditions can be confirmed in the presence of a suboptimal B-mode scan, such as in cases of ectopic kidney, cord insertion in the presence of an omphalocoele, cord cyst, nuchal cord, single umbilical artery and vasa praevia. Careful examination of the position and vasculature of the placenta can aid the detection of placenta praevia, accreta and succenturiate lobes.

Interventional ultrasound guided techniques to obtain fetal tissue

- *Amniocentesis.* This is usually undertaken during the second trimester after 15 weeks for fetal karyotyping; however, it is also done in the third trimester for rhesus incompatibility. A needle is inserted under ultrasound guidance through the maternal abdominal wall and into the amniotic sac and a sample of amniotic fluid collected. Fetal cells in the amniotic fluid are then cultured before testing for chromosomal, biochemical or DNA analysis. There is a procedure-related fetal loss or miscarriage rate of 0.5–1%. The main limitation of amniocentesis is the relatively advanced gestational age at which it is performed and the need to culture cells in the laboratory. Increasingly, fluorescence in situ hybridisation analysis may be used for rapid diagnosis of some cases, particularly in women at an advanced gestational age.

- *Chorionic villus sampling*. CVS can be performed in the first trimester of pregnancy, usually between 11 and 14 weeks of gestation. It can be performed transabdominally, when a needle is passed through the maternal abdominal and uterine wall, or transcervically, when a catheter or biopsy forceps is passed through the cervix into the uterus. Both procedures are performed under ultrasound guidance and the aim of the procedure is to obtain a sample of actively proliferating placental tissue. Both operator preference and the position of the placenta may determine the approach used. DNA analysis, limited cytogenetic analysis and some biochemical studies can be performed on uncultured chorionic villus tissue. Full cytogenetic analysis requires cells to be cultured. Fetal loss rates vary with experience, but are in the region of 1%. CVS is particularly useful where DNA analysis is required, e.g. for Duchenne muscular dystrophy.

- *Fetal blood sampling*. Cordocentesis or percutaneous umbilical blood sampling under ultrasound guidance is a means of obtaining fetal blood cells. These cells can be used for the detection of haematological and some metabolic abnormalities. Chromosome analysis can also be undertaken, and this method may be used to clarify some ambiguous chromosome results on amniocentesis or CVS. The fetal loss rate may vary, depending on the skill and experience of the personnel performing the procedure.

Chromosomal markers

Anatomical 'soft markers' are structural changes detected at ultrasound which may be transient and in themselves have little or no pathological significance, but are thought to be more commonly found in fetuses with congenital abnormalities, particularly chromosomal abnormalities. Common examples are choroid plexus cysts, renal pelvic dilatation, echogenic foci in the fetal heart, short limbs, echogenic bowel and nuchal thickening.

The observation of soft chromosomal markers and their relation to chromosomal abnormalities has been reported since the early 1990s, but there is still controversy regarding the usefulness of these markers. The impact of these soft marker observations has been studied in an unselected population over 6 years.[45] A 4% rise in the detection of fetal malformations was reported; however, there was also a 12-fold increase in the false positive rate. Obvious concerns highlighted were resource implications, risk of pregnancy loss following invasive procedures, and the psychological impact on the expectant parents. In the absence of any conclusive evidence the use of the term 'markers' is discouraged.

Cost-effectiveness of antenatal screening

Two important factors were recognised via systemic review:[46]

1. The skill of the sonographer and the time taken for the scan had a significant influence on the cost-effectiveness of any ultrasound screening programme. Sonographers who are not properly trained may have a detrimental effect on clinical efficacy and cost-effectiveness.
2. Screening for fetal abnormalities in the second trimester is cost-effective, although this result holds only if termination of pregnancy is acceptable.

This review emphasises the need for better research on the costs and cost-effectiveness of screening, and the overall benefit in terms of maternal and fetal mortality and morbidity remains controversial.

Third trimester

Scanning in the third trimester is carried out primarily for fetal surveillance, for clinically small or large for dates gestations, poor obstetric history, multiple pregnancies and maternal conditions such as hypertension and diabetes. It is worth remembering that a one-off morphometric fetal measurement cannot identify the fetus that is constitutionally small for dates, or growth restricted. Serial growth measurements combined with Doppler investigations are needed, along with a fetal non-stress test, and fetal biophysical profile.

From around 1985, Doppler waveform changes were associated with abnormal placental function. Fetal Doppler indices were initially developed for the detection of intrauterine growth restriction and fetal hypoxia. Fetal growth restriction is a significant factor for increasing umbilical artery Doppler indices: it can identify a growth-restricted fetus, which is at higher risk of adverse perinatal outcome. These fetuses are metabolically compromised, with conditions of oxygen and nutrient deprivation. Vascular redistribution occurs in favour of vital organs such as the fetal brain (brain-sparing effect), whereby there is a reduction in the end-diastolic flow velocities in the umbilical arteries and an increase in the fetal cerebral vascular end-diastolic flow. The use of fetal colour power angiography, which demonstrates the hypoperfusion status of various organs, has been reported as useful in the evaluation of circulatory redistribution in the growth-restricted fetus, but there is insufficient evidence to support its use as a routine test.

Oligohydramnios (reduced amniotic fluid), which may be due to ruptured membranes or chronic fetal compromise, and reduction of fetal urine production, intrauterine growth restriction or fetal renal tract anomalies, and polyhydramnios (increased amniotic fluid) due to overproduction of fetal urine or fetal abnormalities concerning the fetal gastrointestinal tract, can be diagnosed by the ultrasonic measurements of either the maximum pool depth, or by an amniotic fluid index where the sum of maximum depth of pools in all four quadrants is calculated.

Placenta praevia can be excluded by the location of placental site in the third trimester, following a low-lying placenta in the second trimester, although only a small percentage (10%) of these remain low at term. A transvaginal approach is often useful to locate the lower edge of a placenta where the low fetal parts prevent clear visualisation of the internal os.

Using a transvaginal approach, cervical length measurements, i.e. the distance between the external and internal os, provide a useful predictor for the risk of early spontaneous preterm delivery in high-risk pregnancies. In cases where the cervical length is 15 mm or less at 28 or 32 weeks, there is an increased risk of preterm labour of respectively 90% and 60%.[47] Other indications for a third trimester scan are fetal weight estimation and fetal presentation.

3D ULTRASOUND IN OBSTETRICS

3D sonography has gained in sophistication and hence significant popularity in prenatal diagnostics. The main advantages in obstetrics are improved assessment of complex anatomical fetal structures, developmental embryology, and the diagnosis of specific malformations such as spina bifida, cleft lip and palate, and limb abnormalities. 4D evaluation of the fetal heart is another emerging application for this technology.[48] Awkward fetal position, maternal habitus and lack

With advances in technology prenatal tests are becoming more accessible, easier, safer, and available much earlier in pregnancy. This may result in informed consent becoming difficult to obtain in a short time, not just for the testing of the fetus but also for 'selective' termination. The diagnosis of a late onset of certain diseases may cause dilemmas in decision making for women, and 'the right to not know' may be the new controversy of the modern age.[49]

PROFESSIONAL ISSUES

In the presence of ever-increasing complexities and the widening scope of ultrasound in all fields of medicine, clinical competence, role extension, appropriate education, ultrasound equipment and safety are all important issues that need to be addressed. It is imperative that sonographers understand their responsibilities and the associated medicolegal implications to ensure safe practice. National and local guidelines and policies are developed to standardise practice; along with regular audit, these ensure the provision of a safe and effective ultrasound service. Where there is an absence of national guidelines in a certain field, it is vital that written local policies and protocols are mutually agreed between all members of the multidisciplinary team to provide a framework in which sonographers can practise. Current literature should be researched to guide the development of such policies, and they should be regularly audited, evaluated and updated. All previous protocols should be archived to allow retrospective reference for medicolegal purposes.

Reporting

Ultrasound examinations are dynamic: interpretations of normality and deviations from the norm are made during the scan. The sonographer undertaking the scan should record all findings and write a report in clear and unambiguous language. The limitations of the scan and the sonographer must be acknowledged, measurements should be reported with reference to normal ranges, and if possible comparison with previous scans should be undertaken with regard to size, and appearances of normal or abnormal observations.

Stored images should represent the scan and provide evidence of what was observed. There should be procedures in place locally for the provision of second opinions or follow-on referrals to more experienced or specialist clinicians in cases of uncertainty. Guidelines have been produced for sonographers in order to maintain standards of reporting, scan content and writing style.[50]

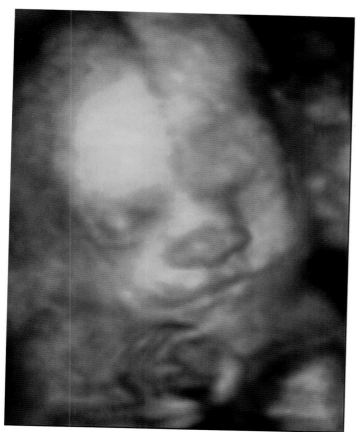

Figure 38.30 3D fetal image.
Reproduced with permission from Ultrasound Now Ltd.

of amniotic fluid around the fetus can all make 3D imaging a challenge.

3D images are difficult both to obtain and to interpret at less than 24 weeks of gestation. There is also a commercial market, which is mainly consumer driven, in non-diagnostic keepsake 3D and 4D images and movie clips of the fetus (Fig. 38.30).

ETHICAL ISSUES

Ultrasound scans are very attractive to parents, enabling early bonding with their babies. They give the parents visual confirmation of pregnancy, to see their baby develop, obtain images and in some cases know the gender of the baby. However, the real purpose of the scan can easily be misunderstood. Women opting for ultrasound scans during pregnancy should be made aware of the medical purpose and the limitations of the scans from the outset.

Prenatal counselling is vital to provide couples with information that will enable them to make an informed choice with respect to their unborn baby. There are potential implications for the psychological and social consequences for pregnant women, such as anxiety, disbelief, negative attitudes towards the fetus, loss of confidence and disappointment when a problem is detected prenatally, or, in cases of false positives, where there are minor anomalies that are of uncertain clinical significance. Conversely, as no screening test is without false negatives, the opposite exists when an abnormality is not detected by ultrasound and there is false reassurance.

FUTURE DEVELOPMENTS

With advancing computer and software technology, ultrasound machines will probably become more dynamic, accessible, portable and sophisticated. Telemedicine enables high-quality care from remote settings, and image quality will be improved further to rival CT and MRI. Transducers will get smaller; more intracavitary applications will be developed to gain better images of internal organs. 3D and 4D ultrasound will be more highly developed and become more accessible.

Wireless technology and voice activation may minimise work-related disorders by enabling sonographers to control the ultrasound machine remotely. All these advances and those as yet unseen will enable ultrasound practices to move further into every field of medicine, not only in diagnostics but also into therapeutic applications.

REFERENCES

1. Department of Health. Activity Statistics, Imaging, & Radiodiagnostics. 2011. http://www.dh.gov.uk/en/Publicationsandstatistics/Statistics/Performancedataandstatistics/HospitalActivityStatistics/DH_077487.

2. Baker J. The history of sonographers. Ultrasound in Medicine 2005;24:1–14.

3. National Institute Health for Clinical Excellence. UTI in Children: Diagnosis, treatment and long term management. Clinical Guidance 2007;54. London.

4. National Institute for Clinical Excellence. Guidance on the use of ultrasound locating devices for placing central venous catheters. Technology Appraisal Guidance 49. London: NICE; 2002.

5. National Screening Committee. Antenatal Screening UK survey of England. Oxford: Institute of Health; 2008.

6. Board of the Faculty of Clinical Radiology. Ultrasound training recommendations for medical and surgical specialties. London: RCR; 2004.

7. Toshiba: Pioneers in ultrasound. Visions Magazine 2003;3:63–9.

8. Watts G. Obituary: John Wild. BMJ 2009;339:b4428.

9. Edler I, Hertz C. The use of ultrasonic reflectoscope for the continuous recording of the movements of heart walls. Clinical Physiology and Functional Imaging 2004;24:118–36.

10. Donald I, et al. Investigation of abdominal masses by pulsed ultrasound. Lancet 1958;1:1188–95.

11. Kasai C, et al. Real time 2 dimensional blood flow imaging using an autocorrelation technique. IEEE TransSonics Ultrasonics 1985;32:458–64.

12. The Society and College of Radiographers. Prevention of Work Related Musculoskeletal Disorders in Sonography. London: 2007.

13. Chiou S, Fox T. Comparing differential tissue harmonic imaging with tissue harmonic and fundamental gray scale imaging of the liver. Journal of Ultrasound in Medicine 2007;26:1557–63.

14. Lewin P. Quo vadis medical ultrasound? Ultrasonics 2004;42:1–7.

15. Dogra V. Advances in Ultrasound. An Issue of Ultrasound Clinics. (The Clinics: Radiology). Saunders; 2010.

16. Benacerraf B, et al. How sonographic tomography will change the face of obstetric sonography: a pilot study. Journal of Ultrasound in Medicine 2005;24:371–8.

17. Wickline S, Lanza G. Nanotechnology for molecular imaging and targeted therapy. Circulation 2003;107:1092–5.

18. Xu H. Contrast-enhanced ultrasound: The evolving applications. World Journal of Radiology 2009;1:15–24.

19. Oyen R. Safety of ultrasound contrast agents. In: Thomsen H, editor. Contrast media Berlin: Springer; 2006.

20. ter Haar G. Safety and bio-effects of ultrasound contrast agents. Medical and Biological Engineering and Computing 2009;47:893–900.

21. ter Haar G, Duck F. The safe use of ultrasound in medical diagnosis. London: British Institute of Radiology; 2000.

22. BMUS. Safety guidelines for the safe use of diagnostic ultrasound equipment. Ultrasound 2010;18:52–9.

23. The Society and College of Radiographers. Industry standards for the prevention of work related musculoskeletal disorders in sonography. London: SCoR; 2006.

24. HSE. Display screen equipment regulations. London: HSE; 1992.

25. NHS abdominal aortic aneurysm screening programme. essential elements in developing an abdominal aortic aneurysm (AAA) screening and surveillance programme. London: NHS; 2011.

26. Gracey D, McClure MJ. The impact of ultrasound in suspected acute appendicitis. Clinical Radiology 2007;62:573–78.

27. Ryan A, Roberts S. Endoscopic ultrasound of the upper gastrointestinal tract and adnexae. British Medical Ultrasound Society Bulletin 2001;9(4):24–9.

28. Solbiati L, et al. Thyroid nodules: which sonographic criteria for differentiation between benign and malignant lesions? British Medical Ultrasound Society Bulletin 2001;9(3):11–9.

29. Sykes C, Connell D. Ultrasound elbows MRI in joint examinations. Diagnostic Imaging Europe 2003;June/July: 31–3.

30. Kurjak A, et al. Preoperative evaluation of pelvic tumours by Doppler and three dimensional sonography. Journal of Ultrasound in Medicine 2001;29(8):829–40.

31. Weber G, et al. A new sonographic scoring system (Mainz score) for the assessment of ovarian tumors using transvaginal ultrasonography Part II. A comparison between the scoring system and the assessment by an experienced sonographer in post menopausal women. Ultrashall in der Medizin 1999;20(1):2–8.

32. Vergote I, et al. Screening for ovarian carcinoma: not quite there yet. Lancet Oncology 2009;10(4):308–9.

33. Jacobs I, et al. Sensitivity of transvaginal ultrasound screening for endometrial cancer in postmenopausal women: a case-control study within the UKCTOCS cohort. Lancet Oncology 2011;12(1):38–48.

34. NHS Fetal Anomaly Screening Programme. Model of best practice: Screening for Down's syndrome: UK NSC Policy recommendations 2007–10. 2010. www.dh.gov.uk/publications.

35. Loughna P, et al. Ultrasound fetal size and dating: charts recommended for clinical obstetric practice. British Medical Ultrasound Society 2009;17:3.

36. Walker J, Shillito J. Early pregnancy assessment units, service and organisational aspects. In: Gradzinskas J, O'Brien P, editors. Problems in early pregnancy, advances in diagnosis and management. London: RCOG Press; 1997.

37. RCOG. Guidelines on ultrasound procedures in early pregnancy. Guideline 25. London: RCOG; 2000.

38. Jauniaux E, et al. The role of ultrasound imaging in diagnosing and investigating early pregnancy failure. Ultrasound in Obstetrics and Gynecology 2005;25:613–24.

39. Condous G, et al. The conservative management of early pregnancy complications: a review of the literature. Ultrasound in Obstetrics and Gynecology 2003;22(4):420–30.

40. Wiebe E, Janssen P. Conservative management of spontaneous abortions. Women's experiences. Canadian Family Physician 1999;45:2355–60.

41. Nicolaides K. Nuchal translucency and other first-trimester sonographic markers of chromosomal abnormalities. American Journal of Obstetrics and Gynecology 2004;191(1):45–67.

42. National Collaborating Centre for Women's and Children's Health. Antenatal care: routine care for the healthy pregnant woman. CG62: full guidance. London: NICE; 2008.

43. de Jong A, et al. Non-invasive prenatal testing: ethical issues explored. European Journal of Human Genetics 2010;18:272–7.

44. Maiz N, et al. Ductus venosus Doppler in screening for trisomies 21, 18 and 13 and Turner syndrome at 11–13 weeks of gestation. Ultrasound in Obstetrics and Gynecology 2009;33(5):512–7.

45. Boyd P, et al. A 6-year experience of prenatal diagnosis in an unselected population in Oxford, UK. Lancet 1998;352(9140):1577–81.

46. Bricker L, et al. Ultrasound screening in pregnancy: a systematic review of the clinical effectiveness, cost effectiveness and women's views. Health Technology Assessment 2000;4(16).

47. Welsh A, Nicolaides K. Cervical screening for preterm delivery. Current Opinion in Obstetrics and Gynecology 2002;14(2): 195–202.

48. DeVore G. Three-dimensional and four-dimensional fetal echocardiography: a new frontier. Current Opinion in Pediatrics 2005;17:592–604.

49. Schwennesen N, et al. Beyond informed choice: prenatal risk assessment, decision-making and trust. Clinical Ethics 2010;5: 207–16.

50. UKAS. Guidelines For professional working standards: Ultrasound practice. London: UKAS; 2008.

Glossary of radiographic terms

Abduction Refers to limbs or digits, when they are moved away from the median sagittal plane or trunk. An abducted thumb is moved away from the rest of the hand.

Adduction Refers to limbs or digits, when they are brought towards the median sagittal plane or trunk. An adducted thumb is moved towards the rest of the hand.

Anatomical position The trunk and limbs are extended fully, with the arms slightly abducted at the side. The palms of the hands face forwards. The front of the patient faces forwards.

Anterior The front of the patient, or body part, when the patient is in the anatomical position.

Anterior oblique An oblique position, when the anterior aspect of the patient is nearest the image receptor *or* a posteroanterior position with an oblique angle applied in a lateral or medial direction.

Anteroposterior A position where the anterior aspect of the patient faces the X-ray tube, and the central ray passes through this aspect and exits through the posterior aspect.

Anthropological baseline Baseline used in radiography of the head (see Ch. 16).

Bucky Antiscatter device.

Caudal Relating to the lower part of the body, or feet. Used mainly in conjunction with beam angulation, meaning to direct the beam towards the feet.

Coronal plane An imaginary line which divides the front and back of the head and trunk vertically. It is perpendicular to the median sagittal plane.

Cranial Relating to the head. Used mainly in conjunction with beam angulation, meaning to direct the beam towards the head.

Craniocaudal Mammographic term used when the breast is placed with its inferior aspect on the image receptor and the X-ray beam directed vertically to enter the breast on its uppermost surface, exiting inferiorly.

Decubitus The patient is in a horizontal position. Used in conjunction with a qualifying term to indicate which aspect of the body is nearest the image receptor, as in 'lateral decubitus', 'prone decubitus'.

Dorsal The back of the patient or body part; sometimes used instead of 'posterior'.

Dorsiflexion Flexion of the hand at the wrist when the dorsum of the hand moves in a posterior direction, or flexion of the foot at the ankle when the dorsal aspect of the foot moves towards the ankle.

Dorsipalmar The hand is placed with its palmar aspect on the image receptor.

Dorsiplantar The foot is placed with its sole on the image receptor.

Dorsum The back of the hand or the top of the foot.

Erect The patient is standing or sitting, with the median sagittal and coronal planes vertical.

Eversion Lateral flexion at the ankle joint. Excessive forced eversion can cause injury in the ankle or other joints.

Extension Typically, effecting 'opening' or straightening of a joint. For example, the extended elbow will place the arm in a position where the forearm and humerus continue in the same plane. Lumbar or thoracic spine: the patient usually bends backwards. Cervical spine: the head is tipped backwards to lift the chin. Foot: the foot is moved at the ankle so that the toes point downwards or posteriorly (although this is sometimes referred to as plantar flexion).

External On the outside/towards the outside/away from the median sagittal plane. Often used in conjunction with describing rotation of a limb, when the big toes or thumbs are turned outwards, away from the trunk or median sagittal plane.

External auditory meatus Surface marking used in radiography of the head (see Ch. 16).

External occipital protuberance Surface marking used in radiography of the head (see Ch. 16).

Flexion Typically, effecting 'closing' of a joint such as bending the knee or elbow and can be described in conjunction with description of the direction of flexion, such as lateral/dorsal/palmar flexion for other body parts, such as the hands and feet. Lumbar or thoracic spine: the patient usually bends forwards but lateral flexion may also be described. Cervical spine: the head is bent forwards to tuck the chin down.

Focus film distance Distance from the focal spot to the image receptor (known as source image distance in some countries).

Focus object distance Distance from the focal spot to the body part (known as source object distance in some countries).

Glossary of radiographic terms

Fronto-occipital Refers to positioning of the head, when the X-ray beam enters the frontal aspect and exits via the occiput.

Glabella Surface marking used in radiography of the head (see Ch. 16)

Grid Antiscatter device.

Image receptor A plate, upon which X radiation impinges and creates a latent image. Can be a film which is placed in a cassette, or a radiosensitive structure which converts the image digitally for reproduction on a display screen (see Chs 2 and 3).

Inferior Below or underneath.

Inferosuperior A position where the inferior aspect of the body part is nearest the X-ray tube and the central ray passes through this aspect, exiting through the superior aspect. Mainly used in examination of limbs and the shoulder girdle.

Internal On the inside/towards the inside/towards the median sagittal plane. Often used in conjunction with describing rotation of a limb, when the big toes or thumbs are turned inwards, towards the trunk or median sagittal plane.

Inversion Medial flexion of the ankle joint. Excessive forced inversion can cause injury in the ankle or other joints.

Lateral The outermost side of the trunk or body part, furthest from the median sagittal plane. Can be used in description of rotation of limbs (see entry for rotation). Also a radiographic position/projection where the side of the trunk or body part faces the X-ray tube.

Lateral oblique Initially a lateral position, the body part is tilted towards the image receptor *or* the lateral patient position is maintained but a tube angle is employed.

Lateromedial A position where the lateral aspect of the body part faces the X-ray tube and the central ray passes through this aspect, exiting via the medial aspect. Mainly used in mammography but can be used in some limb radiography to describe beam direction.

Left anterior oblique An oblique position, when the anterior aspect of the left side lies nearer the image receptor than the right side.

Left posterior oblique An oblique position, when the posterior aspect of the left side lies nearer the image receptor than the right side.

Lordosis/lordotic The patient is leaning back.

Medial Towards or nearest the median sagittal plane. Can be used in description of rotation of limbs (see entry for rotation).

Median sagittal plane An imaginary line which divides the left and right sides of the head and trunk vertically, in the midline.

Mediolateral A position where the medial aspect of the body part faces the X-ray tube and the central ray passes through this aspect, exiting via the lateral aspect. Mainly used in mammography but can be used in some limb radiography to describe beam direction.

Nasion Surface marking used in radiography of the head (see Ch. 16).

Object–film distance Distance from the body part to the image receptor (known as object image distance in some countries).

Oblique The body part position lies between the lateral and anteroposterior or posteroanterior positions. For hands and feet, the palm or sole is raised from the image receptor along one of the lateral aspects.

Occipitofrontal Refers to positioning of the head, when the X-ray beam enters the occipital aspect and exits via the forehead (frontal bone).

Occipitomental Refers to positioning of the head, when the X-ray beam enters the occipital aspect and exits via the chin.

Orbitomeatal baseline Baseline used for skull radiography (see Ch. 16).

Palmar Relating to the palm of the hand.

Plantar Relating to the sole of the foot.

Plantar flexion Flexion of the foot at the ankle when the dorsal aspect of the foot moves away from the ankle.

Posterior The back of the patient or body part, when the patient is in the anatomical position.

Posterior oblique An oblique position, when the posterior aspect of the patient is nearest the image receptor *or* an anteroposterior position with an oblique angle applied in a lateral or medial direction.

Posteroanterior A position where the posterior aspect of the patient faces the X-ray tube and the central ray passes through this aspect and exits through the anterior aspect.

Pronation Used when referring to the position of the hand when it is placed palm down.

Prone The patient is lying horizontally face down.

Right anterior oblique An oblique position, when the anterior aspect of the right side lies nearer the image receptor than the left side.

Right posterior oblique An oblique position, when the posterior aspect of the right side lies nearer the image receptor than the left side.

Rotation Turning the trunk or head laterally in relationship to the median sagittal plane.
External or lateral rotation: turning a limb when the big toes or thumbs are turned outwards, away from the trunk or median sagittal plane.
Internal or medial rotation: when the big toes or thumbs are turned inwards, towards the trunk or median sagittal plane.

Semi-prone One side of the patient is partly raised from the prone position, as in the anterior oblique position.

Semi-recumbent The patient is leaning back, between the erect and supine positions.

Submentovertical A position of the head where the beam enters below the chin and exits via the top of the skull (vertex).

Superior Above or uppermost.

Superoinferior A position where the superior aspect of the body part is nearest the X-ray tube and the central ray passes through this aspect, exiting through the inferior aspect. Mainly used in examination of limbs.

Supine The patient is lying horizontally on their back.

Tilt Tipping the trunk or head away from the median sagittal plane, anteriorly, posteriorly or laterally.

Index

Index

Index